MEDICAL ASSISTING
REVIEW

Passing the CMA, RMA, CCMA, and NCMA Exams

Sixth Edition

Jahangir Moini, M.D., M.P.H.

Former Professor and Director of Allied Health Sciences including the Medical Assisting Program, Everest University, Melbourne, Florida; and Professor of Science and Health, Eastern Florida State College, Palm Bay, Florida

Mc
Graw
Hill
Education

MEDICAL ASSISTING REVIEW: PASSING THE CMA, RMA, CCMA, and NCMA EXAMS, SIXTH EDITION

Published by McGraw-Hill Education, 2 Penn Plaza, New York, NY 10121. Copyright © 2018 by McGraw-Hill Education. All rights reserved. Printed in the United States of America. Previous editions © 2015 and 2012. No part of this publication may be reproduced or distributed in any form or by any means, or stored in a database or retrieval system, without the prior written consent of McGraw-Hill Education, including, but not limited to, in any network or other electronic storage or transmission, or broadcast for distance learning.

Some ancillaries, including electronic and print components, may not be available to customers outside the United States.

This book is printed on acid-free paper.

5 6 7 8 9 LMN 21 20

ISBN 978-1-259-59293-5
MHID 1-259-59293-6

Chief Product Officer, SVP Products & Markets: *G. Scott Virkler*
Vice President, General Manager, Products & Markets: *Marty Lange*
Managing Director: *Chad Grall*
Executive Brand Manager: *William Lawrensen*
Director, Product Development: *Rose Koos*
Senior Product Developer: *Christine Scheid*
Executive Marketing Manager: *Harper Christopher*
Market Development Manager: *Kimberly Bauer*
Digital Product Analyst: *Katherine Ward*
Director, Content Design & Delivery: *Linda Avenarius*
Program Manager: *Angela R. FitzPatrick*
Content Project Managers: *April R. Southwood/Brent dela Cruz*
Buyer: *Laura M. Fuller*
Design: *Tara McDermott*
Content Licensing Specialists: *Lori Hancock/Lori Slattery*
Cover Image: *© Getty Images/fatido*
Compositor: *SPi Global*
Printer: *LSC Communications*

All credits appearing on page or at the end of the book are considered to be an extension of the copyright page.

Library of Congress Cataloging-in-Publication Data
Names: Moini, Jahangir, 1942- author.
Title: Medical assisting review: passing the cma, rma, ccma, and ncma exams / Jahangir Moini, M.D., M.P.H., Former Professor and Director of Allied Health Sciences including the Medical Assisting Program, Everest University, Melbourne, Florida; and Professor of Science and Health, Eastern Florida State College, Palm Bay, Florida.
Description: Sixth edition. | New York, NY: McGraw-Hill Education, [2018] | Includes index.
Identifiers: LCCN 2016051550 | ISBN 9781259592935 (alk. paper)
Subjects: LCSH: Medical assistants—Examinations, questions, etc. | Physicians' assistants—Examinations, questions, etc.
Classification: LCC R728.8 .M653 2018 | DDC 610.73/7—dc23 LC record available at https://lccn.loc.gov/2016051550

The Internet addresses listed in the text were accurate at the time of publication. The inclusion of a website does not indicate an endorsement by the authors or McGraw-Hill Education, and McGraw-Hill Education does not guarantee the accuracy of the information presented at these sites.

mheducation.com/highered

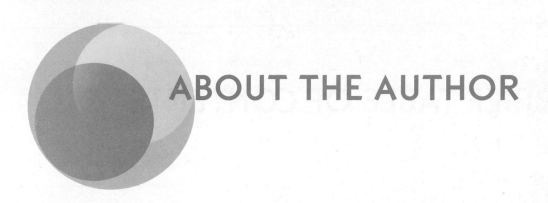

ABOUT THE AUTHOR

Dr. Moini was assistant professor at Tehran University School of Medicine for nine years, teaching medical and allied health students. The author was a professor and former director (for 24 years) of allied health programs at Everest University. Dr. Moini reestablished the Medical Assisting Program in 1990 at Everest University's Melbourne campus. He also established several other new allied health programs for Everest University. He is currently a professor of science and health at Eastern Florida State College.

Dr. Moini was a physician liaison of the Florida Society of Medical Assistants 2000–2008. He has been a marketing strategy team member of the National AAMA and president of the Brevard County chapter of the AAMA. He is currently a board member of the National Healthcareer Association (NHA). He is the author of 19 published allied health textbooks since 1999.

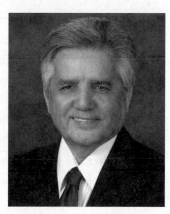

Photo: Courtesy of Dr. Moini/ Crouch Photography

Dedication

To the memory of my Mother,
and
To my wonderful wife,
Hengameh, my two daughters,
Mahkameh and Morvarid,
and also to my precious granddaughters,
Laila Jade and Anabelle Jasmine Mabry.

BRIEF TABLE OF CONTENTS

TABLE OF CONTENTS

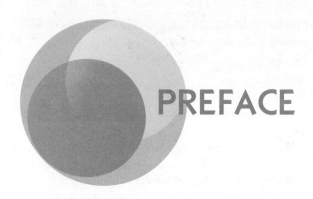

PREFACE

Catching your success has never been easier, with the sixth edition of *Medical Assisting Review: Passing the CMA, RMA, CCMA, and NCMA Exams.* Confidently master the competencies you need for certification with a user-friendly approach and various practice exams. *MA Review* is also now available with McGraw-Hill's revolutionary adaptive learning technology, LearnSmart! Study effectively, spending more time on topics you don't know and less time on the topics you do. Succeed with LearnSmart . . . Join the learning revolution and achieve certified success!

Organization

Medical Assisting Review is divided into three sections, similar to how the certification exams are divided: General Medical Assisting Knowledge (Chapters 1–8); Administrative Medical Assisting Knowledge (Chapters 9–15); and Clinical Medical Assisting Knowledge (Chapters 16–25). Each chapter opens with *Learning Outcomes* to set the stage for the content to come. That list is followed by a table listing the relevant CMA, RMA, CCMA, and NCMA *Medical Assisting Competencies* for that chapter. Throughout the chapters, you will find *At A Glance* tables that summarize key information for quick review. At the beginning and end of most chapters, there are also *Strategies for Success* boxes, which contain tips on study skills and test-taking skills. Each chapter then closes with the *Chapter Review*—10 multiple-choice questions written in the style of CMA, RMA, CCMA, and NCMA exam questions.

New to the Sixth Edition

OVERVIEW

A number of enhancements have been made with the sixth edition to enrich the user's experience with the product:

- Learning Outcomes listed at the beginning of each chapter have been verified, with a few additional ones added. Major chapter heads are numbered to correspond to the numbered learning outcomes.
- NCMA competencies have been added to the competency tables at the beginning of each chapter, along with the CMA, RMA, and CCMA competencies.

- The various competency correlation charts can also be found in the Instructor Resources portion of Connect. This allows us to add additional correlations, organized by learning outcome, to the different standards, including ABHES and CAAHEP. For the recent ABHES update, a correlation guide has been developed. Connect is fully updated to these competencies for the ABHES filter.
- Connect has 12 practice exams, which are divided into three exams each for the CMA, RMA, CCMA, and NCMA. There are four exams included at the back of the book. The existing exams have all been updated to reflect new material in the chapters, and all of the exams have gone through an accuracy review.
- *Medical Assisting Review* is now available on LearnSmart with Smartbook. Ask your Learning Technology Representative how you can obtain it for your students and course.

CHAPTER HIGHLIGHTS

Definitions have been expanded and added in every chapter in direct response to market feedback:

- Chapter 1: Full contact information has been added for the organizations that created the CMA, RMA, CCMA, and NCMA exams. Information about test-taking preparation has been greatly expanded.
- Chapter 2: There is additional text about acceptable and unacceptable abbreviations.
- Chapter 5: The section on microbial control and asepsis has been moved to Chapter 16 for better organization of the text.

- Chapter 6: New information has been added about Lawrence Kohlberg.

- Chapter 7: Information has been updated concerning MyPlate and the Healthy Eating Pyramid. Information has been added about instructing patients with special dietary needs.

- Chapter 8: New information has been added about informed, implied, and expressed consent. Information about public health statutes and compliance has been added.

- Chapter 9: New information about meaningful use, out-guides, and filing guidelines has been added.

- Chapter 10: New information about databases, data management tools, and electronic health records has been added.

- Chapter 13: New information about payroll accounting, disability laws, immigration, and acts related to financial management has been added.

- Chapter 14: Many new definitions have been added, including those related to insurance, legislation, managed care, and health insurance options.

- Chapter 15: New information about medical necessity related to coding has been added.

- Chapter 17: New information has been added about examinations of the respiratory system.

- Chapter 18: New information has been added about thermometers and pulse oximetry.

- Chapter 20: Immunization schedules have been updated.

- Chapter 23: Information about body mechanics, whirlpool baths, chiropractics, acupuncture, and acupressure has been added.

- Chapter 24: Information about the Good Samaritan law has been updated, and information about slings and automated external defibrillators has been added.

- Chapter 25: Information about sedimentation rate, analyzer equipment, incubators, sterilizers, microhematocrit, and occult blood specimens has been added.

For a detailed transition guide between the fifth and sixth editions for all chapters of *Medical Assisting Review,* visit the Instructor Resources in Connect.

Medical Assisting Review Preparation in the Digital World: Supplementary Materials for the Instructor and Student

Instructor Resources

You can rely on the following materials to help you and your students work through the material in this book. All of the resources in the following table are available through the Instructor Resources on the Library tab in Connect.

Supplement	Features
Instructor's Manual	Each chapter has: • Learning Outcomes and Lecture Outline • Overview of PowerPoint Presentations • Teaching Strategies • Answer Keys for End-of-Chapter Questions and two Practice Exams from the back of the book • List of Additional Resources
PowerPoint Presentations	• Key Concepts
Electronic Test Bank (Two Practice Exams)	• TestGen (computerized) • Word version • These two exams are also available in the Library tab of Connect. Both of them, along with 12 additional exams, are available within Connect. • Questions are tagged with learning outcomes, level of difficulty, level of Bloom's taxonomy, feedback, and ABHES and CAAHEP competencies.
Tools to Plan Course	• Transition Guide, by chapter, from Moini, 5e, to Moini, 6e • Correlations of the chapters to the major accrediting bodies (previously included in the book), as well as correlations by learning outcomes to ABHES and CAAHEP • Sample Syllabi • Asset Map—a recap of the key instructor resources, as well as information on the content available through Connect

A few things to note:

- All student content is now available to be assigned through Connect.
- Instructors can share the answer keys and test bank exams available through the Instructor Resources at their discretion.

Need help? Contact McGraw-Hill's Customer Experience Group (CXG). Visit the CXG website at **www.mhhe.com/support.** Browse our FAQs (frequently asked questions) and product documentation and/or contact a CXG representative. CXG is available Sunday–Friday.

Practice Medical Office

Practice Medical Office is a 3-D immersive game that features 12 engaging and challenging modules representing the functional areas of a medical practice: Administrative Check In, Clinical, and Administrative Check Out. As the players progress through each module, they will face realistic situations and learning events, which will test their mastery of critical job-readiness skills and competencies such as professionalism, soft skills, office procedures, application of medical knowledge, and application of privacy and liability regulation. An ideal way to engage, excite, and prepare students to be successful on the job, Practice Medical Office is available for use on tablets and computers. It is perfect for the capstone Medical Assisting Examination Preparation course, and Externship course, or may be used throughout the Medical Assisting program. PMO is accessible through a widget in Connect. For a demo of Practice Medical Office, please go to **http://www.mhpractice.com/products/Practice_Medical_Office** and click on "Play the Demo."

Best-in-Class Digital Support

Based on feedback from our users, McGraw-Hill Education has developed Digital Success Programs that will provide you and your students the help you need, at the moment you need it.

- One-to-One Training: Get ready to drive classroom results with our Digital Success Team—ready to provide in-person, remote, or on-demand training as needed.
- Peer Support and Training: No one understands your needs like your peers. Get easy access to knowledgeable digital users by joining our Connect Community, or speak directly with one of our digital faculty consultants.
- Online Training Tools: Get immediate anytime, anywhere access to modular tutorials on key features through our Connect Success Academy at **www.mhhe.com/support.**

Get started today. Learn more about McGraw-Hill Education's Digital Success Programs by contacting your local sales representative.

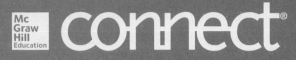

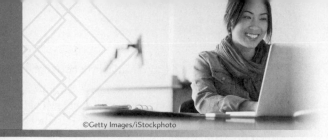

McGraw-Hill Connect®
Learn Without Limits

Connect is a teaching and learning platform that is proven to deliver better results for students and instructors.

Connect empowers students by continually adapting to deliver precisely what they need, when they need it, and how they need it, so your class time is more engaging and effective.

73% of instructors who use **Connect** require it; instructor satisfaction **increases** by 28% when **Connect** is required.

Connect's Impact on Retention Rates, Pass Rates, and Average Exam Scores

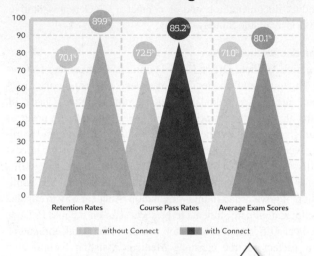

Using **Connect** improves retention rates by **19.8%**, passing rates by **12.7%**, and exam scores by **9.1%**.

Analytics

Connect Insight®

Connect Insight is Connect's new one-of-a-kind visual analytics dashboard that provides at-a-glance information regarding student performance, which is immediately actionable. By presenting assignment, assessment, and topical performance results together with a time metric that is easily visible for aggregate or individual results, Connect Insight gives the user the ability to take a just-in-time approach to teaching and learning, which was never before available. Connect Insight presents data that helps instructors improve class performance in a way that is efficient and effective.

Impact on Final Course Grade Distribution

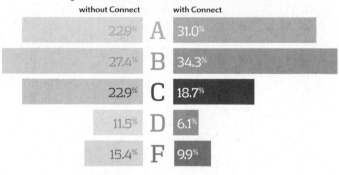

Students can view their results for any **Connect** course.

Mobile

Connect's new, intuitive mobile interface gives students and instructors flexible and convenient, anytime–anywhere access to all components of the Connect platform.

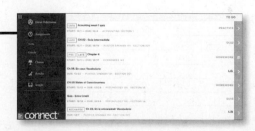

Adaptive

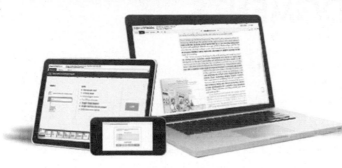

THE **ADAPTIVE** READING EXPERIENCE DESIGNED TO TRANSFORM THE WAY STUDENTS READ

> More students earn **A's** and **B's** when they use McGraw-Hill Education **Adaptive** products.

SmartBook®

Proven to help students improve grades and study more efficiently, SmartBook contains the same content within the print book, but actively tailors that content to the needs of the individual. SmartBook's adaptive technology provides precise, personalized instruction on what the student should do next, guiding the student to master and remember key concepts, targeting gaps in knowledge and offering customized feedback, and driving the student toward comprehension and retention of the subject matter. Available on smartphones and tablets, SmartBook puts learning at the student's fingertips—anywhere, anytime.

> Over **eight billion questions** have been answered, making McGraw-Hill Education products more intelligent, reliable, and precise.

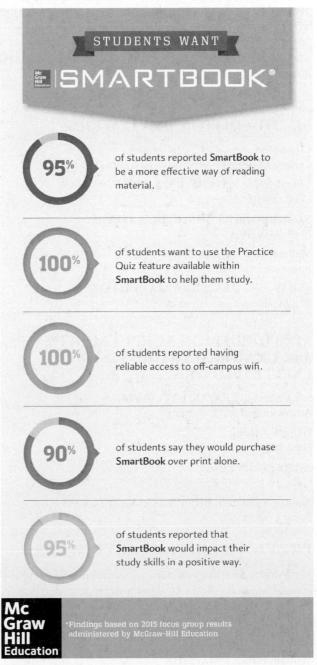

STUDENTS WANT

SMARTBOOK®

95% of students reported **SmartBook** to be a more effective way of reading material.

100% of students want to use the Practice Quiz feature available within **SmartBook** to help them study.

100% of students reported having reliable access to off-campus wifi.

90% of students say they would purchase **SmartBook** over print alone.

95% of students reported that **SmartBook** would impact their study skills in a positive way.

*Findings based on 2015 focus group results administered by McGraw-Hill Education

www.mheducation.com

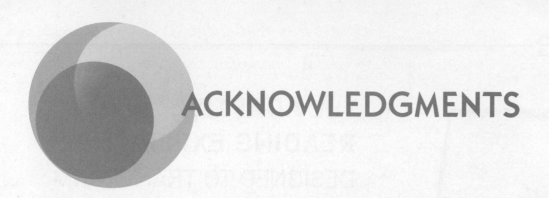

ACKNOWLEDGMENTS

Suggestions have been received from faculty and students throughout the country. This is vital feedback that is relied on for product development. Each person who has offered comments and suggestions has our thanks. The efforts of many people are needed to develop and improve a product. Among these people are the reviewers and consultants who point out areas of concern, cite areas of strength, and make recommendations for change. In this regard, the following instructors provided feedback that was enormously helpful in preparing the manuscript.

SIXTH EDITION REVIEWERS

Elizabeth Cason, CPC, CDC, CMA
Centura College

Cheryl Kolar, AS in HS, RMA, LPN
Cecil College

Sarah Kuzera, BS, AAS, CMA (AAMA)
Bryan University

Melissa Rub, CMA (AAMA)
Rasmussen College

Jodi Wyrick, MBA, BBA, CMA (AAMA)
Bryant and Stratton University

SIXTH EDITION SUPPLEMENTS and LEARNSMART REVISION CONTRIBUTORS

Sue Coleman, LPN, AS, RMA (AMT)
American National University

Danielle Mbadu
Orbis Educaton

Ashita Patel, CPC-A
Wake Technical Community College

Tammy Vannatter, BHSA, CMA (AAMA), RMA, CPC
Baker College

PREVIOUS EDITION REVIEWERS

Many instructors have attended focus groups or reviewed the manuscript while it was in development, providing valuable feedback that has directly impacted the last five editions.

Ramona Atiles
New Life Business Institute

William Butler, RMA, MHA
ECPI University

Elizabeth Cason, CPC, CDC, CMA
Centura College

Amanda Davis-Smith, NCMA, AHI, CPC
Jefferson Community College

Jessica DeLuca
College of Westchester

Kathy Gaeng, AOS in Bus Mgmt, MA, RMA, Red Cross Instructor, Proctor-NCCT, Burdick Cert.
Vatterott College

Henry Gomez
ASA College

Gabriel Holder
Berkeley College

Karlene Jaggan, NRAHA, PN, BIT
Centura College

Cheryl Kolar, AS in HS, RMA, LPN
Cecil College

Sarah Kuzera, BS, AAS, CMA (AAMA)
Bryan Career College

Angela LeuVoy, AAMA, CCMA, CMA, CMRS
Fortis College

Lynnae Lockett, RMA, CMRS, RN
Bryant and Stratton College

Marta Lopez, MD, LM, CPM, RMA, BMO
Miami Dade College

Carrie A. Mack, AS, CMA (AAMA)
Branford Hall Career Institute

Lori Mikell, RMA, AHI
Ridley-Lowell Business and Technical Institute

Nanci Milbrath, AAS, CMA (AAMA)
Pine Technical College

Shauna Phillips, CCMA, CPT, CET, CMT
Fortis College

Dale Schwartz, RMA
Sanford-Brown Institute

Lisa Smith, CMA (AAMA), LXMO
Minnesota School of Business

Kasey Waychoff, CMA, CPT
Centura College

Jodi Wyrick, MBA, BBA, CMA (AAMA)
Bryant and Stratton College

Deborah Zenzal, RN, BSN, MS, CPC, CCS-P, RMA
Penn Foster College

SURVEY RESPONDENTS

Multiple instructors participated in surveys to help guide the early development of the product.

Doris Allen, LPN
Wichita Technical Institute

Annette S. Baer, CMA (AAMA)
Johnicka Byrd, CMA (AAMA), AS
Virginia College

Monica Cox, CMA, BA in HRM, MHA
Virginia College

Todd Farney, BS, DC
Wichita Technical Institute

Kathy Gaeng, AOS in Bus Mgmt, MA, RMA, Red Cross Instructor, Proctor-NCCT, Burdick Cert.
Vatterott College

Cindy Gordon, MBA, CMA (AAMA)
Baker College

Gary L. Hayes, MD
ECPI University

Pamela Hurst, CMA/AC (AAMA), AS
Ridley-Lowell Business and Technical Institute

Christina Ivey, NRCMA, BSHS/M
Centura College

Karlene Jaggan, NRAHA, PN, BIT
Centura College

Hunter Jones, PhD RN
Virginia College

Angela LeuVoy, AAMA, CCMA, CMA, CMRS
Fortis College

G. Martinez, BS (HSO), MS (HA), Cert. Medical Billing
Wichita Technical Institute

M. McGuire, RN
Wichita Technical Institute

Lori Mikell, RMA, AHI
Ridley-Lowell Business and Technical Institute

Mariela Nale, CMA, RPT
Centura College

Sherry Nemconsky, CMA
Ridley-Lowell Business and Technical Institute

Shauna Phillips, CCMA, CPT, CET, CMT
Fortis College

Sharmalan Sathiyaseelan, MD, RMA
Sanford-Brown Institute

Lucy Schultz, BBA, NCICS
Dorsey Schools

Dale Schwartz, RMA
Sanford-Brown Institute

LaShawn Smalls, DC
Virginia College

Kasey Waychoff, CMA, CPT
Centura College

Andrea Weymouth, CMA, NCCT, RMA
Ridley-Lowell Business and Technical Institute

Deborah Wuethrick, MBA/HR, AMT, CPT, CMAA, NHA, BLS, AHA
Computer Systems Institute

Deborah Zenzal, RN, BSN, MS, CPC, CCS-P, RMA
Penn Foster College

TECHNICAL EDITING/ACCURACY PANEL

A panel of instructors completed a technical edit and review of the content in the book page proofs to verify its accuracy.

Annette S. Baer, CMA (AAMA)
Shauna Phillips, CCMA, CPT, CET, CMT
Fortis College

Melissa M. Rub, BA, CMA (AAMA)
Rasmussen College

Deborah Wuethrick, MBA/HR, AMT, CPT, CMAA, NHA, BLS, AHA
Computer Systems Institute

SYMPOSIA

An enthusiastic group of trusted faculty members active in this course area attended symposia to provide crucial feedback.

Sandra Brightwell, RHIA
Central Arizona College

Linda Buchanan-Anderson, RN, BSN, RMA (AMT)
Central Arizona College

William Travis Butler, RMA, MHA
ECPI University

Mohammed Y. Chowdhury, MBBS, MPH, CCA (AHIMA), CBCS (NHA), CAHI (AMT)
Lincoln Technical Institute

Kristy Comeaux, CMA, CPT, EKG
Delta College

Amanda Davis-Smith, NCMA, AHI, CPC
Jefferson Community and Technical College

Marylou de Roma-Ragaza, BSN, MSN, RN
Lincoln Educational Services

Kathy Gaeng, RMA, CAHI
Vatterott College

Karlene Jaggan, PN, NRCAHA, BIT
Centura College

Jennifer B. Kubetin, CEHR
Branford Hall Career Institute

Cheryl A. Kuck, BS, CMA (AAMA)
Rhodes State College

Lynnae Lockett, RN, RMA, MSN
Bryant & Stratton College

Marta Lopez, MD, LM, CPM, RMA, BMO
Miami Dade College – Medical Campus

Carrie A. Mack, CMA (AAMA)
Branford Hall Career Institute

Nanci Milbrath, AAS, CMA (AAMA)
Pine Technical College

Corina Miranda, CMPC-I, CPC
Kaplan College

Angela M. B. Oliva, BS, CMRS
Heald College and Boston Reed College

Debra J. Paul, BA, CMA-AAMA
Ivy Tech Community College

Denise Pruitt, EdD
Middlesex Community College

Wendy Schmerse, CMRS
Charter College

LaShawn D. Sullivan, BSHIM, CPC
Medtech

Gina F. Umstetter
Bachelor in Computer Management, MSIT (ABT)
Instructor, Delta College of Arts & Technology

Lisa Wright, CMA (AAMA), MT, SH
Bristol Community College

Deborah Ann Zenzal, RN BSN MS CCS-P CPC RMA
Penn Foster

SPECIAL THANKS TO THE INSTRUCTORS WHO HELPED WITH THE DEVELOPMENT OF CONNECT AND LEARNSMART. THESE INCLUDE:

Belinda Beeman, M.Ed, CMA (AAMA), PBT (ASCP)
Eastern New Mexico University-Roswell

Kendra Barker, AA, BS
Pinnacle Career Institute

William Travis Butler, RMA, MHA
ECPI University

Susan Cousins, RN, CPC, M.Ed., MBA
Daymar College-Online

Carol Dew, MA-T, CMA-AC (AAMA)
Baker College

Amy Ensign, CMA (AAMA), RMA (AMT)
Baker College

Patti Finney, CMA
Ridley Lowell Business and Technical Institute

Cheryl Kolar, AS in HS, RMA, LPN
Cecil College

Cheryl A. Kuck, BS, CMA (AAMA)
Rhodes State College

Sarah Kuzera, BS, AAS, CMA (AAMA)
Bryan Career College

Marta Lopez, MD, LM, CPM, RMA, BMO
Miami Dade College–Medical Campus

Carrie A. Mack, CMA (AAMA)
Branford Hall Career Institute

Stephanie McGahee, CMA (AAMA)
Augusta Technical College

Nanci Milbrath, AAS, CMA (AAMA)
Pine Technical College

Lori Mikell, RMA, AHI
Ridley-Lowell Business and Technical Institute

Sherry Nemconsky, CMA
Ridley-Lowell Business and Technical Institute

Debra J. Paul, BA, CMA-AAMA
Ivy Tech Community College

Denise Pruitt, Ed.D.
Middlesex Community College; Fisher College

Kristy Royea, MBA, CMA (AAMA)
Mildred Elley College

Dale Schwartz, RMA
Sanford-Brown Institute

Lisa Smith, CMA (AAMA), LXMO
Minnesota School of Business

Sharon L. Vaughan, RN, BSN, RMA (AMT)
Georgia Northwestern Technical College

Kasey Waychoff, CMA, CPT
Centura College

Sten Wiedmeier RMA, BS
Bryan University

ACKNOWLEDGMENTS FROM THE AUTHOR

Sincere thanks go to the following McGraw-Hill staff for their considerable efforts, invaluable assistance, and vital guidance during the development of this book:

Chad Grall, Managing Director for Health Professions; William Lawrensen, Executive Brand Manager; Harper Christopher, Executive Marketing Manager; Christine "Chipper" Scheid, Senior Product Developer; Katie Ward, Digital Product Analyst.

I would also like to thank Danielle Mbadu for her work on revising the Instructor's Manual and PowerPoint presentation, and Tammy Vannatter for her work on revising and updating the Connect materials.

Additionally, I would like to express my appreciation to McGraw-Hill for providing the artwork that helped illustrate this book. Last, I would like to thank Greg Vadimsky, Assistant to the Author, for his help. I would also like to acknowledge the reviewers listed for their time and efforts in aiding me and contributing to this book.

GENERAL MEDICAL ASSISTING KNOWLEDGE

SECTION OUTLINE

THE PROFESSION OF MEDICAL ASSISTING

LEARNING OUTCOMES

1.1 Describe the administrative, clinical, and specialized duties of a medical assistant.

1.2 List the benefits of a Medical Assisting Program.

1.3 Identify the different types of credentials available to medical assistants through examination.

1.4 List the three areas of knowledge included in the CMA and RMA exams.

1.5 Explain the requirements for obtaining and maintaining the CCMA credential.

1.6 Describe the subject areas covered by the NCMA exam.

1.7 Describe the purpose and benefits of the extern experience.

1.8 Describe the personal attributes of a professional medical assistant.

MEDICAL ASSISTING COMPETENCIES

COMPETENCY	CMA	RMA	CCMA	NCMA
General/Legal/Professional				
Respond to and initiate written communications by using correct grammar, spelling, and formatting techniques	X	X	X	X
Recognize and respond to verbal and nonverbal communications by being attentive and adapting communication to the recipient's level of understanding	X	X	X	X
Be aware of and perform within legal and ethical boundaries	X	X	X	X
Demonstrate knowledge of and monitor current federal and state health-care legislation and regulations; maintain licenses and accreditation	X	X	X	X
Exercise efficient time management	X	X	X	X
Project a positive attitude	X	X	X	

MEDICAL ASSISTING COMPETENCIES (cont.)

General/Legal/Professional

Be a "team player"	X	X	X	
Exhibit initiative	X	X	X	
Adapt to change	X	X	X	
Project a responsible attitude	X	X	X	
Be courteous and diplomatic	X	X	X	
Conduct work within scope of education, training, and ability	X	X	X	X
Be impartial and show empathy when dealing with patients	X	X	X	
Understand allied health professions and credentialing	X	X	X	

1.1 The Profession of Medical Assisting

Medical assisting is one of the most versatile health-care professions. Men and women can be equally successful as medical assistants. They are able to work in a variety of administrative and clinical positions within health care. According to the U.S. Department of Labor's *Occupational Outlook Handbook,* medical assisting is one of the 10 fastest growing occupations.

The Duties of a Medical Assistant

Medical assistants are skilled health-care professionals who work primarily in ambulatory settings such as medical offices and clinics. The duties a medical assistant may perform include administrative and clinical duties.

Administrative duties: Administrative medical assisting duties include the following:

- Greeting patients
- Handling correspondence
- Scheduling appointments
- Answering telephones
- Communicating with patients, families, and coworkers
- Creating and maintaining patient medical records
- Handling billing, bookkeeping, and insurance claim form processing
- Performing medical transcription
- Arranging for hospital admissions and testing procedures
- Organizing and managing office supplies
- Explaining treatment procedures to patients
- Educating patients

- Coding for specific procedures and tests when filling out lab requests
- Collection of payments and speaking with patients about collection policies

Clinical duties: Medical assistants' clinical duties vary according to state law. They may include the following:

- Asepsis and infection control
- Preparing the examination and treatment areas
- Interviewing patients and documenting patients' vital signs and medical histories
- Preparing patients for examinations and explaining treatment procedures
- Assisting the physician during examinations
- Disposing of contaminated supplies
- Performing diagnostic tests, such as electrocardiograms (ECGs)
- Giving injections (where allowed by law)
- Performing first aid and cardiopulmonary resuscitation (CPR)
- Preparing and administering medications as directed by the physician, and following state laws for invasive procedures
- Removing sutures or changing wound dressings
- Sterilizing medical instruments
- Assisting patients from diverse cultural backgrounds, as well as patients with hearing or vision impairments or physical or mental disabilities
- Educating patients

Medical assistants' clinical duties may also include processing various laboratory tests. Medical assistants may prepare the patient for the test, collect the sample, complete the test, report the results to the physician, and report information about the test from the physician to the patient. It must be noted that medical assistants are not qualified to make any diagnoses. Specific laboratory duties may include:

- Performing tests, such as a urine pregnancy test, in the physician's office laboratory (POL)
- Performing Clinical Laboratory Improvements Act (CLIA)-waived tests that have a low risk of an erroneous result, which include urinalysis and blood chemistry
- Collecting, preparing, and transmitting laboratory specimens, including blood, body fluids, cultures, tissue samples, and urine specimens
- Teaching specimen collection to patients
- Arranging laboratory services
- Meeting safety standards and fire protection mandates
- Performing as an Occupational Safety and Health Administration (OSHA) compliance officer

Specialization

Medical assistants may choose to specialize in a specific field of health care, in either an administrative or clinical area. For example, ophthalmic medical assistants help ophthalmologists (physicians who provide eye care) by administering diagnostic tests, measuring and recording vision, testing the functioning of a patient's eyes and eye muscles, and performing other duties. Additional training may be required for a medical assistant to specialize in certain areas.

Administrative specialty areas include the following:

- Multiskilled health-care professional
- Medical office administrator
- Dental office administrator
- Medical transcriptionist
- Medical record technologist
- Coding, billing, and insurance specialist

Clinical specialty areas include the following:

- Histologic technician
- Surgical technologist
- Physical therapy assistant
- CPR instructor
- Medical laboratory assistant
- Phlebotomist

1.2 Membership in a Medical Assisting Association

Certification and Registration

Certification or registration is not required to practice as a medical assistant in *most* states. However, for instance, as of July 2013, the state of Washington now requires certification. *Source: http://apps.leg.wa.gov/rcw/default.aspx?cite=18.360&full=true.* You may practice with a high school diploma or the equivalent. However, you will have more career options if you graduate from an accredited school and become certified or registered.

A solid medical assisting program provides the following:

- Facilities and equipment that are up to date
- Job placement services
- A cooperative education program and opportunities for continuing education

1.3 Medical Assisting Credentials

Professional associations set high standards for quality and performance in a profession. They define the tasks and functions of an occupation. They also provide members with the opportunity to communicate and network with one another.

State and Federal Regulations

Certain provisions of the Occupational Safety and Health Act (OSHA) and the Clinical Laboratory Improvements Act of 1988 (CLIA '88) are making mandatory credentialing for medical assistants a logical step in the hiring process. Currently, OSHA and CLIA '88 do not require that medical assistants be credentialed. However, various components of these statutes and their regulations can be met by demonstrating that medical assistants in a clinical setting are certified.

One of the CLIA regulatory categories based on their potential risk to public health is waived tests. Waived tests are "laboratory examination and procedures that have been approved by the Food and Drug Administration (FDA) for home use or that, as determined by the secretary, are simple laboratory examinations and procedures that have an insignificant risk of an erroneous result."

CMA Certification

The Certified Medical Assistant (CMA) credential is awarded by the Certifying Board of the American Association of Medical Assistants (AAMA). The AAMA works to raise the standards of medical assisting to a more professional level.

The AAMA's address is 20 N. Wacker Drive, Suite 1575, Chicago, IL 60606. Phone: 1-312-899-1500 or 1-800-228-2262. Fax: 1-312-899-1259. E-mail: certification@aama-ntl.org. Their website address is: www.aama-ntl.org.

The AAMA Role Delineation Study: In 1996 the AAMA formed a committee. Its goal was to revise and update the standards used for accrediting medical assisting programs. Accreditation is defined as a process in which recognition is granted to an education program. The committee's findings were published in 1997 under the title of the "AAMA Role Delineation Study: Occupational Analysis of the Medical Assisting Profession." Included was a new Role Delineation Chart that outlined the areas of competence entry-level medical assistants must master. The Role Delineation Chart was further updated in 2003. The AAMA's certification examination evaluates the mastery of medical assisting competencies on the basis of the 2003 Role Delineation Study. To take this exam, you must have graduated from a postsecondary accredited program. The National Board of Medical Examiners (NBME) also provides technical assistance in developing the tests. Its website address is www.nbme.org.

The areas of competence listed in the AAMA Role Delineation Study must be mastered by all students enrolled in accredited medical assisting programs. Each of the three areas of competence—administrative, clinical, and general (or transdisciplinary)—contains a list of statements that describe the medical assistant's role.

According to the AAMA, the Role Delineation Chart may be used to:

- Describe the field of medical assisting to other healthcare professionals
- Identify entry-level competency areas for medical assistants
- Help practitioners assess their own current competence in the field
- Aid in the development of continuing education programs
- Prepare appropriate materials for home study

Recertification for the CMA is required every five years. The medical assistant may choose to recertify by taking the examination again, or by obtaining 60 continuing education units (CEUs) over this five-year period.

RMA Certification

The Registered Medical Assistant (RMA) credential is awarded by the American Medical Technologists (AMT), an organization founded in 1939. AMT is accredited by the National Commission for Certifying Agencies (NCCA) and a member of the Institute for Credentialing Excellence.

The AMT's address is 10700 West Higgins Road, Suite 150, Rosemont, IL 60018. Phone: 1-847-823-5169. Fax: 1-847-823-0458. E-mail: mail@americanmedtech.org. The AMT's website address is www.americanmedtech.org.

Professional support for RMAs: The AMT offers many benefits for RMAs. These include:

- Insurance programs, including liability, health, and life
- Membership in the AMT Institute for Education
- State chapter activities
- Annual meeting and educational seminars

Recertification for the RMA is required every three years. Also, 30 hours of continuing education credits are required every year to maintain certification.

The American Registry of Medical Assistants (ARMA)

Medical assistants who become certified by passing a national certification examination (for example, the CMA or RMA) and medics in military service may apply for membership with the American Registry of Medical Assistants (ARMA).

ARMA is a national registry established in 1950 that certifies medical assistants who have provided the necessary documentation to be a qualified medical assistant.

ARMA grants qualified members the credential of RMA for clinical medical assistants and RMA-A for administrative medical assistants. The ARMA's website address is http://arma-cert.org.

1.4 CMA and RMA Exam Topics

The CMA and RMA qualifying examinations are rigorous. Participation in an accredited program, however, will help you learn what you need to know. The examinations cover several distinct areas of knowledge. These include:

- Administrative knowledge, including scheduling appointments, managing mail and office correspondence, medical records management, collections, insurance processing, and HIPAA (Health Insurance Portability and Accountability Act)
- Clinical knowledge, including examination room techniques; pharmacology—the preparation, calculation, and administration of medications; first aid and emergency care; performing ECGs; specimen collection and laboratory testing
- General medical knowledge, including terminology, anatomy and physiology, behavioral science, and medical law and ethics

The CMA exam is computer based and features 200 multiple-choice questions that have "one best answer" from five different answer choices. There are 180 questions that are scored, and 20 that are pretest questions that are not scored. They are formatted as incomplete statements or questions, and the answer choices either complete the statement or answer the question. Some questions require identification of body parts or anatomical regions from illustrations or diagrams. The questions on the exam are administered in four 40-minute segments.

Each person taking the test must achieve a passing score on every section in order to become certified. An *unofficial* "pass" or "fail" is given immediately after the test, but final confirmation is mailed within 12 weeks.

The RMA exam is either computer based or can be taken using pencil and paper. It features 210 multiple-choice questions that have "one best answer" from four different answer choices. Candidates have 2.5 hours to complete the exam. It requires recall of facts, understanding of medical illustrations, solving of problems, and interpretation of information from case studies. The computerized version of the exam offers an immediate pass/fail score. If the pencil-and-paper version is taken, results will arrive by mail within eight weeks. A score of 70 or above is required to pass the exam. Candidates who fail the exam will be given detailed information about areas in which their knowledge was weakest. Anyone retaking the exam must complete the entire examination in full. Like the CMA exam, the RMA covers three areas: general, administrative, and clinical medical assisting knowledge.

1.5 Certified Clinical Medical Assistant (CCMA) Examination

This credential is awarded by the National Healthcareer Association (NHA). The CCMA exam is offered in a written form or by computer via its website. It consists of 150 questions plus 20 pretest questions covering several distinct areas of knowledge. These areas emphasize clinical knowledge, including general assisting, ECG, phlebotomy, and basic lab skills. Also included is preparation of patients, such as taking a medical history, vital signs, physical examination, and patient positioning; biological hazards; emergency first aid; infection control; understanding the structure of a prescription; anatomy and physiology; law and ethics; pharmacology; specimen handling; quality control; use of microscopes; and various laboratory procedures. CCMAs also need 10 hours of continuing education every two years in order to keep their certification. Recertification for the CCMA is required every two years.

The NHA's address is 1161 Overbrook Road, Leawood, KS 66211. Phone: 1-800-499-9092 or 1-913-661-5592. Fax: 1-913-661-6291. E-mail: info@nhanow.com. The website address is http://nhanow.com.

1.6 National Certified Medical Assistant (NCMA) Examination

The NCMA exam is offered by the National Center for Competency Testing (NCCT), a for-profit agency. To take the NCMA exam, candidates must have completed either an approved medical assistant training program or at least two years of on-the-job training that was supervised by a physician. Unlike the other medical assisting exams, the NCMA credential must be renewed every year, and 14 continuing education credits must be earned in order for renewal to be approved. The exam is offered in both computerized and paper forms. It consists of 165 questions, which includes 15 that are not graded. Three hours are allowed to take the exam. The NCMA exam covers a variety of subject areas, which include pharmacology,

medical procedures, patient care, phlebotomy, diagnostic tests, electrocardiogram, general office procedures, medical office general management, financial management, and law and ethics.

The NCCT's address is 7007 College Blvd., Suite 385, Overland Park, KS 66211. Phone: 1-800-875-4404. Fax: 1-913-498-1243. The website address is http://www.ncctinc.com.

Table 1-1 summarizes the various certification examinations and their related information.

1.7 Externships

An externship offers work experience while you complete a medical assisting program. You will practice skills learned in the classroom in an actual medical office environment. A medical assisting extern must be able to accept constructive criticism, be flexible, and also be willing to learn. In an externship, you may be exposed to some procedures that are not performed exactly as you were taught in the classroom or clinical laboratory. Learn as much as possible while on an externship. It is unprofessional to argue with an externship preceptor. Ask your externship preceptor to explain any differences in techniques from what you learned while you were in the classroom.

1.8 Preparing for Employment

Career Services will assist you with your resume, interviewing skills, and learning about positions in your field. It is important to include certification awarded in relation to a position on your resume.

New employee: An initial performance evaluation should be given 90 days after employment.

Personal Attributes

Medical assistants can be more effective and productive if they have the personal qualifications of professionalism, empathy, flexibility, self-motivation, integrity and honesty, and accountability. A neat and professional appearance is also essential.

AT A GLANCE	Medical Assistant Certification Exams		
Organization	Credential	Fees	Notes
American Association of Medical Assistants (AAMA)	CMA (5 years)	$125 recent graduates and members, $250 for others	Not-for-profit. Annual fees $25–$40 for students, up to $107 for others, all based on state.
American Medical Technologists (AMT)	RMA (3 years)	$120	Not-for-profit. Annual fees $50.
National Healthcareer Association (NHA)	CCMA (2 years)	$149	For-profit.
National Center for Competency Testing (NCCT)	NCMA (1 year)	$90 recent graduates; $135 for others	For-profit.

Table 1-1

Professionalism: A medical assistant should demonstrate courtesy, conscientiousness, and a generally businesslike manner at all times. It is essential for medical assistants to act professionally with patients, doctors, and coworkers. Present a neat appearance and show courtesy and respect for peers and instructors.

Professionalism is also displayed in your attitude. The medical assistant is a skilled professional on whom many people, including coworkers and patients, depend. Your attitude can make or break your career. A professional always projects a positive, caring attitude. The medical assistant should avoid using terms of endearment with patients and remain strictly professional.

Empathy: Empathy is the ability to put yourself in someone else's situation—to identify with and understand another person's feelings. Patients who are sick, frustrated, or frightened appreciate empathetic medical personnel. It is always advisable for the medical assistant to ask patients if they need any assistance, including disabled patients.

Flexibility: An attitude of flexibility will allow you to adapt to and handle situations with professionalism. For example, when a physician's schedule changes to include evening and weekend hours, the staff also may be asked to change their schedules. Therefore, you must be flexible and meet the employer's needs.

Self-motivation: You must be self-motivated and offer assistance with work that needs to be done, even if it is not your assigned job. For example, if a coworker is on sick leave or vacation, offer to pitch in and work extra time to keep the office running smoothly.

Integrity and honesty: Medical assistants with integrity hold themselves to high standards. Integrity may be characterized by honesty, dependability, and reliability. The most important elements in providing superior customer service to patients are integrity and honesty. If you make an error, be honest about it. In order to have integrity, you must be dependable and reliable.

Accountability: Legal, mental, or moral responsibility. In medicine, it refers to the responsibility for moral and legal requirements of patient care.

Neat appearance: Medical facilities expect externs and their staff to appear as medical professionals. Most require a uniform that consists of a scrub top and bottom and a lab jacket. Your name tag or badge should always be worn and visible to patients. Visible tattoos must be covered. Your hair should be a natural color and pulled back from your face and off the collar. Perfumes and colognes should be avoided because patients with respiratory conditions or allergies may not be able to tolerate them.

Test-Taking Preparation

It is important to understand all of the content that the examination you choose to take will include. You must create a study schedule and follow it closely. Waiting until the last minute is never a good idea, and may even cause you to fail. Each of these exams is difficult and requires sufficient study in order to pass.

It is suggested that you take as many practice exams as possible prior to taking either the CMA, RMA, CCMA, or NCMA exam. When taking a practice exam, make sure to read all of the answer key content, including the rationales for each correct answer, and each incorrect answer. This will greatly help you to understand the material more deeply, and is a great way to study. The various organizations that offer these certification exams also provide guides and study materials to help you prepare. There are also exam study groups, handbooks, and other materials available via the Internet. Another important suggestion is to practice doing mathematic calculations without the use of a calculator or scratch paper, both of which are not allowed when you take an actual exam.

On the day of the exam, make sure you are well rested, wearing comfortable clothing, wearing a watch if you have one, and have eaten enough so that you do not get hungry during the exam. It is not suggested that you study right up until you leave to take the exam, since it is important to allow yourself a little "buffer time." Then, you will be more prepared to absorb the questions, and take in and process information. Arrive early, and make sure you bring whatever materials are required to enter the examination area. Do not bring anything else that will not be allowed into that area. Once inside, remember not to talk to anyone else taking the exam. Never leave the examination area without the permission of the test administrator. Be ready to get started, and remember that with all of your preparations, you should do very well.

The most important thing to remember when taking one of these exams is to read each question carefully, paying attention to detail. Questions that contain the words "except" or "not" can be tricky if you read them too quickly. Before you look at the answer choices, see if you have the answer already in mind. This way, the answer choices will not influence your selection, and you are less likely to choose incorrectly. Usually, one or more of the answer choices can be easily eliminated. Another tip is to cross off each of these in order to focus on the other remaining choices more effectively. Methods of "marking" various questions vary between computerized versions of the exams, but paper exams are obviously easy to mark up.

Do not spend too much time on each question; instead, circle those that seem more difficult and come back to them. Pace yourself as you move through the various sections of the test. Do not simply go straight through the questions and attempt to answer each of them while not paying attention to the time that you are spending on each.

Make sure you respond to each question. No points will be subtracted for incorrect answers—you are only graded on the amount that you answer correctly. For the more difficult questions, eliminate as many answer choices as possible prior to making your selection. For paper exams, make sure you monitor your answer sheet carefully so that you are filling in the correct area for each question. If you must erase or change an answer, make sure you do it clearly so that your intended answer is obvious. At the end of an exam, or a section of an exam, if you still have extra time, go back over your answers to double check for any errors.

Give your eyes a break during your exam by looking away from the computer monitor or the test paper briefly, every 10–15 minutes. Excessive concentration while focusing on them can cause eye strain, resulting in a headache.

CHAPTER 1 REVIEW

Instructions:
Answer the following questions.

1. Accreditation may be defined as
   - A. a contract that specifies an agreement.
   - B. permission to engage in a profession.
   - C. permission to be licensed.
   - D. an assessment of an individual's performance.
   - E. a process in which recognition is granted to an education program.

2. Which of the following organizations offers the Registered Medical Assistant credential?
   - A. AMA
   - B. AAMA
   - C. AMT
   - D. CDC
   - E. NBME

3. The CMA and RMA examinations cover all of the following distinct areas of knowledge *except*
   - A. calculations for preparing medications.
   - B. HIPAA.
   - C. criminal justice.
   - D. medical records.
   - E. behavioral science.

4. Which of the following professional attributes indicates the ability to identify with someone else's situation?
   - A. empathy
   - B. professionalism
   - C. self-motivation
   - D. integrity
   - E. flexibility

5. After you become a certified clinical medical assistant, how often is recertification required?
   - A. every year
   - B. every two years
   - C. every three years
   - D. every five years
   - E. every seven years

6. Which of the following terms describes behaving courteously, conscientiously, and in a generally businesslike manner?
   - A. self-motivation
   - B. professionalism
   - C. job description
   - D. ethics
   - E. morals

7. Which of the following constitutes unprofessional behavior when interacting with an externship preceptor?
   - A. accepting criticism
   - B. arguing
   - C. being flexible
   - D. listening to instructions
   - E. having references

8. Which of the following is the correct website address for the National Board of Medical Examiners?
   - A. www.nbme.org
   - B. www.nbme.gov
   - C. www.nbm.com
   - D. www.meboard.com
   - E. www.medexam.com

9. Which of the following is *not* an example of a medical assistant's clinical duties?
   - A. preparing patients for examinations
   - B. interviewing patients and documenting their vital signs
   - C. performing diagnostic tests
   - D. explaining treatment procedures to patients
   - E. diagnosing communicable diseases

10. A patient with a physical disability comes to the office. The most appropriate response by the medical assistant is to
    - A. express sympathy regarding the disability.
    - B. tell your supervisor.
    - C. ask the patient whether assistance is needed.
    - D. ask the patient how the disability occurred.
    - E. assume that the patient needs assistance and begin giving aid.

MEDICAL TERMINOLOGY

LEARNING OUTCOMES

2.1 Identify and define common roots, suffixes, and prefixes.

2.2 Demonstrate proper spelling of common medical terms in singular, plural, and possessive forms.

2.3 Identify abbreviations commonly used in medical practice.

2.4 Define medical terms used in relation to diseases and body systems.

2.5 Describe unacceptable abbreviations as outlined by the Joint Commission.

MEDICAL ASSISTING COMPETENCIES

COMPETENCY	CMA	RMA	CCMA	NCMA
General/Legal/Professional				
Use appropriate medical terminology	X	X	X	X

▶ *Study Skills*

Organize and manage!
Organize your notes after class. Doing so will not only help you review material but also make it easier to understand your notes when you go back to them to study for an exam. Organizing your notes right away will also give you plenty of time to ask your instructor to clarify something you didn't understand.

2.1 Word Building

Root: The main part of a word that gives the word its central meaning. The root is the basic foundation of a word.

Prefix: A structure at the beginning of a word that modifies the meaning of the root. Not all medical words have a prefix. For a list of common prefixes, see Table 2-1.

Suffix: A word ending that modifies the meaning of the root. Not all words have a suffix. For a list of common suffixes, see Table 2-2.

Combining vowels: When a medical term is formed from many different word parts, these parts are often joined by a vowel. This vowel is usually an *o* and occasionally an *i*. The

AT A GLANCE **Common General Prefixes**

Prefix	Meaning	Example	Definition
a-	Without	Aphonia	Inability to produce sound
ab-	From, away from	Abduct	To move away from the midline of the body
ad-, ac-, af-, ag-, al-, ap-, ar-, as-, at-	Toward, increasing	Adduct	To move toward the midline of the body
alb-	White	Albinism	Whiteness of skin, hair, and eyes caused by the absence of pigment
ambi-	Both	Ambidextrous	Able to use both hands effectively
ana-	Up, upward	Anaphylactic	Characterized by an exaggerated reaction to an antigen or toxin
ante-	Before	Antepartum	Before childbirth
anti-	Against	Antibiotic	Acting against microorganisms
auto-	Self	Autodermic	Of the patient's own skin (said of skin grafts)
bi-	Two, both	Bilateral	Pertaining to both sides
bio-	Life	Biology	Study of life
broncho-	Bronchus, bronchi	Bronchorrhaphy	Suturing a wound of the bronchus
circum-	Around	Circumcision	Removal of the skin around the tip of the penis
con-, col-, com-, cor-	Together, with	Congenital	Accompanying birth, present at birth
contra-	Against	Contraceptive	Preventing conception
de-	Away from, down, not	Decalcify	To decrease or remove calcium
dia-	Through	Diagnosis	Knowledge through testing
dis-	Apart, separate	Dislocation	Removal of any part of the body from its normal position

Table 2-1

Prefix	Meaning	Example	Definition
dys-	Bad, difficult, painful, poor	Dysuria	Painful urination
ec-	Out, away	Ectopic	Pertaining to something outside its normal location
ecto-	Outside	Ectoplasm	Outermost layer of cell protoplasm
en-, em-	In	Endemic	Occurring continuously in a population
		Empyema	Pus in a body cavity
endo-	Within	Endoscope	Instrument to examine something from within
epi-	Upon, over	Epidermal	Upon the skin
eu-	Good	Eupnea	Normal, good breathing
ex-, e-	Out, away	Exhale	To breathe out
		Emanation	Something given off
hemi-	Half	Hemicardia	Half of the heart
hyper-	Excessive, beyond	Hyperlipemia	Condition of excessive fat in the blood
hypo-	Below, under	Hypoglycemia	Low blood sugar
in-, il-, im-, ir-	Not	Impotence	Inability to achieve erection
infra-	Below, under, beneath	Inframammary	Below the breast
inter-	Between	Intercellular	Between cells
intra-	Within	Intravenous	Within a vein
iso-	Equal	Isometric	Of equal dimension
juxta-	Near, beside	Juxtaarticular	Near a joint
mal-	Bad	Malaise	Discomfort
mega-, megal- / o	Large	Megacephaly	Abnormal enlargement of the head
mes- / o	Middle	Mesoderm	Middle layer of the skin
meta-	Beyond, after	Metastasis	Spread of disease from one part of the body to another
micro-	Small	Microscope	Instrument used to view small organisms
milli-	One-thousandth	Milliliter	One-thousandth of a liter
mono-	One, single	Mononuclear	Having only one nucleus
multi-	Many	Multidisciplinary	Pertaining to many areas of study
neo-	New, recent	Neonatal	Pertaining to the period after birth
non-	Not	Noninvasive	Not invading the body through any organ, cavity, or skin (said of a diagnostic or therapeutic technique)
para-	Near, beside, beyond, opposite, abnormal	Paramedic	Person who provides emergency medical care (alongside other medical personnel)

Table 2-1, continued

AT A GLANCE | Common General Prefixes

Prefix	Meaning	Example	Definition
per-	Through	Percutaneous	Through the skin
peri-	Around, surrounding	Perianal	Around the anus
poly-	Many	Polyarthritis	Inflammation of many joints
post-	After	Postmortem	After death
pre-	Before	Premature	Before maturation
primi-	First	Primiparous	Having given birth for the first time
re-	Again, back	Reactivate	To make active again
retro-	Back, backward, behind	Retrograde	Going backward
rube-	Red	Rubella	Viral disease characterized by red rashes, among other things
sacro-	Sacrum	Sacroiliac	Pertaining to the sacrum and iliac bones
sarco-	Flesh	Sarcoma	A malignant tumor arising from connective tissues
semi-	Half	Semiconscious	Half conscious
sub-	Under, below	Sublingual	Under the tongue
super-	Above, excessive	Superficial	Near or above the surface
supra-	Above, over	Suprapubic	Above the pubic area
syn-, sym-	Together	Symbiosis	Mutual interdependence
tri-	Three	Triceps	Muscle with three heads
ultra-	Beyond, excessive	Ultrasound	Sound with a very high frequency, used to obtain medical images
uni-	One	Unicellular	One-celled

Table 2-1, concluded

AT A GLANCE | Common General Suffixes

Suffix	Meaning	Example	Definition
-ac	Pertaining to	Cardiac	Pertaining to the heart
-ad	Toward	Cephalad	Toward the head
-al	Pertaining to	Thermal	Pertaining to the production of heat
-ar	Pertaining to	Articular	Pertaining to a joint
-desis	Binding	Arthrodesis	Surgical binding or fusing of a joint
-e	Noun marker	Dermatome	Instrument used to cut the skin
-ectomy	Excision, removal	Hysterectomy	Removal of the entire uterus
-emesis	Vomit	Hyperemesis	Excessive vomiting

Table 2-2

Suffix	Meaning	Example	Definition
-form	Resembling, like	Vermiform	Shaped like a worm
-genic	Beginning, originating, producing	Toxigenic	Producing toxins
-gram	Record	Electrocardiogram	Record of the variations in electrical potential caused by the heart muscle
-graph	Instrument for recording	Electrocardiograph	Instrument for making electrocardiograms
-graphy	Process of recording	Electrocystography	Process of recording the changes of electric potential in the urinary bladder
-iasis	Condition, formation	Lithiasis	Formation or presence of stones
-iatric	Pertaining to medical treatment	Pediatric	Pertaining to the treatment of children
-iatry	Study or field of medicine	Psychiatry	Study of the human psyche
-ic	Pertaining to	Thoracic	Pertaining to the thorax
-ical	Pertaining to	Neurological	Pertaining to nerves
-ism	Condition	Cryptorchidism	Condition of undescended testes
-ist	Specialist	Otorhinolaryngologist	Physician who specializes in the ear, nose, and larynx
-itis	Inflammation	Appendicitis	Inflammation of the appendix
-logist	Specialist in the study of	Microbiologist	Biologist who specializes in the study of microorganisms
-logy	Study of	Microbiology	Study of microorganisms
-lysis	Destruction, breaking down	Hemolysis	Breaking down of blood
-megaly	Enlargement	Cardiomegaly	Enlargement of the heart
-meter	Instrument used to measure	Scoliosometer	Instrument for measuring the curves of the spine
-oma	Tumor	Carcinoma	Cancerous, malignant tumor
-ory	Pertaining to	Auditory	Pertaining to hearing
-osis	Condition, disease	Leukocytosis	Condition of increased leukocytes in the blood
-pathy	Disease	Hemopathy	Disease of the blood
-penia	Abnormal reduction	Leukocytopenia	Decrease in the number of white blood cells
-philia	Attraction	Necrophilia	Attraction to dead bodies
-phobia	Abnormal fear	Photophobia	Fear of light
-plasia	Development	Dysplasia	Faulty formation
-plasty	Molding, surgical repair	Rhinoplasty	Surgical repair of the nose
-ptosis	Drooping, prolapse, falling	Mastoptosis	Drooping of the breast
-rrhage, -rrhagia	Excessive flow, discharge	Hemorrhage	Bursting forth of blood
-rrhea	Discharge, flow	Amenorrhea	Absence of menstrual flow

Table 2-2, continued

Suffix	Meaning	Example	Definition
-rrhexis	Rupture	Cardiorrhexis	Rupture of the heart
-scope	Instrument used to view	Oscilloscope	Instrument that displays visual representation of electrical variations
-scopy	Process of viewing with a scope	Opthalmoscopy	Process of examining the interior of the eye by using an opthalmoscope
-stasis	Stoppage, balance, control	Hemostasis	A stopping of the flow of blood
-stomy	Surgical creation of a new opening	Colostomy	Creation of an opening between the colon and the surface of the body
-tomy	Incision, cutting	Phlebotomy	Incision into a vein

Table 2-2, concluded

vowel *o* is the most common combining vowel. The combining vowel is used to ease pronunciation.

Guidelines for using combining vowels include the following:

- When a root and a suffix beginning with a vowel are connected, a combining vowel is usually not used.
- Connecting a word root and a suffix that starts with a consonant usually requires a connecting vowel.
- When two roots are connected, a combining vowel is most often used even if vowels are present at the junction.
- Most common prefixes can be connected to other word parts without a combining vowel.

2.2 Spelling

Spelling: Some commonly misspelled words are:

- Abscess
- Accessible
- Aerobic
- Agglutinate
- Analyses
- Analysis
- Aneurysm
- Asepsis
- Asthma
- Auxiliary
- Benign
- Capillary
- Chancre
- Changeable
- Clavicle
- Conscious
- Defibrillator
- Desiccation
- Dissect
- Epididymis
- Fissure
- Glaucoma
- Hemorrhoid
- Homeostasis
- Humerus
- Hyperglycemia
- Hypoglycemia
- Irrelevant
- Ischium
- Occlusion
- Osseous
- Pamphlet

- Parenteral
- Parietal
- Perineum
- Perseverance
- Precede
- Predictable
- Principle
- Sizable
- Specimen
- Surgeon
- Tranquility
- Vaccine
- Vacuum

To correct a misspelled word in a patient's chart, you must draw a single line through the word.

Plural forms: Here are some general rules. Remember, there are almost always exceptions.

- Add an *s* or *es* to most singular nouns to make them plural.
- When a medical term in the singular form ends in *is,* drop the *is* and add *es* to make it plural (metastasis/metastases).
- When the term ends in *um* or *on,* drop the *um* or *on* and add *a* (atrium/atria, ganglion/ganglia).
- When the term ends in *us,* drop the *us* and add *i* (bronchus/bronchi). Exceptions to this rule mainly involve certain words of Latin origin (corpus/corpora, genus/genera, sinus/sinuses, virus/viruses).
- When the term ends in *ma,* add *ta* (stoma/stomata).
- When the term otherwise ends in *a,* drop the *a* and add *ae* (vertebra/vertebrae).

Possessive forms: For singular nouns and plural nouns that do not end in *s,* add an apostrophe and an *s.* For plural nouns that end in *s,* just add an apostrophe but no additional *s.*

2.3 Common Medical Abbreviations

Abbreviations: The most common abbreviations used in association with medical care facilities are presented in Table 2-3. The most common medical record abbreviations are listed in Table 2-4, abbreviations associated with the metric system are

AT A GLANCE Medical Care Facility Abbreviations

Abbreviation	Meaning	Abbreviation	Meaning
CCU	Coronary care unit	OR	Operating room
ED	Emergency department	PAR	Postanesthetic recovery
ER	Emergency room	postop	Postoperative
ICU	Intensive care unit	preop	Preoperative
IP	Inpatient	RTC	Return to clinic
OP	Outpatient	RTO	Return to office
OPD	Outpatient department		

Table 2-3

AT A GLANCE Medical Record Abbreviations

Abbreviation	Meaning	Abbreviation	Meaning
AIDS	Acquired immunodeficiency syndrome	GYN	Gynecology
a.m.a.	Against medical advice	H & P	History and physical
BP	Blood pressure	HEENT	Head, ears, eyes, nose, throat
bpm	Beats per minute	HIV	Human immunodeficiency virus
C	Celsius, centigrade	Ht	Height
CBC	Complete blood count	Hx	History
C.C.	Chief complaint	I & D	Incision and drainage
CNS	Central nervous system	inj	Injection
c/o	Complains of	IV	Intravenous
CP	Chest pain	L	Left
CPE	Complete physical examination	L & W	Living and well
CV	Cardiovascular	lab	Laboratory studies
D & C	Dilation and curettage	MM	Mucous membrane
Dx	Diagnosis	N & V	Nausea and vomiting
ECG/EKG	Electrocardiogram	NP	New patient, Nurse practitioner
ED, ER	Emergency room	P	Pulse
F	Fahrenheit	Pap	Pap smear
FH	Family history	PE	Physical examination
Fl/fl	Fluid	pH	Hydrogen concentration (acidity/alkalinity)
GBS	Gallbladder series	PI	Present illness
GI	Gastrointestinal	PMH	Past medical history
GU	Genitourinary	PMS	Premenstrual syndrome

Table 2-4, continued

Abbreviation	Meaning	Abbreviation	Meaning
PNS	Peripheral nervous system	stat	Immediately
pt	Patient	STD	Sexually transmitted disease
PT	Physical therapy	surg	Surgery
Px	Physical examination	T	Temperature
R	Right	TPR	Temperature, pulse, respirations
re✓	Recheck	Tx	Treatment
ref	Referral	UCHD	Usual childhood diseases
R/O	Rule out	US	Ultrasound
ROS/SR	Review of systems/systems review	VS	Vital signs
Rx	Prescription	WDWN	Well-developed and well-nourished
subq.	Subcutaneously	WNL	Within normal limits
sig	Sigmoidoscopy	Wt	Weight
SOB	Shortness of breath	y.o.	Year old
S/R	Suture removal		

Table 2-4, concluded

listed in Table 2-5, and common prescription abbreviations are listed in Table 2-6. Tables of relevant abbreviations are also included for each body system.

Pharmaceutical Abbreviations

Metric system: A system of measurement based on the decimal system. Its units include the meter, gram, and liter. It is the most commonly used system of measurement in health care.

For a list of common abbreviations used in the metric system, see Table 2-5.

Conversion factors for the metric system: The meter (m), used for length, equals approximately 39.37 inches; the liter (L or l), used for volume, equals approximately 1.056 U.S. quarts; and the gram (g or gm), used for weight, equals approximately 0.035 ounce.

Apothecaries' system: An old system of measurement in which the weight measure is based on one grain of wheat and

Abbreviation	Meaning	Abbreviation	Meaning
cm	Centimeter (2.5 cm = 1 inch)	deca-	× 10
km	Kilometer	hect-	× 100
mL	Milliliter (1 mL = 1 cc)	kilo-	× 1000
mm	Millimeter	deci-	÷ 10
g, gm	Gram	centi-	÷ 100
kg	Kilogram (1 kg = 1000 gm = 2.2 pounds)	milli-	÷ 1000
L or l	Liter = 1000 mL (1 gallon = 4 quarts = 8 pints = 3.785 L; 1 pint = 473.16 mL)	micro-	÷ 1,000,000

Table 2-5

Abbreviation	Meaning	Abbreviation	Meaning
a	Before	p.o., PO	By mouth
a.c.	Before meals	PR	Through the rectum
ad lib.	As desired	p.r.n., PRN	As needed
AM, a.m.	Morning	PV, vag.	Through the vagina
amt	Amount	q	Every
aq	Water	qh	Every hour
b.i.d., BID	Twice a day	q2h	Every 2 hours
buc	Buccal	q.i.d., QID	Four times a day
$\bar{c}$	With	®	Right, registered trademark
cap	Capsule	Rx	Prescription, take
d	Day	$\bar{s}$	Without
Fl.	Fluid	sub-Q, subcu	Subcutaneous
h, hr	Hour	Sig:	Instruction to patient
h.s.*	At bedtime, at the hour of sleep	soln.	Solution
ID	Intradermal	sp.	Spirits
IM	Intramuscular	$\overline{ss}$	One half
IV	Intravenous	stat	Immediately
noc., n.	Night	supp., suppos	Suppository
NPO	Nothing by mouth	syr.	Syrup
oint., ung.	Ointment	T	Topical
$\bar{p}$	After	tab	Tablet
p.c.	After meals	t.i.d., TID	Three times a day
per	By, through	x	Times, for
PM, p.m.	After noon		

Table 2-6

*Though this abbreviation is on the JCAHO's *Do Not Use List*, it is still in common usage.

the liquid measure is based on one drop of water. The apothecaries' system measures weight by grains (gr), scruples (scr), drams (dr), ounces (oz), and pounds (lb). It uses minims (min), fluidrams (fl dr), fluid ounces (fl oz), pints (pt), quarts (qt), and gallons (gal) to measure volume. In the apothecary system, dosage quantities are written in lowercase Roman numerals (i = 1, ii = 2, iv = 4, v = 5, vi = 6, ix = 9, x = 10, xi = 11, xx = 20, xl = 40, l = 50, lx = 60, xc = 90, c = 100, cx = 110, cc = 200, d = 500, m = 1000, mm = 2000, etc.). A bar written above a numeral multiplies its value by 1000:

$$(\bar{v} = 5000, \bar{c} = 100,000, \overline{m} = 1,000,000, \overline{ss} = \tfrac{1}{2}, \text{etc.})$$

Conversion factors for the apothecaries' system: There are approximately 60 milligrams to a grain, and 15 grains to a gram.

grains × 60 = milligrams

grains ÷ 15 = grams

2.4 Medical Terminology in Practice

Common Terms Related to Disease

AT A GLANCE	Common Terms Related to Disease
Term	**Meaning**
Benign	Noncancerous
Convalescent	The period of recovery after an illness, injury, or surgery
Declining	Gradually deteriorating, weakening, or wasting
Degeneration	Change of tissue to a less functionally active form
Etiology	Cause of a disease
Incubation period	The time between exposure to an infectious organism and the onset of symptoms of illness
Malaise	Not feeling well (the first indication of illness)
Malignant	Cancerous
Prodromal	Pertaining to early symptoms that may mark the onset of a disease
Prognosis	Prediction about the outcome of a disease
Prophylaxis	Protection against disease
Remission	Cessation of signs and symptoms

Table 2-7

Integumentary System

AT A GLANCE	Integumentary System—Common Combining Forms		
Combining Form	**Meaning**	**Example**	**Definition**
adip / o	Fat	Adipose tissue	Layer of fat beneath the skin
albin / o	White	Albinism	Condition caused by the lack of melanin pigment in the skin, hair, and eyes
cry / o	Cold	Cryosurgery	Surgery that uses liquid nitrogen to freeze tissue
cutane / o	Skin	Subcutaneous	Beneath the skin
dermat / o	Skin	Dermatitis	Inflammation of the skin
erythr / o	Red	Erythrodermatitis	Inflammation of the skin marked by redness and scaling
hidr / o	Sweat	Hidradenitis	Inflammation of a sweat gland
hist / o	Tissue	Histology	Study of tissues
kerat / o	Hard skin, horny tissue, keratin	Keratosis	Lesion formed from an overgrowth of the horny layer of skin
leuk / o	White	Leukoplakia	Raised, white patches on the mouth or vulva
lip / o	Fat	Lipoma	Common benign tumor of the fatty tissue
onych / o	Nail	Onycholysis	Separation of the nail from its bed

Table 2-8

AT A GLANCE — Integumentary System—Common Combining Forms

Combining Form	Meaning	Example	Definition
pachy / o	Thick	Pachyonychia	Abnormal thickness of fingernails or toenails
seb / o	Sebum (oil)	Seborrhea	Excessive secretion of sebum
squam / o	Scale	Squamous	Scale-like
trich / o	Hair	Trichopathy	Any disease of the hair
xanth / o	Yellow	Xanthoma	Yellow deposit of fatty material in the skin
xer / o	Dry	Xerosis	Abnormal dryness of the eye, skin, and mouth

Table 2-8

AT A GLANCE — Integumentary System—Suffixes

Suffix	Meaning	Example	Definition
-malacia	Softening	Onychomalacia	Softening of the nails
-phagia	Eating, swallowing	Dysphagia	Difficulty swallowing, painful swallowing

Table 2-9

AT A GLANCE — Integumentary System—Abbreviations

Abbreviation	Meaning
Bx	Biopsy
Derm	Dermatology
SC, sub-Q, SQ, subcu, subq	Subcutaneous

Table 2-10

Musculoskeletal System

AT A GLANCE — Musculoskeletal System—Common Combining Forms

Combining Form	Meaning	Example	Definition
ankyl / o	Stiff	Ankylosis	Complete loss of movement in a joint
arthr / o	Joint	Arthralgia	Pain in the joint
bucc / o	Cheek	Buccinator	Cheek muscle
burs / o	Bursa	Bursolith	Stone in a bursa
calc / o	Calcium	Hypercalcemia	Excessive amount of calcium in the blood
carp / o	Wrist	Carpal	Pertaining to the wrist
cervic / o	Neck	Cervical	Pertaining to the neck

Table 2-11, continued

Combining Form	Meaning	Example	Definition
chondr / o	Cartilage	Osteachondroma	Benign bone tumor
cost / o	Rib	Intercostal	Between the ribs
crani / o	Cranium (skull)	Cranial	Pertaining to the skull
dors / o	Back	Dorsal	Pertaining to the back
fasci / o	Band of fibrous tissue	Fasciotomy	Operation to relieve pressure on the muscles by making an incision into the fascia
fibr / o	Fiber	Fibroma	Benign tumor of the connective tissues
kyph / o	Hump	Kyphosis	Excessive curvature of the spine, "humpback"
lamin / o	Lamina	Laminectomy	Surgical removal of the lamina
lei / o	Smooth muscle	Leiomyoma	Benign tumor of smooth muscle
lord / o	Curve	Lordosis	Inward curvature of the spine, "swayback"
my / o	Muscle	Myalgia	Muscle pain
myos / o	Muscle	Myositis	Inflammation of muscle tissue
oste / o	Bone	Osteoporosis	Condition in which bones become porous and fragile
pector / o	Chest	Pectoral	Pertaining to the chest
rhabd / o	Striated, skeletal muscle	Rhabdomyolysis	Destruction of muscle tissue accompanied by the release of myoglobin
spondyl / o	Vertebra	Spondylitis	Inflammation of the joints between the vertebrae in the spine
synov / i	Synovia	Synovial membrane	Membrane lining the capsule of a joint
ten / o, tend / o, tendin / o	Tendon	Tendinitis	Inflammation of the tendons

Table 2-11, concluded

Suffix	Meaning	Example	Definition
-asthenia	Weakness	Myasthenia gravis	Disorder of neuromuscular transmission marked by weakness
-clasia	Breaking	Arthroclasia	Artificial breaking of adhesions of an ankylosed joint
-desis	Binding	Arthrodesis	Surgical binding or fusing of a joint
-physis	Growth	Metaphysis	The growing portion of a long bone
-schisis	Splitting	Rachischisis	Failure of vertebral arches and neural tube to fuse
-trophy	Development	Hypertrophy	Excessive development

Table 2-12

AT A GLANCE — Musculoskeletal System—Abbreviations

Abbreviation	Meaning
C1, C2, . . . C7	Individual cervical vertebrae (first through seventh)
Ca	Calcium
CTS	Carpal tunnel syndrome
EMG	Electromyography
fx	Fracture
L1, L2, . . . L5	Individual lumbar vertebrae (first through fifth)
ortho	Orthopedics
ROM	Range of motion
SLE	Systemic lupus erythematosus
T1, T2, . . . T12	Individual thoracic vertebrae (first through twelfth)

Table 2-13

AT A GLANCE — Actions of Muscles

Motion	Meaning
Abduction	Movement away from the midline
Adduction	Movement toward the midline
Circumduction	Movement in a circular motion
Depression	Act of lowering a body part from a joint
Dorsiflexion	Act of pointing the foot upward
Elevation	Act of raising a body part from a joint
Eversion	Act of turning outward
Extension	Increase in the angle of a joint
Flexion	Decrease in the angle of a joint
Hyperextension	Increase in the angle of a joint beyond what is normal
Inversion	Act of turning inward
Plantar flexion	Act of pointing the foot downward
Pronation	Act of turning downward or inward
Protraction	Movement of a body part anteriorly
Retraction	Movement of a body part posteriorly
Rotation	Act or process of turning on an axis
Supination	Act of turning upward or outward

Table 2-14

AT A GLANCE Nervous System—Common Combining Forms

Combining Form	Meaning	Example	Definition
cerebell / o	Cerebellum	Cerebellar	Pertaining to the cerebellum
cerebr / o	Cerebrum	Cerebral cortex	Outer layer of the cerebrum
dur / o	Dura mater	Subdural hematoma	Bleeding between the dural and arachnoidal membranes
encephal / o	Brain	Encephalitis	Inflammation of the brain
mening / o	Membrane	Meningomyelocele	Protrusion of the spinal cord through a defect in the vertebral column
myel / o	Spinal cord, bone marrow	Myelogram	Radiographic study of the spinal subarachnoid space
neur / o	Nerve	Neuralgia	Pain in a nerve
poli / o	Gray matter	Poliodystrophy	Wasting of gray matter
psych / o	Mind	Psychosomatic	Pertaining to the influence of the mind on the body

Table 2-15

AT A GLANCE Nervous System—Prefixes

Prefix	Meaning	Example	Definition
hemi-	Half	Hemihypesthesia	Diminished sensation in one side of the body
tetra-	Four	Tetraparesis	Weakness of all four extremities

Table 2-16

AT A GLANCE Nervous System—Suffixes

Suffix	Meaning	Example	Definition
-algesia	Excessive sensitivity to pain	Analgesia	Without a sense of pain
-algia	Pain	Neuralgia	Nerve pain
-esthesia	Feeling sensation	Anesthesia	Loss of sensation
-kinesia	Movement	Bradykinesia	Decrease in spontaneity and movement
-kinesis	Movement	Hyperkinesis	Excessive muscular activity
-lepsy	Seizure	Epilepsy	Chronic brain disorder, often characterized by seizures
-paresis	Slight paralysis	Hemiparesis	Weakness on one side of the body
-phasia	Speech	Aphasia	Impairment of language ability
-plegia	Paralysis	Hemiplegia	Paralysis of one side of the body
-praxia	Action	Apraxia	Impairment of purposeful movement

Table 2-17

Abbreviation	Meaning
ALS	Amyotrophic lateral sclerosis
CAT	Computed axial tomography
CNS	Central nervous system
CP	Cerebral palsy
CSF	Cerebrospinal fluid
CT	Computed tomography
CVA	Cerebrovascular accident (stroke)
EEG	Electroencephalogram
LP	Lumbar puncture
MRI	Magnetic resonance imaging
MS	Multiple sclerosis
TIA	Transient ischemic attack

Table 2-18

Cardiovascular System

AT A GLANCE   Cardiovascular System—Common Combining Forms

Combining Form	Meaning	Example	Definition
angi / o	Vessel	Angiogram	X-ray image of a blood vessel
aort / o	Aorta	Aortic stenosis	Narrowing of the aorta
arter / i	Artery	Arteriectomy	Surgical removal of a portion of an artery
arter / o, arteri / o	Artery	Arteriosclerosis	Thickening of arterial walls
atri / o	Atrium	Atrial	Pertaining to an atrium
bas / o	Base	Basophil	Cell with granules that stain specifically with basic (alkaline) dyes
cardi / o	Heart	Cardiomegaly	Enlargement of the heart
coagul / o	Clotting	Anticoagulant	Drug that prevents clotting of the blood
coron / o	Crown, circle	Coronary arteries	Blood vessels encircling the heart
cyt / o	Cell	Cytology	Study of cells
hem / o, hem / a, hemat / o	Blood	Hemorrhage	Abnormal discharge of blood
		Hematology	Study of blood
is / o	Same, equal	Anisocytosis	Abnormality of red blood cells that are of unequal size
kary / o	Nucleus	Eukaryote	Cell that contains membrane-bound nucleus with chromosomes
lymph / o	Lymph	Lymphadenitis	Inflammation of the lymph nodes

Table 2-19, continued

AT A GLANCE — Cardiovascular System—Common Combining Forms

Combining Form	Meaning	Example	Definition
phleb / o	Vein	Phlebotomy	Incision in vein to draw blood
plasm / o	Plasma	Plasmapheresis	Removal of plasma from the body, separation and extraction of specific elements, and reinfusion
thromb / o	Clot	Thrombolysis	Dissolving of a clot
valv / o, valvul / o	Valve	Valvoplasty	Surgical reconstruction of a cardiac valve
vas / o	Vessel	Vasoconstriction	Narrowing of the blood vessels
ven / o	Vein	Venous	Pertaining to a vein

Table 2-19, concluded

AT A GLANCE — Cardiovascular System—Suffixes

Suffix	Meaning	Example	Definition
-apharesis	Removal	Plasmapheresis	Removal of plasma from the blood with a centrifuge
-blast	Immature stage, germ, bud	Myoblast	Immature muscle cell
-clast	Breakdown	Osteoclast	Bone breakdown
-crit	Separation	Hematocrit	Percentage of volume of a blood sample that is composed of cells
-cytosis	Abnormal condition of cells	Poikilocytosis	Presence of large, irregularly shaped blood cells
-globin	Protein	Hemoglobin	Protein of red blood cells

Table 2-20

AT A GLANCE — Cardiovascular System—Abbreviations

Abbreviation	Meaning
AED	Automatic external defibrillator
AF	Atrial fibrillation
AS	Aortic stenosis
ASD	Atrial septal defect
BP	Blood pressure
CAD	Coronary artery disease
CHD	Coronary heart disease
CHF	Congestive heart failure
ECG, EKG	Electrocardiogram
ECHO	Echocardiography

Table 2-21

AT A GLANCE — Cardiovascular System—Abbreviations

Abbreviation	Meaning
HTN	Hypertension
MI	Myocardial infarction (heart attack)
MVP	Mitral valve prolapse
PDA	Patent ductus arteriosus
PVC	Premature ventricular contraction
VT	Ventricular tachycardia

Table 2-21

Respiratory System

AT A GLANCE — Respiratory System—Common Combining Forms

Combining Form	Meaning	Example	Definition
adenoid / o	Adenoid	Adenoidectomy	Operation to remove adenoid growths
alveol / o	Air sac	Alveolar	Pertaining to a small cell or cavity
bronch / i, bronch / o	Bronchus	Bronchitis	Inflammation of the mucous membrane of the bronchial tubes
capn / o	Carbon dioxide	Hypercapnia	Excessive carbon dioxide in the blood
coni / o	Dust	Pneumoconiosis	Pulmonary disease caused by prolonged inhalation of fine dust
cyan / o	Blue	Cyanosis	Bluish discoloration of the skin caused by a deficiency of oxygen in the blood
laryng / o	Larynx	Laryngitis	Inflammation of the mucous membrane in the larynx
lob / o	Lobe of the lung	Lobectomy	Excision of a lobe
nas / o	Nose	Paranasal sinuses	Accessory sinuses in the bones of the face that open into the nasal cavities
ox / o, ox / i	Oxygen	Hypoxia	Deficiency of oxygen in tissue cells
phon / o	Voice, Sound	Dysphonia	Hoarseness, difficulty speaking
phren / o	Diaphragm	Phrenohepatic	Pertaining to the diaphragm and liver
pneum / o, pneum / a, pneumat / o	Lung, air	Pneumatosis	Abnormal presence of air or other gas
pneum / o, pneumon / o	Lung	Pneumonia	Inflammation of the lung parenchyma
pulmon / o	Lung	Pulmonary	Pertaining to the lungs
rhin / o	Nose	Rhinorrhea	A watery discharge from the nose
spir / o	Breathing	Spirometer	Gasometer used to measure respiration
tonsill / o	Tonsil	Tonsillectomy	Removal of the tonsil

Table 2-22

Suffix	Meaning	Example	Definition
-ema	Condition	Empyema	Condition of having pus in a body cavity as a result of a lung infection
-oxia	Oxygen	Anoxia	Absence of oxygen from blood or tissues
-pnea	Breathing	Apnea	Inability to breathe
-ptysis	Spitting	Hemoptysis	Coughing up and spitting out blood
-sphyxia	Pulse	Asphyxia	Impairment of oxygen intake
-thorax	Chest	Hemothorax	Blood in the pleural cavity

Table 2-23

AT A GLANCE Respiratory System—Abbreviations

Abbreviation	Meaning
ARDS	Acute respiratory distress syndrome
COPD	Chronic obstructive pulmonary disease
CPR	Cardiopulmonary resuscitation
CXR	Chest X-ray
PFT	Pulmonary function test
TB	Tuberculosis
URI	Upper respiratory infection

Table 2-24

AT A GLANCE Digestive System—Common Combining Forms

Combining Form	Meaning	Example	Definition
an / o	Anus	Perianal	Located around the anus
append / o	Appendix	Appendectomy	Surgical removal of the appendix
bucc / o	Cheek	Buccalabial	Pertaining to the cheek and lip
cec / o	Cecum	Cecal	Pertaining to the cecum
cheil / o	Lip	Cheilosis	Dry scaling and fissuring of lips
chol / o, chol / e	Bile	Choledochus	Bile duct
cholecyst / o	Gallbladder	Cholecystectomy	Surgical removal of the gallbladder
col / o	Colon	Colostomy	Creation of an artificial opening into the colon
colon / o	Colon	Colonic	Pertaining to the colon

Table 2-25

AT A GLANCE Digestive System—Common Combining Forms

Combining Form	Meaning	Example	Definition
enter / o	Intestine	Enteropathy	Intestinal disease
epigastr / o	Above the stomach	Epigastrorrhaphy	Suturing the region above the stomach
gastr / o	Stomach	Gastritis	Inflammation of the stomach
gingiv / o	Gum	Gingivitis	Inflammation of the gums
gloss / o	Tongue	Hypoglossal	Below the tongue
hepat / o	Liver	Hepatitis	Inflammation of the liver
lapar / o	Abdomen	Laparoscopy	Examination and often surgery of the abdominal cavity with a laparoscope
or / o	Mouth	Oral	Pertaining to the mouth
peritone / o	Peritoneum	Peritonitis	Inflammation of the peritoneum
rect / o	Rectum	Rectocele	Prolapse of the rectum
stomat / o	Mouth	Stomatitis	Inflammation of the mouth

Table 2-25

Digestive System

AT A GLANCE Digestive System—Suffixes

Suffix	Meaning	Example	Definition
-ase	Enzyme	Amylase	Class of digestive enzymes that act on starch
-chezia	Defecation	Hematochezia	Passage of bloody stools
-iasis	Abnormal condition	Choledocholithiasis	Stones in the common bile duct
-pepsia	Digestion	Dyspepsia	Upset stomach
-prandial	Meal	Postprandial	Following a meal
-rrhaphy	Repair or suture	Hepatorrhaphy	Repair of a wound or rupture in the liver.

Table 2-26

AT A GLANCE Digestive System—Abbreviations

Abbreviation	Meaning
BE	Barium enema
EGD	Esophagogastroduodenoscopy
EUS	Endoscopic ultrasound
GERD	Gastroesophageal reflux disease
GI	Gastrointestinal
IBS	Irritable bowel syndrome

Table 2-27

AT A GLANCE | Endocrine System—Common Combining Forms

Combining Form	Meaning	Example	Definition
aden / o	Gland	Adenectomy	Excision of a gland
adrenal / o, adren / o	Adrenal gland	Adrenalectomy	Removal of one or both adrenal glands
andr / o	Male	Androgen	Hormone produced by the testes in males and by the adrenal cortex in males and females
calc / i	Calcium	Hypercalcemia	Elevated concentration of calcium in the blood
cortic / o	Cortex, outer region	Corticosteroid	Steroid produced by the adrenal cortex
crin / o	Secretion	Endocrinologist	Physician who specializes in endocrinology
dips / o	Thirst	Polydipsia	Prolonged excessive thirst
epinephr / o	Adrenal gland	Epinephritis	Inflammation of an adrenal gland
glyc / o	Sugar	Hyperglycemia	High blood sugar
gonad / o	Sex gland	Gonadotropin	Hormone that promotes gonadal growth
home / o	Like, similar	Homeostasis	State of bodily equilibrium
hormon / o	Hormone	Hormonal	Pertaining to hormones
kal / i	Potassium	Hypokalemia	Lack of potassium in the blood as a result of dehydration, excessive vomiting, and diarrhea
lact / o	Milk	Prolactin	Hormone that stimulates milk production during pregnancy
natr / i	Sodium	Hyponatremia	Low concentration of sodium in the blood
parathyroid / o	Parathyroid gland	Parathyroidectomy	Excision of the parathyroid gland
somat / o	Body	Somatotropic	Having a stimulating effect on body growth
ster / o	Solid structure	Steroid	Pertaining to the steroids, some of which increase muscle mass
thyr / o	Thyroid gland	Thyrotropin hormone	Hormone that stimulates growth of the thyroid gland
thyroid / o	Thyroid gland	Thyroiditis	Inflammation of the thyroid gland

Table 2-28

AT A GLANCE | Endocrine System—Prefixes

Prefix	Meaning	Example	Definition
oxy-	Rapid, sharp	Oxytocin	Hormone that influences contractions of the uterus
pan-	All	Panhypopituitarism	State of inadequate or absent secretion of pituitary hormones
tri-	Three	Triiodothyronine	Hormone secreted by the thyroid gland that regulates metabolism

Table 2-29

AT A GLANCE   Endocrine System—Suffixes

Suffix	Meaning	Example	Definition
-agon	Assemblage, a gathering together	Glucagon	Hormone produced by the pancreas that causes an increase in blood sugar
-in, -ine	A substance	Epinephrine	Stress hormone secreted by the adrenal gland
-uria	Urine condition	Glycosuria	Urinary excretion of sugar

Table 2-30

AT A GLANCE   Endocrine System—Abbreviations

Abbreviation	Meaning
ACTH	Adrenocorticotropic hormone
BMR	Basal metabolic rate
Ca	Calcium
DI	Diabetes insipidus
DM	Diabetes mellitus
FBS	Fasting blood sugar
FSH	Follicle-stimulating hormone
GH	Growth hormone
GTT	Glucose tolerance test
IDDM	Insulin-dependent diabetes mellitus
K	Potassium
Na	Sodium
NIDDM	Non-insulin-dependent diabetes mellitus
PRL	Prolactin
TFT	Thyroid function test

Table 2-31

Sensory System
The Eye

AT A GLANCE   The Eye—Common Combining Forms

Combining Form	Meaning	Example	Definition
aque / o	Water	Aqueous	Containing, or like water
blephar / o	Eyelid	Blepharitis	Inflammation of the eyelids
conjunctiv / o	Conjunctiva	Conjunctivitis	Inflammation of the conjunctiva, pinkeye
cor / o, core / o	Pupil	Corepraxy	Procedure to centralize a pupil that is abnormally situated
dacry / o	Tear, tear duct	Dacryoadenitis	Inflammation of the lacrimal gland

Table 2-32, continued

Combining Form	Meaning	Example	Definition
dipl / o	Double	Diplopia	Condition in which one object is perceived as two objects (double vision)
glauc / o	Gray	Glaucoma	Eye disease that may result in blindness
ir / o	Iris	Iritis	Inflammation of the iris
lacrim / o	Tear	Lacrimal	Pertaining to tears
mi / o	Smaller, less	Miosis	Contraction of the pupil
nyct / o, noct / o	Night	Nyctalopia	Poor night vision
ocul / o	Eye	Intraocular	Inside the eye
ophthalm / o	Eye	Ophthalmologist	Physician who specializes in treating eyes
opt / o	Vision	Optometer	Instrument for determining refraction of the eye
palpebr / o	Eyelid	Palpebral	Pertaining to the eyelid
phot / o	Light	Photophobia	Fear and avoidance of light
presby / o	Old age	Presbyopia	Loss of accommodation in the eye resulting from aging
pupill / o	Pupil	Pupillary	Pertaining to the pupil
retin / o	Retina	Retinitis	Inflammation of the retina
scot / o	Darkness	Scotoma	Blind spot in which vision is absent or depressed
uve / o	Vascular layer of the eye	Uveitis	Inflammation of the uveal tract
vitre / o	Glassy	Vitreous humor	Fluid component of the transparent vitreous body

Table 2-32, concluded

AT A GLANCE The Eye—Suffixes

Suffix	Meaning	Example	Definition
-opia	Vision	Hyperopia	Farsightedness
-tropia	A turning	Estropia	Inward turning of the eye, toward the nose

Table 2-33

AT A GLANCE The Eye—Abbreviations

Abbreviation	Meaning
ast	Astigmatism
IOP	Intraocular pressure
OD*	Right eye
OS*	Left eye

Table 2-34

AT A GLANCE The Eye—Abbreviations

Abbreviation	Meaning
OU*	Each eye, both eyes
PERRLA	Pupils equal, round, reactive to light and accommodation
REM	Rapid eye movement
VA	Visual acuity
VF	Visual field

Table 2-34

The Ear

AT A GLANCE The Ear—Common Combining Forms

Combining Form	Meaning	Example	Definition
acou, acous / o	Hearing	Acoustic	Pertaining to hearing
audi / o	Hearing	Audiometer	Instrument for measuring hearing
audit / o	Hearing	Auditory	Pertaining to the sense or organs of hearing
aur / i	Ear	Aural	Pertaining to the ear
cochle / o	Cochlea	Cochlear	Pertaining to the cochlea
mastoid / o	Mastoid process	Mastoiditis	Inflammation of the mastoid process
myring / o	Tympanic membrane	Myringoplasty	Surgical repair of damaged tympanic membrane
ot / o	Ear	Otic	Pertaining to the ear
tympan / o	Eardrum	Tympanoplasty	Operation on a damaged middle ear

Table 2-35

AT A GLANCE The Ear—Suffixes

Suffix	Meaning	Example	Definition
-cusis, -acousia	Hearing	Presbycusis, presbyacousia	Nerve deafness caused by aging
-otia	Ear condition	Macrotia	Enlarged ears

Table 2-36

AT A GLANCE The Ear—Abbreviations

Abbreviation	Meaning
AD*	Right ear
AS*	Left ear
AU*	Both ears
EENT	Eyes, ears, nose, and throat
oto	Otology

Table 2-37

AT A GLANCE Urinary System—Common Combining Forms

Combining Form	Meaning	Example	Definition
albumin / o	Protein	Albuminuria	Protein in the urine
bacteri / o	Bacterium, bacteria	Bacteriuria	Bacteria in the urine
cali / o	Calix (calyx)	Caliectasis	Dilation of the calices
cyst / o	Urinary bladder	Cystitis	Inflammation of the urinary bladder
ket / o	Ketone bodies	Ketosis	Enhanced production of ketone bodies
lith / o	Stone	Nephrolithiasis	Presence of a renal stone or stones
meat / o	Opening, passageway	Meatoscope	Speculum for examining the urinary meatus
nephr / o	Kidney	Nephromegaly	Enlargement of the kidney
olig / o	Scanty, few	Oliguria	Scanty urine production
pyel / o	Renal pelvis	Pyelolithotomy	Operation to remove a stone from the kidney
ren / i, ren / o	Kidney	Renography	Radiography of the kidney
ur / o, urin / o	Urine, urinary tract	Urodynia	Pain on urination
vesic / o	Urinary bladder	Perivesical	Surrounding the urinary bladder

Table 2-38

AT A GLANCE Urinary System—Suffixes

Suffix	Meaning	Example	Definition
-tripsy	Crushing	Lithotripsy	Crushing of a stone in the renal pelvis, ureter, or bladder
-uria	Urination	Dysuria	Difficulty or pain in urinating

Table 2-39

AT A GLANCE Urinary System—Abbreviations

Abbreviation	Meaning
ADH	Antidiuretic hormone; vasopressin
ARF	Acute renal failure
BUN	Blood urea nitrogen
Cath	Catheter
CRF	Chronic renal failure

Table 2-40

AT A GLANCE — Urinary System—Abbreviations

Abbreviation	Meaning
ESRD	End-stage renal disease
HD	Hemodialysis
IVP	Intravenous pyelogram
KUB	Kidney, ureter, and bladder
PKU	Phenylketonuria
UA	Urinalysis
UTI	Urinary tract infection

Table 2-40

Reproductive System

AT A GLANCE — Reproductive System—Common Combining Forms

Combining Form	Meaning	Example	Definition
amni / o	Amnion	Amniocentesis	Aspiration of amniotic fluid for diagnosis
balan / o	Glans penis	Balanitis	Inflammation of the glans penis
cervic / o	Cervix, neck	Endocervicitis	Inflammation of the mucous membrane of the cervix
colp / o	Vagina	Colposcopy	Examination of the cervix using a colposcope
crypt / o	Hidden	Cryptorchism	Failure of one or both testes to descend
culd / o	Cul-de-sac	Culdocentesis	Aspiration of fluid from the cul-de-sac
epididym / o	Epididymis	Epididymitis	Inflammation of the epididymis
galact / o	Milk	Galactorrhea	Abnormal, persistent discharge of milk
gon / o	Generation, genitals	Gonorrhea	Contagious inflammation of the genital mucous membrane
gynec / o	Female	Gynecology	The study of the female reproductive system
hyster / o	Uterus	Hysterectomy	Removal of the uterus
lact / i, lact / o	Milk	Lactation	Production of milk
mamm / o	Breast	Mammogram	Breast X-ray
mast / o	Breast	Mastectomy	Excision of the breast
men / o	Menses	Amenorrhea	Absence or abnormal cessation of menses
metr / o	Uterus	Metrorrhagia	Irregular bleeding from the uterus between periods
nat / i	Birth	Neonatal	Pertaining to the first month of life
orchi / o, orchid / o	Testis, testicle	Orchiectomy	Removal of one or both testes

Table 2-41, continued

Reproductive System—Common Combining Forms

Combining Form	Meaning	Example	Definition
ov / o	Egg	Ovum	Female sex cell, or egg
prostat / o	Prostate gland	Prostatitis	Inflammation of the prostate gland
terat / o	Monster	Teratoma	Neoplasm composed of tissues not normally found in the organ
test / o	Testis, testicle	Testicular	Pertaining to the testes
vagin / o	Vagina	Vaginitis	Inflammation of the vagina
vas / o	Vessel, duct	Vasectomy	Removal of a section of the vas deferens
vert / i, vers / i	A turning	Cephalic version	Turning of the fetus so that the head is correctly positioned for delivery

Table 2-41, concluded

Reproductive System—Suffixes

Suffix	Meaning	Example	Definition
-arche	Beginning	Menarche	Time of the first menstrual period
-gravida	Pregnant	Primigravida	Woman in her first pregnancy
-one	Hormone	Testosterone	Hormone related to masculinization and reproduction
-pause	Cessation	Menopause	The cessation of menses
-pexy	Fixation, fastening	Orchiopexy	Surgical treatment of an undescended testicle
-stomy	(New) opening	Vasostomy	Surgical procedure of making a new opening into the vas deferens
-tocia	Labor, birth	Dystocia	Difficult childbirth

Table 2-42

Reproductive System—Abbreviations

Abbreviation	Meaning
AB	Abortion
AIDS	Acquired immunodeficiency syndrome
BPH	Benign prostatic hyperplasia/benign prostatic hypertrophy
CS, C-section	Cesarean section
CX	Cervix
D & C	Dilation and curettage
ECC	Endocervical curettage

Table 2-43

Abbreviation	Meaning
EMB	Endometrial biopsy
FHT	Fetal heart tones
FSH	Follicle-stimulating hormone
GYN	Gynecology
HCG	Human chorionic gonadotropin
HIV	Human immunodeficiency virus
HSV	Herpes simplex virus
LH	Luteinizing hormone
Multip	Multipara
Pap smear	Papanicolaou smear (test for cervical or vaginal cancer)
PMS	Premenstrual syndrome
PSA	Prostate-specific antigen
STI	Sexually transmitted infection

Table 2-43

STRATEGIES TO SUCCESS

▶ *Test-Taking Skills*

Think success!
Approach the exam with confidence. It's unlikely that you will get all the questions right. Don't panic or become stressed when you can't answer a question. Relax, and imagine yourself doing wonderfully. A positive attitude will help you stay in control and allow you to focus on all the questions that you do know.

2.5 Unacceptable Abbreviations

Unacceptable Abbreviations: Today, there are certain abbreviations that the Joint Commission recommends medical professionals to avoid. Table 2-44 includes examples of unacceptable abbreviations. The Joint Commission's complete list of these abbreviations can be found at http://www.jointcommission.org/topics/patient_safety.aspx.

Terms	Do Not Use	What You Should Do
Daily	qd	Write out
Discontinue and discharge	D/C, dc, DC	Write out
Every other day	qod	Write out
International units	IU	Write out
Magnesium sulfate	MgSO4	Write out
Microgram	μg	Use mcg or write out
Morphine sulfate	MS, MSO4	Write out
Related to the ears	AD, AS, AU	Write out
Related to the eyes	OD, OS, OU	Write out
Subcutaneous	SC, SQ	Use subQ or subC
Units	U or u	Write out

Table 2-44

CHAPTER 2 REVIEW

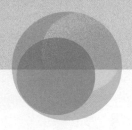

Instructions:

Answer the following questions.

1. A prefix is
   A. the first part of a word.
   B. a word structure at the end of a term that modifies the root.
   C. a word structure at the beginning of a term that modifies the root.
   D. found on all medical terms.
   E. the last part of a word that gives the word its root meaning.

2. Which of the following suffixes means "inflammation"?
   A. -iasis
   B. -trophy
   C. -itis
   D. -osis
   E. -desis

3. Which of the following prefixes is matched correctly with its meaning?
   A. hypo / above
   B. peri / around
   C. antero / back
   D. endo / over
   E. micro / large

4. The combining vowel is used to
   A. give a central meaning.
   B. ease pronunciation.
   C. modify the root.
   D. divide word meanings.
   E. connect longer medical terms.

5. Which of the following words is misspelled?
   A. abscess
   B. homostasis
   C. venous
   D. prostate
   E. integumentary

6. Which of the following abbreviations means "four times a day"?
   A. b.i.d.
   B. q.e.d.
   C. t.i.d.
   D. q.d.
   E. q.i.d.

7. The suffix -stasis means
   A. condition.
   B. stoppage.
   C. destruction.
   D. discharge.
   E. unchanged.

8. Nephr / o and ren / o both refer to which of the following?
   A. the lungs
   B. the heart
   C. the bladder
   D. the kidney
   E. the rectum

9. The underlined portions of the words _pneumonia_ and _pneumoconiosis_ represent which of the following word parts?
   A. prefix
   B. root
   C. suffix
   D. combining form
   E. combining vowel

10. The prefix _retro-_ means
    A. behind.
    B. around.
    C. below.
    D. before.
    E. above.

ANATOMY AND PHYSIOLOGY

LEARNING OUTCOMES

3.1 Describe the organizational levels of the body.

3.2 Identify the organelles and division of cells, and the movement of substances across cell membranes.

3.3 Recognize the terminology related to the chemical composition of the body.

3.4 Describe the composition and types of body tissues and membranes.

3.5 Identify the types of divisional planes and locations of the body cavities.

3.6 Recall the structures and functions of the integumentary system.

3.7 Recall the structures and functions of the muscular and skeletal systems of the body.

3.8 Identify the divisions of the nervous system, and the structures and functions of each division.

3.9 Describe the functions of the organs associated with each of the five senses.

3.10 Identify the composition and functions of the blood, blood vessels, heart, and lymphatic system.

3.11 Explain how the body oxygenates the cells and removes carbon dioxide.

3.12 Describe the process in which the digestive organs change food to be used by the body.

3.13 Identify the glands of the body and the hormones they secrete to coordinate body functions.

3.14 Describe how the urinary system removes waste, salt, and excess water from the body.

3.15 Identify the structures and functions of the male and female reproductive systems.

MEDICAL ASSISTING COMPETENCIES

COMPETENCY	CMA	RMA	CCMA	NCMA
General/Legal/Professional				
Conduct work within scope of education, training, and ability	X	X	X	
Use appropriate medical terminology	X	X	X	X

► *Study Skills*

Find a good place to study!
Think about what atmosphere you study best in. Are you distracted by the slightest noise? Do you like a certain level of noise to keep you going and focused? Do you like studying alone or in groups? Also consider how comfortable you want to be. Do you find yourself drifting off when you study on your bed or in a comfortable chair? Is studying at a desk too uncomfortable? There's no right place or way to study. Some people pace the halls whereas others find a secluded place in their house where their family and friends can't bother them. We do suggest that you find a place that is well lighted. Unnecessary eye strain could cause you to become tired too soon. Whatever place you pick, make sure it's right for you and make it a habit to study there regularly.

3.1 Levels of Organization

Anatomy: The structure of organisms.
Physiology: The functions and activities of organisms.
The human body is composed of atoms that join together to form molecules at the chemical level.

The human body is structurally organized beginning with cells, and continuing with tissues, organs, organ systems, and the body as a whole. The other levels of organization of the body are shown in Figure 3-1.

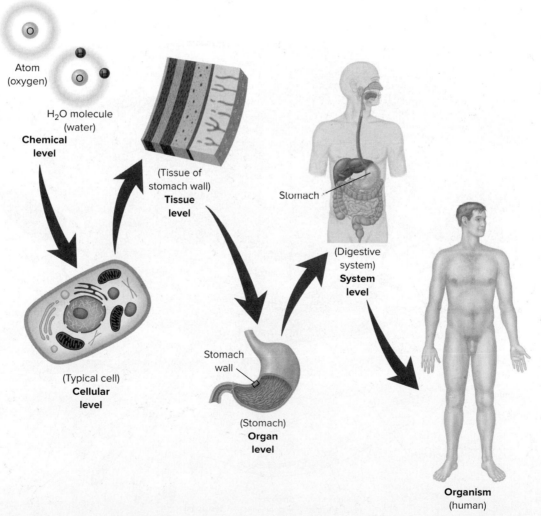

Atom
(oxygen)

H₂O molecule
(water)
**Chemical
level**

(Tissue of
stomach wall)
**Tissue
level**

Stomach

(Digestive
system)
**System
level**

(Typical cell)
**Cellular
level**

Stomach
wall

(Stomach)
**Organ
level**

Organism
(human)

Figure 3-1 *The human body is organized in levels, beginning with the chemical level and progressing to the cellular, tissue, organ, system, and organism (whole body) levels.*

3.2 Cell Structure

Cell: The basic structural unit of all organisms. Cells have three main parts: the cell membrane, the cytoplasm, and the nucleus. See Figure 3-2.

1. **Cell membrane:** A bilayer of phospholipid and protein molecules that controls the passage of materials in and out of the cell. It is also known as *ectoplasm*.

2. **Cytoplasm:** The medium for chemical reactions in the cell. It contains water, dissolved ions, nutrients, and different organelles. The cytoplasm surrounds the nucleus and is encircled by the cell membrane.

3. **Nucleus:** The largest and innermost organelle in the cell. It contains DNA, which regulates the cell's activities. The nucleus is the *control center* of the cell. The plural of *nucleus* is *nuclei*.

DNA: Deoxyribonucleic acid. DNA consists of long chains of chemical bases along a sugar-phosphate backbone; this pattern of bases carries genetic information that directs all cell activities.

Gene: A segment of DNA that is responsible for physical and inheritable characteristics; also, the structure of a protein and an RNA molecule.

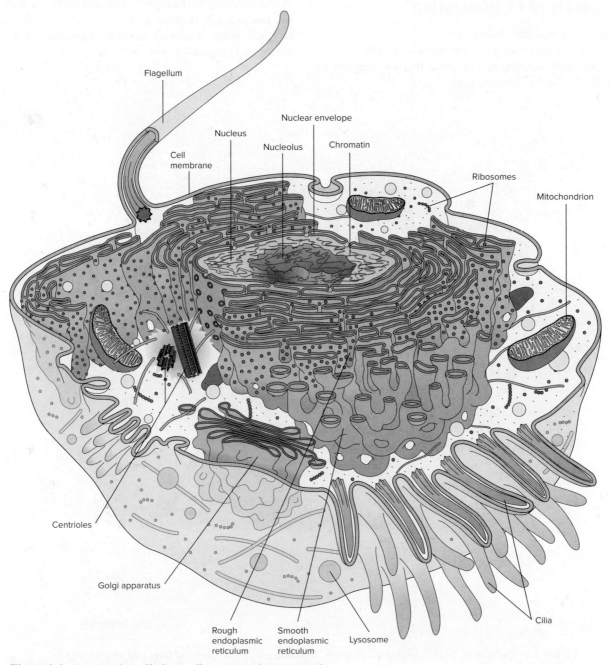

Flagellum

Nuclear envelope

Nucleus

Cell membrane

Nucleolus

Chromatin

Ribosomes

Mitochondrion

Centrioles

Golgi apparatus

Rough endoplasmic reticulum

Smooth endoplasmic reticulum

Lysosome

Cilia

Figure 3-2 *A composite cell. Organelles are not drawn to scale.*

Chromatin: The genetic material contained in the nucleus of a nondividing cell. It consists primarily of chromosomes, made of strands of DNA bound in clumps to proteins.

Chromosome: An organized structure of DNA and protein in cells that contains many genes, regulatory elements and other nucleotide sequences, and DNA-bound proteins.

Autosome: Any chromosome not considered to be a sex chromosome, or not involved in sex determination.

Nucleolus: A dense body within the nucleus, also known as the little nucleus, composed of DNA, RNA, and protein molecules. It is the site for synthesis of ribosomal RNA (rRNA).

RNA: Ribonucleic acid. RNA consists of long, single chains of chemical bases along a sugar-phosphate backbone. RNA molecules are transported from the nucleus into the cytoplasm, where they direct the formation of proteins.

Organelle: A specialized part of a cell that performs a particular function.

Organelles

Ribosome: A granular cytoplasmic organelle composed of RNA. Ribosomes provide enzymes that link amino acids for protein synthesis.

Mitochondrion: A small, rod-shaped organelle that serves as the power plant of the cell because it provides energy. Adenosine triphosphate (ATP) is produced here.

Lysosome: Cytoplasmic particle that digests material that comes into the cell. It breaks down nutrient molecules and foreign particles.

Endoplasmic reticulum: A network of tubules that transports material through the cytoplasm and aids in the synthesis of proteins and lipids.

Golgi apparatus: A small membranous structure found in most cells that forms the carbohydrate side chains of glycoproteins. It is also called the Golgi body or Golgi complex. It primarily functions as a storage unit for newly formed secretory proteins.

Cytoskeleton: The cytoplasmic elements that coordinate the movement of organelles.

Centriole: An intracellular, rod-shaped body involved with cell division and organizing mitotic spindles.

Cilium: One of numerous small, hairlike extensions that move substances across the surface of a cell.

Flagellum: A long, whiplike extension from a cell that aids in movement. The only human cell with a tail (flagellum) is sperm. Otherwise, flagellum is usually associated with a parasite.

Cell Division

Mitosis: The division of a somatic cell to form two new cells, each identical to the parent cell. The four stages of mitosis are *prophase* (early and late), *metaphase, anaphase,* and *telophase.*

Meiosis: A type of nuclear division in which the number of chromosomes is reduced to half the number found in a normal body cell. It results in the formation of an egg or sperm.

Cytokinesis: Separation of the cytoplasm into two cells after nuclear division has occurred.

Movement of Substances Across the Cell Membrane

Diffusion: The movement of molecules from a region of higher concentration to a region of lower concentration, a concentration gradient.

Osmosis: The diffusion of water through a selectively permeable membrane in response to the concentration gradient.

Facilitated diffusion: Diffusion through a membrane by means of proteins acting as carrier molecules.

Filtration: The movement of fluid through a membrane in response to hydrostatic pressure.

Active transport: The movement of substances against a concentration gradient, from a region of lower concentration to a region of higher concentration. It requires a carrier molecule and uses energy.

Endocytosis: The formation of vesicles in the cell membrane to transfer particles and droplets from the outside into the cell. Phagocytosis (ingestion of solids) and pinocytosis (ingestion of liquids) are two such processes.

Exocytosis: The discharge from a cell of particles too large to pass through the cell membrane by diffusion.

Isotonic solution: A solution that has the same concentration (osmotic pressure) as the fluids within a cell.

Hypertonic solution: A solution that has a higher concentration (osmotic pressure) than the fluids within a cell.

Hypotonic solution: A solution that has a lower concentration (osmotic pressure) than the fluids within a cell.

3.3 Chemistry

Element: The simplest form of matter with unique chemical properties. Oxygen, iron, gold, and other elements cannot be broken down into different substances by ordinary chemical means. All matter, living and nonliving, is composed of elements.

Atom: The smallest particle of an element, consisting of electrons surrounding a nucleus composed of protons, neutrons, and other entities.

Atomic number: The number of protons in the nucleus of the atom. The hydrogen atom, for example, has one proton and its atomic number is 1. Carbon has six protons and its atomic number is 6.

Atomic weight: The relative weight of an atom, determined by the number of protons and neutrons together and compared with the standard carbon atom (which has a mass of 12 and an atomic weight of 12).

Ionic bond: A relatively weak attraction formed when one or more electrons are transferred from one atom to another. It is easily disrupted in water.

Covalent bond: The chemical bond formed when two atoms share a pair of electrons. It is the strongest type of chemical bond.

Ion: An atom that has acquired a charge through the gain or loss of one or more electrons.

Anion: A negatively charged ion.

Cation: A positively charged ion.

Compound: A molecule composed of two or more different elements, such as carbon dioxide (CO_2).

Mixture: A combination of substances that are not chemically combined and can be separated by physical means.

Suspension: A mixture in which a solid is distributed but not dissolved. It will separate unless it is shaken.

Electrolyte: A substance that permits the transfer of electrons in solution. Common electrolytes include acids, bases, and salts.

pH: The number used to indicate the exact strength of an acid or base.

pH scale: A scale, ranging from 0 to 14, that measures the hydrogen ion concentration of a solution.

Acid: A substance with a pH less than 7.0 that ionizes in water to release hydrogen ions. Because a hydrogen ion consists of a proton, an acid is referred to as a *hydrogen ion donor* or a *proton donor*.

Base: A substance with a pH greater than 7.0. It is referred to as a *hydrogen ion acceptor* or a *proton acceptor*. Bases contain higher concentrations of hydroxyl ions (OH^-), whereas acids contain higher concentrations of hydrogen ions (H^+).

Buffer: A substance that prevents or reduces changes in pH and counterbalances the addition of an acid or base.

Buffer system: A system that uses chemical reactions occurring in body fluids to maintain a particular pH. The acid-base balance is regulated by two buffer systems in the body: the lungs and the kidneys.

ATP: The abbreviation for adenosine triphosphate. ATP is the primary provider of energy for a cell.

Neutral: A pH between 6.5 and 7.5, which is close to the pH of pure water (7.0).

3.4 Tissues of the Body

Histology: The microscopic study of tissues.

Tissue: A collection of similar cells acting together to perform a particular function. Types include epithelial (see Table 3-1), connective, muscular, and nervous.

Gland: An organ that contains special cells that secrete substances. Some glands lubricate; others produce hormones (see Table 3-2).

Unicellular glands: Glands that consist of only one cell.

Multicellular glands: Glands that may be classified on the basis of structure (simple or compound), type of secretion (mucous, serous, or mixed), presence or absence of ducts (exocrine or endocrine), characteristics of secreting units (alveolar or acinar), and manner of secretion (merocrine, apocrine, or holocrine).

Goblet cell: The only unicellular exocrine gland. Goblet cells produce mucus in digestive, respiratory, urinary, and reproductive tracts.

Connective tissue: Tissue that connects, protects, supports, and forms a framework for all body structures. Connective tissue includes loose fibrous tissue, adipose tissue, dense fibrous tissue, cartilage, bone, and blood.

Loose fibrous tissue: Tissue that fills spaces in the body and binds structures together.

Adipose tissue: A specialized form of loose fibrous tissue that provides insulation; it is commonly called fat.

Dense fibrous tissue: Connective tissue that forms tendons and ligaments.

Cartilage: A hard, dense connective tissue consisting of cells embedded in a matrix that can withstand considerable pressure and tension. It provides support, a framework, and attachment; protects underlying tissues; and forms structural models for many developing bones. Cartilage does not contain any nerves or blood supply. There are three types of cartilage: hyaline, fibrous, and elastic.

Bone: A hard, connective tissue consisting of specialized cells embedded in a matrix of hardened mineral salts. It is the most rigid connective tissue. Its fundamental, functional unit is called an osteon, or Haversian system.

Blood: The only type of connective tissue that is liquid, composed of cells suspended in a fluid matrix called plasma.

Nervous tissue: Tissue found in the brain, spinal cord, and nerves.

Muscle tissue: Tissue that provides movement, maintains posture, and produces heat. Muscle tissue is composed of elongated muscle fibers that can contract and thereby move body parts. There are three types of muscle tissue: skeletal, smooth, and cardiac. Skeletal muscles attach to bones and are controlled voluntarily. Smooth muscles, which lack the striations of skeletal muscles, line the walls of hollow internal organs. Cardiac muscles, which are striated, are found only in the heart. Both smooth and cardiac muscles are controlled involuntarily.

Sarcoma: A malignant tumor that forms in connective tissue.

AT A GLANCE	Types of Epithelial Tissue	
Type	**Description**	**Location**
Simple squamous	Single layer of thin, flat cells	Alveoli of lungs, capillary walls
Simple cuboidal	Single layer of cube-shaped cells	Ovary, thyroid gland
Simple columnar	Single layer of tall cells	Intestines, stomach
Stratified squamous	Several layers of cells with flat cells at the free surface	Skin, vagina, anus
Transitional	Tissue specialized to change in response to increased tension; cells become thinner when distended	Urinary bladder

Table 3-1

Secretion Mode	Meaning	Examples
Merocrine	Pertaining to a secretory cell that remains intact during secretion	Salivary glands, certain sweat glands, pancreatic glands
Apocrine	Pertaining to a secretory cell that contributes part of its protoplasm to the secretion	Mammary glands and certain sweat glands
Holocrine	Pertaining to a secretory cell that produces secretions consisting of altered cells of the same gland	Sebaceous glands

Table 3 2

Body Membranes

Membrane: A layer of tissue that lines body cavities, covers organs, or separates structures.

Cutaneous membrane: The membrane that covers the body. It is also known as the skin.

Epithelial membranes: Mucous and serous membranes.

Serous membranes: The pleura, pericardium, and peritoneum.

Connective tissue membranes: Synovial membranes and the meninges.

Meninx: One of three connective tissue coverings, or meninges, around the brain and spinal cord. The three layers, from the outermost to the innermost, are the dura mater, arachnoid, and pia mater. The plural of meninx is *meninges.*

Adenoma: A benign tumor of glandular epithelial cells.

Adenocarcinoma: A malignant tumor originating in glandular epithelium.

3.5 Division Planes and Body Cavities

Division Planes

Division plane: Imaginary planes (frontal, sagittal, midsagittal, and transverse) used as references in describing positions of the body or of parts of the body. See Figure 3-3.

Frontal plane: A plane that divides the body into front and back halves. This plane is also referred to as the coronal plane.

Sagittal plane: A plane that divides the body into left and right portions. This plane is also referred to as the lateral plane.

Midsagittal plane: A plane that passes along the midline and divides the body into equal left and right halves. This plane is also referred to as the median plane.

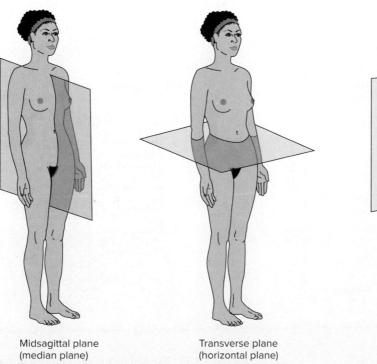
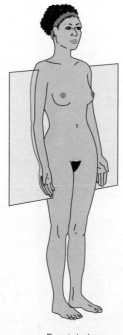

Midsagittal plane (median plane)
Transverse plane (horizontal plane)
Frontal plane (coronal plane)

Figure 3-3 *Sectioning the body along various planes.*

Transverse plane: A plane that divides the body into upper and lower halves. This plane is also referred to as the horizontal plane.

Body Cavities

Body cavity: Either of two main cavities in the body, the dorsal and the ventral. See Figure 3-4.

Dorsal cavity: The main body cavity consisting of the cranial cavity, which contains the brain; and the spinal cavity, which contains the spinal cord.

Ventral cavity: The main body cavity consisting of the thoracic, the abdominal, and the pelvic cavities. It is much larger than the dorsal cavity.

The division of the abdominal area: The two most common ways to subdivide the abdominal area are into either nine regions or four quadrants. See Figure 3-5.

3.6 Integumentary System

Integumentary system: The skin and its derivatives. Functions of the skin include protection, the regulation of body temperature, sensory reception, and the synthesis of vitamin D.

Cutaneous membrane: The medical term for skin. It consists of three layers: the epidermis, the dermis, and subcutaneous tissue. See Figure 3-6.

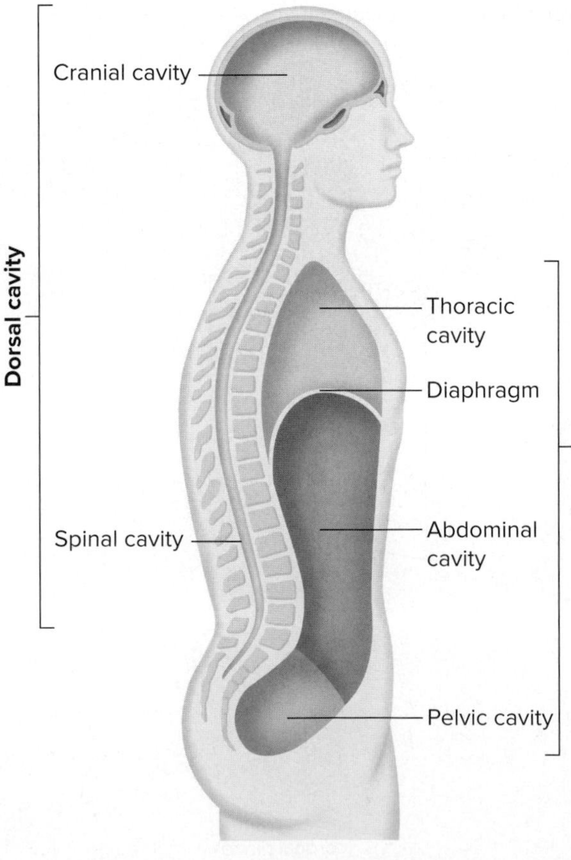

Epidermis: The outermost layer of the skin. It contains no blood vessels, but it does contain melanin, which gives skin its characteristic color, and keratin, which is a waterproof barrier against pathogens and chemicals. Specialized cells in the epidermis called melanocytes produce melanin. The more melanin in skin, the darker its color. The epidermis consists of five layers, or strata. They are, from outermost to innermost, the stratum corneum, the stratum lucidum, the stratum granulosum, the stratum spinosum, and the stratum germinativum.

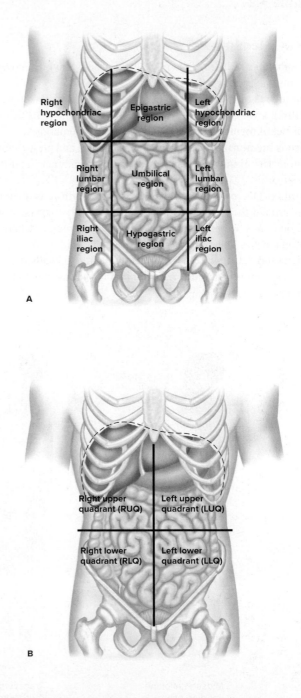

Figure 3-5 *(A) The abdominal area divided into nine regions and (B) the abdominal area divided into four quadrants.*

Figure 3-4 *The two main body cavities are dorsal and ventral.*

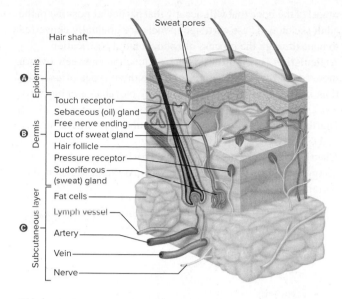

Figure 3-6 *The skin consists of three layers. A. The epidermis (outer layer) is made entirely of epithelial cells. B. The dermis (middle layer) contains connective tissue, nerve endings, hair follicles, and the sweat and oil glands. C. The subcutaneous (innermost) layer contains fat cells, loose connective tissue, and blood and lymph vessels.*

Dermis: The layer of skin containing hair follicles, nails, glands (that secrete oil or sebum), fibers, sense receptors, and blood vessels. It is also called true skin.

Subcutaneous tissue: The bottom layer of the cutaneous membrane, beneath the true skin.

Stratum lucidum: A translucent band that is seen best in thick, glabrous (smooth, hairless) skin.

Stratum corneum: Dead, keratinized cells located on the outer surface of the epidermis.

Keratinization: A process by which epithelial cells lose their moisture, which is replaced by keratin (protein).

Sebaceous gland: An oil gland, associated with hair follicles. Sebaceous glands secrete sebum and are abundant in the scalp, external ear, face, nose, mouth, and anus.

Sweat gland: A gland that secretes sweat, either directly to the skin's surface (eccrine type) or indirectly through hair follicles (apocrine type). Also called sudoriferous glands, sweat glands are widely distributed over the body, except for the lips, nipples, and parts of the external genitalia.

Hydrosis: The formation and excretion of sweat.

3.7 Musculoskeletal System

Skeletal System

Bone: An individual unit of osseous tissue, part of the body's supporting framework. Although they appear hard and lifeless because of the calcium contained in them, bones are living tissue. Bones also produce blood cells, act as a storage area for calcium, and protect delicate organs of the body.

Types: There are two types of bone tissue: compact and spongy bone tissue. The three types of cells in bone are osteoblasts, osteoclasts, and osteocytes.

Classification: Bones are classified into four types according to their shape: long, short, flat, and irregular. The femur, radius, and humerus are long bones. The carpals and tarsals are short bones. The ribs, scapula, skull, and sternum are flat bones. The vertebrae, sacrum, and mandible are irregular bones. The adult human skeleton is made up of 206 named bones. See Figure 3-7 and Table 3-3.

Diaphysis: The shaft of a long bone, located between the epiphyses.

Epiphysis: Spongy bone tissue, located at either end of a long bone.

Endochondral ossification: During development, most bones originate as hyaline cartilages. Each cartilage is a miniature

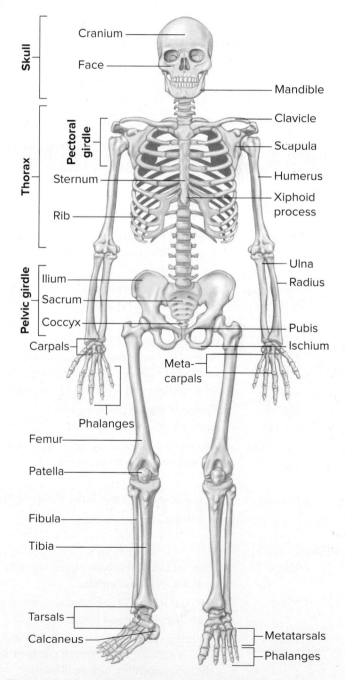

Figure 3-7 *The skeletal system is composed of bones, joints, and related connective tissue.*

Axial skeleton	80 bones
Skull, consisting of:	28 bones, as follows:
a. Cranial bones	8
b. Facial bones	14
c. Auditory ossicles	6
Thoracic cage	**25 bones**
Appendicular skeleton:	126 bones, as follows:
a. Upper extremity	60
b. Lower extremity	60
c. Pelvic girdle	2
d. Pectoral girdle	4

Table 3-3

model of the bone that will occupy that particular position in the adult skeleton. These cartilage models are gradually converted to bone through the process of endochondral ossification.

Articulation, or joint: A place of junction between two or more bones of the skeleton. There are three types of articulation: immovable (synarthrosis), slightly movable (amphiarthrosis), and freely movable (diarthrosis).

Diarthrosis joints are the most common type in the human body.

Classification of synovial joints: Synovial joints are classified according to the shapes of their parts and the movements they permit:

- Ball-and-socket joint
- Condyloid joint
- Gliding joint
- Hinge joint
- Pivot joint
- Saddle joint

Table 3-4 summarizes these types of joints.

Type of Joint	Description	Possible Movements	Examples
Fibrous	Articulating bones are fastened together by a thin layer of dense connective tissue.	None	Suture between bones of skull, joint between the distal ends of tibia and fibula
Cartilaginous	Articulating bones are connected by hyaline cartilage or fibrocartilage.	Limited movement, as when back is bent or twisted	Joints between the bodies of vertebrae, symphysis pubis
Synovial	Articulating bones are surrounded by a joint capsule of ligaments and synovial membranes; ends of articulating bones are covered by hyaline cartilage and separated by synovial fluid.	Allow free movement (see the following list)	
1. Ball-and-socket	Ball-shaped head of one bone articulates with cup-shaped cavity of another.	Movements in all planes and rotation	Shoulder, hip
2. Condyloid	Oval-shaped condyle of one bone articulates with elliptical cavity of another.	Variety of movements in different planes, but no rotation	Joints between the metacarpals and phalanges
3. Gliding	Articulating surfaces are nearly flat or slightly curved.	Sliding or twisting	Joints between various bones of wrist and ankle, sacroiliac joints, joints between ribs 2–7 and sternum
4. Hinge	Convex surface of one bone articulates with concave surface of another.	Flexion and extension	Elbow, joints of phalanges
5. Pivot	Cylindrical surface of one bone articulates with ring of bone and ligament.	Rotation around a central axis	Joint between the proximal ends of radius and ulna
6. Saddle	Articulating surfaces have both concave and convex regions; the surface of one bone fits the complementary surface of another.	Variety of movements	Joint between the carpal and metacarpal of thumb

Table 3-4

Hyoid bone: A U-shaped bone in the neck that supports the tongue. This bone does not articulate directly with any other bone.

Vertebral column, or spinal column: The portion of the skeleton consisting of vertebrae (26 in the human adult) and intervertebral disks. There are four curvatures: cervical curve, thoracic curve, lumbar curve, and sacral curve.

Atlas: The first cervical vertebra. It articulates with the occipital bone and the axis.

Axis: The second cervical vertebra, with which the atlas bone articulates. This articulation allows the head to be turned (rotated), extended, and flexed.

Coccyx: The last bone at the base of the vertebral column. The coccyx, also called the tailbone, attaches to the end of the sacrum.

Sternum: The bone that forms the anterior portion of the thoracic cage. It consists of the manubrium, the body (or gladiolus), and the xiphoid process. It supports the clavicles and articulates directly with the first seven pairs of the ribs.

True ribs: Seven pairs of ribs, which attach to the sternum directly by their individual costal cartilages.

False ribs: Ribs in pairs 8 through 10, which attach to the sternum indirectly.

Floating ribs: Ribs in pairs 11 and 12, which do not attach to the sternum.

Pectoral girdle: The skeletal structure consisting of the two clavicles (collarbones), and the two scapulae (shoulder blades).

Clavicle: One of the pair of long bones that form the anterior part of the pectoral girdle. It is commonly called the collarbone.

Scapula: One of the pair of large, flat, triangular bones that form the dorsal part of the pectoral girdle. It is commonly called the shoulder blade.

Olecranon process: A projection on the ulna that forms the bony point of the elbow.

Styloid process: A projection on the temporal bone.

Pelvic girdle: The skeletal structure consisting of the ilium, the sacrum, and the coccyx.

Femur: The thigh bone, which is the longest and strongest bone in the skeleton.

Acetabulum: The deep depression on the lateral surface of the hipbone, on which the ball-shaped head of the femur articulates.

Obturator foramen: A large opening on each side of the lower part of the hipbone.

Patella: A flat, triangular bone at the front of the knee joint. It is also called the kneecap.

Malleolus: A rounded bony process on each side of the ankle.

Muscular System

Muscle: Connective tissue made up of contractile cells or fibers that produce movement. There are three types of muscle: skeletal (voluntary); smooth, also called visceral, or involuntary; and cardiac (involuntary). There are two types of proteins in muscle tissue: actin and myosin. For a list of some of the main muscles of the human body, see Figure 3-8.

Skeletal muscle: A muscle composed of cylindrical, multinucleated, and striated fibers that works together with bones to enable movement. Skeletal muscles are characterized by contractility, elasticity, excitability, and extensibility. There are more than 600 skeletal muscles in the human body. See Table 3-5 for examples of skeletal muscles and their actions. Skeletal muscles are also called striated or voluntary muscles.

Smooth muscle: A spindle-shaped, involuntary muscle that causes the contraction of blood vessels and viscera such as the intestines and the stomach.

Cardiac muscle: A special striated muscle of the myocardium that pumps blood through the heart and blood vessels. Its contraction is not under voluntary control.

Muscle fiber: Any individual muscle cell.

Myofibril, or **myofibrilla:** A slender, striated strand of contractile fiber within skeletal and cardiac muscle cells.

Epimysium: The fibrous sheath that surrounds muscle tissue. It may also fuse with a fascia that attaches a muscle to a bone.

Endomysium: The fibrous sheath that surrounds each individual muscle cell.

Fascia: A sheet of fibrous connective tissue that covers, separates, or supports muscle.

Tendon: A band of dense fibrous connective tissue, generally white in color, that attaches muscle to bone.

Ligament: A band or sheet of fibrous tissue that connects two or more bones, cartilages, or other structures.

Sarcoplasm: The cytoplasm of muscle fiber.

Sarcolemma: The cell membrane of a muscle fiber.

Sarcomere: The smallest functional unit of a myofibril.

Neuromuscular junction: The region of contact between the ends of an axon and a skeletal muscle fiber.

Excitability: The ability of muscle tissue to react and respond to stimulation.

Contractility: The ability of muscle tissue to shorten, or contract, in response to a stimulus.

Elasticity: The capacity of tissues to return to their original shape and length after contraction or extension.

Contraction: A shortening or tightening of a muscle. Skeletal muscles need actin, myosin, calcium, ATP, and neurotransmitters to contract. All other muscles need only ATP and calcium.

Actin: A protein that forms the thin fibrils in muscle fibers.

Myosin: A skeletal and cardiac muscle protein that interacts with actin to cause muscle contraction.

Muscle tone: The continual state of slight contraction present in muscles. It is also called tonus.

Flexion: A bending that decreases the angle between two bones of a joint.

Extension: A straightening that increases the angle between two bones of a joint.

3.8 Nervous System

Nervous system: One of the body's regulatory systems. It controls all body activities by responding to internal and external stimuli and sending out signals or impulses to other nerves and various body organs. The brain, the spinal cord, and the nerves make up the nervous system, which is divided into two groups: the central nervous system and the peripheral nervous system. See Figure 3-9.

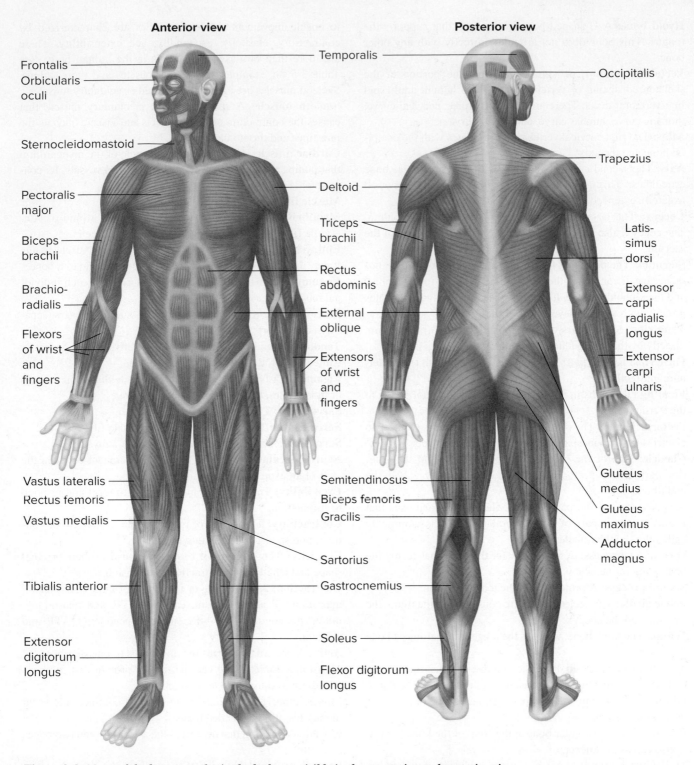

Anterior view

Frontalis
Orbicularis oculi
Sternocleidomastoid
Pectoralis major
Biceps brachii
Brachio-radialis
Flexors of wrist and fingers
Vastus lateralis
Rectus femoris
Vastus medialis
Tibialis anterior
Extensor digitorum longus

Temporalis
Deltoid
Triceps brachii
Rectus abdominis
External oblique
Extensors of wrist and fingers
Semitendinosus
Biceps femoris
Gracilis
Sartorius
Gastrocnemius
Soleus
Flexor digitorum longus

Posterior view

Occipitalis
Trapezius
Latis-simus dorsi
Extensor carpi radialis longus
Extensor carpi ulnaris
Gluteus medius
Gluteus maximus
Adductor magnus

Figure 3-8 *Many of the large muscles in the body are visible in these anterior and posterior views.*

Nerve Cells and Neurotransmitters

Neuron: A nerve cell, the basic unit of the nervous system. It consists of a cell body, one or more dendrites, and a single axon. The two forms of neurons are sensory and motor.

Cell body of a neuron: The main part of the neuron. It is also called the soma.

Dendrite: A nerve cell process that conducts impulses to the cell body.

Axon: A nerve cell process that conducts impulses away from the cell body.

Sensory neuron: A neuron that carries impulses to the spinal cord and the brain. It is also known as an afferent neuron.

Motor neuron: A neuron that carries impulses from the central nervous system out to muscles and glands. It stimulates a muscle to contract or a gland to secrete. It is also known as an efferent neuron.

Skeletal Muscle	Action
Masseter	Closes the jaw
Temporalis	Closes the jaw
Sternocleidomastoid	Flexes and rotates the head
Trapezius	Extends the head and moves the scapula
Pectoralis major	Adducts and flexes the arm
Deltoid	Abducts the arm
Biceps	Flexes and supinates the forearm
Triceps	Extends the forearm
Brachioradialis	Flexes the forearm
Brachialis	Flexes the forearm
Gluteus maximus	Extends the thigh
Gluteus medius	Abducts and rotates the thigh
Quadriceps femoris	Extends the leg
Sartorius	Flexes the thigh; flexes and rotates the leg
Hamstring	Flexes the leg and extends the thigh
Gastrocnemius	Flexes the foot

Table 3-5

Myelin: A white, fatty substance, largely composed of phospholipids and protein, that surrounds many nerve fibers.

Synapse: The junction between two neurons.

Neuroglia cell: A type of nerve cell that supports, protects, and nourishes the neuron. There are four kinds: astrocytes, microglia, ependymal cells, and oligodendrocytes.

Astrocyte: A large, star-shaped cell that provides nutrition.

Microglion: One of many small interstitial cells in the brain and spinal cord that serve as phagocytic cells and respond to inflammation.

Ependymal cell: A columnar cell located in the brain that produces cerebrospinal fluid.

Oligodendrocyte: A type of neuroglial cell that produces myelin, the white matter of the nervous system.

Nerve impulse: The electrochemical process involved in neural transmission.

Action potential: The sudden electrical charge transmitted across the cell membrane of a nerve fiber.

Neurotransmitter: A chemical substance that is released from synaptic knobs into synaptic clefts. Neurotransmitters include acetylcholine, dopamine, norepinephrine, epinephrine, serotonin, histamine, and gamma-aminobutyric acid (GABA).

Central Nervous System

Central nervous system: The part of the nervous system consisting of the brain and the spinal cord.

The Brain

Brain: The part of the central nervous system contained within the cranium. The brain consists of four major parts: the cerebrum, the cerebellum, the diencephalon, and the brainstem. See Figure 3-10.

Cerebrum: The largest and uppermost portion of the brain. The cerebrum is divided into two hemispheres, right and left, and five lobes: frontal, parietal, occipital, temporal, and insular (central).

Right hemisphere: The portion of the brain responsible for controlling the left side of the body. It also controls hearing and tactile and spatial perception.

Left hemisphere: The portion of the brain responsible for controlling the right side of the body. It is also responsible for verbal, analytical, and computational skills.

Frontal lobe: The part of the brain responsible for complex concentration, planning, and problem solving. It also contains the olfactory cortex, which interprets smells.

Parietal lobe: The part of the brain responsible for interpretation of sensory input other than sight, sound, and smell. It contains the gustatory area responsible for taste.

Occipital lobe: The part of the brain responsible for visual recognition.

Temporal lobe: The part of the brain responsible for the interpretation of sensory experiences such as hearing and smell. It is also said to be the center for emotion, memory, and personality.

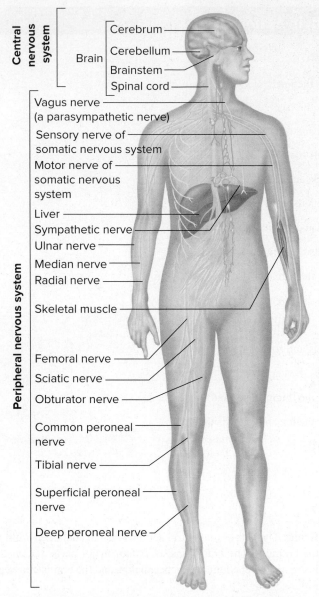

Central nervous system
- Brain
  - Cerebrum
  - Cerebellum
  - Brainstem
- Spinal cord

Peripheral nervous system
- Vagus nerve (a parasympathetic nerve)
- Sensory nerve of somatic nervous system
- Motor nerve of somatic nervous system
- Liver
- Sympathetic nerve
- Ulnar nerve
- Median nerve
- Radial nerve
- Skeletal muscle
- Femoral nerve
- Sciatic nerve
- Obturator nerve
- Common peroneal nerve
- Tibial nerve
- Superficial peroneal nerve
- Deep peroneal nerve

Figure 3-9 *The main organs of the nervous system are the brain, the spinal cord, and the nerves. The spinal nerves originate in the spinal cord, whereas the cranial nerves (for example, the vagus nerve) originate in the brain.*

Insular lobe, or **central lobe:** The part of the brain responsible for visceral or primitive emotions, drives, and reactions.

Broca's area: The part of the brain responsible for motor speech and for controlling the muscular actions of the mouth, tongue, and larynx (located in the left frontal lobe).

Wernicke's area: The part of the brain responsible for language comprehension (located in the right frontal lobe).

Corpus callosum: A large and transverse band of myelinated nerve fibers that connect the cerebral hemispheres. It is the largest commissure of the brain.

Basal ganglion: One of four islands of gray matter located in the white matter of the cerebrum: the lentiform nucleus, the caudate nucleus, the amygdaloid nucleus, and the claustrum. One function of the basal ganglia is to initiate and regulate muscular activity.

Diencephalon: The centrally located portion of the brain surrounded by the cerebrum that contains the thalamus and hypothalamus.

Thalamus: The subdivision of the diencephalon that sorts sensory impulses and directs them to the appropriate areas in the brain. It is basically a relay station for sensory impulses.

Hypothalamus: The subdivision of the diencephalon that assists in controlling body temperature, water balance, sleep, appetite, emotions of fear and pleasure, and involuntary functions.

Brainstem: The portion of the brain, located between the diencephalon and the spinal cord, that controls vital visceral activities. It consists of the midbrain, the pons, and the medulla oblongata.

Midbrain: The section of the brainstem that controls visual and auditory reflexes, such as turning to listen to a loud noise.

Pons: The section of the brainstem that relays sensory impulses and regulates the rate and depth of breathing in coordination with the medulla oblongata.

Medulla oblongata: The section of the brainstem that contains the cardiac center (which controls heart rate), the vasomotor center (which controls blood pressure), and the respiratory center (which controls the rate, rhythm, and depth of breathing).

Cerebellum: The second largest portion of the brain, located below the occipital lobes of the cerebrum. The cerebellum coordinates skeletal muscle activity. Damage to this area can result in tremors, loss of muscle tone, and loss of equilibrium.

Ventricle: One of four small interconnected cavities within the brain filled with cerebrospinal fluid.

The Spinal Cord

Spinal cord: A part of the central nervous system that conducts sensory and motor impulses, through nerves to the trunk and limbs, and serves as a center for reflex activities. Located in the vertebral canal, it extends from the foramen magnum at the base of the skull to the lumbar region. It is covered by three layers of meninges (the dura mater, the arachnoid mater, and the pia mater).

Peripheral Nervous System

Peripheral nervous system: The portion of the nervous system outside the central nervous system, consisting of the cranial nerves, the spinal nerves, and ganglia. It can be subdivided into the somatic and the autonomic nervous systems.

Somatic Nervous System

Somatic nervous system: The part of the peripheral nervous system consisting of the cranial and spinal nerves that connect the central nervous system with the skin and skeletal muscles. The somatic nervous system is responsible for conscious activities.

Cranial nerves: Twelve pairs of nerves that emerge from the brainstem. Three pairs have only sensory fibers. See Table 3-6.

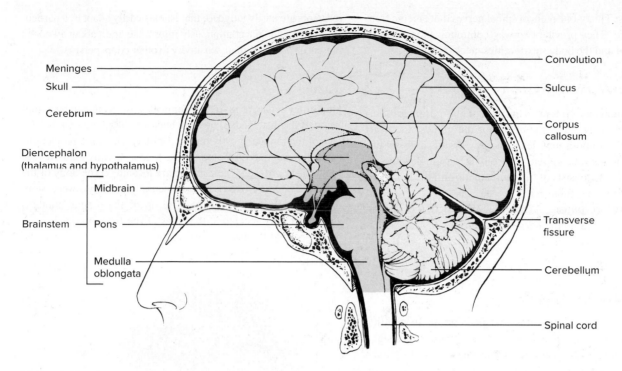

Figure 3-10 *The major portions of the brain include the cerebrum, the cerebellum, and the brainstem.*

AT A GLANCE	The Cranial Nerve Branches and Functions	
Cranial Nerve (Number)	**Branch**	**Primary Function**
Olfactory (I)		Special sensory
Optic (II)		Special sensory
Oculomotor (III)		Motor
Trochlear (IV)		Motor
	Ophthalmic	
	Maxillary	Mixed
Trigeminal (V)	Mandibular	Sensory
Abducens (VI)		Motor
Facial (VII)		Mixed
Vestibulocochlear (VIII)	Cochlear	Special sensory
	Vestibular	
Glossopharyngeal (IX)		Mixed
Vagus (X)		Mixed
Accessory (XI)	Internal	Motor
	External	
Hypoglossal (XII)		Motor

Table 3-6

Spinal nerves: Thirty-one pairs of spinal nerves that emerge from the spinal cord. They provide two-way communication between the spinal cord and the body's extremities, neck, and trunk.

Autonomic Nervous System

Autonomic nervous system: The part of the peripheral nervous system that regulates the action of the glands, the heart muscle, and the smooth muscles of hollow organs and vessels. The autonomic nervous system controls unconscious activities such as reflexes. It consists of the sympathetic and the parasympathetic systems. See Table 3-7.

Fight-or-flight response: A reaction in which the sympathetic part of the autonomic nervous system acts as an accelerator for organs whose functions are needed to meet a stressful situation.

3.9 Sensory System

Sense: A general faculty of physical perception. In addition to the commonly recognized "five senses" (smell, taste, sight, hearing, and touch and pressure), important senses in human beings include position, equilibrium, proprioception, temperature, hunger and thirst, and pain. They are found throughout the body and are therefore referred to as somatic senses.

Smell

Olfaction: The sense of smell.

Nose: The organ of smell. It also moistens, warms, and filters air that passes through it.

Olfactory receptor: A receptor, located in the upper portions of the nose, that is sensitive to gases and dissolved chemicals. Olfactory receptors are easily fatigued; that is, they easily adapt to a particular smell and do not continuously inform the brain about an odor's presence. However, their sensitivity to other odors persists.

Taste

Gustatory sense, or **taste:** A chemical sense produced by stimulation of the taste buds. The taste buds are distributed on the surface of the tongue, mostly on the papillae, which are projections of the tongue mucosa that make the tongue slightly abrasive (see Figure 3-11). Most of the papillae are located on the body of the tongue. There are five basic taste sensations: salty, sweet, sour, bitter, and umami (delicious). The tip of the tongue contains sweet and salty receptors, the sides of the tongue contain sour receptors, and the back of the tongue contains bitter receptors.

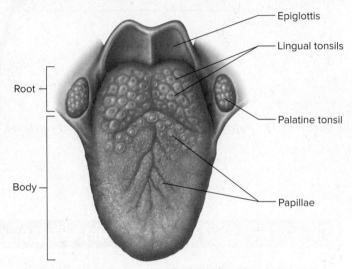

Figure 3-11 *The taste receptors of the tongue.*

AT A GLANCE	Effects of the Sympathetic and Parasympathetic Systems on Selected Visceral Effectors	
Visceral Effector	**Sympathetic Action**	**Parasympathetic Action**
Pupil of the eye	Dilation	Constriction
Sweat glands	Stimulation	No effect
Heart	Increase in heart rate	Decrease in heart rate
Bronchi	Dilation	Constriction
Digestive gland	Decrease in secretion of enzymes	Increase in secretion of enzymes
Digestive tract	Decrease in peristalsis	Increase in peristalsis
Digestive tract sphincter	Stimulation (closing of sphincter)	Inhibition (opening of sphincter)
Urinary bladder	Closing of sphincter	Opening of sphincter
Penis	Ejaculation	Erection
Adrenal medulla	Stimulation	No effect
Liver	Increase in release of glucose	No effect

Table 3-7

The taste reception of umami is linked to all of the other four taste receptors, and has no specific location on the tongue. The root makes up the posterior one-third of the tongue and contains the lingual tonsils. The epiglottis is a cartilage that is almost totally covered by a mucosa that contains taste buds. Each palatine tonsil lies within the walls of the oropharyngeal mucosa.

Sight

Eye: A group of specialized tissues that permits sight. Tears, lashes, eyelids, muscle, and fatty tissue surround and protect the eye.

Eyeball: The globe of the eye. It is made up of concentric coats, or tunics. The outer layer is the fibrous tunic. The middle layer, or uvea, consists of the choroid, the ciliary body, and the iris. The innermost coat of the eye is called the nervous tunic, or retina. The bulb of the eye is composed of two cavities separated by a crystalline lens. See Figure 3-12.

Fibrous tunic: The outermost, external protective layer of the eye. It consists of the white, opaque sclera and the transparent cornea.

Cornea: The transparent outer layer of the eye.

Sclera: The white outer layer of the eye.

Choroid: The part of the uvea that absorbs excess light rays.

Ciliary body: The part of the uvea that changes the shape of the lens.

Iris: The part of the uvea that regulates the size of the pupil and gives the eye its color.

Pupil: The dark opening of the eye, surrounded by the iris, through which light rays pass.

Retina: The light-sensitive nerve cell layer of the eye that contains the rods and cones.

Rod: A photoreceptor for black-and-white vision. Rods are essential for vision in dim light and for peripheral vision.

Cone: A photoreceptor for color vision and visual acuity. The three types of color suggested to be distinguished by the cones are blue, red, and green.

Aqueous humor: A clear, watery fluid that fills the anterior cavity of the eye and circulates in the anterior and posterior chambers.

Vitreous humor: A transparent jellylike substance that fills the posterior cavity of the eye, between the lens and the retina. It is the main component of the vitreous body; the two terms are used synonymously. It helps maintain sufficient intraocular pressure to prevent the eyeball from collapsing.

Accommodation: The adjustment of the eye for close or distant vision, which is primarily achieved through changing the curvature of the lens.

Hearing

Ear: The organ of hearing. It consists of three parts: the external, the middle, and the inner ear. This complex organ also aids in balance. See Figure 3-13.

External ear: The part of the ear consisting of the auricle and the external auditory meatus. It ends at the tympanic membrane.

Tympanic membrane: The eardrum, which separates the external from the middle ear, covers the auditory canal, and transmits sound vibrations to the inner ear by the auditory ossicles.

Middle ear: The part of the ear containing the auditory ossicles, the oval window, and the round window. It is also called the tympanic cavity.

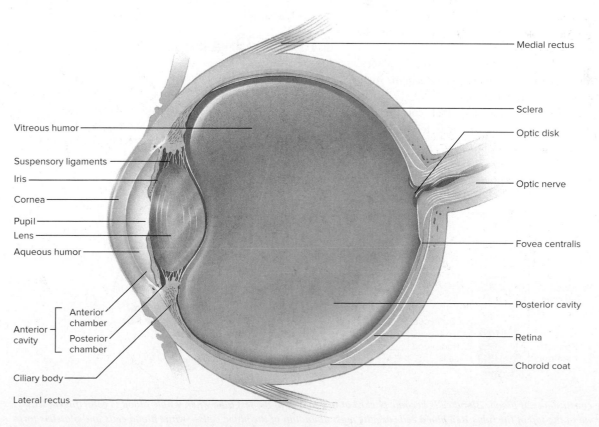

Figure 3-12 *Transverse section of the left eye (superior view).*

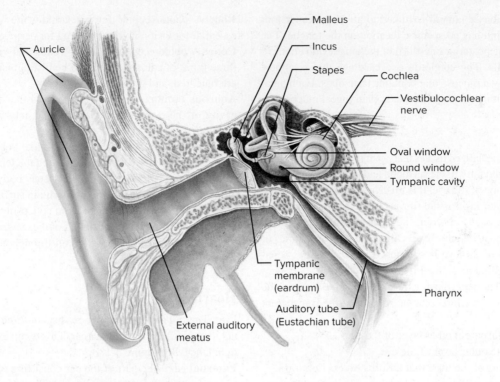

Figure 3-13 *Major parts of the ear.*

Eustachian tube: A tube that joins the nasopharynx and the middle ear cavity. This tube is also called the auditory tube.

Auditory ossicles: The three tiny bones in the middle ear: the malleus (hammer), the incus (anvil), and the stapes (stirrup). These bones transmit and amplify vibrations, and are the smallest bones in the body.

Inner ear: The part of the ear consisting of the vestibule, the semicircular canals, and the cochlea.

Vestibule: The middle part of the inner ear, involved in balance.

Semicircular canal: One of three curved passages in the inner ear that detect motion and govern balance.

Cochlea: The snail-shaped, spiral tube that contains the organ of Corti, the receptor for hearing. It is located in the inner ear.

Labyrinth: Those passages of the vestibule, the semicircular canals, and the cochlea that contain receptors for hearing and equilibrium. The term is loosely used as a synonym for the inner ear.

Cerumen: A waxy substance secreted by the external ear. It is also called ear wax.

3.10 Cardiovascular System

The Blood

Blood: A type of connective tissue that contains cellular and liquid components. The blood volume of the adult human is about five liters and accounts for 8% of body weight. About 55% of blood is plasma, and 45% is formed elements. See Figure 3-14.

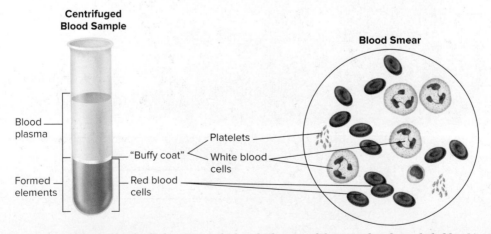

Figure 3-14 *The constituents of blood. Blood cells become packed at the bottom of the test tube when whole blood is centrifuged, leaving the fluid plasma at the top of the tube. Red blood cells are the most abundant of the blood cells—white blood cells and platelets form only a thin, light-colored "buffy coat" at the interface between the packed red blood cells and the plasma.*

Arterial blood: Highly oxygenated, bright red blood that travels from the heart to the capillaries and carries nutrients to the cells.

Venous blood: Dark red, carbon-dioxide-rich blood that travels from the capillaries to the heart and carries waste away from cells.

Formed element: An erythrocyte, a leukocyte, or a thrombocyte.

Hemocytoblast: The stem cell from which all formed elements of the blood develop. It is found in bone marrow and in lymphatic tissue. See Figure 3-15.

Plasma: The liquid portion of blood, made up of 90% water and 10% solutes.

Albumin: The most abundant plasma protein, essential for maintaining the osmotic pressure of the blood. (Osmotic pressure is the pressure that must be applied to a solution to prevent a solvent from passing into it.)

Globulin: One of a number of simple plasma proteins, which are classified in three groups: alpha, beta, and gamma.

Gamma globulin: An antibody obtained from pooled human plasma.

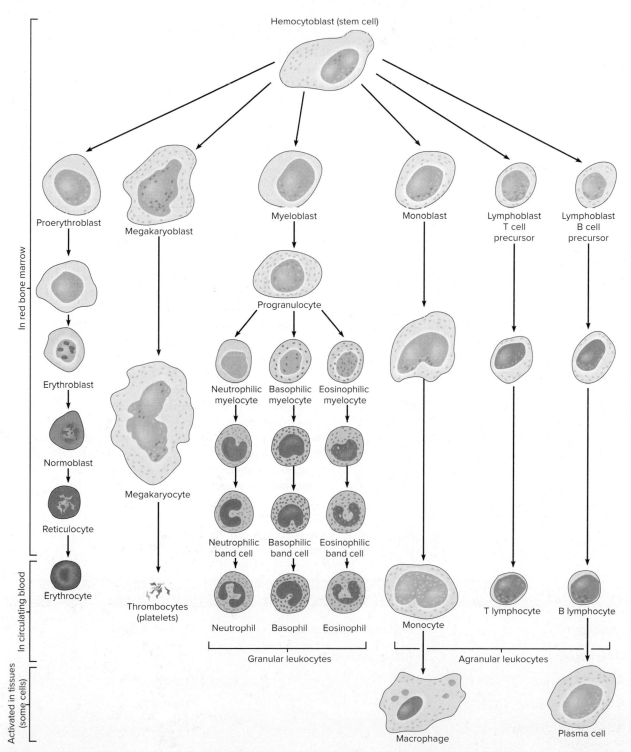

Figure 3-15 *Origin and development of blood cells from a hemocytoblast (stem cell) in bone marrow.*

Fibrinogen: The smallest fraction of plasma protein, which functions to form blood clots.

Erythropoietin: A glycoprotein hormone released from the kidney that regulates the formation of red blood cells (RBCs).

Fibrin: An insoluble fibrous protein formed by the action of thrombin on fibrinogen during blood coagulation.

Prothrombin: A plasma protein that leads to the formation of blood clots.

Thrombus: A blood clot that remains at its formation site in a blood vessel.

Embolus: A piece of thrombus or fragment of a clot that moves in a blood vessel.

Hemoglobin: A complex protein-iron compound in the blood that carries oxygen to the cells from the lungs and carbon dioxide away from the cells to the lungs. Hemoglobin is found in red blood cells.

Hemostasis: The stoppage of bleeding.

Hematocrit: A measure of the packed cell volume of RBCs, expressed as a percentage of the total blood volume.

Agglutinin: An antibody in plasma.

Agglutination: The clumping of RBCs.

Agglutinogen: A genetically determined antigen on the cell membrane of an RBC that determines blood types.

Blood typing: The identification of genetically determined RBC antigens and antibodies related to RBCs. See Table 3-8.

Blood group: A genetically determined pattern of antigen distribution on the surface of an RBC. In the ABO system, there are four blood groups: A, B, AB, and O. The ABO group is important in establishing compatibility in blood transfusions. The Rhesus (Rh) blood group system is important in obstetrics.

Rh factor: A type of protein (antigen) on the surface of red blood cells. Most people with this factor are "Rh-positive," and those without are "Rh-negative." To treat immune thrombocytopenic purpura in patients with Rh-positive blood, the Rho(D) immune globulin is injected, preventing death of the fetus.

Type A blood: Blood that has the A antigen on the surface of RBCs and anti-B antibodies in plasma.

Type B blood: Blood that has the B antigen on the surface of RBCs and anti-A antibodies in plasma.

Type O blood: Blood that has neither A nor B antigens on the surface of RBCs and has both anti-A and anti-B antibodies in plasma. Type O is referred to as the *universal donor* blood group.

Type AB blood: Blood that has both A and B antigens on the surface of RBCs and has neither anti-A nor anti-B antibodies in plasma. Type AB is referred to as the *universal recipient* blood group.

Rh⁺ blood: Blood in which the Rh factor is present.

Rh⁻ blood: Blood from which the Rh factor is absent. When a woman with Rh⁻ blood is pregnant with a fetus with Rh⁺ blood, the interaction between the two blood types will create anti-Rh agglutinin in the woman's blood. In subsequent pregnancies, these Rh antibodies may cross the placenta and destroy fetal cells.

Universal donor: A person with blood type O, Rh⁻.

Universal recipient: A person with blood type AB, Rh⁺.

Blood Cell Types

Erythrocyte, or **red blood cell (RBC):** A type of blood cell that has no nucleus and usually survives for 120 days, after which it is destroyed by the liver and the spleen. RBCs contain hemoglobin, which contains iron and carries oxygen from the lungs to the body and carries carbon dioxide from the body tissues to the lungs.

Erythrocytosis: An increased number of red cells in the blood, also called polycythemia.

Anisocytosis: A condition in which there is excessive inequality in the size of blood cells.

Reticulocyte: An immature RBC.

Poikilocytosis: Variation in the shape of RBCs (sickle cells, spherocytes, elliptocytes, etc.).

Leukocyte, or **white blood cell (WBC):** A part of the body's defense against infection. Leukocytes do not have hemoglobin, and they move through capillary walls by diapedesis. They are classified into two groups: granulocytes and agranulocytes.

Granulocyte, or **granular leukocyte:** A leukocyte that has large granules in its cytoplasm, which stain in different colors under a microscope. Granular leukocytes include neutrophils, basophils, and eosinophils.

Neutrophil: The most frequently occurring leukocyte (55% to 70% of all WBCs). Neutrophils are phagocytic in acute inflammatory response.

Basophil: A granulocyte that mediates allergic reactions. In the tissues, a basophil is called a mast cell. These cells produce heparin and histamine.

Eosinophil: A granulocyte that functions as defense against helminthic and protozoan infections and also participates in allergic reactions.

Phagocyte: A cell that ingests bacteria, foreign particles, and other cells.

AT A GLANCE Blood Typing

RBC Antigen	Plasma Antibodies	Donor Types
Type O (no antigens)	Anti-A and Anti-B	O
Type A (type A antigen)	Anti-B	O and A
Type B (type B antigen)	Anti-A	O and B
Type AB (type AB antigen)	None	O, A, B, and AB

Table 3-8

Phagocytosis: The process by which special cells engulf and destroy cellular debris and microorganisms. It is also called cell eating.

Pinocytosis: The process by which extracellular fluid is taken into a cell. It is also known as cell drinking.

Agranulocyte: A leukocyte that lacks granules. Nongranular leukocytes include lymphocytes and monocytes.

Lymphocyte: The smallest WBC. These cells travel from the blood to the lymph and lymph nodes and back into circulation. They are the main means of providing the body with immunity. They recognize antigens, produce antibodies, prevent excess tissue damage, and become memory cells. Type B lymphocytes produce antibodies. Type T lymphocytes regulate type B lymphocytes and macrophages.

Monocyte: The largest of the WBCs. Monocytes and neutrophils are largely phagocytic.

Macrophage: A monocyte that has left circulation and settled in tissue. Along with neutrophils, macrophages are the major phagocytic cells of the immune system. They recognize and digest all antigens and also process and present these antigens to T cells, activating the specific immune response.

Thrombocyte: A cell fragment and the smallest formed element of blood. It is also called a platelet. Thrombocytes are essential in blood coagulation.

The Heart and Blood Vessels

Heart: A muscular organ, about the size of a closed fist, that acts as the pump of the circulatory system. It is made up of three layers: the epicardium, the myocardium, and the endocardium. See Figure 3-16.

Circulatory system: The system responsible for transporting materials throughout the entire body. It includes the heart, blood, and blood vessels. The movement of blood and its materials is known as circulation. The circulatory system also circulates lymph as well as blood. Transported materials include nutrients, oxygen, carbon dioxide, and hormones.

Endocardium: The innermost layer of the heart.

Myocardium: The middle layer of the heart and the most important structure of the heart. It contains the heart muscles that can regulate cardiac output.

Epicardium: The outermost layer of the heart.

Pericardium: The double membranous sac that envelops and protects the heart.

Atrium: A thin-walled chamber that receives blood from the veins. There are two atria in the heart, the right atrium and the left atrium.

Right atrium: The chamber that receives deoxygenated blood from systemic veins (superior and inferior vena cava).

Left atrium: The chamber that receives oxygenated blood from the pulmonary veins.

Ventricle: A thick-walled chamber that pumps blood out of the heart. There are two ventricles in the heart, the right ventricle and the left ventricle.

Right ventricle: The chamber that pumps blood to the lungs.

Left ventricle: The chamber that pumps blood to the tissues of the whole body. It is the largest and the most powerful of the four chambers.

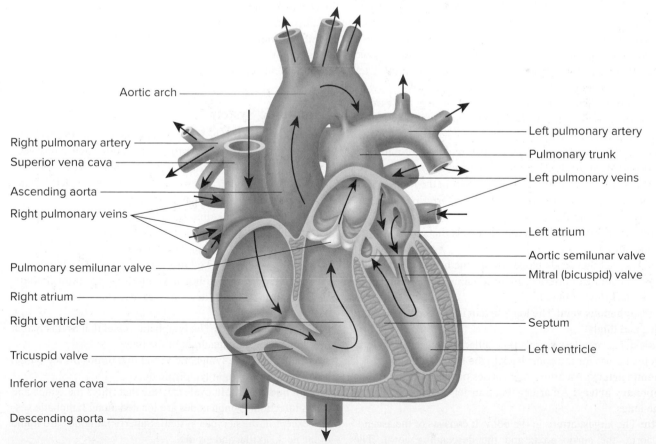

Figure 3-16 *The heart has four main chambers: left and right atria and left and right ventricles. This figure shows the pathway of blood through the heart.*

Valve: A membranous structure that temporarily closes to permit the flow of fluid through a passage in only one direction. The four valves in the heart are the bicuspid (or mitral) valve, the tricuspid valve, the aortic valve, and the pulmonary valve.

Cardiac cycle: The contraction and relaxation of the ventricles, known as systole and diastole. At a normal heart rate, one cardiac cycle lasts 0.8 second.

Systole: The contraction phase of the ventricles of the heart.

Diastole: The relaxation phase of the ventricles of the heart.

Cardiac center: The control center of the heart located in the medulla oblongata. It has both sympathetic and parasympathetic components.

Cardiac conduction system: A system consisting of specialized cardiac muscle cells. Its components are the sinoatrial (SA) node, the atrioventricular (A-V) node, the A-V bundle (bundle of His), the bundle branches, and the Purkinje fibers (see Chapter 21).

Cardiac output: The volume of blood pumped per minute by the heart, which increases during exercise.

Stroke volume: The amount of blood that the ventricle discharges with each heartbeat.

Pulse pressure: The pressure exerted by the circulating volume of blood on the walls of the blood vessels. It is proportional to stroke volume.

Myocardial oxygen demand: The demand for oxygen by the heart muscle. It is raised by increases in diastolic blood pressure, contractility, heart rate, and heart size.

Contractility: The force of left ventricular ejection.

Diastolic blood pressure: The blood pressure during diastole (relaxation phase), the period of least pressure in the arterial vascular system.

Systolic blood pressure: The blood pressure during systole (contraction phase), the period of greatest pressure in the arterial vascular system.

Heart sound: A normal noise produced during the cardiac cycle by the closure of the mitral and tricuspid valves and of the aortic and pulmonic valves.

Murmur: Abnormal heart sound. The three types of murmurs are systolic, diastolic, and continuous murmurs.

Artery: A vessel that carries blood away from the heart.

Arteriole: A small arterial branch; terminal arterioles are continuous with the capillary network.

Capillary: One of many very small vessels that connect arteries and veins.

Vein: A vessel that sends blood toward the heart. Its walls are thinner than those of arteries, and it contains valves, which prevent the backflow of blood.

Great saphenous vein: The longest vein in the body, located in the leg and thigh.

Venules: The smallest vessels that collect deoxygenated blood from the tissues for transport back to the heart.

Systemic artery: An artery that carries oxygenated blood.

Pulmonary artery: An artery that transfers low-oxygen blood to the lungs.

Aorta: The largest artery in the body. It consists of the ascending aorta, the aortic arch, and the descending aorta. The descending aorta consists of the thoracic aorta and the abdominal aorta.

Coronary artery: One of a pair of vessels that supply blood to the myocardium. The coronary arteries are the only vessels that branch from the ascending aorta.

Aortic arch: A part of the aorta from which three vessels branch: the brachiocephalic trunk (or innominate artery), the left common carotid artery, and the left subclavian artery.

External iliac artery: An artery that provides the blood supply for the lower extremities.

Internal iliac artery: An artery that supplies blood to the pelvic organs.

Internal carotid artery: One of the primary vessels that provide blood to the brain.

Vertebral artery: One of the primary vessels that provide blood to the brain.

Internal jugular vein: One of the primary vessels that drain blood from the brain.

Vertebral vein: One of the primary vessels that drain blood from the brain.

Azygous vein: One of the seven veins in the thorax. It drains blood from the thoracic and abdominal walls and empties into the superior vena cava.

Umbilical cord: The attachment connecting a fetus with the placenta. First formed during the fifth week of pregnancy, it contains two arteries and one vein.

Ductus venosus: The vascular channel in the fetus that is a continuation of the umbilical vein to the inferior vena cava. It becomes the ligamentum venosum of the liver.

Ductus arteriosus: A vascular channel in the fetus located between the pulmonary artery and the aorta. It becomes the ligamentum arteriosum.

Fetal circulation: The pathway of blood circulation in the fetus. Oxygenated blood from the placenta is carried through the umbilical vein to the fetal heart.

Lymphatic System

Lymphatic system: The body system that returns excess interstitial fluid to the blood and protects the body against disease.

Lymph: A thin, watery fluid in the lymphatic vessels that is filtered by the lymph nodes and contains chyle, RBCs, and WBCs, most of which are lymphocytes.

Chyle: A milklike alkaline fluid consisting of digestive products and absorbed fats.

Gastrectasia: Stretching of the stomach.

Lymphatic vessel: A vessel that carries lymph. Lymphatic vessels resemble veins, but they have more valves, thinner walls, and lymph nodes, and they carry excess fluid away from the tissues.

Right lymphatic duct: The lymphatic vessel that drains lymph from the upper right quadrant of the body.

Thoracic duct: The lymphatic vessel that drains all the lymph not drained by the right lymphatic duct.

Lymph node: A small, oval structure that filters the lymph and fights infection. Lymph nodes are located along lymphatic vessels except in the nervous system. Superficial nodes are found in the neck, axilla, and groin.

Spleen: The lymph organ that filters and also serves as a reservoir for blood.

Thymus: A gland essential to the maturation and development of the immune system. T lymphocytes mature in this gland.

3.11 Respiratory System

Respiratory system: The body system that provides oxygen to cells and removes carbon dioxide from them. The organs of the respiratory system include the nose, the pharynx, the larynx, the trachea, the bronchi, and the lungs. See Figure 3-17.

Bronchi: Two main branches of the trachea that pass into the lungs, further dividing into bronchioles and alveoli. The singular form of the word is *bronchus.*

Respiratory center: A group of nerve cells in the medulla oblongata and pons of the brain that control the rhythm of breathing in response to changes in oxygen and carbon dioxide levels in the blood and cerebrospinal fluid.

Nose: The projection that serves as the entrance to the nasal cavities. Hairs and cilia in the nose help trap dust, bacteria, and other particles and keep them from entering the body. The nose also warms and moistens the air, and it is involved with the sense of smell.

Larynx: The organ at the upper end of the trachea that contains the vocal cords, which vibrate to make speech.

Trachea: The tube that extends from the larynx and branches into two bronchi that lead to the lungs. It is also called the windpipe.

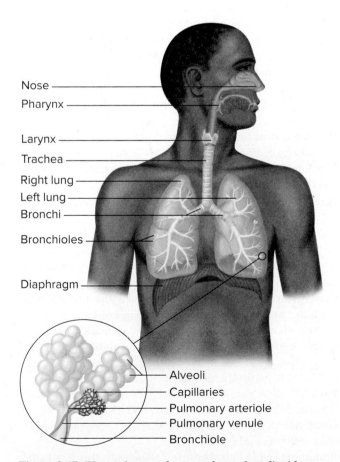

Figure 3-17 *The exchange of oxygen for carbon dioxide between the air and blood occurs within the lungs, where the alveoli and the capillaries are in intimate contact.*

Lung: A spongy organ in the thorax used for breathing. The two highly elastic lungs are the main component of the respiratory system. The left lung is divided into two lobes, and the right lung is divided into three lobes.

Alveolus: One of many clusters of air sacs at the end of the bronchioles in the lungs. The exchange of gases occurs in the alveoli.

Inspiration: The process of letting air into the lungs, also known as inhalation. The major muscle of inspiration is the diaphragm, the contraction of which creates a negative pressure in the chest.

Diaphragm: The musculomembranous partition separating the abdominal and thoracic cavities. It serves as a major muscle aiding inhalation.

Expiration: Breathing out, the process of letting air out of the lungs, which is normally a passive process. It is also called exhalation.

External respiration: The exchange of oxygen and carbon dioxide between the air in the lungs and the blood in the surrounding capillaries.

Internal respiration: The exchange of gases between the tissue cells and the blood in the tissue capillaries.

Carbon dioxide transport: A process that moves carbon dioxide from the tissues to the lungs in three forms: as bicarbonate, bound to hemoglobin; as carbaminohemoglobin; and as dissolved carbon dioxide.

Oxygen transport: The transfer of oxygen in the blood. Approximately 3% of oxygen is transported as a dissolved gas in the plasma; 97% is carried by hemoglobin molecules.

Surfactant: Any of certain lipoproteins that are produced by the lungs and that reduce the surface tension within the alveoli, keeping them inflated. Artificial surfactants are administered to premature infants to help prevent their lungs from collapsing.

Spirometer: An instrument that measures and records the volume of air that moves in and out of the lungs.

Spirogram: A chart with recorded volumetric information. See Figure 3-18.

Spirometry: Laboratory evaluation of the air capacity of the lungs by means of a spirometer.

Pulmonary function test: The assessment that provides information about airflow, lung volume, and the diffusion of gas.

3.12 Digestive System

Digestive system: The group of organs that change food so that it can be used by the body. The organs of the digestive system include the mouth, the pharynx, the esophagus, the stomach, and the small and large intestines. See Figure 3-19.

Digestive tract, or **alimentary canal:** The digestive tube, running from the mouth to the anus. The wall consists of four layers, or tunics: the mucosa, the submucosa, the muscular layer, and the serous layer, or serosa.

Serosa: The outermost layer of the digestive tract. It is composed of connective tissue. Above the diaphragm, it is known as the adventitia.

Saliva: A fluid that moistens food and begins the chemical breakdown of carbohydrates. It is produced by the salivary glands.

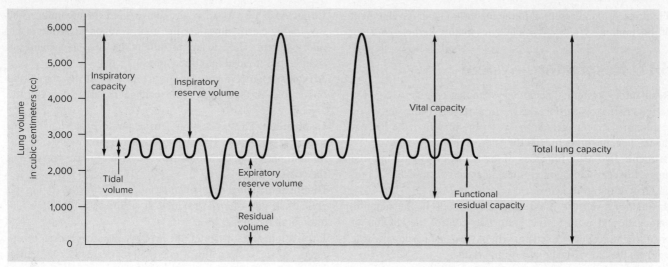

Figure 3-18 *A spirogram showing lung volumes and capacities.* *A lung capacity is the sum of two or more lung volumes. The vital capacity, for example, is the sum of the tidal volume, the inspiratory reserve volume, and the expiratory reserve volume. Note that residual volume cannot be measured with a spirometer because it is air that cannot be exhaled. Therefore, the total lung capacity (the sum of the vital capacity and the residual volume) also cannot be measured with a spirometer.*

Salivary gland: A gland that secretes saliva. There are three pairs of glands secreting into the mouth: the parotid glands, the sublingual glands, and the submandibular glands.

Parotid gland: The largest salivary gland, which secretes serous fluid.

Sublingual gland: The smallest salivary gland, which secretes mucus.

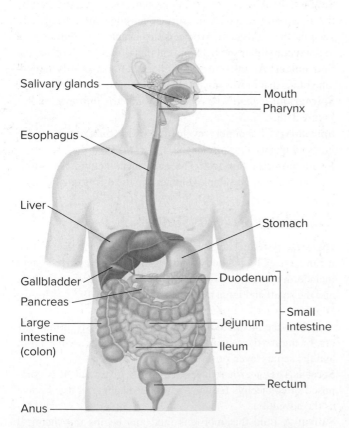

Figure 3-19 *The main organs and accessory organs of the digestive system change food into a form the body can use.*

Submandibular gland: A salivary gland located in the floor of the mouth. It secretes both mucus and serous fluid.

Uvula: A structure of soft tissue hanging down from the soft palate in the mouth.

Tooth: A dental structure that develops in the jaws, consisting of the crown (which projects above the gum), the neck (between the crown and the root), and the root.

Enamel: The hardest substance in the body, covering the crown and consisting mainly of calcium salts.

Dentin: The bulk of the tooth.

Pulp cavity: The interior part of a tooth, containing dental pulp, which consists of cells, nerves, and blood vessels or lymph vessels.

Deciduous dentition: The set of teeth that appear in the mouth first, also called deciduous or primary teeth.

Esophageal sphincter: The sphincter located in the lower portion of the esophagus. It is also called the cardiac sphincter.

Peristalsis: Rhythmic contractions that move food. This action occurs throughout the digestive tract.

Stomach: A muscular J-shaped organ that stores, churns, and further digests food. The stomach produces strong acids and enzymes that, combined with the churning action, begin the chemical breakdown of food.

Pyloric sphincter: The sphincter located at the junction of the stomach and the duodenum of the small intestine.

Gastric gland: One of the glands in the stomach mucosa that secrete hydrochloric acid, mucin, and pepsinogen. Four different types of cells make up the gastric glands: mucous cells (goblet cells), parietal cells, chief cells, and endocrine cells.

Parietal cell: A gastric cell that secretes hydrochloric acid and intrinsic factor, which aids in the absorption of vitamin B_{12}.

Chief cell: A gastric cell that secretes pepsinogen, an active form of the enzyme pepsin.

Endocrine cell: In the digestive system only, this is a gastric cell that secretes the hormone gastrin, which regulates gastric activity. See Table 3-9.

AT A GLANCE	Hormones of the Digestive System	
Secretion	**Source**	
Gastrin	Stomach	
Secretin	Small intestine	
Cholecystokinin	Small intestine	

Table 3-9

Chyme: A mixture of partially digested food, water, and digestive juices that forms in the stomach and passes through the pylorus into the duodenum.

Intestine: One of two long, tubular organs distinguished by the difference in their diameters.

Small intestine: The longest part of the digestive tract. The chemical digestion of fats and the final breakdown of carbohydrates and proteins take place here. Most of the nutrients in food are absorbed in the small intestine. The small intestine is divided into three parts: the duodenum, the jejunum, and the ileum.

Villus: One of many small, fingerlike projections, or villi, on the surface of the membrane in the small intestine through which digested food is absorbed. Villi increase the surface area of the small intestine.

Cholecystokinin: A hormone that is secreted from the mucosa of the upper small intestine and stimulates contraction of the gallbladder to release bile and pancreatic enzymes.

Large intestine: The large intestines joined to the small intestine at the ileum and extends to the anus. It consists of the cecum, the colon, the rectum, and the anal canal. It is divided into ascending, transverse, descending, and sigmoid portions. The large intestine is responsible for making vitamin K and some B vitamins, absorbing water and electrolytes, and storing and eliminating undigested waste.

Anal canal: The final portion of the digestive tract, between the rectum and the anus. The internal anal sphincter is under involuntary control. The external anal sphincter can be controlled voluntarily.

Additional Organs and Processes Involved with Digestion

Kupffer cell: A cell in the liver responsible for cleansing the blood.

Hepatocyte: A liver cell responsible for storage, synthesis of bile salts, detoxification, synthesis of plasma proteins, and metabolism of carbohydrates, proteins, and lipids.

Liver: An organ of the digestive system whose main role is to produce bile.

Bile: The fluid responsible for excreting bile pigments and cholesterol from the breakdown of hemoglobin. Bile helps the body digest and absorb fat.

Gallbladder: The reservoir for bile on the posteroinferior surface of the liver.

Pancreas: An organ that produces enzymes that digest fats, proteins, and carbohydrates. Pancreatic substances also neutralize the acids produced by the stomach.

Metabolism: The physical and chemical processes that take place in a living organism, resulting in growth, production of energy, elimination of wastes, and other body functions. The fundamental metabolic processes are anabolism and catabolism.

Basal metabolism: The minimal energy that is necessary to maintain the body's functions at a low level.

Anabolism: The conversion of simple compounds into more complex substances needed by the body and living matter.

Catabolism: The breakdown of substances into simple compounds that liberates energy for use in work and heat production. It produces carbon dioxide, water, and energy.

Thermogenesis: The production of heat needed to utilize food, especially within the human body.

Core temperature: The temperature around the internal organs.

Shell temperature: The temperature near the body surface.

3.13 Endocrine System

Endocrine system: A system of glands whose secretions coordinate many body functions. Its response to change is slower and more prolonged than that of the nervous system. See Figure 3-20.

Endocrine gland: A ductless gland that secretes hormones directly into the bloodstream. See Table 3-10.

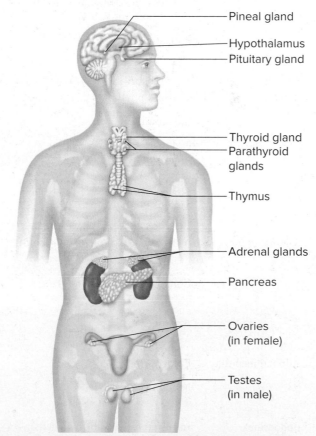

Pineal gland
Hypothalamus
Pituitary gland
Thyroid gland
Parathyroid glands
Thymus
Adrenal glands
Pancreas
Ovaries (in female)
Testes (in male)

Figure 3-20 *The endocrine system produces hormones that affect activities such as growth, metabolism, and reproduction.*

Gland	Hormones	Major Functions
Hypothalamus	Releasing and inhibiting hormones (TRH—Thyrotropin-releasing hormone, CRH—Corticotropin-releasing hormone, GnRH—Gonadotropin-releasing hormone, GHRH—Growth hormone-releasing hormone)	These hormones control the release of anterior pituitary hormones. Vasopressin and oxytocin are *stored* in the posterior pituitary.
	Vasopressin (antidiuretic hormone)	Vasopressin increases reabsorption of water in kidney tubules and stimulates smooth muscle tissue in blood vessels to constrict.
	Oxytocin	Oxytocin increases the contractility of the uterus and causes milk ejection.
Anterior pituitary (adenohypophysis)	Thyroid-stimulating hormone (TSH)	TSH stimulates the thyroid gland to produce thyroid hormones (T_3 and T_4 secretion).
	Adrenocorticotropic hormone (ACTH)	ACTH stimulates the adrenal cortex to produce cortisol.
	Growth hormone (GH)	GH promotes growth of bone and soft tissue.
	Follicle-stimulating hormone (FSH)	FSH stimulates follicular growth and secretion of estrogen; it also stimulates growth of the testes and promotes development of sperm cells.
	Luteinizing hormone (LH; in males, called interstitial cell-stimulating hormone, or ICSH)	LH causes development of a corpus luteum at the site of a ruptured ovarian follicle in females; also it can stimulate secretion of testosterone in males.
	Prolactin	Prolactin promotes breast development in females and stimulates milk secretion.
Thyroid	Thyroid hormone (thyroxine or T_4, and triiodothyronine or T_3)	Thyroxine increases metabolic rate; it is essential for normal growth and nerve development.
	Calcitonin	Calcitonin decreases plasma calcium concentrations.
Parathyroid	Parathyroid hormone	Parathyroid hormone regulates the exchange of calcium between the blood and bones, and it increases the calcium level in the blood.
Thymus	Thymosin	Thymosin enhances the proliferation and function of T lymphocytes.
Adrenal cortex	Aldosterone (a mineralocorticoid)	Aldosterone increases Na^+ reabsorption and K^+ secretion in kidney tubules.
	Cortisol (a glucocorticoid)	Cortisol increases blood glucose at the expense of protein and fat stores; it also contributes to stress adaptation.
	Androgens	Androgens are responsible for stimulating development of secondary sex characteristics.
Adrenal medulla	Epinephrine	Epinephrine increases blood pressure and heart rate.
	Norepinephrine	Norepinephrine reinforces the sympathetic nervous system.
Endocrine pancreas (islets of Langerhans)	Insulin (produced by beta cells)	Insulin promotes cellular uptake and is required for cellular metabolism of nutrients, especially glucose; it also decreases blood sugar levels.

Gland	Hormones	Major Functions
	Glucagon (produced by alpha cells)	Glucagon stimulates the liver to release glucose and increase blood sugar levels.
Ovaries	Estrogens (e.g., estradiol)	Estrogens promote follicular development, which is responsible for development of secondary sex characteristics; it also stimulates uterine and breast growth.
	Progesterone	Progesterone prepares the uterus for pregnancy.
Testes	Testosterone	Testosterone stimulates the production of spermata and their maturation; it also is responsible for development of secondary sex characteristics.

Table 3-10

Hormone: A protein or steroid carried through the blood to a target organ. Secretion is regulated by other hormones, through a negative feedback system, or by neurotransmitters.

Steroid hormone: A hormone derived from cholesterol. Steroid hormones include the adrenal cortex hormones, androgens, and estrogens.

Control of Hormonal Secretions

Hormone secretion is precisely regulated by the hypothalamus, the anterior pituitary gland, and other groups of glands that respond to the hypothalamus and pituitary glands.

3.14 Urinary System

Urinary system: The system that removes waste products, salts, and excess water from the blood and eliminates them from the body. The organs of the urinary system are the kidneys, the ureters, the urinary bladder, and the urethra. See Figure 3-21.

Body Fluids

Body fluid: Any of several fluids, primarily intracellular and extracellular fluids, that make up 60% of the adult's body weight.

Extracellular fluid: Fluid outside a cell. Extracellular fluids are composed of intravascular and interstitial fluids.

Intracellular fluid: Fluid within cells. Intracellular fluids contain potassium and phosphates.

Organs and Function of the Urinary System

Kidney: One of a pair of organs that perform the main functions of the urinary system. The kidneys help maintain balance in the volume of body fluid and in the levels of potassium, sodium, and chloride. The functions of the kidneys, which are governed by hormones, involve the processes of glomerular filtration, tubular reabsorption, and tubular secretion. See Table 3-11.

Glomerular filtration: A process in which plasma components cross the filtration membrane from the glomerulus into the glomerular capsule.

Glomerulus: A small ball of capillaries in the nephron where capillary filtration occurs.

Tubular reabsorption: A process that moves substances from the filtrate into the blood. About 65% of the reabsorption takes place in the proximal convoluted tubule.

Tubular secretion: A process in which the kidney tubules selectively add some toxic waste products to the quantity already filtered by the process of tubular reabsorption.

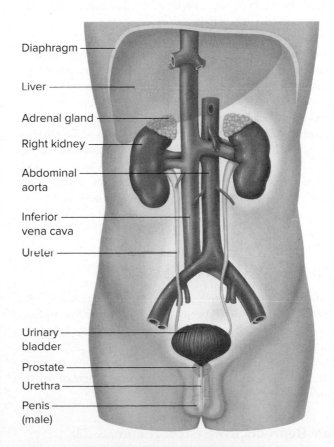

Diaphragm

Liver

Adrenal gland

Right kidney

Abdominal aorta

Inferior vena cava

Ureter

Urinary bladder

Prostate

Urethra

Penis (male)

Figure 3-21 *The urinary system, also known as the excretory system, removes waste products from the body and maintains the proper balance of body fluids and their chemistry.*

Hormone	Stimulus
Vasopressin (ADH)	Increases plasma osmolarity and increases blood volume
Aldosterone	Increases blood volume via angiotensin II and decreases plasma potassium ions
Angiotensin II	Increases blood volume via renin
Parathyroid hormone	Increases plasma calcium ions

Table 3-11

Nephron: The functional unit of the kidney forms urine by the processes of filtration, reabsorption, and secretion. Nephrons filter water and waste products from the blood and create urine.

Renal corpuscle: A part of the nephron, consisting of a glomerulus enclosed within Bowman's capsule.

Renal tubule: A structure that carries fluid away from the glomerular capsule, consisting of three regions: the proximal convoluted tubule, the nephron loop (loop of Henle), and the distal convoluted tubule.

Juxtaglomerular apparatus: A structure that monitors blood pressure and secretes renin. The formation of angiotensin II in the bloodstream involves several organs and includes multiple actions that conserve sodium and water, resulting in an increased blood volume.

Ureter: One of two long, slender tubes that extend from the kidneys to the urinary bladder.

Urinary bladder: The expandable organ that temporarily stores urine. Stretch receptors in the bladder create the urge to urinate. Urination is also called voiding urine or micturition.

Ruga: A ridge, wrinkle, or fold, as in a mucous membrane. Rugae line the urinary bladder and the stomach.

Detrusor muscle: The smooth muscle of the urinary bladder wall.

Trigone: A triangular area on the internal floor of the bladder between the opening of the two ureters and the internal urethral orifice.

Urethra: The tube through which urine leaves the body.

Buffer system: A physical or physiological system that tends to maintain constancy. For example, the kidneys act as a buffer system to help regulate blood pH.

3.15 Reproductive System

Genitalia: The reproductive organs of males and females.

Gonad: One of the two types of primary reproductive organs, the ovary and the testis, or testicle. Ovaries and testes produce gametes and hormones.

Follicle-stimulating hormone (FSH): The hormone produced by the anterior pituitary that stimulates development of ova in the ovary and spermatozoa in the testes.

Male Reproductive System (Figure 3-22)

Testis: The male gonad. There are two testes, normally situated in the scrotum, which produce sperm cells and male sex hormones.

Lobule: One of two layers that surround each testis: an outer mesothelial layer (tunica vaginalis) and an inner white capsule (tunica albuginea).

Spermatogonium: A male germ cell that gives rise to a spermatocyte early in spermatogenesis.

Spermatocyte: A male germ cell, or gamete, that arises from a spermatogonium.

Spermatozoon: A mature male gamete that develops in the seminiferous tubules of the testes, consisting of a head, a midpiece, and a tail.

Acrosome: A caplike structure over the head of the spermatozoon that helps the sperm to penetrate the ovum during fertilization. It is also called the acrosomal cap.

Ejaculatory duct: The passage formed by the junction of the duct of the seminal vesicles and ductus deferens through which semen enters the urethra.

Seminal vesicle: One of a pair of saclike accessory glands located posterior to the urinary bladder in the male that provide nourishment for sperm.

Prostate: A gland, located below the neck of the bladder in males, that surrounds the proximal portion of the urethra. It is a firm structure composed of muscular and glandular tissue that secretes alkaline phosphatase.

Cowper's gland: One of two pea-sized glands near the base of the penis in the male. It is also called a bulbourethral gland.

Semen, or **seminal fluid:** A thick, whitish secretion of the male reproductive organs discharged from the urethra on ejaculation.

Epididymis: One of the pair of long, tightly coiled tubules along the posterior margin of each testis that store and carry sperm from the testis to the vas deferens.

Glans penis: The bulbous end of the penis.

Prepuce, or **foreskin:** A fold of loose skin that covers the glans penis.

Emission: A discharge or release of seminal fluid into the urethra.

Tunica albuginea: A white capsule that surrounds each testis in the male.

Phimosis: A tightness and narrowing of the prepuce on the penis that prevents the retraction of the foreskin over the glans penis. It may obstruct urine flow and is usually congenital, although it may be caused by infection.

Impotence: The inability to achieve penile erection or to ejaculate after achieving an erection.

Circumcision: Surgical removal of the foreskin, or prepuce of the penis, commonly performed on newborn males.

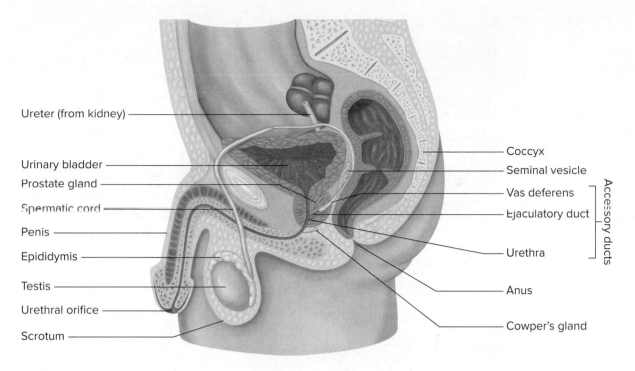

Ureter (from kidney)

Urinary bladder

Prostate gland

Spermatic cord

Penis

Epididymis

Testis

Urethral orifice

Scrotum

Coccyx

Seminal vesicle

Vas deferens

Ejaculatory duct

Urethra

Anus

Cowper's gland

Accessory ducts

Figure 3-22 *The male reproductive system produces sperm and delivers them in a form that keeps them viable long enough to fertilize an egg.*

Vasectomy: Surgical removal of the bilateral part or all of the ductus (vas) deferens for male sterilization.

Female Reproductive System (Figure 3-23)

Ovary: The female gonad, located in the pelvic cavity, in which the ova, or germ cells, are formed. There are two ovaries; each is covered with a single layer of epithelium. The ovarian follicle walls secrete estrogen.

Oogonium: A female germ cell that gives rise to an oocyte.

Oocyte: A female germ cell, or gamete, that arises from an oogonium.

Ovum: A mature female gamete.

Graafian follicle: A vesicular follicle of the ovary containing an oocyte.

Oogenesis: The process of cell division, growth, and maturation of the ova.

Ovulation: The expulsion and release of a mature ovum from a follicle in the ovary as a result of cyclic ovarian and pituitary endocrine function, usually about two weeks before the next menstrual period.

Corpus luteum: A yellow-bodied spheroid formed from an ovarian follicle after ovulation. It secretes estrogen, as did the follicle, and also secretes progesterone.

Progesterone: A hormone that maintains the uterine endometrium in the richly vascular state necessary for implantation and pregnancy.

Corpus albicans: A pale white scar tissue on the surface of the ovary that arises from the corpus luteum if conception does not occur.

Broad ligament: The largest peritoneal ligament that supports the uterus. It is also called the ligamentum latum uteri.

Mons pubis: A pad of fatty tissue that overlies the pubic symphysis in females. After puberty, it is covered with pubic hair.

Perineum: External area between the vulva and the anus.

Menstrual cycle: The recurring 28-day cycle of change in the endometrium during which the decidual layer of the endometrium is shed, then regrows and proliferates. The uterine phases of the cycle are the proliferative phase, the secretory phase, and the menstrual phase.

Menarche: The first menstruation in females, which usually occurs between the ages of 9–17.

Fertilization: The union of a secondary oocyte and a sperm cell.

Zygote: A cell produced when an oocyte and sperm fuse.

Cleavage: Early successive division of the zygote into a ball of progressively smaller cells.

Menopause: The cessation of the reproductive cycle. Menstrual cycles stop naturally with the decline of cyclic hormonal production between the ages 35–60.

Fetus: The developing organism in the uterus. In humans, the term is applied after the eighth week of gestation.

Gestation: The period of development of the fetus from the time of fertilization to birth. It is another name for pregnancy.

Umbilical cord: A cordlike structure containing one vein and two arteries that connects the fetus to the placenta.

Ductus venosus: The blood vessel that connects the umbilical vein and the inferior vena cava in a fetus.

Prenatal: Beginning with fertilization and ending at birth.

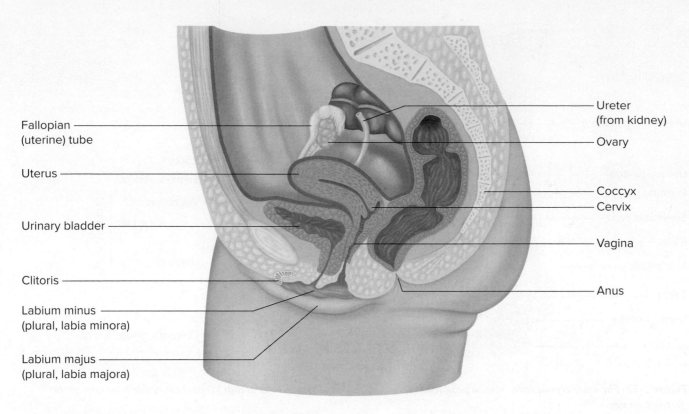

Figure 3-23 *The female reproductive system produces eggs for fertilization and provides the place and means for a fertilized egg to develop.*

Embryonic stage: The stage of development from conception until the eighth week of pregnancy.
Fetal stage: Beginning at the end of the eighth week of development and lasting until birth.
Foramen ovale: An opening in the interatrial septum of the fetal heart.
Homozygous: The presence of identical alleles (variants) of a gene in an individual.

Heterozygous: The presence of two different alleles of a gene in an individual.
Ante partum: Before delivery.
Parturition: The process of giving birth to a child, or delivery.
Neonatal: Pertaining to the first four weeks after birth.
Postnatal: Beginning at birth and ending at death.

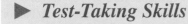

STRATEGIES FOR SUCCESS

▶ *Test-Taking Skills*

Read and understand the directions!
Before you begin, quickly look over the exam and read all the directions carefully. Ask questions if you don't understand all the procedures.

CHAPTER 3 REVIEW

Instructions:

Answer the following questions.

1. The energy that is necessary to keep the body functioning at a minimal level is known as
    A. thermogenesis.
    B. catabolism.
    C. metabolite.
    D. metabolic reaction.
    E. basal metabolism.

2. The portion of the brain that coordinates skeletal muscle activity is the
    A. cerebellum.
    B. pons.
    C. medulla oblongata.
    D. thalamus.
    E. hypothalamus.

3. The part of the eye responsible for peripheral vision is the
    A. iris.
    B. cone.
    C. rod.
    D. aqueous humor.
    E. conjunctiva.

4. The abdomen is divided into how many regions?
    A. three
    B. five
    C. seven
    D. nine
    E. eleven

5. The universal donor blood group is
    A. type A.
    B. type O.
    C. type B.
    D. type AB.
    E. none of these

6. An expandable organ that stores urine is the
    A. urinary bladder.
    B. kidney.
    C. urethra.
    D. ureter.
    E. nephron.

7. Which of the following bones in the neck is U-shaped?
    A. hyoid bone
    B. atlas
    C. axis
    D. coccyx
    E. none of these

8. All of the following are neurotransmitters *except*
    A. histamine.
    B. dopamine.
    C. renin.
    D. serotonin.
    E. norepinephrine.

9. Which of the following terms means "cell eating"?
    A. pinocytosis
    B. phagocytosis
    C. exocytosis
    D. endocytosis
    E. cytokinesis

10. Which of the following is *not* a glandular manner of secretion?
    A. transitional
    B. merocrine
    C. holocrine
    D. apocrine
    E. all of these

CHAPTER 4

PATHOPHYSIOLOGY

LEARNING OUTCOMES

4.1 Recall the terms associated with the mechanisms of disease.

4.2 Describe the body's immune response and the different types of immunity.

4.3 Identify common hereditary and congenital diseases and conditions.

4.4 Recognize and describe the many types of benign and malignant neoplasms.

4.5 Recall infectious diseases that are common to the human body.

4.6 Identify major diseases and disorders of the human body and the body systems affected.

MEDICAL ASSISTING COMPETENCIES

COMPETENCY	CMA	RMA	CCMA	NCMA
General/Legal/Professional				
Provide patients with methods of health promotion and disease prevention	X	X	X	X
Use appropriate medical terminology	X	X	X	X

4.1 Mechanisms of Disease

Pathology: The study of the characteristics, causes, and effects of disease. Also, a condition produced by disease.

Etiology: The study of all factors that cause a disease. Also, the cause of a disease. The causes of disease may be intrinsic (such as age, inheritance, or sex) or extrinsic (such as infectious agents, or behaviors that include inactivity, illegal drug use, or smoking).

Nosocomial: Pertaining to an infection acquired in a hospital or other medical care facility at least 72 hours after admission.

Acute: Characterized by sudden onset and short duration, with marked intensity or sharpness.

Chronic: Developing gradually and persisting for a long period, often for the remainder of a person's lifetime.

Aplastic: Lacking new development, or pertaining to the failure of a tissue to produce normal cell division.

Hypertrophy: An increase in the size of individual cells or an organ, resulting in an enlarged tissue mass. The cells of the heart, kidney, and prostate are particularly prone to hypertrophy.

Ischemia: Inadequate oxygenated blood supply to an organ or tissue, often marked by pain and organ dysfunction.

Infarction: An area of dead cells that results from a lack of oxygen.

Gangrene: An area of necrotic (dead) tissue caused by an invasion of bacteria or loss of blood supply (ischemia). The extremities are most often affected, but it can occur in the intestines or gallbladder.

4.2 Immunology

Immunity: The quality of being resistant to a disease, often because of the presence of antibodies. Immunity can be acquired in a variety of different ways. See Table 4-1.

Immune system: Includes two major components: nonspecific immune mechanisms and specific immune mechanisms.

Antigen: A marker on the surface of a cell that identifies the cell as self or nonself. A nonself (foreign) antigen stimulates an immune response.

Immunodeficiency disorders: Health conditions caused by a deficiency of the immune system in which individuals are more susceptible to infections and chronic diseases. These diseases may be congenital or acquired, or they may result from therapeutic intervention for transplants.

Nonspecific Defense Mechanism

Nonspecific defense mechanism: The body's initial response to any threat, whether it be trauma, organisms, or chemicals. Nonspecific defense mechanisms include mechanical barriers, chemical defenses/barriers, fever, inflammation, and genetic barriers.

Phagocyte: A cell that has the ability to ingest and destroy pathogens such as bacteria and protozoa, as well as cells, cell debris, and dust particles.

Macrophages: The main phagocytic cells of the immune system. They have the ability to recognize and ingest all foreign antigens. These antigens are then destroyed by lysosomes.

AT A GLANCE — Ways of Acquiring Immunity

Active Immunity	Passive Immunity
The body produces its own antibodies. Provides long-term immunity.	Antibodies produced outside the body are introduced into the body. Provides temporary immunity.
Natural Active Immunity	**Natural Passive Immunity**
Results from exposure to disease-causing organism.	Results when antibodies from the mother cross the placenta to the fetus.
Artificial Active Immunity	**Artificial Passive Immunity**
Results from the administration of a vaccine with killed or weakened organisms.	Results from immunization with antibodies to a disease-causing organism.

Table 4-1

Macrophages also serve a vital role in processing antigens and presenting them to T cells, thereby activating a specific immune response. Macrophages are present in the lymph nodes, liver, spleen, lungs, bone marrow, and connective tissue and in the blood as monocytes.

Kupffer cells: The fixed macrophages of the liver.

Neutrophil: A granular leukocyte that is responsible for much of the body's protection against infection. Neutrophils destroy antigens by phagocytosis, and they play a vital role in inflammation and the nonspecific immune response.

Interferons: Antiviral, soluble glycoproteins produced by cells infected with viruses, chlamydiae, rickettsiae, and protozoa (e.g., malaria). They inhibit virus production within the cells and mark infected cells to be destroyed by T cells.

Specific Immune Response

Specific immune mechanisms: Mechanisms required if the nonspecific immune response cannot cope with the invasion or injury to the body. These defenses are directed and controlled by T cells and B cells. They are highly changed after exposure to a pathogen. They can "remember" pathogens such that the next time they invade the body, the specific immune response is quicker and specifically directed at the pathogen.

Cell-mediated immune response: An immune response involving the production of lymphocytes by the thymus (T cells) in response to antigen exposure. This response is important in the rejection of transplants, malignant growths, hypersensitivity, and some infections.

Humoral immune response: An immune response involving the production of plasma lymphocytes (B cells), leading to subsequent antibody formation. This response can produce immunity and hypersensitivity.

Antibody: An immunoglobulin produced by the lymphocytes in response to foreign antigens, such as those on bacteria and viruses.

Autoantibody: An antibody produced in response to a self-antigen. An autoantibody attacks the body's own cells. Autoantibodies are the basis for autoimmune diseases such as rheumatoid arthritis.

Hypersensitivity: An abnormal condition characterized by an exaggerated response of the immune system to an antigen. The four types of hypersensitivity are shown in Table 4-2.

Organs and Tissues of the Immune System

Thymus: The gland located in the mediastinum. It is the site of the maturation and proliferation of the T lymphocytes.

Lymphatic tissue: Tissue containing many lymphocytes that remove foreign matter. Examples include the spleen, tonsils, lymph nodes, thymus, bone marrow, and the lymphoid tissue of the digestive system.

Bone marrow: Soft material that fills the cavity of the bones. Bone marrow is the source of stem cells and lymphocytes, and it is the site where B lymphocytes mature.

4.3 Hereditary and Congenital Diseases and Conditions

Hereditary diseases: Diseases caused by an error in the individual's genetic or chromosomal makeup. These diseases may or may not be apparent at birth. Hereditary diseases require a gene from one or both parents, depending on whether the gene is dominant or recessive.

Congenital anomaly: Any abnormality present at birth, which may be inherited or acquired during gestation. It is also called a birth defect.

Hereditary Diseases and Conditions

Albinism: A genetic condition that results in the lack of melanin pigment in the body, increasing the chance of sunburn and skin cancer.

Classic hemophilia: A hereditary bleeding disorder caused by a deficiency of clotting factors. Hemophilia is an X-linked genetic disorder in males.

Color blindness: The hereditary inability to distinguish between certain colors, generally red and green. Color blindness is more common in males.

Galactosemia: An inherited disorder in which the patient lacks the enzyme that converts galactose to glucose. Galactose accumulates in the blood and interferes with development of the brain, liver, and eyes and can lead to anorexia, vomiting, diarrhea, and even death if it goes untreated.

Phenylketonuria (PKU): A hereditary congenital disease in which the newborn child is unable to oxidize an amino acid because of a defective enzyme. If not treated early, this condition results in brain damage and severe mental retardation.

AT A GLANCE	Types of Hypersensitivity

Type	Example
I	Hay fever, anaphylaxis, asthma, eczema
II	Transfusion reactions, drug reactions, erythroblastosis fetalis, autoimmune disorders, glomerulonephritis
III	Serum sickness
IV	Tuberculin reaction, contact dermatitis, transplant rejection

Table 4-2

Sickle cell anemia: An inherited disorder that primarily affects Africans and African Americans. Red blood cells become crescent-shaped, rigid, sticky, and fragile and cause chronic anemia, tissue hypoxia, weakness, and fatigue.

Tay-Sachs disease: A fatal hereditary congenital disease that primarily affects people of Ashkenazic (Eastern European) Jewish origin. An enzyme deficiency causes abnormal lipid metabolism in the brain, which leads to mental and physical retardation. Individuals affected with Tay-Sachs disease die at a very young age.

Congenital Conditions

Achondroplasia: Defective cartilage formation in the fetus. As a result, the long bones of the arm and legs are short, the trunk of the body is normal in size, and the head is large.

Down syndrome: A congenital condition caused by trisomy 21 (the presence of an extra autosomal chromosome 21). It results in varying degrees of mental retardation and distinctive physical features.

Klinefelter's syndrome: A congenital endocrine condition caused by the presence of an extra X chromosome, in which the individual appears to be male but has small testes and enlarged breasts.

Polydactyly: A congenital anomaly characterized by the presence of extra fingers or toes.

Turner's syndrome: A congenital endocrine disorder caused by the lack of a second X chromosome in females. The individual appears to be female, but the ovaries do not develop.

Ventricular septal defect: The most common congenital cardiac disease, in which a defect in the septum allows blood to be shunted between the left and right ventricles.

Coarctation of the aorta: Narrowing of the aortic arch, which creates increased left ventricular pressure and decreased blood pressure distal to the narrowing. Signs include left ventricular failure with pulmonary edema, dyspnea, and tachycardia.

Patent ductus arteriosus (PDA): A defect in which the ductus arteriosus, a fetal blood vessel, fails to close after birth. This condition often results in heart failure.

Tetralogy of Fallot: The most common cyanotic cardiac defect, of which there are four symptoms: ventricular septal defect, dextroposition of the aorta, pulmonary stenosis, and right ventricular hypertrophy.

Cyanosis: A bluish or grayish discoloration of the skin due to decreased amounts of hemoglobin, which carries oxygen, in the blood.

Cerebral palsy: A motor function disorder caused by a permanent, nonprogressive brain defect or lesion present at birth or shortly thereafter.

Spina bifida: A congenital neural tube defect in which there is incomplete closure of the vertebral column.

Myelomeningocele: A developmental defect of the central nervous system in which a hernial cyst containing meninges and part of the spinal cord protrudes through a congenital cleft in the vertebral column.

Hydrocephalus: A pathologic condition characterized by an abnormal accumulation of cerebrospinal fluid, usually under increased pressure, within the cranial vault, and subsequent dilation of the ventricles.

Muscular dystrophy: A progressive degeneration and weakening of the skeletal muscles.

Duchenne's muscular dystrophy: The form of muscular dystrophy that accounts for 50% of all cases, mostly affects males, and primarily involves the muscles of the shoulders, hips, and thighs. It is an X-linked condition that usually causes death within 10 to 15 years of symptom onset.

Phimosis: A narrowing of the opening of the foreskin.

Congenital pyloric stenosis: A narrowing of the pyloric sphincter at the exit of the stomach. A symptom of this disease is projectile vomiting after feeding that starts at two–three weeks of age.

Hirschsprung's disease: The congenital absence of autonomic ganglia in the smooth muscle wall of the distal part of the colon that causes poor or absent peristalsis, resulting in fecal accumulation and bowel dilation.

4.4 Neoplasia

Neoplasia: The new and abnormal growth of cells, which may be benign or malignant.

Neoplasm: Literally, a new growth, commonly called a tumor.

Hyperplasia: An increase in the number of cells in a body part that results from an increased rate of cellular division that can cause the formation of a tumor.

Malignant: Invasive and capable of metastasis.

Benign: Not recurrent or progressive; nonmalignant.

Metastasis: Development of a tumor away from the site of origin. It occurs when tumor cells spread to distant parts of the body through lymphatic circulation or the bloodstream and implant in lymph nodes or other organs.

Anaplasia: Reversion of cells to an immature (or less differentiated) form, such as that which occurs in malignant tumor cells.

Dysplasia: Alteration in size, shape, and organization of adult cells.

Cancer: A neoplasm characterized by the uncontrolled growth of abnormal cells that invade surrounding tissue and metastasize to distant body sites. As shown in Table 4-3, cancer is second only to heart disease as a cause of mortality in the United States. Possible causes of cancer include smoking; viruses; hormones; radiation; excessive alcohol consumption; genetic predisposition; chemicals used in industry, food, cosmetics, and plastic; and air and water pollution. See Table 4-4 for the most common types of cancer in men, women, and children. See Table 4-5 for the most common types of cancer that result in death for men and women.

AT A GLANCE	Common Causes of Death in the United States
1. Heart disease	
2. Cancer	
3. Chronic lower respiratory disease	
4. Cerebrovascular diseases	

Table 4-3

Men	Women	Children
Prostate	Breast	Leukemia
Lung	Lung	Brain and other nervous system
Colon	Colon	

Table 4-4

AT A GLANCE	Most Common Lethal Cancers	
Male	**Female**
Lung	Lung
Prostate	Breast
Colon and rectum	Colon and rectum
Pancreas	Ovary

Table 4-5

Carcinogen: A substance or agent that causes cancer or increases the incidence of cancer.

Carcinoma: A malignant tumor of the epithelial cells. This neoplasm tends to infiltrate and metastasize through the lymphatic system or the bloodstream. It develops most often in the skin, large intestine, lungs, stomach, prostate, cervix, or breast.

Sarcoma: A malignant neoplasm of the connective tissues, such as bone or muscle. This type of cancer might affect the bones, bladder, kidneys, liver, lungs, or spleen.

Teratoma: A congenital tumor composed of different kinds of tissue, none of which normally occur together or at the site of the tumor. It is most common in the ovaries or testes.

Leukemia: A primary cancer of the bone marrow with proliferating leukocyte precursors. Its cause is generally unknown, but environmental risk factors include exposure to radiation and to certain chemicals.

Lymphoma: A cancer of the lymph nodes and lymphoid tissue that usually responds to treatment. The two main kinds are Hodgkin's disease and non-Hodgkin's lymphoma.

Renal carcinoma: A cancer of the kidneys, also called hypernephroma. Painless hematuria is common with this condition. Metastasis to the lungs, liver, bones, and brain is possible.

Prostate cancer: A slowly progressive adenocarcinoma of the prostate that affects males after the age of 50. It is the second leading cause of cancer death among men in the United States. The cause is unknown, but it is believed to be hormone related.

Bladder cancer: The most common cancer of the urinary tract, it occurs more often in men than in women. The risk of bladder cancer increases with cigarette smoking and exposure to aniline dyes and to materials used in the petroleum, paint, plastics, and timber industries.

Cancer of the mouth: A malignancy that may develop in the gums, in the cheeks, or on the roof of the mouth. In men, it is common to see a cancer of the lower lip, which may be related to pipe smoking.

Colorectal cancer: A malignancy of the large intestine, characterized by a change in bowel habits and the passing of blood. This cancer usually occurs in people older than 50. The risk of colorectal cancer is increased in patients with chronic ulcerative colitis, Crohn's disease, villous adenomas, and familial adenomatous polyposis of the colon.

Colonoscopy: The examination of the mucosal lining of the colon with a colonoscope. This procedure is performed under conscious sedation.

Laryngeal cancer: A cancer of the larynx that occurs most frequently in those 50–70 years of age. Persistent hoarseness or dysphonia are usually the only symptoms.

Lung cancer: A pulmonary malignancy attributable in the majority of cases to cigarette smoking. Other predisposing factors are exposure to arsenic, asbestos, coal products, ionizing radiation, mustard gas, and petroleum. It is the leading cause of cancer death, in both sexes, in the United States. Metastasis is to the brain, bone, and skin.

Cervical cancer: A malignancy of the uterine cervix that can be detected in the early, curable stage by the Papanicolaou (Pap) test. Risk factors include coitus at an early age, relations with many sexual partners, genital herpes virus infections, multiparity, and poor obstetric and gynecological care.

Endometrial cancer: An adenocarcinoma of the endometrium of the uterus. It is the most prevalent malignancy of the female reproductive system, most often occurring in the fifth or sixth decade of life. Some of the risk factors include infertility; anovulation; late menopause; administration of exogenous estrogen; and a combination of diabetes, hypertension, and obesity.

Ovarian carcinoma: A malignant neoplasm of the ovaries rarely detected in the early stage. It occurs commonly in the fifth decade of life. Risk factors include infertility, nulliparity or low parity, delayed childbearing, repeated spontaneous abortion, endometriosis, and group A blood type.

Adenocarcinoma of the vagina: A rare vaginal cancer that begins in the adenomatous cells, and may occur in young women. It has occasionally been linked to use of the hormone diethylstilbestrol (DES) by the mothers of women who develop this cancer.

Breast cancer: The most common cancer in North American women and the leading cause of death in females 35–54 years of age. This adenocarcinoma commonly metastasizes to the lungs, liver, brain, and bone.

Testicular cancer: A malignant neoplastic disease of the testis occurring most frequently in men 20–35 years of age. Patients with early testicular cancer are often asymptomatic, and metastases may be present in lymph nodes, the lungs, and the liver.

Pancreatic cancer: A type of cancer beginning in pancreatic tissues that has a poor prognosis due to its rapid spread; it is usually discovered once it has become quite advanced, and is a leading cause of cancer death.

Oncologist: A physician who specializes in the treatment of patients with cancer.

4.5 Common Infectious Diseases

Influenza: Also known as the flu or grippe, an acute respiratory infection characterized by the sudden onset of fever, chills, headache, and muscle pain or tenderness. Inflammation of the nasal mucous membrane, cough, and sore throat are common. The incubation period is one–three days.

Mumps (parotitis): The inflammation of one or both parotid glands caused by viral infection, with an incubation period of two–three weeks. Complications may include meningoencephalitis, pericarditis, deafness, arthritis, nephritis, and sterility in men.

Chickenpox (varicella): A highly contagious, acute viral infection characterized by spots and an elevated temperature. The incubation period is two–three weeks. Complications may include encephalitis, meningitis, Reye's syndrome, pneumonia, and conjunctival ulcer. The virus may reemerge later as shingles. Chickenpox can be severely damaging to a fetus.

Measles (rubeola): An acute, highly contagious viral disease. The incubation period is 7–14 days. The condition is characterized by spots and a rash. Complications may include otitis media, pneumonia, and encephalitis.

German measles (rubella): Also called three-day measles, a highly communicable viral disease that has an incubation period of 14–21 days. It is characterized by spots. Rubella poses great danger to the fetus.

Meningitis: Any infection or inflammation of the membranes covering the brain and spinal cord. The most common causes for different age groups are summarized in Table 4-6. Aseptic meningitis may be caused by nonbacterial agents such as chemical irritants, viruses, or neoplasms.

Infectious mononucleosis: An acute infectious disease that causes changes in the leukocytes. It is also called glandular fever and the "kissing disease." Mononucleosis is caused by the Epstein-Barr virus and is usually transmitted by direct oral contact. It is rare in those older than 35 years of age.

Epiglottitis: An inflammation of the epiglottis that commonly occurs in children three–seven years of age. The most common cause is *Haemophilus influenzae* type B bacteria.

Genital lesion: A symptom that usually accompanies a sexually transmitted disease such as herpes or syphilis. It is found in the genital region of either males or females.

Botulism: A severe form of food poisoning from botulinus toxins produced by the *Clostridium botulinum* bacterium.

Gastroenteritis: Stomach and intestinal inflammation caused by a food-borne or water-borne virus.

Tetanus: An infection of the central nervous system caused by the tetanus bacillus, *Clostridium tetani*. The symptoms include sudden, extremely painful muscle contractions and stiffness of certain muscles such as the neck and the jaw. It is commonly called lockjaw.

Tapeworm: A species of parasitic worm that can infect the intestines when ingested with uncooked meat containing the larvae.

Ringworm: A fungal infection of the skin characterized by patches of rough, reddened skin; it is more common in males than females. It is caused by the fungi known as *Tinea*.

4.6 Major Diseases and Disorders

Integumentary System

Viral infections of the skin: Infections that include chickenpox and shingles (varicella), measles (rubeola), German measles (rubella), and warts (condyloma acuminata).

AT A GLANCE	Meningitis	
Age Group		**Most Common Infective Causes**
Neonates		*Streptococcus, Escherichia coli*
Infants		*Haemophilus influenzae*
Adults		*Neisseria meningitidis*
Elderly individuals		*Streptococcus pneumoniae*
Overall		*Haemophilus influenzae*

Table 4-6

Bacterial infections of the skin: Infections that include scarlet fever (erysipelas), impetigo (a type of pyoderma), folliculitis (carbuncles), and anthrax (woolsorter's disease).

Fungal infections of the skin: Infections that include ringworm (tinea), dermatophytosis, and dermatomycosis.

Herpes: A group of viruses (*Herpesviridae*) that cause latent or lytic infections, including facial cold sores, genital herpes, chickenpox, shingles, mononucleosis, and others. Species of the herpesvirus include HSV-1, HSV-2, varicella zoster, Epstein-Barr, and cytomegalovirus.

Shingles: A reactivation in adults of the varicella (chickenpox) provirus, *Herpes zoster,* marked by inflammation of segments of the spinal or cranial peripheral nerves and painful eruption along the course of the nerve.

Scarlet fever: A contagious disease characterized by sore throat, strawberry tongue, fever, rash, and rapid pulse.

Wart: An elevation of skin on a rough surface, caused by a local virus. Warts commonly appear on the hands, face, neck, and knees. Genital warts, also known as condyloma accuminata, are contagious. A wart is also referred to as *verruca vulgaris.*

Impetigo: A skin infection beginning as focal erythema, and progressing to pruritic vesicles, erosions, and honey-colored crusts. It is caused by *Staphylococcus aureus, Streptococcus pyogenes,* or both.

Carbuncle: A large site of staphylococcal infection containing purulent matter in deep, interconnecting subcutaneous pockets.

Seborrheic dermatitis: A skin disease that is most commonly found on the scalp of infants and is referred to as "cradle cap."

Tinea corporis: A superficial fungal infection of the nonhairy skin of the body, usually caused by species of *Trichophyton* or *Microsporum.*

Tinea capitis: A superficial fungal infection of the scalp, most common in children, usually caused by species of *Trichophyton.*

Tinea cruris: A superficial fungal infection of the groin caused by species of *Trichophyton* or *Epidermophyton.* Also called *jock itch.*

Tinea pedis: A chronic superficial fungal infection of the foot, usually caused by *Trichophyton* or *Epidermophyton.* Also called *athlete's foot.*

Dermatophytosis: A fungal infection of the skin of the hands and feet, especially between the toes.

Dermatomycosis: A skin infection caused by certain fungi.

Acne: An inflammatory disease of the sebaceous glands and hair follicles of the skin.

Eczema: Acute or chronic inflammation of the skin.

Psoriasis: A chronic skin disorder characterized by circumscribed red patches, covered by thick, dry silvery adherent scales.

Vitiligo: A skin condition characterized by patches that lack pigmentation surrounded by normally pigmented skin.

Wheal: A small, swollen skin lesion that usually occurs from an insect bite, or reaction to a medication or allergen; also known as a "welt."

Musculoskeletal System

Atrophy: A decrease in the size of cells, resulting in reduced tissue mass. A skeletal muscle may undergo atrophy as a result of lack of physical exercise or neurological disease.

Crepitation: A grating sound made by movement of some joints or broken bones.

Exostosis: A projection arising from a bone that develops from cartilage.

Myalgia: Muscle pain.

Herniated disk: A protrusion of a degenerated or fragmented intervertebral disk that causes compression of the nerve root.

Arthritis: Inflammation of the joints characterized by swelling, redness, warmth, pain, and limited movement.

Osteoarthritis: The most common form of arthritis, affecting the weight-bearing joints.

Rheumatoid arthritis: The most crippling form of arthritis, characterized by chronic systemic inflammation of joints and synovial membranes.

Gout: A hereditary metabolic form of acute arthritis.

Tendinitis or **tendonitis:** Inflammation of a tendon.

Scoliosis: Abnormal sideways curvature of the spine.

Kyphosis: Abnormal outward curvature of the spine. This condition is also known as a humpback.

Lordosis: Abnormal inward curvature of the spine, known as swayback.

Fracture: A break or crack in a bone. Table 4-7 lists the types of fractures. See Figure 4-1.

Fibromyalgia: A fairly common condition that results in chronic pain, primarily in joints, muscles, and tendons.

Myasthenia gravis: A condition in which affected persons experience muscle weakness.

Arthroplasty: The surgical reconstruction or replacement of a painful, degenerated joint (caused by osteoarthritis), to restore mobility.

Arthrostomy: Establishment of a temporary opening into a joint cavity.

Bursitis: Inflammation of a bursa (a fluid-filled sac that cushions tendons). It occurs most commonly in the elbow, knee, shoulder, and hip.

Carpal tunnel syndrome: A condition that occurs when the median nerve in the wrist is excessively compressed.

Osteogenesis imperfecta: A disease characterized by decreased amounts of collagen in the bones, leading to very fragile bones. This disease is more commonly called brittle-bone disease.

Osteoporosis: A condition in which bones become thinned over time.

Paget's disease: A disease that causes bones to enlarge and become deformed and weak.

Nervous System

Dysphasia: Difficulty in speaking.

Delirium: A state of mental confusion due to disturbances in mental function.

Dementia: A progressive organic mental disorder characterized by chronic personality, disintegration, confusion, disorientation, and deterioration of intellectual capacity and function.

Encephalitis: Inflammation of the brain, commonly caused by a viral infection. Secondary encephalitis may develop from viral childhood diseases such as measles, mumps, or chickenpox.

Sleeping sickness: A type of encephalitis characterized by lethargy, oculomotor paralysis, delirium, stupor, coma, and reversal of sleep rhythm.

AT A GLANCE Types of Fractures

Fracture	Description
Closed (simple)	Ends of fractured bone do not break through skin.
Open (compound)	Ends of fractured bone break through skin.
Complete	Bone is completely broken into two or more pieces.
Incomplete	Bone is partially broken.
Greenstick	Bone is bent on one side and has an incomplete fracture on the opposite side. This type of fracture is very common in children.
Hairline	Bone has fine cracks but bone sections remain in place.
Comminuted	Bone is broken into three or more pieces.
Displaced	Ends of fractured bone move out of the normal position.
Nondisplaced	Ends of fractured bone stay in the normal position.
Impacted	Piece of broken bone is forced into a space of another bone fragment.
Depressed	Fractured bone forms a concavity; mostly seen in skull fractures.
Linear	Fracture is parallel to the long axis of the bone.
Transverse	Fracture is perpendicular to the long axis of the bone.
Oblique	Fracture runs diagonally across the bone.
Spiral	Fracture spirals around long axis of bone, usually the result of twisting a bone.
Colles	Fracture is at the distal end of radius and ulna.
Pott	Fracture is at the distal end of tibia or fibula.

Table 4-7

Rabies: An infectious, acute, fatal disease of the brain and spinal cord caused by an RNA virus that is transmitted by the saliva of an infected animal, often through a bite. The incubation period is long, 40–60 days or more. Rabies is also called hydrophobia (fear of water).

Multiple sclerosis (MS): A chronic, progressive inflammatory disease of unknown origin that usually affects young adults between the ages 20–40. Symptoms include changes in vision and muscle weakness. It is difficult to diagnose and has no specific treatment.

Amyotrophic lateral sclerosis (ALS): Also known as Lou Gehrig's disease, a chronic, terminal neurological disease that causes progressive muscular atrophy. The cause is unknown. It occurs most commonly in people in their 50s and 60s, and it is slightly more common in males than in females.

Alzheimer's disease: Diffuse cortical atrophy of the brain characterized by confusion, memory failure, disorientation, and hallucination. The most common form occurs in people older than 65.

Parkinson's disease: A brain degeneration that appears gradually and progresses slowly. It is also known as shaking palsy. Signs of Parkinson's disease include slowness of movement, resting tremor, and rigidity. The degeneration occurs in the basal ganglia. There is dopamine depletion.

Cerebral hemorrhage: Hemorrhage in epidural, subdural, or subarachnoid spaces in the meninges. The major cause of this condition is hypertension.

Concussion: An immediate loss of consciousness caused by a violent blow to the head or neck. It may last from a few seconds to several minutes.

Contusion: Bruising of the brain, a more serious head injury than a concussion. Permanent damage to the brain may result. It is commonly associated with skull fracture.

Diplegia: Paralysis of both sides of any body part or of the same parts on the opposite sides of the body.

Monoplegia: Paralysis of only one extremity.

Paraplegia: Paralysis of motor or sensory abilities of the lower trunk and lower extremities. The individual may lose bowel and bladder control, and sexual dysfunction is common.

Quadriplegia: Paralysis of the lower and upper extremities (the arms, legs, and trunk) that results from injury to the spinal cord at the fifth, sixth, or seventh cervical vertebra. A major cause of death is respiratory failure. It is also known as *tetraplegia*.

Hemiplegia: Paralysis on one side of the body.

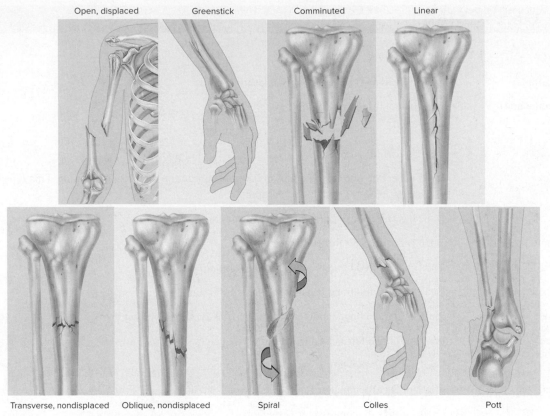

| Open, displaced | Greenstick | Comminuted | Linear |

| Transverse, nondisplaced | Oblique, nondisplaced | Spiral | Colles | Pott |

Figure 4-1 *Some types of bone fractures.*

Epilepsy: A chronic brain disorder associated with abnormal and sudden discharge of electrical activity in the brain, which results in seizures. There are two major types of seizures: partial seizures and generalized. A simple partial seizure was originally called Jacksonian epilepsy. Generalized seizures include absence (petit mal) and tonic–clonic (grand mal).

Bell's palsy: A paralysis of the facial nerve that results from trauma to the nerve, compression of the nerve by a tumor, or an unknown infection. It commonly occurs 20–60 years of age. It is usually self-limiting (temporary paralysis).

Trigeminal neuralgia: Also called tic douloureux, a condition that involves pain in the fifth cranial nerve. Paroxysmal episodes of the pain may last for hours.

Migraine: A type of periodic headache, which may or may not be accompanied by aura or neurological dysfunction. Pain is usually confined to one side, but it can be bilateral.

Cardiovascular System

Arteriosclerosis: A disease of the arterial vessels characterized by thickening, hardening, and loss of elasticity in the arteries. This is due to yellowish plaques of cholesterol, or other lipids, and various cellular debris, in the arterial walls.

Atherosclerosis: The most common form of arteriosclerosis, marked by cholesterol, lipid, and calcium deposits in arterial linings.

Angina pectoris: A paroxysmal chest pain caused by a temporary oxygen insufficiency as a result of atherosclerosis, spasms of the coronary arteries, or thrombosis.

Myocardial infarction: Necrosis of a portion of cardiac muscle caused by an obstruction in a coronary artery, resulting from atherosclerosis, a thrombus (heart attack), or a spasm.

Congestive heart failure: A slowly developing condition in which the heart weakens over time. In time, the heart is no longer able to pump enough blood to meet the body's needs.

Coronary thrombosis: A blood clot in a coronary artery, the most common cause of myocardial infarction.

Myocarditis: Inflammation of the myocardium. It is commonly caused by viruses, bacteria, fungi, or protozoa.

Endocarditis: Inflammation of the inner lining and valves of the heart due to an invasion of microorganisms or an abnormal immunological reaction. There are several types of endocarditis.

Acute endocarditis: Inflammation of the lining and valves of the heart caused by *Staphylococcus aureus* and group A beta-hemolytic streptococci.

Subacute endocarditis: Inflammation of the lining and valves of the heart commonly caused by *Escherichia coli* or *Streptococcus viridans*.

Pericarditis: Inflammation of the pericardium. It may be caused by myocardial infarction, viral uremia, bacteria, fungi, parasites, or rheumatic fever. There are three types: fibrinous, serous, and suppurative.

Rheumatic fever: A systemic, inflammatory autoimmune disease involving the heart and the joints. There are two types: acute rheumatic fever and rheumatic heart disease.

Acute rheumatic fever: Rheumatic fever caused by beta-hemolytic streptococci and characterized by polyarthritis, erythema, subcutaneous nodules, chorea, and carditis. It is more common in children.

Rheumatic heart disease: A disease that causes stenosis or insufficiency of the mitral valve.

Cardiac tamponade: Accumulation of fluid, such as blood, in the pericardial sac.

Cardiogenic shock: Shock resulting from extensive myocardial infarction.

Aneurysm: A dilation or saclike formation in a weakened blood vessel wall. A common cause is atherosclerotic plaque. Other causative agents include trauma, inflammation or infection, and congenital factors.

Abdominal aortic aneurysm: The most common form of aneurysm.

Thrombophlebitis: Also called phlebitis, the inflammation of a vein, often accompanied by the formation of a clot. It occurs most commonly in the lower legs.

Varicose vein: An enlarged, twisted superficial vein, usually in the lower leg, caused by incompetent valves. It is very common, especially in women.

Buerger's disease (thromboangiitis obliterans): An occlusion and inflammation of the peripheral vascular circulation, usually in the leg or foot. The primary cause is a long history of smoking tobacco.

Raynaud's disease: Episodic vasospasm of the small cutaneous arteries, usually occurring in the fingers. It is often aggravated by cold temperatures.

Iron-deficiency anemia: The most common type of anemia. It results from greater demand on stored iron than can be supplied. RBC count may be normal, but there is insufficient hemoglobin.

Pernicious anemia: Chronic anemia caused by decreased hydrochloric acid in the stomach, lack of intrinsic factor, and a vitamin B_{12} deficiency. It can also be caused by regional enteritis (Crohn's disease).

Aplastic anemia: A congenital form of anemia, also called Fanconi syndrome. The bone marrow stops producing erythrocytes, leukocytes, and platelets. It is caused by exposure to excessive radiation, certain drugs, and industrial toxins.

Sickle cell anemia: A condition in which abnormal hemoglobin causes RBCs to change to a sickle (crescent) shape. These sickle-shaped red blood cells get stuck in capillaries.

Polycythemia: An increase in the number of circulating erythrocytes and the amount of hemoglobin. There are three types: polycythemia vera, secondary polycythemia, and relative polycythemia. Complications may include thrombosis, cerebrovascular accident, peptic ulcers, leukemia, and hemorrhage.

Agranulocytosis: Also called neutropenia, a condition in which the number of leukocytes is very low.

Lymphedema: An abnormal collection of lymph, commonly in the extremities. Congenital lymphedema is known as Milroy's disease.

Lyme disease: A tick-borne disease characterized by skin lesions, malaise, fatigue, arthritis, carditis, encephalitis, meningitis, loss of memory, numbness, and facial palsy. The incubation period is 3–33 days after a tick bite.

Hemolysis: The destruction of red blood cells.

Toxoplasmosis: A systemic protozoan disease that results in fever, lymphadenopathy, lymphocytosis, pneumonia, rashes, myocarditis, and death. The primary infection may be asymptomatic.

Respiratory System

Common cold: A viral infection of the upper respiratory tract, signified by runny nose, sore throat, cough, watery eyes, sneezing, and congestion. It is caused by more than 100 different viruses, and usually resolves within one–two weeks.

Pharyngitis: Inflammation of the pharynx most often caused by a viral infection.

Epiglottitis: An acute infection usually caused by the bacterial organism *Haemophilus influenzae* type B. It is common in children between the ages of three–seven years.

Anosmia: The loss or impairment of the sense of smell. Nasal polyps and allergic rhinitis are the most common cause.

Rhinitis: Inflammation of the nasal mucosa, causing nasal congestion, sneezing, and itching of the nose.

Allergic rhinitis: Hay fever.

Bronchitis: Inflammation of the lining of the bronchial tubes, which may be either acute or chronic. It often develops from a cold or other respiratory infection, may be linked to smoking, and is a potential component of COPD.

Bronchiectasis: Chronic dilation and distention of the bronchial walls. It is irreversible. Complications are lung abscess, pneumonia, and empyema.

Atelectasis: A collapsed or airless state of the lung that results in hypoxia. Dyspnea may be the only symptom.

Pneumonia: Inflammation of the lungs caused by viral or bacterial infection. Bacterial pneumonia is commonly caused by pneumococci, staphylococci, *Klebsiella pneumoniae,* or group A hemolytic streptococci. *Streptococcus pneumoniae* is the most common cause in all age groups. It is the fifth leading cause of death in the United States.

Chronic obstructive pulmonary disease (COPD): A group of common chronic respiratory disorders that are characterized by progressive tissue loss and obstruction in the airways of the lungs. It includes emphysema and chronic bronchitis.

Emphysema: A chronic pulmonary disease characterized by an abnormal increase in the size of air spaces distal to the terminal bronchiole, with destructive changes in their walls. Patients have increased levels of carbon dioxide and decreased levels of oxygen.

Asthma: A respiratory disorder characterized by recurring episodes of paroxysmal dyspnea, wheezing on expiration and inspiration caused by constriction of the bronchi, coughing, and viscous mucoid bronchial secretions. The episodes may occur as a result of inhalation of allergens or pollutants, infection, cold air, vigorous exercise, or emotional stress.

Cystic fibrosis: An inherited autosomal-recessive disorder of the exocrine glands, which causes the production of abnormally thick secretions of mucus, the elevation of sweat electrolytes, and an increase in the enzymes of saliva. The glands most affected are those in the pancreas and respiratory system and the sweat glands.

Hemoptysis: Coughing and spitting up of blood from the respiratory tract. In true hemoptysis, the sputum is bright red and frothy with air bubbles.

Legionnaires' disease: A type of pneumonia caused by *Legionella pneumophila.* Predisposing factors include smoking, alcoholism, and physical debilitation.

Histoplasmosis: A type of pneumonia that may become a systemic disease. It is caused by inhalation of dust containing spores of *Histoplasma capsulatum,* a fungus commonly found in the Mississippi and Ohio River valleys. It is also called Darling's disease, and it clinically resembles tuberculosis.

Anthracosis: A lung disease caused by inhalation of coal dust. It is also called coal-miner's lung or black lung.

Asbestosis: A form of pneumoconiosis caused by exposure to asbestos. It is the most common type of dust disease.

Silicosis: Long-term inhalation of the dust of an inorganic compound, silicon dioxide, which is found in sands, quartzes, and flints. It is also called grinder's disease.

Pleurisy: Inflammation of the pleural membranes.

Pneumothorax: Entrance of air or gas into the pleural space, resulting in a collapsed lung.

Hemothorax: Blood in the pleural cavity caused by trauma to or erosion of a pulmonary vessel. It can also cause the lung to collapse.

Pulmonary edema: A condition wherein fluid collects in the alveoli and interstitial area. This accumulation of fluid reduces the amount of oxygen diffusing into the blood and interferes with lung expansion.

Pulmonary embolus: A blood clot or a mass of other material that obstructs the pulmonary artery or one of its branches. This blocks the flow of blood through the lung tissue.

Flail chest: A loss of stability in the chest wall, due to a multiple fracture of each affected rib, that produces a characteristic movement pattern during respiration.

Diphtheria: A potentially fatal childhood disease, caused by *Corynebacterium diphtheriae,* that begins with a sore throat and affects the mucous membranes of the respiratory tract. Complications may include myocarditis, heart failure, pneumonia, otitis media, and pulmonary emboli.

Tuberculosis: An infectious disease caused by *Mycobacterium tuberculosis.* Tuberculosis is transmitted through inhalation of airborne droplets, prolonged direct contact with infected individuals, consumption of contaminated milk, or contact with infected cattle.

Whooping cough: Also called pertussis, an infectious disease caused by *Bordetella pertussis,* a gram-negative, encapsulated coccobacillus. It produces both an endotoxin and an exotoxin.

Aspiration: The passage of food or fluid, vomitus, drugs, or other foreign materials into the trachea and lungs.

Digestive System

Gingivitis: Inflammation and swelling of the gums, often the result of poor oral hygiene.

Oral leukoplakia: A precancerous disease that results in the thickening and hardening of a part of the mucous membranes in the mouth. It is more common in elderly individuals.

Esophagitis: Inflammation of the mucosal lining of the esophagus. Its most common cause is a backflow of gastric juice from the stomach.

Gastroesophageal reflux disease (GERD): A condition characterized by the return of stomach contents into the esophagus, causing a burning sensation or heartburn.

Gastritis: Inflammation of the lining of the stomach, caused by aspirin; excessive coffee, tobacco, or alcohol intake; or an infection. It can be acute or chronic.

Peptic ulcers: Ulcers of the stomach or duodenum. They are also called gastric ulcers, and they may be acute or chronic. *Helicobacter pylori* is a bacterium that may cause peptic ulcers.

Regional enteritis (Crohn's disease): A condition of the intestinal tract characterized by patches of inflammation, and even ulceration. This condition most typically occurs in the ileum portion.

Ulcerative colitis: A chronic, inflammatory and ulcerative disease arising in the clonic mucosa and rectum. It typically begins at the anorectal junction and extends proximally. Complications can include perforation of the bowel, septicemia, and death. There is a high risk of a colon malignancy.

Intussusception: The prolapse of one segment of the intestine into the lumen of another segment, causing intestinal obstruction. The cause is usually unknown. It is one of the most common causes of intestinal obstruction in infants.

Volvulus: The torsion of a loop of intestine, causing intestinal obstruction with or without strangulation. It occurs most often in the ileum, the cecum, or the sigmoid colon in infants and some elderly adults.

Diverticula: Abnormal pockets in the gastrointestinal tract.

Diverticulosis: The presence of diverticula in the colon. There is no inflammation.

Diverticulitis: Inflammation and perforation of diverticula. Chronic diverticulitis can cause complications such as abscesses, fistulas, and adhesions.

Enteritis: Inflammation of the intestine, particularly the small intestine.

Food poisoning: An illness that results from the ingestion of foods containing poisonous substances. Symptoms of poisoning include nausea, cramping, vomiting, and diarrhea.

Enteric fevers: Systemic infections caused by pathogens that enter the gastrointestinal tract and are absorbed through the intestinal mucosa into the bloodstream. Examples of causative pathogens include *Escherichia coli, Vibrio cholerae,* some *Salmonella,* and some *Shigella.*

Giardiasis: Also called traveler's diarrhea, an infection of the small intestine caused by *Giardia lamblia,* a flagellate protozoon that produces cysts. The source of infection is usually untreated contaminated water.

Appendicitis: Inflammation of the appendix.

Hepatitis: Infectious inflammation of the liver most commonly caused by either the type A or type B hepatitis virus.

Hernia: Protrusion of a part from its normal location. See Table 4-8 for types of hernia.

Hematemesis: Vomiting of bright red blood, indicating rapid upper GI bleeding.

AT A GLANCE | Types of Hernia

Type	Description
Hiatal	A part of the stomach protruding upward through the diaphragm
Incarcerated	A hernia that is swollen and fixed within a sac, creating an obstruction
Inguinal	A loop of the intestine protruding through the abdominal wall in the inguinal region
Strangulated	A hernia that is so constricted (cut off from circulation) that it may become gangrenous
Umbilical	A part of the intestine protruding through the abdominal wall around the umbilicus

Table 4-8

Endocrine System

Hypoglycemia: Low blood sugar.

Hyperglycemia: High blood sugar.

Ketosis: The accumulation of ketone bodies in the blood and urine as a result of abnormal utilization of carbohydrates.

Gigantism: Excessive size and stature of the body, usually caused by the hypersecretion of growth hormone. It is usually the result of a tumor (adenoma) of the anterior pituitary and generally occurs before puberty.

Acromegaly: A disease caused by an excess of growth hormone in an adult. The bones of the hands, feet, and face can be enlarged. It is generally due to a tumor.

Dwarfism: A growth hormone deficiency that results in the abnormal underdevelopment of the body, or hypopituitarism, mainly in children. It causes extreme shortness of stature.

Hyperthyroidism: Hypersecretion of the thyroid gland that results in protrusion of the eyeballs, tachycardia, goiter, and tumor.

Hypothyroidism: Hyposecretion of the thyroid gland that results in sluggishness, slow pulse, and obesity.

Goiter: An enlargement of the thyroid gland, possibly due to a lack of iodine in the diet, thyroiditis, inflammation from infection, tumors, or hyperfunction or hypofunction of the thyroid gland.

Graves' disease: A condition of severe hyperthyroidism, possibly with an autoimmune base. A sudden exacerbation of symptoms may signal thyrotoxicosis.

Thyrotoxicosis: A toxic condition caused by hyperactivity of the thyroid gland and characterized by rapid heartbeat, tremors, nervous symptoms, and weight loss.

Hashimoto's disease: An inflammatory autoimmune disease that attacks the thyroid gland. It is more common in women and is the leading cause of nonsimple goiter and hypothyroidism.

Myxedema: The acquired form of severe hypothyroidism. It is more common in females and occurs in adulthood.

Cretinism: A congenital condition characterized by severe hypothyroidism and often associated with other endocrine abnormalities.

Cushing's syndrome: Hyperactivity of the adrenal cortical gland that develops from an excess of the glucocorticoid hormone. The individual experiences fatigue, weakness, fat deposits in the scapular area (buffalo humps), protruding abdomen, hypertension, edema, and hyperlipidemia.

Addison's disease: A life-threatening condition resulting from chronic hypoadrenalism. Symptoms include weakness, nausea, abdominal discomfort, anorexia, and weight loss, among many others.

Diabetes insipidus: A metabolic disorder caused by injury to the neurohypophyseal system. The disease results from antidiuretic hormone deficiency.

Diabetes mellitus: A chronic disorder of carbohydrate, fat, and protein metabolism resulting from inadequate production of insulin by the pancreas. This disorder results in hyperglycemia, which is characterized by polyurea, thirst, and polyphagia. Type 1 is insulin-dependent, and Type 2 is generally not insulin-dependent.

Gestational diabetes: A type of diabetes that occurs during pregnancy and often resolves after the birth of the baby.

Hyperinsulinism: A condition resulting from excessive insulin in the blood, causing hypoglycemia, fainting, and convulsions.

Sensory System
The Eye

Myopia: A severe form of nearsightedness that results when light rays entering the eye focus in front of the retina. Myopia occurs when the eyeball is abnormally long.

Hyperopia: A severe form of farsightedness that occurs when light rays entering the eye focus behind the retina. The eyeball is abnormally short.

Presbyopia: The inability to focus with the lens because of loss of its elasticity. It commonly develops with advancing age, usually beginning in the mid 40s.

Nystagmus: A constant involuntary, rhythmic movement of one or both eyes. Brain tumors or cerebrovascular lesions may cause nystagmus.

Astigmatism: An irregular focusing of the light rays entering the eye. The cornea is not spherical, and vision is typically blurred.

Strabismus: A disorder in which the visual axes of the eyes are not directed at the same point. Hence, the eyes are crossed. The main symptom is diplopia.

Conjunctivitis: Inflammation of the conjunctiva caused by bacterial or viral infection, allergy, or environmental factors. Red eyes, thick discharge, and sticky eyelids in the morning are the most common signs and symptoms.

Hordeolum: Also called stye, an infection of the hair follicles of the eyelids.

Cataract: A clouding of a normally clear lens of the eye. The most common cause is aging.

Glaucoma: One of the most common and severe ocular diseases, characterized by increased intraocular pressure, which can result in damage to the optic nerve. It is more common in people 60 and older.

Retinal detachment: An elevation of the retina from the choroid. Extremely nearsighted people are more susceptible to retinal detachments.

Uveitis: Inflammation of the uveal tract, including the iris, ciliary body, and choroid.

The Ear

Otalgia: Earache.

External otitis: Also known as swimmer's ear, an infection of the ear canal, commonly caused by *Escherichia coli, Pseudomonas aeruginosa, Proteus vulgaris, Staphylococcus aureus,* or *Aspergillus* (a genus of fungi).

Otitis media: An infection of the middle ear. It is most common in children younger than eight.

Tympanitis: Inflammation of the eardrum.

Conductive hearing loss: Loss of hearing caused by an interruption in the transmission of sound waves to the inner ear.

Sensorineural hearing loss: Hearing loss caused by damage to the inner ear, to the nerve from the ear to the brain, or to the brain itself, so that the brain does not perceive sound waves as sound.

Anacusis: Total hearing loss.

Tinnitus: Ringing or buzzing in the ear.

Vertigo: Dizziness.

Rinne tuning-fork testing: A method of distinguishing conductive from sensorineural hearing loss. The base of a vibrating tuning fork is placed against the patient's mastoid bone.

Audiometry: The testing of the sensitivity of the sense of hearing, using a variety of tests.

Urinary System

Dysuria: Painful urination.

Enuresis: Involuntary discharge of urine, most often due to a lack of bladder control.

Incontinence: Involuntary discharge of urine, feces, or semen.

Urethritis: Inflammation of the urethra.

Cystitis: Inflammation of the urinary bladder. It is more common in women.

Urinary tract infection (UTI): Bacteria or other organisms in the urethra and bladder, causing dysuria and malaise.

Renal failure: In acute cases a sudden and severe reduction in renal function. Causes include complications from surgery, shock after an incompatible blood transfusion, severe dehydration, and trauma or kidney disease. Renal failure results in uremia, and increases blood urea nitrogen (BUN).

Uremia: Excess of urea and other waste in the blood as a result of kidney failure.

Glomerulonephritis: Inflammation of the glomerulus in the kidney. There are three types: acute, chronic, and subacute. It results in uremia.

Acute glomerulonephritis: A common disease, primarily affecting children and young adults, marked by protein and blood in the urine and edema with no pus formation. It is a type of allergic disease caused by an antigen-antibody reaction.

Chronic glomerulonephritis: A slowly progressive, noninfectious disease that may result in irreversible renal damage and renal failure. Uremia is common with this condition.

Nephrotic syndrome: Referred to as the protein-losing kidney, a condition characterized by protein in the urine, hypoalbuminemia, hypertension, and hyperlipidemia.

Pyelonephritis: A diffuse pyogenic infection of the renal pelvis. It is the most common type of renal disease, and it may be acute or chronic. It is commonly caused by infection, calculi, pregnancy, tumors, or benign prostatic hypertrophy.

Hydronephrosis: Distention of the pelvis and calyces of the kidney by urine that cannot flow past an obstruction in the ureter. The obstruction may be a result of urinary calculi, a tumor, an enlarged prostate gland, or pregnancy.

Polycystic renal disease: A congenital anomaly that affects children and adults and results in kidney failure due to the presence of multiple cysts in the kidney tubules.

Renal calculus: A deposit that can block urine flow in the ureter, resulting in renal colic with chills, fever, hematuria, and a frequent need to urinate. If the stones don't pass and they continue to block urine flow, surgery must be performed, or the stones can be destroyed with ultrasound.

Prostate cancer: The second most common cancer in men. It is referred to as a "silent killer" because it lacks symptoms until the disease is late in its progression. Males age 50 or older should have annual prostate examinations.

Micturition: Urination.

Reproductive System

Gonorrhea: A contagious inflammation of the genital mucous membrane of both sexes caused by the gram-negative gonococcus bacterium. It may also affect other parts of the body, including the heart, rectum, and joints, and in women it may cause pelvic inflammatory disease.

Genital warts: An infection caused by any of a group of human papillomaviruses (HPVs). In women, genital warts may be associated with cancer of the cervix.

Chlamydial infection: The most prevalent sexually transmitted disease in the United States. It is a leading cause of pelvic inflammatory disease in women. Chlamydia is caused by the *Chlamydia trachomatis* bacterium, and it is sometimes called the silent STD because the symptoms may be very mild. Chlamydia left untreated can lead to infertility and sterility.

Syphilis: One of the most serious sexually transmitted diseases. The causative organism is a spirochete, *Treponema* *pallidum*. Infection in pregnant women can cause congenital defects in the fetus (such as mental retardation, physical deformities, deafness, and blindness), the death of the fetus, and spontaneous abortion.

Genital herpes: A very painful, recurring, incurable viral disease that involves the mucous membranes of the genital tracts. During pregnancy, it can cause spontaneous abortion and premature delivery, and it can be transmitted to the newborn. It can also develop into cervical cancer and spread to the lungs, brain, liver, and spleen.

HIV: The human immunodeficiency virus, which is transferable by direct sexual contact (homosexual or heterosexual), by contaminated intravenous needles and syringes, and by blood transfusion with contaminated blood or other blood products. It is also transplacental and can be transferred from mother to child. As the disease progresses, there is a steady drop in the number of T cells in the blood. Diagnosis is determined by the detection of HIV antibodies in the blood. HIV/AIDS is actually classified as both a reproductive disorder and an immune disorder.

AIDS: Acquired immunodeficiency syndrome, the ultimate result of infection with HIV. It is currently a fatal disease of the immune system. AIDS is marked by opportunistic infections that would otherwise be eliminated by a healthy individual's immune responses. These infections include candidiasis, herpes, Kaposi's sarcoma, recurrent pneumonia, and lymphoma. The typical course of HIV is defined by three phases: primary infection phase, usually lasting between a few days and two weeks; chronic asymptomatic or latency phase, lasting an average of 10 years; and overt AIDS phase, which can lead to death (without antiretroviral therapy) within two–three years.

Female Reproductive System

Pelvic inflammatory disease: Inflammation and serious infection of organs in the pelvic cavity, including the fallopian tubes, ovaries, and endometrium. The infection can occur after miscarriage, childbirth, or abortion, but it is most common in young nulliparous females and is not necessarily related to a pregnancy.

Vaginitis: An inflammation and/or infection of the vaginal tissues. It is common in all age groups and is characterized by various discharges, depending on the causative agent, from clear and odorless to copious, greenish yellow, and foul smelling.

Toxic shock syndrome: An acute, systemic infection with exotoxin-producing strains of *Staphylococcus aureus*. The syndrome has been associated with menstruating females who use tampons.

Menopause: The cessation of menstrual periods. Many women experience the onset of menopause between the ages of 45 and 55. Hot flashes and night sweats often are reported.

Cervical cancer: A malignancy of the uterine cervix. The biggest risk factor for development of invasive cervical carcinoma is lack of regular cervical Pap smear screening. The other major risk factor is exposure to oncogenic types of HPV, such as 16, 18, 31, and 45. Women should be encouraged to have regular cervical Pap smear screening.

Ovarian cancer: A malignancy that accounts for more deaths than any other gynecological malignancy. Most ovarian cancers occur in women between the ages 40–65.

Endometrial cancer: A malignancy of the lining of the uterus, which undergoes cyclic changes as a result of hormonal stimulation. It is the most common gynecological cancer in women over age 45.

Hydatidiform moles: Tumors of the uterine lining, most of which are benign, that develop after pregnancy or in association with an abnormal pregnancy. These tumors consist of multiple cysts that resemble a bunch of grapes.

Fibroadenoma: The most common benign tumor of the breast. It is a single, movable nodule that occurs at any age. It is painful at the time of the menstrual period.

Amenorrhea: The absence of the onset of menstruation at puberty or the cessation or interruption of menstruation in adulthood.

Menorrhagia: Excessive uterine bleeding that occurs between menstrual periods. Its causes include uterine tumors, pelvic inflammatory disease, and abnormal conditions of pregnancy.

Metrorrhagia: Uterine bleeding at any time other than during menstruation.

Endometriosis: Proliferation of endometrial tissue outside of the uterus. Endometriosis may cause dysmenorrhea, sterility, and dyspareunia.

Ectopic pregnancy: Implantation of the fertilized ovum outside of the uterus, most commonly in the fallopian tubes, rather than on the inside wall of the uterus. It is also called extrauterine pregnancy.

Miscarriage: A spontaneous abortion, commonly as a result of a genetic abnormality.

Preeclampsia: A pathological condition of late pregnancy characterized by edema, protein in the urine, and hypertension. It is also known as the first phase of the toxemia of pregnancy.

Eclampsia: Toxemia of pregnancy resulting in convulsions and coma. It is a potentially life-threatening disorder characterized by severe hypertension, edema, and protein in the urine.

Placenta previa: Implantation of the placenta in the lower uterine segment on the internal cervical os, which causes painless bleeding.

Abruptio placentae: Premature separation of the placenta from the uterine wall too early in a pregnancy of 20 weeks or more, or during labor before delivery of the fetus. Bleeding from the site of separation causes abdominal pain, uterine tenderness, and tetanic uterine contraction. Bleeding may be concealed within the uterus, sometimes as sudden massive hemorrhage.

Male Reproductive System

Orchitis: Infection of the testis caused by viral or bacterial infection or injury. It may affect one or both testes, causing swelling, tenderness, and acute pain.

Prostatitis: Acute or chronic inflammation of the prostate gland. It is more common in men older than 50. The cause of inflammation of the prostate is usually infection but is not always known.

Impotence: Failure to initiate or maintain an erection until ejaculation.

Benign prostatic hyperplasia: Enlargement of the prostate gland. It is common in men over the age of 50. This condition usually progresses to the point of causing compression of the urethra with urinary obstruction.

Testicular cancer: A malignancy of the testicle that is one of the most curable solid neoplasms. Nearly all testicular tumors are germ cell tumors. These tumors are most common in males between the ages 20–35.

Cryptorchidism: The failure of the testes to descend into the scrotum from the abdominal cavity. Undescended testes atrophy and may become the potential site of cancer.

Specific to Children

Colic: Abdominal distress of unknown cause in newborns or young infants.

Reye's syndrome: A combination of encephalopathy and fatty infiltration of the internal organs that may follow acute viral infections, most commonly in children under 15 years of age. The condition sometimes arises following infection with influenza A or B viruses or chickenpox and has been linked to the use of aspirin during these infections.

Sudden infant death syndrome (SIDS): Also called crib death, a syndrome that occurs in infants younger than 1 year of age. Death occurs within seconds during sleep. The cause is unknown. However, there are several risk factors, such as stomach sleeping, soft mattress, loose bed covers, room temperature too warm, and low birth weight.

Erythroblastosis fetalis: A type of hemolytic anemia in newborns that results from maternal fetal blood group incompatibility, specifically involving the Rh factor and the ABO blood groups. Common symptoms include anemia, jaundice, kernicterus, splenomegaly, and hepatomegaly. It is sometimes called hydrops fetalis.

Wilms' tumor: Also called nephroblastoma, a highly malignant neoplasm of the kidney that affects children younger than five years. It is the most common kidney tumor of childhood.

Child abuse: The Federal Child Abuse Prevention and Treatment Act states that all threats to a child's physical and/or mental welfare must be reported. These include trauma to the nervous system; old healed fractures; internal abdominal pain; discolorations or bruising on the buttocks, back, abdomen, elbow, wrist, and shoulder; poor hygiene; malnutrition; and obvious dental neglect.

STRATEGIES FOR SUCCESS

 ### *Test-Taking Skills*

No tricks, just focus!
Always read all the responses to a question before answering. If you choose an answer too hastily, you might miss the best answer. Don't make any assumptions about the questions and how the writer of the question might be trying to trick you. Use only the information provided in the question and choose the best answer based on your knowledge of the subject matter.

Instructions:

Answer the following questions.

1. Chronic glomerulonephritis and renal failure may both result in

   A. dehydration.
   B. cystitis.
   C. uremia.
   D. an enlarged prostate.
   E. Hirschsprung's disease.

2. What is the name of the condition caused by hypersecretion of growth hormone before puberty?

   A. myxedema
   B. acromegaly
   C. dwarfism
   D. gigantism
   E. hyperthyroidism

3. Which of following sexually transmitted diseases is sometimes called the silent STD?

   A. syphilis
   B. AIDS
   C. genital warts
   D. moles
   E. chlamydial infection

4. Failure of the testes to descend into the scrotum from the abdominal cavity is called

   A. orchitis.
   B. epididymitis.
   C. varicocele.
   D. cryptorchidism.
   E. Peyronie's disease.

5. Which of the following is the most common disease or condition of the urinary system?

   A. hydronephrosis
   B. renal failure
   C. pyelonephritis
   D. renal atrophy
   E. nephrotic syndrome

6. Vitiligo is a condition that affects which of the following body systems?

   A. respiratory
   B. reproductive
   C. endocrine
   D. integumentary
   E. digestive

7. Tetanus is commonly called

   A. lockjaw.
   B. sleeping sickness.
   C. hydrophobia.
   D hydronephrosis.
   E. lockjaw and hydrophobia.

8. Which of the following is *not* an obvious sign of Parkinson's disease?

   A. tremor
   B. rigidity
   C. seizure
   D. slowness of movement
   E. all of these

9. The absence of the onset of menstruation at puberty is called

   A. metrorrhagia.
   B. amenorrhea.
   C. dysmenorrhea.
   D. miscarriage.
   E. eclampsia.

10. Undescended testes may become the potential site of

    A. infection.
    B. lymphedema.
    C. gangrene.
    D. polyposis.
    E. cancer.

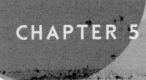

CHAPTER 5

MICROBIOLOGY

LEARNING OUTCOMES

5.1 Identify microorganisms including bacteria, viruses, fungi, and protozoa.

5.2 Recognize terminology used in relation to the growth of microbes.

5.3 Recall the different types of microbes and the role they play in the cycle of infection.

MEDICAL ASSISTING COMPETENCIES

COMPETENCY	CMA	RMA	CCMA	NCMA
Clinical				
Apply principles of aseptic techniques and infection control, including hand washing	X	X	X	X
Practice standard precautions	X	X	X	X
General/Legal/Professional				
Use appropriate medical terminology	X	X	X	X

5.1 Microorganisms

Microbiology: The study of very small living organisms, including bacteria, algae, fungi, protozoa, and viruses; often called microbes, germs, or single-celled organisms.

Microscope: An instrument used to obtain an enlarged image of a small object and to reveal details of a structure otherwise not distinguishable.

Microorganisms: Tiny microscopic entities that are able to carry on all the processes of life, including metabolism, reproduction, and motility.

Saprophyte: An organism that obtains its nutrients from dead organic matter. Many bacteria and fungi are saprophytes.

Eukaryote: An organism that has cells containing a membrane-bound nucleus, with chromosomes.

Prokaryote: A unicellular organism that does not contain a true nucleus surrounded by a double membrane, such as a bacterium.

Bacteria

Bacteria: Vary in size, shape, and cell arrangement and include bacilli, cocci, spirilla, diplobacilli, streptobacilli, and coccobacilli. See Figure 5-1. There are three basic forms of bacteria: bacilli, cocci, and spirilla.

Bacilli: Rod-shaped bacteria, such as *Bacillus anthracis,* tubercle bacilli, and typhoid bacilli.

Cocci: Spherical bacteria. Pathogenic cocci are staphylococci, streptococci, and diplococci. See Table 5-1.

Spirilla: Spiral-shaped bacteria.

Diplococci: Any of the spherical or coffee-bean-shaped bacteria that usually appear in pairs.

Streptobacilli: Bacteria in which the rods or filaments tend to fragment into chains.

Coccobacilli: Short bacilli that are thick and somewhat ovoid.

Characteristics of bacteria: Bacteria are classified according to morphology, motility, growth, staining reactions, metabolic activities, pathogenicity, antigen-antibody reactions, and genetic composition.

Stain: A substance used to impart color to tissue or cells in order to study and identify microscopic organisms.

Gram's stain: A staining procedure in which bacteria are stained with crystal violet, treated with strong iodine solution, and decolorized with ethanol. Microorganisms that retain the stain are said to be gram positive, and those that lose the crystal violet stain by decolorization but stain with a counterstain are said to be gram negative.

Gram-positive bacteria: Bacteria with cell walls that are composed of peptidoglycan and teichoic acid. Some of the most important pathogenic gram-positive bacteria are listed in Table 5-2. Gram-positive bacteria retain a crystal violet stain.

Gram-negative bacteria: Bacteria with cell walls that are composed of a thin layer of peptidoglycan covered by an outer membrane of lipoprotein and lipopolysaccharide. Table 5-3 is a summary of some gram-negative bacteria. Gram-negative bacteria do not retain a crystal violet stain.

Gram stain limitations: The following organisms do not Gram stain well: rickettsia, mycoplasma, treponema, chlamydia, mycobacteria, and *Legionella pneumophila.*

Streptococci: A genus of gram-positive bacteria that occur in chains.

Staphylococci: A genus of gram-positive bacteria made up of spherical microorganisms arranged in grapelike clusters. See Table 5-4.

Intermediate organisms: Obligate intracellular parasites, which can reproduce only in living cells. There are three groups: rickettsia, chlamydia, and mycoplasma.

Rickettsia: Any of several small intracellular parasites of the genus *Rickettsia* that require a vector (such as fleas, ticks, or lice) to spread disease.

Chlamydia: A gram-negative nonmotile obligate intracellular parasite that is totally dependent on the host cell for energy. The genus *Chlamydia* comprises three species: *C. trachomatis, C. psittaci,* and *C. pneumoniae.* See Table 5-5.

Mycoplasma: A group of bacteria considered to be the smallest free-living organisms. Unlike most other bacteria, they lack a cell wall. Some are saprophytes, some are parasites, and many are pathogens. They cause primary atypical pneumonia and many secondary infections.

Mycobacterium: A genus of bacteria distinguished by a high lipid content that produces resistance to drying, acids, and various germicides. Several are highly significant human pathogens that cause tuberculosis, leprosy, granuloma, and skin ulcers.

Legionella pneumophila: The bacterium that causes Legionnaires' disease. Primarily intracellular, it stains by silver stain.

Viruses

Viruses: Infectious agents that are even simpler in nature than bacteria. They are usually not considered cellular.

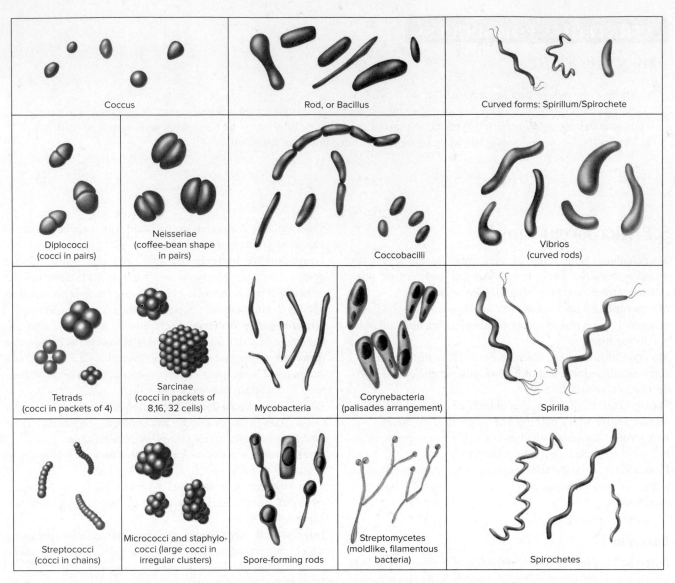

Figure 5-1 *Bacterial shapes and arrangements (not necessarily shown to exact scale).*

Arrangement	Description	Pathogenic Form
Diplococci	Pairs	*Neisseria gonorrhoeae*
Streptococci	Chains	*Streptococcus pyogenes*
Staphylococci	Clusters	*Staphylococcus aureus*

Table 5-1

Viruses are composed of a small amount of DNA or RNA wrapped in a protein covering. A virus is visible only with an electron microscope. Viruses are the smallest of all microorganisms.

Virion: A virus that exists outside a host cell.

Bacteriophage or **phage:** A virus that has a bacterial host.

Fungi

Fungi: Eukaryotic organisms with cellulose or chitin cell walls that include mushrooms, molds, and yeasts. Spores, the means of reproduction for fungi, can be carried great distances by the wind and are resistant to heat, cold, acids, bases, and other chemicals.

AT A GLANCE — Some Important Pathogenic Gram-Positive Bacteria

Bacterium	Type	Diseases Caused
Corynebacterium diphtheriae	Rod, nonmotile	Diphtheria
Staphylococcus aureus	Cocci in clusters	Carbuncles, septicemia, pneumonia, boils
Streptococcus pyogenes	Cocci in chains	Strep throat, rheumatic fever, septicemia, scarlet fever
Streptococcus pneumoniae	Diplococcus	Pneumonia
Mycobacterium tuberculosis	Rod	Tuberculosis
Mycobacterium leprae	Rod	Leprosy
Clostridium tetani	Noncapsulate, sporing, motile	Tetanus
Clostridium botulinum	Spore-forming rod, noncapsulate, motile	Botulism (food poisoning)
Clostridium perfringens	Spore-forming rod, nonmotile, noncapsulate	Gas gangrene, wound infections

Table 5-2

AT A GLANCE — Some Important Pathogenic Gram-Negative Bacteria

Bacterium	Type	Diseases Caused
Escherichia coli	Rod	Urinary infections
Haemophilus influenzae	Rod	Meningitis or pneumonia
Haemophilus ducreyi	Rod	Chancroid
Klebsiella pneumoniae	Rod	Pneumonia
Neisseria gonorrhoeae	Diplococci	Gonorrhea
Neisseria meningitidis	Diplococci	Meningitis
Rickettsia rickettsii	Rod	Rocky Mountain spotted fever
Salmonella typhi	Rod	Typhoid fever
Shigella species	Rod	Shigellosis (bacillary dysentery)
Treponema pallidum	Spirochete	Syphilis
Vibrio cholerae	Curved rod	Cholera

Table 5-3

Mushrooms: A class of true fungi.

Mycelium: A network of filaments or strands in mushrooms.

Molds: Multicellular fungi that are the main source of antibiotics. Some are used to produce large quantities of enzymes (amylases) and citric acid. Molds can also be harmful, and some are toxic.

Aflatoxin: A toxin produced by *Aspergillus* mold on peanuts and cottonseed. Aflatoxin is extremely toxic to humans and farm animals, and it is also carcinogenic.

Yeasts: Single-celled microscopic eukaryotes that produce vitamins and proteins.

Candida albicans: A type of pathogenic yeast that causes candidiasis. Types of candidiasis include antibiotic candidiasis, candidal vulvovaginitis, diaper candidiasis, oral candidiasis, perianal candidiasis, and systemic candidiasis.

Dimorphism: The ability to live in two different forms, such as the few fungi, usually pathogens, that can live either as molds or as yeasts depending on growth conditions.

AT A GLANCE Staphylococci

Type	Diseases Caused
S. aureus	Skin infections
	Osteopyelitis
	Food poisoning
	Endocarditis
	Toxic shock syndrome
S. epidermidis	Infections following instrumentation or implantation
S. saprophyticus	Urinary tract infection

Table 5-4

AT A GLANCE Chlamydia

Type	Diseases Caused	Treatment
C. trachomatis	Urethritis	Tetracycline; ophthalmic antibiotic solution for newborns
C. psittaci (found in bird feces)	Psittacosis	Tetracycline or doxycycline
C. pneumoniae	Pneumonia, bronchitis, sinusitis	Tetracycline or erythromycin

Table 5-5

Protozoa

Protozoa: Unicellular eukaryotic organisms of diverse types, once believed to be the lowest forms of animal life. Protozoa have the ability to move, and they are found in water and soil. Protozoa include free-living forms, such as amoebas and paramecia, as well as parasites. These pathogens are summarized in Table 5-6. (The singular form is *protozoon* or *protozoan*.)

5.2 Microbial Growth

Fermentation: The decomposition of complex substances through the action of enzymes produced by microorganisms.
Photosynthesis: A process by which the energy of light is used to produce organic molecules. Some bacteria are capable of photosynthesis.
Aerobe: A microorganism that lives and grows in the presence of free oxygen. The majority of microbes are aerobes.
Anaerobe: A microbe that grows and lives in the absence of oxygen.
Obligate anaerobe: A microbe that lives only in the absence of oxygen.

Heterotrophs: Organisms that obtain carbon from organic material.
Autotrophs: Organisms that use inorganic carbon dioxide (CO_2) as their basic carbon source.
Chemotrophs: Organisms that use chemical substances as a source of energy.
Phototrophs: Organisms that use light as a source of energy.
Exotoxin: A potent toxin that is secreted or excreted by living microorganisms as the result of bacterial metabolism. Exotoxins are the most poisonous substances known to human beings. Bacteria of the genus *Clostridium* are the most frequent producers of exotoxins.

5.3 Microbes and the Human Body

Medical microbiology: The study of pathogens and the disease process, including epidemiology, diagnosis, treatment, infection control, and immunology. A list of major diseases, including the causative organisms, routes of transmission, and signs and symptoms, is provided in Tables 5-7 through 5-12.
Normal (resident) flora: Bacteria that are permanent and generally beneficial residents in the human body.

AT A GLANCE — Protozoal Pathogens and Infections

Pathogen	Diseases Caused
Entamoeba histolytica	Amebic dysentery
Dientamoeba fragilis	Diarrhea, fever
Trypanosoma gambiense	Sleeping sickness
Trichomonas vaginalis	Infections of the male and female genital tracts
Giardia lamblia	Gastroenteritis (intestinal infection)
Plasmodium species	Malaria
Pneumocystis carinii	Severe secondary infections in persons with suppressed immune systems (such as those who have AIDS)

Table 5-6

AT A GLANCE — Microbial Disease—Integumentary System

Disease	Causative Organism	Route of Transmission	Signs and Symptoms
Anthrax	*Bacillus anthracis*	Inhalation or ingestion of spores; consumption of contaminated food	Fever, chills, night sweats, cough, shortness of breath, fatigue, muscle aches, sore throat
Skin infections	*Staphylococcus aureus*	Direct contact of individuals colonized or infected with this bacteria; hand hygiene is the single most important step in controlling spread of these bacteria	Minor: pimples, boils Major: septicemia, surgical wound infection, necrotizing fasciitis

Table 5-7

Source: Centers for Disease Control, Health Topics A to Z. Atlanta, Georgia, 2013. www.cdc.gov/health/default.htm

AT A GLANCE — Microbial Disease—Respiratory System

Disease	Causative Organism	Route of Transmission	Signs and Symptoms
Pneumonia	*Haemophilus influenzae* *Streptococcus pneumoniae* *Mycoplasma pneumoniae*	Direct contact with respiratory droplets	Fever, decreased breath sounds, shortness of breath, increased heart rate (tachycardia), increased respiratory rate (tachypnea)
Legionellosis • Legionnaires' disease (severe form) • Pontiac fever (mild form)	*Legionella pneumophila*	Breathing water mists contaminated with *Legionella* bacteria (spa, air conditioner, shower)	Fever, chills, and a cough; muscle aches, headache, tiredness, loss of appetite, and occasionally diarrhea

Table 5-8, continued

Disease	Causative Organism	Route of Transmission	Signs and Symptoms
Tuberculosis	*Mycobacterium tuberculosis*	Respiratory droplet spread	A bad cough that lasts longer than 2 weeks, pain in the chest, coughing up blood or sputum (phlegm from deep inside the lungs), weakness, fatigue, weight loss, lack of appetite, chills, fever, and night sweats
Pertussis	*Bordetella pertussis*	Contact with respiratory droplets	Typically manifested in children with paroxysmal spasms of severe coughing, whooping, and posttussive vomiting
Diphtheria	*Corynebacterium diphtheriae*	Person-to-person spread through respiratory tract secretions	Sore throat, low-grade fever, adherent membrane of the tonsils, pharynx, or nose, neck swelling
Influenza	Influenza A and B virus	Respiratory droplet spread	Fever (usually high), headache, extreme tiredness, dry cough, sore throat, runny nose, and muscle aches; gastrointestinal symptoms include nausea, vomiting, and diarrhea
Common cold	Rhinoviruses	Respiratory droplet spread	Runny nose, sneezing, sore throat, mild, hacking cough
Severe acute respiratory syndrome (SARS)	SARS-associated coronavirus (SARS-CoV)	Close person-to-person contact	High fever (temperature greater than 100.4°F [38.0°C]), headache, overall feeling of discomfort, body aches, dry cough, pneumonia

Table 5-8, concluded

Source: Centers for Disease Control, Health Topics A to Z. Atlanta, Georgia, 2013. www.cdc.gov/health/default.htm

AT A GLANCE Microbial Disease—Gastrointestinal System

Disease	Causative Organism	Route of Transmission	Signs and Symptoms
Salmonellosis	*Salmonella enteritidis*	Consumption of contaminated food (raw eggs, chicken, or beef)	Fever, abdominal cramps, diarrhea beginning 12–72 hours after consuming a contaminated food or beverage
Typhoid fever	*Salmonella typhi*	Fecal oral	Sustained high fever (103°–104°F), weakness, stomach pains, headache, loss of appetite
E.coli diarrhea	*Escherichia coli O157:H7*	Eating contaminated foods (ground beef, raw milk)	Severe bloody diarrhea, abdominal cramps
Cholera	*Vibrio cholerae*	Drinking contaminated water or eating contaminated food	Profuse watery diarrhea, vomiting, leg cramps, dehydration, shock
Botulism	*Clostridium botulinum*	Consuming improperly canned food contaminated with botulinum	Double vision, blurred vision, drooping eyelids, slurred speech, difficulty swallowing, dry mouth, muscle weakness
Mumps	*Mumps virus (paramyxovirus)*	Airborne and direct contact with infected respiratory droplets	Fever, headache, muscle ache, swelling of the lymph nodes close to the jaw

Table 5-9

Disease	Causative Organism	Route of Transmission	Signs and Symptoms
Hepatitis A	Hepatitis A virus	Hepatitis A: fecal oral	Symptoms are similar for each: jaundice, fatigue, abdominal pain, loss of appetite, nausea, diarrhea, fever, joint pain, dark urine
Hepatitis B	Hepatitis B virus	Hepatitis B: blood and body fluids	
Hepatitis C	Hepatitis C virus	Hepatitis C: blood and body fluids	

Table 5-9

Source: Centers for Disease Control, Health Topics A to Z. Atlanta, Georgia, 2013. www.cdc.gov/health/default.htm

AT A GLANCE Microbial Disease—Genitourinary System

Disease	Causative Organism	Route of Transmission	Signs and Symptoms
Chlamydia	*Chlamydia trachomatis*	Sexual contact	Usually silent; can have mild symptoms of abnormal vaginal discharge or a burning sensation when urinating
Gonorrhea	*Neisseria gonorrhea*	Sexual contact	Mucopurulent endocervical or urethral exudates
Syphilis	*Treponema pallidum*	Sexual contact; also can be passed to the fetus from an infected woman	Single sore, usually firm, round, small, and painless, that appears at the spot where syphilis entered the body
Chickenpox	*Varicella zoster* (Human herpesvirus type 3 [HHV-3])	Droplets spread through coughing and sneezing	Skin rash of blisterlike lesions, usually on the face, scalp, or trunk
Shingles	*Varicella zoster* (Human herpesvirus type 3 [HHV-3])	Previous outbreak of chickenpox that reactivates	Inflammation of segments of spinal or cranial peripheral nerves and painful eruption along the course of the nerve
Genital herpes	*Herpes simplex viruses* type 1 (HSV-1) and type 2 (HSV-2)	HSV-1: oral-and-genital contact HSV-2: sexual contact	Genital sores: flulike symptoms, including fever, swollen glands

Table 5-10

Source: Centers for Disease Control, Health Topics A to Z. Atlanta, Georgia, 2013. www.cdc.gov/health/default.htm

AT A GLANCE Microbial Disease—Nervous System

Disease	Causative Organism	Route of Transmission	Signs and Symptoms
Meningitis	*Neisseria meningitidis* *Streptococcus pneumoniae* *Haemophilus influenzae*	Direct contact with respiratory secretions from a carrier	High fever, headache, stiff neck, nausea, vomiting, photophobia, confusion, sleepiness
Toxoplasmosis	*Toxoplasma gondii*	Accidental ingestion of cat feces; ingestion of contaminated raw or undercooked meat, or contaminated water	Swollen lymph glands or muscle aches and pains that last for a month or more
Poliomyelitis	*Polioviruses* 1, 2, and 3	Person-to-person, fecal or oral	Ranges from asymptomatic to symptomatic, including acute flaccid paralysis, quadriplegia, respiratory failure, and, rarely, death
Rabies	*Rabies virus*	Bite of a rabid animal	Fever, headache, confusion, sleepiness, or agitation

Table 5-11

Source: Centers for Disease Control, Health Topics A to Z. Atlanta, Georgia, 2013. www.cdc.gov/health/default.htm

Disease	Causative Organism	Route of Transmission	Signs and Symptoms
Plague	*Yersinia pestis*	Flea-borne from infected rodents to humans; respiratory droplets from cats and humans with pneumonic plague	Bubonic plague: enlarged, tender lymph nodes, fever, chills, prostration Septicemic plague: fever, chills, prostration, abdominal pain, shock, bleeding into skin and other organs Pneumonic plague: fever, chills, cough, and difficulty breathing; rapid shock
Rocky Mountain spotted fever	*Rickettsia rickettsii*	Tick-borne ixodid ticks infected with *R. rickettsii*	Fever, nausea, vomiting, severe headache, muscle pain, lack of appetite, rash, abdominal pain, joint pain, diarrhea
Lyme disease	*Borrelia burgdorferi*	Tick-borne deer ticks infected with *B. burgdorferi*	Fever, headache, fatigue, myalgia
Mononucleosis	Epstein-Barr virus	Contact with saliva of infected person	Fever, sore throat, swollen lymph glands
HIV/AIDS	Human immunodeficiency virus	Blood and body fluids	The following *may be* warning signs of infection with HIV: rapid weight loss; dry cough; recurring fever or profuse night sweats; profound and unexplained fatigue; swollen lymph glands in the armpits, groin, or neck; diarrhea that lasts for more than one week; white spots or unusual blemishes on the tongue, in the mouth, or in the throat; pneumonia; red, brown, pink, or purplish blotches on or under the skin or inside the mouth, nose, or eyelids; memory loss, depression, and other neurological disorders
Malaria	*Plasmodium: P. falciparum, P. vivax, P. ovale,* or *P. malariae*	Mosquito-borne from Anopheles mosquito infected with *P. malariae*	Fever and influenza-like symptoms, including chills, headache, myalgias, and malaise

Table 5-12

Source: Centers for Disease Control, Health Topics A to Z. Atlanta, Georgia, 2013. www.cdc.gov/health/default.htm

Host: An organism in which another, usually parasitic, organism is nourished and harbored.

Symbiosis: The living together of two organisms of different species.

Mutualism: A relationship in which both organisms benefit. For example, certain normal flora living in the human intestine synthesize vitamin K, biotin, riboflavin, pantothenate, and pyridoxine.

Commensalism: A one-sided relationship in which one member benefits and neither is harmed. Yeast, *Candida albicans,* is one of the normal flora that has a *commensal* relationship with the skin (meaning that it benefits from contact with the skin but does not harm it).

Parasitism: A one-sided relationship between a host and a parasite.

Parasite: An organism that lives in, on, or at the expense of another organism without contributing to the host's survival.

Obligate intracellular parasite: A parasite that is completely dependent on its host and must be in a living cell in order to reproduce.

Opportunism: A relationship in which a usually harmless organism becomes pathogenic when the host's resistance is impaired.

Opportunistic microbe: A harmless microorganism that causes disease only if it invades the body when the immune system is weakened and unable to defend against it.

Pathogens: Disease-causing microorganisms. Only a small percentage of microbes are pathogenic; the others are considered harmless or beneficial.

Pathogenicity: The ability of a pathogenic agent to cause a disease.

Virulence: The degree of pathogenicity or relative power of a microorganism to produce a disease.

Infective dose: The number of organisms required to cause a disease in a susceptible host.

Contagious disease: A disease that is transmitted from one person to another. The following factors influence the cycle involved in the spread of infectious disease: means of transmission, means of entrance, susceptible host, reservoir host, and means of exit. To prevent infection any part of this cycle must be broken. The cycle of infection begins with the reservoir host. See Figure 5-2.

Breaking the cycle of infection: Medical assistants can help break the cycle of infection by proper hand washing, maintaining strict housekeeping standards, adhering to government guidelines to protect against diseases, and educating patients about hygiene, health promotion, and disease prevention.

Vector: A living organism that carries microorganisms from an infected organism to another. See Table 5-13.

Biological vector: An animal in which the infecting organism multiplies or develops before becoming infectious.

Resistance: The body mechanisms that oppose infection. The host's state of health and other factors, including race, age, sex, and occupation, affect the ability of a pathogen to cause disease. Resistance is also the ability of a microorganism to live in the presence of antibiotics, antimicrobial agents, and phages.

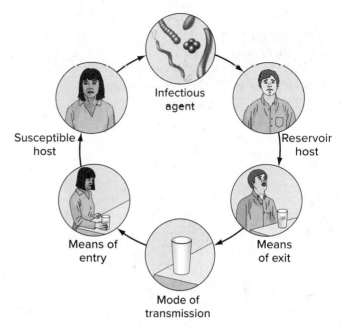

Figure 5-2 *The cycle of infection must be broken at some point to prevent the spread of disease.*

AT A GLANCE　Vectors

Carrier	Diseases
Dogs, raccoons	Rabies
Mosquitoes	Malaria, encephalitis
Ticks	Rocky Mountain spotted fever, Lyme disease

Table 5-13

STRATEGIES FOR SUCCESS

▶ *Test-Taking Skills*

After you're finished, review!
When you are finished with the exam, go back and review any questions you skipped earlier or ones that you were unsure about. Change your answer only when you are positive that it's wrong. Change obvious mistakes, but keep in mind that first guesses often turn out to be the right ones. Before you turn in your exam, make sure that you answered all the questions and erase any stray marks on the exam.

Instructions:

Answer the following questions.

1. Which of the following microorganisms is a grapelike cluster?
   A. streptococci
   B. spirochete
   C. *Neisseria gonorrhoeae*
   D. *Vibrio cholerae*
   E. staphylococci

2. Which of the following organisms requires a vector?
   A. chlamydia
   B. mycoplasma
   C. rickettsia
   D. saprophyte
   E. diplococcus

3. The smallest organisms are called
   A. viruses.
   B. chlamydia.
   C. rickettsia.
   D. acidophiles.
   E. bacteria.

4. If a virus has a bacterial host, it is called
   A. a bacteriophage.
   B. bacteriostatic.
   C. bactericidal.
   D. bacteriostatic or bactericidal.
   E. none of these

5. Any close relationship that exists between two different species is known as
   A. sebum.
   B. symbionts.
   C. syncope.
   D. synergism.
   E. symbiosis.

6. Which of the following is *not* true of the Gram stain procedure?
   A. It works for all bacteria.
   B. The stain used is crystal violet.
   C. It differentiates between gram-positive and gram-negative bacteria.
   D. Some bacteria lose the stain by decolorization.
   E. An iodine solution is used.

7. Spiral-shaped bacteria are called
   A. cocci.
   B. spirilla.
   C. bacilli.
   D. diplococci.
   E. sarcinae.

8. Streptococci appear in
   A. clusters of cocci.
   B. pairs of cocci.
   C. chains of cocci.
   D. spirilla.
   E. capsulate and spore forms.

9. The bacterium *Escherichia coli* can cause
   A. urinary infections.
   B. pneumonia.
   C. gonorrhea.
   D. chancroid.
   E. arthritis.

10. Which of the following words is misspelled?
    A. chlamydia
    B. myecobacteria
    C. staphylococci
    D. eukaryote
    E. rickettsia

CHAPTER 6

GENERAL PSYCHOLOGY

LEARNING OUTCOMES

6.1 Recognize terminology used in relation to the principles of psychology.

6.2 Describe the differences and similarities between motivation and emotions.

6.3 Describe personality and the theoretical beliefs of Sigmund Freud and Carl Jung.

6.4 Explain the humanistic beliefs regarding psychological motivation, affiliation, fear of success, and Maslow's hierarchy of needs.

6.5 Explain the theory of learning through operant conditioning.

6.6 Identify and define common psychological disorders.

6.7 Describe Erik Erikson's stages of psychosocial development and Elisabeth Kübler-Ross's stages of grief.

6.8 Define grief and its adaptive processes.

6.9 Identify behaviors and techniques to decrease stress and promote wellness.

6.10 Describe substance abuse and withdrawal and their psychological and emotional effects on the human body.

MEDICAL ASSISTING COMPETENCIES

COMPETENCY	CMA	RMA	CCMA	NCMA
General/Legal/Professional				
Recognize and respond to verbal and nonverbal communications by being attentive and adapting communication to the recipient's level of understanding.	X	X	X	X
Instruct individuals according to their needs.	X	X	X	X
Provide patients with methods of health promotion and disease prevention.	X	X		
Be impartial and show empathy when dealing with patients.	X	X		

6.1 Basic Principles

Psychology: The science of behavior and mental processes. Psychology is considered to be a science because psychologists attempt to understand people through careful, controlled observation.

Subfields: The broad nature of psychology has given rise to subfields. They are related to one another and share the common purpose of understanding behavior. The subfields are easier to identify if you are able to look at the basic premise about behavior that they address.

Scientific method: A systematic approach applied by psychologists to question the world around them and to gain knowledge. The scientific method has three steps: (1) identify the problem, (2) formulate a rationale, and (3) perform supportive research.

Theories: Wide-ranging predictions or explanations of everyday behavior or phenomena. Theories can show relationships among otherwise unorganized facts. Psychologists use the "Theories of Personalities" to explain why people do what they do.

Hypothesis: A prediction that has its origins in a theory and is written in such a way to allow for testing and further research. Simply put, we have broad theories about life, and then, because of these theories, we predict behavior through a hypothesis. The following is an example of a hypothesis originating in a theory: All women are happy and smiling, which indicates happiness (theory); then, all women we will meet will be smiling (hypothesis). When we meet one woman who is not smiling, then we have nullified our hypothesis, making the theory questionable and in need of modification.

Thanatology: The study of death and dying.

6.2 Motivation and Emotion

Motivation

Motivation: Psychologists who study motivation seek to discover a person's particular desired goals. Motivation is closely related to the topic of emotions. The term *emotion* refers to a positive or negative feeling, generally in reaction to stimuli that are accompanied by physiological arousal and related behavior. This consists of the factors that direct and energize the behavior of humans and other organisms.

Behavior: A person's overt actions that others can directly observe, such as walking, speaking, and writing.

Mental processes: Private thoughts, emotions, feelings, and motives that others cannot directly observe. Observers can only draw inferences about these.

Emotions

Emotions: Feelings or effects that often have physical as well as cognitive and behavioral elements.

Empathy: The experiencing of another person's emotional state by viewing the situation through that person's eyes. It is commonly stated as, "walking in another person's shoes."

Sympathy: An emotion by which the person feels sad for another person, usually because of his or her own identification with the situation.

Fear: An emotion that invokes a physiological, cognitive, and behavioral response, such as the fight-or-flight syndrome.

6.3 Personality

Personality: The sum total of the typical ways of acting, thinking, and feeling that makes each person unique.

Freud

Psychodynamic theory of personality: The original pioneer of the psychodynamic approach was Sigmund Freud. His psychoanalytical theory stated that unconscious forces act as determinants of personality.

Unconscious: A part of the personality of which a person is not aware and that is a potential determinant of behavior.

Freud's mind: The division by Freud of the mind into three parts: the id, the ego, and the superego. Each part is different but related.

The id: One of Freud's personality components, consisting of our basic instincts and our psychic energy. It is unconscious. The id has no contact with reality and works on the *pleasure principle,* the impulse to seek pleasure and avoid pain (regardless of how harmful it might be to others).

The ego: The personality component based in reality. The ego works on the *reality principle,* that is, the mind's attempt to bring pleasure and sexual impulses, and to balance the impulses of the id with the norms of society. The ego is partly conscious and helps us test reality to see how far we can go before we run into trouble or harm.

The superego: The personality component, not based in reality, that questions whether an act is right or wrong. The superego is our moral barometer, commonly called *our conscience.* Freud suggested that the superego is the part of the personality that represents the rights and wrongs of society, developing from direct teaching and from the models of parents, teachers, and other significant individuals.

Defense mechanisms: Coping skills that Freud believed were formed to help the ego reduce anxiety and help a person cope with daily life. Anxiety occurs because the superego and the id are both unrealistic. This unrealistic view can make it difficult for the ego to live in reality because the ego is caught between impulses from the id ("I want what I want now") and the superego ("I judge everything"). Because of this struggle, the ego is said to form defense mechanisms to reduce the anxiety by unconsciously changing reality. See Table 6-1.

Freud's theory on developing personality: Freud's theory on the development of personality in childhood through a series of stages. The theory is unique in focusing each stage on a major biological function, such as pleasure, in each given period. See Table 6-2.

Jung

Carl Jung's theories: Jung's theories are based on extroversion, introversion, personal unconscious, and collective unconscious.

Extroversion: According to Jung, the tendency of some individuals to be friendly and open to the world.

Defense Mechanism	Meaning	Example
Repression	Unacceptable impulses are pushed back into the subconscious.	A rape victim cannot recall the crime.
Rationalization	A self-justifying explanation is substituted for an unacceptable one.	An athlete who did not win the game says, "It makes you a better player to lose."
Projection	Unwanted feelings are attributed to someone else.	A person who has aggressive tendencies accuses others of starting fights.
Denial	An anxiety-producing event is not accepted as reality.	A compulsive gambler refuses to believe his behavior is hurting anyone.
Regression	In order to face stress, an earlier developmental period is sought.	An older sibling starts to suck his thumb when a newborn is brought home.
Displacement	Feelings toward an unacceptable object are shifted onto a more acceptable one.	A father is angry at his boss but cannot yell at him, so he yells at his children when he comes home.
Sublimation	An unacceptable impulse is replaced by a more acceptable impulse.	An aggressive person becomes a boxer.
Reaction formation	An unacceptable motive is changed to the exact opposite.	A person who fears his violent behavior becomes a religious zealot.

Table 6-1

Introversion: According to Jung, the tendency of some individuals to be shy and to focus their attention on themselves.
Personal unconscious: According to Jung, the motives, conflicts, and information that are repressed by a person because they are threatening to that individual.
Collective unconscious: According to Jung, the shared content of the unconscious mind with which all humans are born.

6.4 Humanistic Theory of Personality

Humanistic theory of personality: This theory asserts that humans are striving to reach their full potential and that, with encouragement and unconditional positive regard, they can achieve it. The founders of humanistic psychology include Carl Rogers, Abraham Maslow, Victor Frankl, and others.

Age	Stage	Characteristics
Birth to 12–18 months	Oral	Interest in oral gratification (sucking, eating, mouthing, biting), in which an infant's center of pleasure is the mouth
12–18 months to 3 years	Anal	Gratification by withholding and expelling feces and getting used to society's controls regarding toilet training, in which a child's pleasure is centered on the anus
3 to 5–6 years	Phallic	Interest in the genitals and coming to terms with the Oedipal conflict (which leads to identification with the same-sex parent); a child's pleasure focuses on the genitals
5–6 years to adolescence	Latency	Unimportance of sexual concerns; children's sexual concerns are temporarily put aside
Adolescence to adulthood	Genital	Reemergence of sexual interests; mature sexual relationships are established, or the period from puberty until death, marked by mature sexual behavior (such as sexual intercourse)

Table 6-2

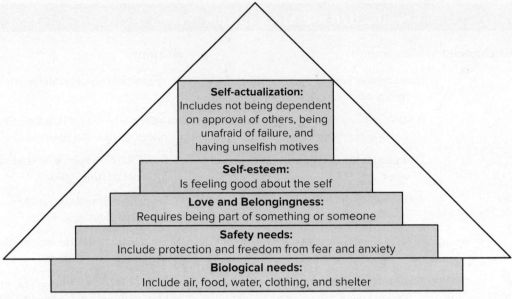

Figure 6-1 *A pyramid illustrates Maslow's hierarchy of human needs.*

Humanists believe that humans possess an internal force, an *inner-directedness,* that pushes them to grow, to improve, and to become the best individuals that they are capable of being. People have the freedom to make choices, and they are generally pretty good at making intelligent choices that further their personal growth.

Psychological motives: Motives that are not directly related to the biological survival of the individual. They are "needs" in the sense that the individual's happiness and well-being depend on these motives.

Motive for affiliation: The need to be with other people and to have personal relationships.

Fear of success: The fear of the consequences of success, particularly the envy of others.

Maslow's hierarchy of needs: Abraham Maslow believed that the basic needs of humans must be met before upper-level functioning can occur. Maslow's pyramid details how the basics of life are of first concern, and then safety, love, belonging, and esteem must be met before humans can begin to become fully actualized. If lower needs in the hierarchy are not met for the most part, then higher motives will not operate. Higher needs lie dormant until the individual has a chance to satisfy immediately pressing lower needs, such as hunger, thirst, and safety. See Figure 6-1.

Personality and culture: Psychologists are accepting the idea that sociocultural factors, such as ethnicity, race, gender, sexual preference, and physical challenges, are important in understanding human personality. One new focus of cross-cultural research has been on the validity of North American concepts of personality in other cultures.

6.5 Behavioral/Learning Theory of Personality

Behavioral/learning theory of personality: Learning through operant conditioning (consequences cause a change). Positive reinforcement is achieved when a reward is given. Negative or positive behavior can be reinforced, thereby causing it to be repeated. Other schedules can cause increased learning, such as random intermittent reinforcement schedule, which explains why people gamble. The reward is random and definitely intermittent, which causes the person who has won in the past to try for the reinforcer against all odds. Extinction of the behavior occurs when the reinforcers are no longer given.

Adaptation: The adjustment of a person's sensory capacity after prolonged exposure to a stimulus. For example, viewing excessive violence over a longer period of time does not bring on the same response as during the original sighting.

Behavior modification: A technique used to promote the frequency of a desired behavior while decreasing an undesirable behavior.

Biofeedback: A process whereby the person learns to control internal physiological systems, such as blood pressure, pulse, and respirations, by the use of conscious thought.

Cognitive theory: The theory that a person's emotions are a result of how that person interprets stimuli through his or her belief system. For example, if two people associate the color green with money, the person with the positive belief system about money will be happy when shown the color green. On the contrary, a person who has a negative view of money may react sadly when shown the color green.

Cognitive development: The process through which an infant becomes an intelligent person, acquiring knowledge with growth and improving his or her ability to think, learn, reason, and abstract. Jean Piaget demonstrated the orderly sequence of this process from early infancy through childhood.

Cognition: The intellectual processes through which information is obtained, transformed, stored, retrieved, and otherwise used.

Language: A symbolic code used in communication.

Intelligence: The cognitive abilities of an individual to learn from experience, to reason well, and to cope with the demands of daily living.

Cognitive: Pertaining to the mental processes of comprehension, judgment, memory, and reasoning, as contrasted with emotional and volitional processes.

Cognitive dissonance: The tension that occurs when a person holds two conflicting attitudes about the same event. The anxiety that is generated by the contradictory views causes the person to either change his or her mind about how the event occurred or to deny how he or she really feels about it. One of the typical areas of cognitive dissonance is medical advice. A patient may enjoy smoking but still know that it can cause cancer. With these two contradictory facts, the patient may modify one or both of the cognitions, as follows: modification of one cognition (e.g., "I hardly smoke at all"), addition of cognitions (e.g., "I eat healthily so I am relatively strong"), or outright denial (e.g., "Not all people who smoke get cancer").

6.6 Psychological Disorders

Psychological disorders: A mental disorder or disturbance of thought or emotion. It is a disorder of the brain that results in a disruption in a person's thinking, feeling, moods, and ability to relate to others.

Anxiety disorders: Psychological disorders that involve excessive levels of negative emotions, such as nervousness, tension, worry, fright, and anxiety; the occurrence of anxiety without an obvious external cause, affecting daily functioning.

Depression: Emotional state characterized by feelings of sadness, lack of energy, and feelings of hopelessness and despair. It is also known as *major depression, major depressive disorder*, and *clinical depression*. Types of depression include *manic, reactive, endogenous,* and *involutional*.

Seasonal depression: A common form of depression in which depressive feelings occur at the same time every year, most commonly in the winter. It is also known as *seasonal affective disorder*.

Phobias: Intense, irrational fears of specific objects or situations. Common phobias include fear of spiders, snakes, heights, death, dogs, and confined spaces.

Generalized anxiety disorder: The experience of long-term, persistent anxiety and worry; an uneasy sense of general tension and apprehension that makes the individual highly uncomfortable because of prolonged presence. Sometimes the individual's concerns are about identifiable issues involving family, money, work, or health.

Panic anxiety disorder: A pattern of anxiety in which long periods of calm are broken by an intensely uncomfortable attack of anxiety.

Obsessive-compulsive disorders: Disorders that involve obsessions (anxiety-provoking thoughts that will not go away). Obsessions and compulsions are two separate problems, but they often occur together in the same individuals. Compulsions are irresistible urges to engage in behaviors such as repeatedly touching a spot on one's shoulder or repeatedly washing one's hands.

Dissociative disorders: Disorders that involve the apparent, abrupt, and repeated shifting from one "personality" to another. Formerly, a dissociative disorder was known as *multiple personality*.

Personality disorders: Psychological disorders that are believed to result from personalities that developed improperly during childhood. A number of personality disorders differ widely from one another, but share several characteristics:

- All personality disorders begin early in life.
- They are disturbing to the person and to others.
- They are very difficult to treat.

Somatoform disorders: Disorders in which the individual experiences symptoms of health problems that have psychological rather than physical causes. They are more common in women than in men. They take the form of chronic and recurrent aches, pains, tiredness, and other symptoms of somatic (body) illnesses.

Hypochondriasis: A disorder in which people have a constant fear of illness and a preoccupation with their health.

Conversion disorder: A major somatoform disorder that involves an actual physical disturbance, such as the inability to use a sensory organ or the complete or partial inability to move an arm or leg.

Schizophrenia: A psychological disorder involving cognitive disturbances (delusions and hallucinations), disorganization, and reduced enjoyment and interests. Schizophrenia is an uncommon disorder that affects about 1% of the general population.

Mania: An extended state of intense elation. People experiencing mania feel intense happiness, power, invulnerability, and energy. They may become involved in wild schemes, believing they will succeed at anything they attempt.

Bipolar disorder: A disorder in which a person alternates between periods of euphoric feelings and mania and periods of depression. Bipolar disorder and major depression are among the most common mood disorders.

Attention deficit disorder: A disorder primarily affecting children and adolescents, characterized by the inability to focus attention, leading to behavior problems and learning disabilities. ADD is more common in boys than in girls and is usually treated with psychotherapy and stimulant drugs. ADD is one type of attention deficit hyperactivity disorder (ADHD).

Attention deficit hyperactivity disorder: A common behavioral disorder that affects boys three times as often as girls, and that is signified by impulsive actions, hyperactivity, and difficulty focusing. There are three types: ADHD-1 (also known as ADD), ADHD-2 (primarily hyperactive, impulsive), and ADHD-3 (inattentive, hyperactive, impulsive).

Autism: A mental disorder characterized by extreme withdrawal and an abnormal absorption in fantasy, accompanied by delusions, hallucinations, and the inability to communicate verbally or otherwise relate to people. Schizophrenic children are often autistic.

6.7 Aging and Dying

Erikson's stages of psychosocial development: Erikson believed that as people age, they also go through psychosocial changes. He described a struggle between two forces at each milestone of development; the resolution of this struggle results in either positive or negative outcomes. Whichever way a person resolves each conflict, his or her identity is formed:

- Infancy (Birth–1.5 years)—the conflict is trust vs. mistrust
  - Positive outcome—ability to trust
  - Negative outcome—fear of others
- Early Childhood (1.5–3 years)—the conflict is autonomy vs. shame and doubt
  - Positive outcome—self-sufficiency
  - Negative outcome—lack of independence, self-doubt of one's own abilities
- Preschool/ Play Age (3–5 years)—the conflict is initiative vs. guilt
  - Positive outcome—initiation of actions
  - Negative outcome—guilt from actions and thoughts
- School Age (6–12 years)—the conflict is industry vs. inferiority
  - Positive outcome—sense of competence
  - Negative outcome—feelings of inferiority
- Adolescence (12–18 years)—the conflict is identity vs. role confusion
  - Positive outcome—awareness of one's own uniqueness
  - Negative outcome—inability to identify appropriate roles in life
- Young adulthood (18–40 years)—the conflict is intimacy vs. isolation
  - Positive outcome—development of loving sexual relationships and close friends
  - Negative outcome—fear of relationships
- Middle adulthood (40–65 years)—the conflict is generativity (independent creativity) vs. stagnation
  - Positive outcome—contribution to the continuity of life
  - Negative outcome—feeling that acts are trivial for future generations
- Maturity (65+ years)—the conflict is ego-integrity vs. despair
  - Positive outcome—sense of unity with life's accomplishments
  - Negative outcome—regrets over lost opportunities of life

Lawrence Kohlberg's theories of moral development: Lawrence Kohlberg theorized that moral development and ethical behavior depended upon an individual's age and ability to solve problems. He based his work on the work of developmental psychologists such as Piaget, and defined three major stages of development. Kohlberg believed an individual's moral development was based on his or her cognitive or thinking capacity, and exposure to different ideas and human experiences. Kohlberg's three stages are as follows:

- Preconditional stage—young children learn to behave based on rewards and punishments.
- Conventional stage—right and wrong is determined by other people, and is "approved" behavior. Later, the individual recognizes law and order as well as fixed rules and regulations.
- Postconventional or "principled" stage—human rights are part of greater social requirements, and the individual follows universal principles of good behavior and ethics.

Elisabeth Kübler-Ross's stages of grief: Elisabeth Kübler-Ross, a psychiatrist in the late 1960s and early 1970s, gave great insight into the death and dying process. She theorized that people pass through five distinct stages when they learn of their impending deaths and expanded it to include the death of a loved one. However, she cautioned that the dying process has very individual reactions and that anyone involved with the dying person should not try to force how he or she experiences the process. The five stages Dr. Kübler-Ross constructed after hundreds of interviews with dying patients are as follows:

1. **Denial:** There are several ways a person may manifest denial of a terminal diagnosis. The person may seek other opinions or say that the doctors and tests are wrong. This is also the stage when a person may seek a "miracle cure" and could fall into a scam or exhaust savings to try to find the "magic pill." Denial is so powerful that the person may simply look as though he or she has ignored the diagnosis and act as if nothing has changed. Denial is a defense mechanism that patients commonly use to shield themselves from the intense anxiety that can be produced in the medical field.

2. **Anger:** This stage occurs as the denial begins to break down. A common statement that a patient might make is, "Why me?" The patient could also be highly irritable, resentful, and envious of others who are happy.

3. **Bargaining:** After the denial and anger have subsided and the person is beginning to deal with the fact that he or she will die, the patient makes a last attempt to change the inevitable. This attempt is to bargain. The bargains are usually religious in nature, and deals are made to extend one's life: "I will faithfully attend church and donate money to the poor if I can live another year."

4. **Depression:** When the bargaining does not come to fruition and the inevitability of the situation sinks in, the patient may lapse into a deep depression. The sense of hope is gone, and the feelings of guilt may overtake the person. The person may regret things he or she has done or said to loved ones and feel guilty over leaving them.

5. **Acceptance:** As the depression lifts, the person gains a sense of peace that death will happen and a quiet state

of recognition that all living things die and that this is the person's time. This time is not a happy time, but rather is marked with exhaustion yet free of negative emotions.

Note that these grief stages vary and do not always occur in the same order.

6.8 Grief

Grief is defined as a group of intense psychological and physical responses that occur after a loss of some kind. Grief is a natural adaptive response to loss. The adaptive processes of grief include *mourning* (when grief is expressed, and the loss is integrated and resolved) and *bereavement* (the period that follows the death of a loved one). The stages of grief include *shock, reality,* and *recovery.* There are also various types of grief, which include *uncomplicated, anticipatory, dysfunctional,* and *disenfranchised* grief.

6.9 Promoting Health and Wellness

Compliance: Strategies to increase compliance are as follows:

- Provide clear instructions to patients regarding medication schedules.
- Maintain good rapport between patients and medical staff.
- Be honest.
- Keep the patient well informed.
- Frame messages in a positive manner to help the patient with early detection of a disease.
- Frame messages in a negative manner to motivate the patient to prevent disease.

Stress: A person's response to threatening or challenging events. Most people will have a degree of stress when visiting a doctor's office. When a patient is under a high level of stress, he or she may become ill and may be less likely to recover from an illness. It may make the patient less capable of coping with future stressors.

Coping with stress: The ways that a patient attempts to lessen stress through different strategies, such as defense mechanisms. Also, some patients may use alcohol or drugs to cope with stress.

General adaptation syndrome (GAS): Hans Selye's theory that persons under stress experience the same set of physiological reactions regardless of the source of the stress. There are three stages that a person will move through when faced with stress:

- First stage: alarm and mobilization. The patient becomes aware of the stressor, and the nervous system becomes energized.
- Second stage: resistance. If the stress continues, then the patient prepares to fight the stressors. This technique can cause the patient physiological and psychological harm.

- Third stage: exhaustion. If the stressor continues and the patient is unable to adapt or remove the stressor, then the patient will develop negative consequences of physical and psychological symptoms.
- Aftermath: The patient will be able to lessen the stressor through the exhaustion stage by avoidance. If a person is ill, then he or she can avoid the activity that caused the stress. For example, a person who is overloaded at work cannot go to work if he or she is in the hospital or suffering with a severe condition at home.

Psychophysiological disorders: Disorders that are real medical conditions influenced by physical, emotional, and psychological difficulties.

Psychophysiological conditions: Common conditions, such as high blood pressure, headaches, backaches, and skin rashes, that may have a link to or are worsened by stress or other psychological difficulties.

Cataclysmic event stressor: Events that happen suddenly and affect many people, simultaneously causing strong stressors for all. For example, the terrorist attacks in New York and the destruction of New Orleans from Hurricane Katrina were cataclysmic events.

Personal stressors: Major events in one's personal life. Life events, whether positive or negative, can cause a great deal of stress, such as death of a spouse, losing one's job, going to war, moving, abuse, having a baby, or getting married. Some victims of high stressors suffer from post-traumatic stress disorder (PTSD), which is the re-experiencing of a traumatic event, and without help can find themselves so overwhelmed that they may harm themselves or others.

Background stressors: Daily annoyances, such as traffic jams, waiting in line, and irritations at work. Alone, these stressors have the least impact on a person but, coupled with other stressors or multiple daily stressors, can result in psychological and physical problems (e.g., colds, flu, backaches, irritability, agitation, and distractibility).

Uplifts: Stress reducers. Minor positive events that can make a person feel good.

6.10 Substance Abuse

Substance abuse: In this context, a *substance* is a legal or illegal drug that may cause physical or mental impairment. The reversible effect of a substance upon the central nervous system is referred to as *intoxication*. The misuse, improper use, or excessive use of a substance, when avoidance of the substance does not cause symptoms of withdrawal, is termed *abuse*. When a person can no longer avoid using a substance without symptoms of withdrawal, he or she has developed *dependence on (addiction to)* the substance. If an addicted person tries to stop using the substance, there will be functional impairment, physical withdrawal symptoms, and/or psychological cravings. *Withdrawal symptoms* may include anxiety, sleep disturbances, tremors, sweating, hypertension, hallucinations, tachycardia, vomiting, and varying disorientation. Factors related to substance abuse include genetics, family patterns, lifestyle, environmental factors, and developmental factors.

Instructions:

Answer the following questions.

Questions one–three relate to Mr. Martin. He is a 70-year-old male who has been diagnosed with late-stage cancer of the stomach. He probably will only live three–six months. You are the medical assistant at the primary care doctor's office.

1. Mr. Martin has just been told of his diagnosis of cancer and the probability that he will not live too long. According to Kübler-Ross's stages of grief, what do you expect to hear from the patient?

   A. a rationalization
   B. a statement of denial
   C. a positive attitude
   D. a sublimation

2. A month later, Mr. Martin returns to the office and snaps back at the receptionist who comments on the nice day. Mr. Martin meets you and is very argumentative and annoyed when you try to help him to get up from the chair. According to Kübler-Ross's stages, what do you think is happening?

   A. Mr. Martin is grumpy because the staff is annoying.
   B. Mr. Martin is annoyed because he had to wait.
   C. Mr. Martin is realizing that he is dying and is angry.
   D. Mr. Martin has reached an acceptance of death and feels an inner peace with his fate.

3. Mr. Martin is facing death in his late adulthood and is reviewing his life. According to Erikson's stages of development, what conflict is he trying to resolve?

   A. identity vs. role confusion
   B. industry vs. inferiority
   C. trust vs. mistrust
   D. integrity vs. despair

4. Which statement is true about stress?

   A. All stress is from negative sources.
   B. Background stressors are events that happen suddenly.
   C. Stress can affect the body's ability to fight off illness.
   D. All stress causes physiological disorders.

5. Your patient was asked to exercise her neck for three minutes, six times a day. She told the medical assistant that she could not do the exercises because she had to go to work. Which of the following defense mechanisms is she using?

   A. regression
   B. rationalization

   C. repression
   D. projection
   E. displacement

6. A 38-year-old woman who has advanced breast cancer becomes extremely upset with family members when they even talk about the disease. The patient refuses to talk about the diagnosis and even acts as if she has a minor problem. This patient is using which of the following defense mechanisms?

   A. rationalization
   B. denial
   C. displacement
   D. sublimation
   E. projection

7. Major depression and bipolar disorder are most characteristic of which of the following psychological conditions?

   A. dissociative disorder
   B. impulse-control disorder
   C. mood disorder
   D. personality disorder
   E. cognitive disorder

8. A person with a preoccupation toward inner thoughts and a lack of responsiveness to others has which of the following conditions?

   A. paranoia
   B. mania
   C. autism
   D. dysphoria
   E. dyslexia

9. Which of the following is a major life event that commonly causes a high level of stress?

   A. death of spouse
   B. getting a raise
   C. being single
   D. painting your house
   E. meeting new friends

10. The terms *extroversion, introversion, personal unconscious,* and *collective unconscious* are attributed to

   A. Freud.
   B. Skinner.
   C. Bantura.
   D. Maslow.
   E. Jung.

CHAPTER 7

NUTRITION AND HEALTH PROMOTION

LEARNING OUTCOMES

7.1 Identify terminology commonly used in relation to nutrition.

7.2 Describe the functions and effects of water in the human body.

7.3 Recall the classifications, functions, and types of carbohydrates.

7.4 Identify the sources, functions, and types of lipids in the human body.

7.5 Recall the composition, classifications, sources, and functions of proteins.

7.6 Identify the different types of water-soluble and fat-soluble vitamins and their benefits for the human body.

7.7 Recall major minerals and trace elements.

7.8 Recall the dietary guidelines and the food plate developed by the U.S. Department of Agriculture.

7.9 Identify food-related diseases.

MEDICAL ASSISTING COMPETENCIES

COMPETENCY	CMA	RMA	CCMA	NCMA
General/Legal/Professional				
Instruct individuals according to their needs	X	X	X	X
Provide patients with methods of health promotion and disease prevention	X	X	X	
Use appropriate medical terminology	X	X	X	X

7.1 Nutrition

Nutrients: Chemical substances that are necessary for growth, normal functioning, and maintaining life. There are six basic groups of nutrients: carbohydrates, fats, proteins, vitamins, minerals, and water.

Overweight: Having a body weight that is between 10% and 20% greater than the standard for the person's age, height, and body type.

Obesity: Excessive accumulation of fat in the body. Also, weight that is at least 20% higher than that considered desirable for the person's age, height, and bone structure. The focus of treatment for obesity, and diseases associated with obesity, is referred to as *bariatrics*.

Body mass index (BMI): A number calculated from a person's weight and height. BMI provides a good indicator of the amount of body fat.

Malnutrition: Poor nutrition caused by poor diet or by poor utilization of food that may result from an unbalanced, insufficient, or excessive diet.

Metabolism: The chemical changes that take place inside living cells. As a result of metabolism, an organism may grow, maintain body functions, release or store energy, produce and eliminate waste, digest nutrients, and destroy toxins.

7.2 Water

Water: Water has no caloric value but contributes about 65% of an individual's body weight, helps maintain fluid balance, dissolves chemicals and nutrients, transports nutrients, lubricates, aids in digestion, flushes out wastes, and regulates body temperature through perspiration.

Amount of water in human cells: Water is the largest single component of the body. Total body water is higher in athletes than in nonathletes and decreases significantly with age because of diminished muscle mass.

Amount of water needed: On average, people should drink six–eight glasses (48–64 ounces, or three–four pints) of water a day to maintain a healthy water balance.

Thirst: Water intake is controlled mainly by thirst. Thirst control centers are located in the hypothalamus.

Effects of water loss: The loss of 20% of body water may cause death, and the loss of only 10% causes severe disorders. In moderate weather, adults can live up to 10 days without water; children can live up to five days. By contrast, it is possible to survive without food for several weeks.

Dehydration: Excessive loss of body water that usually is accompanied by electrolyte balance changes.

Water intoxication: The presence of excess water that causes cells, particularly brain cells, to swell, leading to headache, nausea, vomiting, convulsion, and death. Water intoxication may result from the excessive administration of water when the antidiuretic hormone and the kidney cannot respond, such as after surgery, trauma, or another condition that causes salt and water loss.

7.3 Carbohydrates

Carbohydrate: The body's primary source of energy. Carbohydrates provide heat, help metabolize fat, and help reserve protein for uses other than supplying energy. One gram of carbohydrate yields four kilocalories of energy. Excess carbohydrates are stored in the liver and muscles as glycogen. Carbohydrates should provide 55%–60% of an individual's total calorie intake.

Starch: A complex carbohydrate that is a major source of energy from plant foods.

Dietary fiber: A nondigestible carbohydrate found in plant cells. It provides bulk and stimulation for the intestines. The main dietary fiber components are cellulose, pectin, lignin, and gums. Dietary fiber is used to treat and prevent constipation, hemorrhoids, diverticular disease, and irritable bowel syndrome.

7.4 Lipids

Fats: Also called lipids, fats are not soluble in water but are soluble in some solvents such as alcohol. They provide energy and heat, carry fat-soluble vitamins, protect and support organs and bones, insulate from cold, and supply essential fatty acids. Each gram of fat provides nine kilocalories of energy. Fats are classified as saturated or unsaturated; unsaturated fats are either monounsaturated or polyunsaturated.

Saturated fats: Fats generally derived from animal sources and usually solid at room temperature. Found in meat, butter, egg yolks, whole milk, and coconut and palm oil, they tend to raise blood cholesterol levels.

Unsaturated fats: Fats that are usually liquid at room temperature and can be monounsaturated or polyunsaturated. They tend to lower blood cholesterol levels.

Monounsaturated fats: Examples include oil from olives, avocados, or cashew nuts.

Polyunsaturated fats: Examples include cooking oils made from sunflower seeds, peanuts, or safflower seeds.

Ketones: Chemical substances that are broken down by fatty acids in the liver.

Ketosis: The abnormal collection of ketones in the blood as a result of excessive breakdown of fats caused by an insufficiency of glucose available for energy.

Cholesterol: A waxy lipid found almost exclusively in foods of animal origin and continuously synthesized in the body. Produced by the liver, cholesterol is essential for the production of vitamin D and bile acid. Because the body produces cholesterol, it is not essential in the diet. Cholesterol is measured by means of a blood test. See Table 7-1.

High-density lipoprotein (HDL): Called "good" cholesterol. It helps transport cholesterol to the liver where it is disposed. It may serve to stabilize very low-density lipoprotein.

Low-density lipoprotein (LDL): Called "bad" cholesterol. A high concentration may result in atherosclerosis and thus puts patients at risk of heart disease. LDL carries cholesterol from the liver to the arterial endothelium.

Cholesterolemia: The presence of an excessive amount of cholesterol in the blood.

Triglyceride: One of several combinations of fatty acids and glycerol that circulate in the blood with HDL and LDL. High levels are associated with atherosclerosis.

7.5 Protein

Protein: The primary function of protein is to build and repair body tissues. It is the only substance that can make new cells and rebuild tissue. They are important components of hormones and enzymes. They maintain fluid balance, are essential for the development of antibodies, and can provide energy. Each gram of protein provides four kilocalories of energy. Proteins are not as efficient as carbohydrates and fats in providing energy.

Amino acids: Nitrogen-containing compounds that make up proteins, also called the building blocks of protein.

Classification of amino acids: There are about 80 amino acids, of which 20 are necessary for human metabolism and growth. The adult body does not produce nine of them, which must be provided in the diet and are known as essential amino acids. See Table 7-2 for a list of the essential and nonessential amino acids.

Complete protein: Contains all the essential amino acids and consequently is of high biological value. Casein (milk protein) and egg whites are examples of complete proteins.

Sources of protein: Meat, fish, poultry, eggs, and milk, which are complete proteins, and nuts, dry beans, grains, and vegetables, which are incomplete proteins.

Adequate protein intake: Learning to combine foods containing incomplete proteins in order to obtain all nine essential amino acids is especially important for people who follow vegetarian diets.

7.6 Vitamins

Vitamin: An organic compound that does not provide energy but helps in the metabolism of protein, carbohydrates, and fat. Vitamins act as catalysts and body regulators for the bones, skin, glands, nerves, brain, and blood, and they protect against diseases caused by nutritional deficiencies. There are two types of vitamins: water soluble and fat soluble. See Table 7-3.

Water-Soluble Vitamins

Vitamin B$_1$ (thiamine): Plays a role in carbohydrate metabolism and is essential for normal metabolism of the nervous system, heart, and muscles. Thiamine also promotes good appetite. Sources include lean pork, wheat germ, lean meat, egg yolk, and fish. Deficiency causes loss of appetite, irritability,

AT A GLANCE — **Common Nutrition-Related Blood Tests**

Test	Normal Range in Adults
Cholesterol	Total: 150–200 mg/dL
	HDL: 25–90 mg/dL
	LDL: 85–200 mg/dL
Glucose	90–120 mg/dL
Iron	50–175 µg/dL
Triglycerides	200–300 mg/dL

Table 7-1

AT A GLANCE — **Amino Acids**

Essential	Nonessential
Arginine (in young children)	Alanine
Histidine	Arginine (in adults)
Isoleucine	Asparagine
Leucine	Aspartic acid
Lysine	Cysteine
Methionine	Glutamic acid
Phenylalanine	Glutamine
Threonine	Glycine
Tryptophan	Proline
Valine	Serine
	Tyrosine

Table 7-2

AT A GLANCE | Classification of Vitamins

Table 7-3

Water-Soluble Vitamins	Fat-Soluble Vitamins
Vitamin B complex:	Vitamin A
Thiamine (vitamin B_1)	Vitamin D
Riboflavin (vitamin B_2)	Vitamin E
Niacin (vitamin B_3)	Vitamin K
Pyridoxine (vitamin B_6)	
Folic acid (vitamin B_9)	
Cyanocobalamin (vitamin B_{12})	
Pantothenic acid	
Biotin (formerly vitamin H)	
Vitamin C	

tiredness, sleep disturbance, nervous disorders, beriberi, loss of coordination, paralysis, and Wernicke-Korsakoff syndrome in people severely dependent on alcohol. Deficiency is often associated with alcoholism.

Vitamin B_2 (riboflavin): Is essential for certain enzyme systems in the metabolism of fats and proteins. It can be sensitive to light. Sources include milk, cheddar cheese, cottage cheese, organ meats, and eggs. Deficiency causes impaired growth, weakness, lip sores and cracks at the corners of the mouth, cheilosis, photophobia, cataracts, anemia, and glossitis.

Vitamin B_3 (niacin): Part of two enzymes that regulate energy metabolism. Also called nicotinic acid and nicotinamide, it maintains the health of the skin, tongue, and digestive system. Sources include lean meats, poultry, fish, and peanuts. Deficiency causes pellagra, gastrointestinal disturbance, and mental disturbances.

Vitamin B_6 (pyridoxine): Aids enzymes in the synthesis of amino acids and is essential for proper growth and maintenance of body functions. Sources include yeast, wheat germ, pork, bananas, and oatmeal. Deficiency causes anemia, neuritis, anorexia, nausea, depressed immunity, and dermatitis.

Vitamin B_9 (folic acid): Is essential for cell growth and the reproduction of RBCs. Also called folacin, it functions in the formation of hemoglobin and aids in metabolism of protein. It is also essential for fetal development, particularly of the neural tube. Sources include liver, kidney beans, lima beans, and fresh dark-green leafy vegetables. Deficiency causes anemia and may cause spina bifida in a fetus.

Vitamin B_{12} (cyanocobalamin): Aids in hemoglobin synthesis, is essential for normal functioning of all cells, and is important in energy metabolism. Sources include liver, kidney, milk, eggs, fish, and cheese. Deficiency causes pernicious anemia and neurological disorders.

Pantothenic acid: A part of the vitamin B complex that is essential for fatty acid metabolism, the manufacture of sex hormones, the utilization of other vitamins, the functioning of the nervous system and the adrenal glands, and normal growth and development. Sources include egg yolks, kidney, liver, and yeast. Deficiency causes fatigue, headaches, nausea, abdominal pain, numbness, tingling, muscle cramps, and susceptibility to respiratory infections and peptic ulcers.

Biotin (formerly vitamin H): A water-soluble B-complex vitamin essential for the breakdown of fatty acids and carbohydrates and for the excretion of the waste products of protein breakdown. Good sources include kidney, liver, egg yolks, soybeans, and yeast.

Vitamin C: Also called ascorbic acid, it protects the body against infections and helps heal wounds. Best sources are fruits and vegetables, especially citrus fruits and tomatoes. Deficiency causes scurvy, lowered resistance to infections, joint tenderness, dental caries, bleeding gums, delayed wound healing, bruising, hemorrhage, and anemia. Vitamin C is lost in cooking fresh foods but not in cooking frozen foods.

Fat-Soluble Vitamins

Vitamin A (retinol, carotene): Contributes to the maintenance of epithelial cells and mucous membranes and is important for night vision. Retinol is also necessary for normal growth, development, and reproduction as well as an adequate immune response. Sources include liver, beef, sweet potato, spinach, milk, and egg yolks. Deficiency causes retarded growth, susceptibility to infection, dry skin, night blindness, xeropthalmia, abnormal gastrointestinal function, dry mucous membranes, and degeneration of the spinal cord and peripheral nerves.

Vitamin D: Is essential for the normal formation of bones and teeth. It aids in the reabsorption of calcium and phosphorus and regulates blood levels of calcium. There are two major forms of vitamin D: vitamin D_2, formed in plants, and vitamin D_3, formed in humans from cholesterol in the skin exposed to sunlight or other ultraviolet radiation. Best sources are butter, cream, egg yolks, liver, and fish liver oils. Deficiency causes rickets and osteomalacia.

Vitamin E: An antioxidant, also called tocopherol. It prevents oxidative destruction of vitamin A in the intestine, and it is essential for normal reproduction, muscle development, and resistance of RBCs to hemolysis. Vitamin E also helps maintain normal cell membranes. Sources include seed oil, fruits, vegetables, and animal fats.

Vitamin K: Is essential to blood clotting. There are several fat-soluble compounds of vitamin K. Vitamin K_2 is synthesized in the intestine by bacteria and is also found in animal foods. Vitamin K is found in large amounts in green leafy vegetables (especially broccoli, cabbage, and lettuce) and in fruits. Vitamin K can be used as an antidote for an overdose of an anticoagulant. Deficiency causes hemorrhage.

Conditions Associated with Vitamins

Avitaminosis: Deficiency of vitamins in the diet that causes a disease such as scurvy, rickets, or beriberi. See Table 7-4 for symptoms and diseases caused by vitamin deficiency.

Vitamin	Symptoms and Diseases
Vitamin A	Retarded growth, susceptibility to infection, dry skin, night blindness, xeropthalmia, abnormal gastrointestinal function, dry mucous membranes, degeneration of the spinal cord and peripheral nerves
Vitamin B_1	Loss of appetite, irritability, tiredness, nervous disorders, sleep disturbance, beriberi, loss of coordination, paralysis, Wernicke-Korsakoff syndrome
Vitamin B_2	Impaired growth, weakness, lip sores and cracks at the corners of the mouth, cheilosis, photophobia, cataracts, anemia, glossitis (Riboflavin deficiency is believed to be the most common vitamin deficiency in the United States.)
Vitamin B_3	Pellagra, characterized by dermatitis, diarrhea, dementia, and death; gastrointestinal and mental disturbances
Vitamin B_6	Anemia, neuritis, anorexia, nausea, depressed immunity, dermatitis
Vitamin B_9 (folic acid)	Anemia, spina bifida in fetal development
Vitamin B_{12}	Pernicious anemia, neurological disorders
Pantothenic acid	Fatigue, headaches, nausea, abdominal pain, numbness, tingling, muscle cramps, susceptibility to respiratory infections and peptic ulcers
Vitamin C	Scurvy, characterized by gingivitis, loose teeth, and slow healing of wounds; lowered resistance to infections; joint tenderness; dental caries; bleeding gums; delayed wound healing; bruising; hemorrhage; anemia
Vitamin D	Rickets and osteomalacia
Vitamin K	Hemorrhage (Extensive oral antibiotic therapy may cause vitamin K_2 deficiency.)

Table 7-4

Hypervitaminosis: A condition caused by an overdose of vitamins, especially fat-soluble vitamins. The main symptoms are loss of hair, severe itching, skin lesions, and abnormal tissue growth.

Excessive intake of vitamin A: Can result in a condition called hypervitaminosis A, the symptoms of which include headache, tiredness, nausea, loss of appetite, diarrhea, dry and itchy skin, hair loss, a yellow discoloration, and irregular menstrual periods. Excessive intake during pregnancy may cause birth defects.

Excessive intake of vitamin B_6: May cause neuritis.

7.7 Minerals

Minerals: Natural, inorganic substances that the body needs to help build and maintain body tissues and to carry on life functions. There are two separate classes of minerals: major minerals and trace elements. Diseases and symptoms associated with mineral deficiencies are listed in Table 7-5. Deficiencies of calcium, iron, and iodine are the three most common mineral deficiencies.

Electrolytes: Compounds, particularly salts, that break up into their separate component particles in water. The particles are called ions, which are electrically charged atoms. Sodium, potassium, and chloride are commonly called electrolytes. Minerals help keep the body's water and electrolytes in balance.

Major Minerals

Calcium (Ca): The body requires calcium for the transmission of nerve impulses, muscle contraction, blood coagulation, and cardiac functions. Calcium also helps build strong bones and teeth and may prevent hypertension. Normal daily requirement: 800–1,200 mg. The following factors enhance the absorption of calcium: adequate vitamin D, large quantities of calcium and phosphorus in diet, and the presence of lactose. A lack of physical activity reduces the amount of calcium absorption.

Phosphorus (P): Essential for the metabolism of protein, calcium, and glucose. It helps to build strong bones and teeth and aids in maintaining the body's acid-base balance. Phosphorus is found in dairy foods, animal foods, fish, cereals, nuts, and legumes.

Chloride (Cl): Involved in the maintenance of fluid and the body's acid-base balance. Disturbances in the acid-base balance can result in possible growth retardation and memory loss.

Sodium (Na): Plays a key role in the maintenance of the body's acid-base balance. It transmits nerve impulses and helps control muscle contractions. Toxic levels may cause hypertension and

Mineral	Symptoms and Diseases
Calcium	Rickets, osteomalacia (adult rickets), tetany, osteoporosis
Copper	Anemia, bone disease (Copper deficiency is very rare in adults.)
Fluoride	Tooth decay, possibly osteoporosis
Iodine	Goiter, cretinism (congenital myxedema) (Goiter is more common among women. A thyroid gland dysfunction can cause acquired myxedema, commonly known as hypothyroidism, in adults.)
Iron	Iron-deficiency anemia, nutritional anemia
Phosphorus	Weight loss, anemia, anorexia, fatigue, abnormal growth, bone demineralization (mineral loss)
Potassium	Impaired growth, hypertension, bone fragility, renal hypertrophy, bradycardia, death
Zinc	Dwarfism, delayed growth, hypogonadism, anemia, decreased appetite

Table 7-5

renal disease. The kidney is the chief regulator of sodium levels in body fluids.

Potassium (K): Important in protein synthesis, correction of imbalance in acid-base metabolism, and glycogen formation. It transmits nerve impulses and helps control them. It also promotes regular heartbeat and is needed for enzyme reactions.

Magnesium (Mg): Helps build strong bones and teeth and activates many enzymes. It helps regulate heartbeat and is essential for metabolism and many enzyme activities. It is stored in bone and is excreted mainly by the kidneys.

Trace Elements

Iodine (I): A component of the thyroid hormone thyroxine. Iodine is also used as a contrast medium for blood vessels in computed tomography (CT) scans.

Zinc (Zn): Essential for several enzymes, growth, glucose tolerance, wound healing, and taste acuity. Best sources are protein foods.

Iron (Fe): A component of hemoglobin and myoglobin. The major role of iron is to deliver oxygen to the body tissues.

Ferrous sulfate (*Feosol*): The most inexpensive and most commonly used form of iron supplement.

Iron dextran (*Imferon*): An injectable form of iron supplement.

Hemochromatosis: Excessive absorption of iron.

Copper (Cu): An element most concentrated in the liver, heart, brain, and kidneys. It is essential for several important enzymes and for good health. It aids in the formation of hemoglobin. Copper helps in the transportation of iron to bone marrow.

Wilson's disease: A hereditary disease that causes copper accumulation in various organs and can result in degeneration of the brain, cirrhosis of the liver, psychic disturbances, and progressive weakness.

Fluoride: An element that increases resistance to tooth decay. It protects against osteoporosis and periodontal (gum) disease. Excessive amounts of fluoride in drinking water may cause the discoloration of teeth.

7.8 Nutrition and Diet Needs

Dietary guidelines: Developed by the U.S. Department of Agriculture and the U.S. Department of Health and Human Services, recommendations to encourage people to eat a balanced diet. Table 7-6 lists the guidelines.

MyPlate and Healthy Eating Pyramid: MyPlate is a diagram introduced by the U.S. Department of Agriculture to show the quantities of food people should consume daily from each of the basic food groups. See Figure 7-1. Also see Table 7-7, which provides information on serving sizes. Some patients may have special dietary preferences or choices. Vegetarians do not eat meat, poultry, and fish. Figure 7-2 shows the Harvard Healthy Eating Pyramid, which illustrates the foods that should be consumed in the daily diet in appropriate quantities.

Therapeutic nutrition: Also referred to as medical nutrition therapy or a therapeutic diet. It may be necessary in order to maintain or improve nutritional status; to correct nutritional

Eat a variety of foods to get the energy, protein, vitamins, minerals, and fiber you need for good health.

Balance the food you eat with physical activity.

Choose a diet with plenty of grain products, vegetables, and fruits.

Choose a diet low in fat, saturated fat, and cholesterol.

Choose a diet moderate in sugars.

Choose a diet moderate in salt and sodium.

If you drink alcoholic beverages, do so in moderation.

Table 7-6

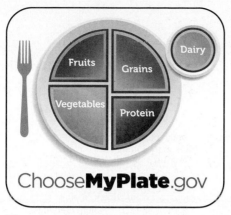

Figure 7-1 *The U.S. Department of Agriculture's Food Guide MyPlate can be used to plan a nutritious, well-balanced diet.* Source: Choose MyPlate.gov. U.S. Department of Agriculture.

deficiencies; to maintain, decrease, or increase body weight; or to eliminate particular foods that may cause allergies.

Nutrition during pregnancy: The protein requirement is increased by 20% for pregnant women. An increase is also recommended in calcium, iron, and folic acid intake. The average energy allowance during the first trimester is 2,200 Kcal per day. Lactating women during the first six months need 2,700 Kcal per day. Doctors recommend that pregnant women gain 24–35 pounds during their pregnancy.

Breastfeeding: The mother's milk provides the infant with temporary immunity to many infectious diseases. It is free from germs and is easy to digest. It usually does not cause allergic reactions. Breastfeeding also stimulates an emotional bond between mother and infant. The American Academy of Pediatrics recommends breastfeeding for at least one year, and the World Health Organization recommends two years. In most

AT A GLANCE   Recommended Serving Sizes

Food Group	Food and Quantity
Grains	1 slice bread
	1 oz. dry cereal
	½ cup cooked rice, pasta, or cereal
Vegetables	1 cup raw leafy vegetable
	½ cup cut-up raw or cooked vegetable
	½ cup vegetable juice
Fruits	1 medium fruit
	¼ cup dried fruit
	½ cup fresh, frozen, or canned fruit
	½ cup fruit juice
Fat-free or low-fat milk and milk products	1 cup milk or yogurt
	½ oz. cheese
Lean meats, poultry, and fish	1 oz. cooked meats, poultry, or fish
	1 egg
Nuts, seeds, and legumes	⅓ cup or 1½ oz. nuts
	2 Tbsp. peanut butter
	2 Tbsp. or ½ oz. seeds
	½ cup cooked legumes (dried beans, peas)
Fats and oils	1 tsp. soft margarine
	1 tsp. vegetable oil
	1 Tbsp. mayonnaise
	1 Tbsp. salad dressing

Nutrition and Your Health: Dietary Guidelines for Americans, 5th ed. (Washington, DC: U.S. Department of Agriculture and U.S. Department of Health and Human Services, 2010).

Table 7-7

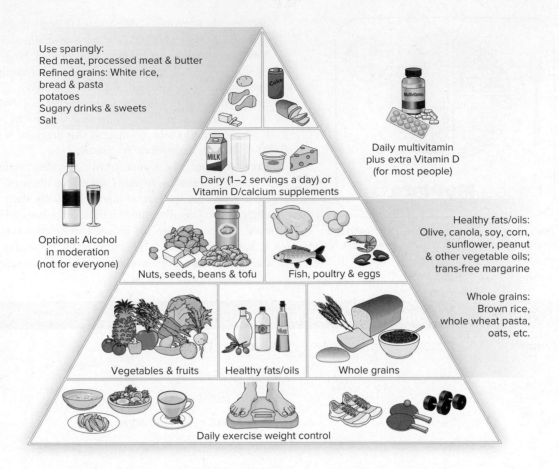

Figure 7-2 *The Healthy Eating Pyramid established by the Department of Nutrition, Harvard School of Public Health.*
Source: Adapted from The Healthy Eating Pyramid, Department of Nutrition, Harvard School of Public Health.

cases breastfeeding is the best source of milk for a growing child.

Mechanical soft diet: A diet that consists of soft but otherwise normal foods. It is used by individuals who have difficulty chewing because of a lack of dentures or teeth, inflammation of the oral cavity, or severe dental decay that may cause pain in chewing.

Liquid diet: A diet used by individuals who cannot tolerate solid foods or by patients whose gastrointestinal tract must be free of solid foods. The diet consists of tea, coffee, cream soups, fruit juices, clear broths, and eggnog.

Tube feeding: A diet used for patients with indications such as esophageal obstruction, burns, gastric surgery, or anorexia nervosa.

Bland diet: A diet that is nonirritating to the gastrointestinal tract. It is often prescribed in the treatment of peptic ulcer, ulcerative colitis, gallbladder disease, diverticulitis, and gastritis. This diet consists of milk, cream, mashed potatoes, and hot cereal.

High-fiber diet: A diet that may be prescribed for atonic constipation, diverticulosis, therapy of gastric ulcers, cancer of the colon, hypercholesterolemia, diabetes, or obesity.

Diabetic diet: A diet prescribed in the treatment of diabetes mellitus. It usually contains limited amounts of simple sugars and increased amounts of proteins, complex carbohydrates, and unsaturated fats. This diet is carefully calculated for each patient to minimize the occurrence of hyperglycemia and hypoglycemia, to maintain body weight, and to promote good health.

Dumping syndrome diet: A diet used for patients who have had a partial gastrectomy or gastric bypass surgery. This diet is low in concentrated sweets and limits fluids at mealtimes to avoid dumping the stomach contents into the small intestine, which results in diarrhea.

Restricted-fat diet: A diet used for patients with diseases of the liver, gallbladder, and pancreas. Generally 40–50 grams of fat per day is an adequate and realistic restriction.

Low-cholesterol diet: A diet often recommended for patients with elevated blood cholesterol levels, those with atherosclerosis, and those with elevated triglycerides and low HDL cholesterol.

High-fat diet: A diet that may be indicated for purposes of weight gain. Ideally, the fat should be monounsaturated. The maximum fat intake is generally 35%–40% of kilocalories.

Restricted-sodium diet: A diet that is very common for patients with hypertension, renal disease with edema, congestive heart failure, and cirrhosis of the liver with ascites.

Increased-sodium diet: A diet that may be useful in treating Addison's disease.

Restricted-potassium diet: A diet that may be necessary for patients with renal disease.

Increased-potassium diet: A diet used for patients who are on diuretics. Sources of potassium in the diet are whole grains, meat, legumes, fruit (bananas), and vegetables.

High-iron diet: A diet to treat iron-deficiency anemia.

High-calcium and high-phosphorus diets: An increase in calcium and phosphorus intake is desirable in a patient with rickets, osteomalacia, tetany, dental caries, or acute lead poisoning.

Restricted-copper diet: A diet to treat Wilson's disease, oliguria, and anuria.

Vegetarian diet: A diet that focuses on plants for food and excludes all types of meat. Types of vegetarian diets include *lacto-vegetarian* (which includes dairy products), *lacto-ovo vegetarian* (which includes dairy products and eggs), *ovo-vegetarian* (which includes eggs but excludes dairy products), and *vegan* (which includes only plant foods).

Instructing a patient with special dietary needs: Many patients have specific dietary needs that are based on medical conditions. Medical assistants should instruct patients with such needs using appropriate brochures and other types of information. Examples of patients with special dietary needs include those with hypertension, congestive heart failure, or diabetes, as well as women who are pregnant or breastfeeding.

7.9 Food-Related Diseases

Food poisoning: An illness usually caused by human ignorance or carelessness. Food is generally contaminated with harmful microorganisms or chemical poisons. The most common food illnesses are caused by *Salmonella* bacteria, *Clostridium perfringens, Staphylococcus aureus,* and protozoa. Examples of food illnesses include botulism and trichinosis.

Trichinosis: Infestation with the parasitic roundworm *Trichinella spiralis.* It is transmitted by eating raw or undercooked pork from infected pigs.

Botulism: Caused by the toxin produced by the spores of the *Clostridium botulinum* bacterium. It is the most deadly of all food poisonings. Home-canned foods are generally the source of botulism. The antitoxin must be administered as soon as possible.

Food allergies: Usually develop as a reaction to proteins. Allergies to specific substances are not inherited, but the tendency to develop allergies is inherited. Allergic individuals seem most prone to allergic reactions during periods of stress.

Anorexia nervosa: An eating disorder in which people starve themselves because they fear that otherwise they will become grossly overweight. It is most common among women in their teens and early 20s.

Bulimia: An eating disorder in which people eat a large amount of food in a short time, then attempt to counter the effects by self-induced vomiting, the use of laxatives or diuretics, and/or excessive exercise.

Binge eating: Eating a large amount of food in a short time without subsequent purging.

STRATEGIES FOR SUCCESS

▶ *Test-Taking Skills*

Use your time wisely!
Learn to budget your time while taking the exam. When you practice answering the questions at the back of this book set a timer for 60 minutes and see whether you can answer 60 questions in that length of time. If you can't answer a question right away, don't panic. Move on to the next question, and come back at the end of the exam to any questions you've left blank. Sometimes other questions may jog your memory and help you get those elusive answers.

Instructions:

Answer the following questions.

1. Which of the following nutrients are the body's primary source of energy?

   A. proteins
   B. vitamins
   C. amino acids
   D. fats
   E. carbohydrates

2. One gram of carbohydrate yields _____ Kcal.

   A. four
   B. six
   C. eight
   D. nine
   E. 10

3. Which of the following is called "good" cholesterol?

   A. HDL
   B. LDL
   C. VLDL
   D. triglycerides
   E. none of these

4. How many amino acids are essential to include in a person's diet because they cannot be produced by the adult human body?

   A. 9
   B. 11
   C. 20
   D. 22
   E. 30

5. Olive oil is an example of a

   A. polyunsaturated fat.
   B. protein.
   C. saturated fat.
   D. vitamin.
   E. monounsaturated fat.

6. The best source of vitamin C (ascorbic acid) is

   A. liver.
   B. fruits.
   C. soybeans.
   D. egg yolk.
   E. yogurt.

7. Zinc deficiency may result in all of the following *except*

   A. dwarfism.
   B. delayed growth.
   C. hypogonadism.
   D. anemia.
   E. acromegaly.

8. Calcium deficiency may result in all of the following disorders *except*

   A. tetany.
   B. rickets.
   C. renal hypertrophy.
   D. osteomalacia.
   E. osteoporosis.

9. Iodine deficiency may cause

   A. cretinism (congenital myxedema).
   B. anemia.
   C. rickets.
   D. osteoporosis.
   E. hypertension.

10. Vitamin D deficiency can cause

    A. dry skin.
    B. rickets.
    C. night blindness.
    D. osteomalacia.
    E. rickets and osteomalacia.

MEDICAL LAW AND ETHICS

LEARNING OUTCOMES

8.1 Recognize the types of law and terminology related to the court and legal systems, including violations of the law.

8.2 Recall the legal requirements in medicine, including confidentiality, protecting patient privacy, malpractice, records management, and HIPAA.

8.3 Identify common ethical issues in the medical field, including abortion, and organ and tissue donation and transplantation.

8.4 Identify medical and legal issues related to death and dying.

MEDICAL ASSISTING COMPETENCIES

COMPETENCY	CMA	RMA	CCMA	NCMA
Prepare, organize, and maintain medical records	X	X	X	X
General/Legal/Professional				
Demonstrate proper telephone techniques	X	X	X	X
Identify and respond to issues of confidentiality by maintaining confidentiality at all times and following appropriate guidelines when releasing records or information	X	X	X	X
Be aware of and perform within legal and ethical boundaries	X	X	X	X
Determine the needs for documentation and reporting, and document accurately and appropriately	X	X	X	X
Demonstrate knowledge of and monitor current federal and state health-care legislation and regulations; maintain licenses and accreditation	X	X	X	X
Follow established policy in initiating or terminating medical treatment	X	X	X	X
Perform risk management procedures	X	X	X	
Be courteous and diplomatic	X	X	X	

MEDICAL ASSISTING COMPETENCIES (cont.)

General/Legal/Professional

Conduct work within scope of education, training, and ability	X	X	X	X
Be impartial and show empathy when dealing with patients	X	X	X	
Use appropriate medical terminology	X	X	X	X
Receive, organize, prioritize, and transmit information appropriately	X	X	X	X
Understand allied health professions and credentialing	X	X	X	

STRATEGIES FOR SUCCESS

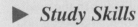 **Study Skills**

Set goals!
The CMA, RMA, and CCMA exams cover a lot of material, and it's not uncommon to feel stressed in trying to review it all. Try to make your workload easier by prioritizing and setting goals. Create a schedule to review material and set aside time to practice answering exam questions. If there is a certain topic you know you have difficulty with, make sure that you devote more time to review it and less time to something you know you already understand.

8.1 Law

Law: A body of regulations that govern society and that people are obligated to observe.

Sources of law: The U.S. Constitution divides the federal government into three equal branches: the legislative branch, which passes laws; the executive branch, which implements laws; and the judicial branch, which interprets laws.

Types of Law

Common law: Law that derives authority from ancient usages and customs affirmed by court judgments and decrees. It is created by the judicial branch through decisions in court cases.

Criminal law: Law dealing with criminal offenses and their punishments.

Private law: The legal rights defining the relationship between private entities.

Public law: The legal rights defining the relationship between the government and the governed.

Case law: Law established by judicial decision in legal cases and used as legal precedent.

Civil law: Rules that govern private rights and remedies, as well as disputes between individuals regarding contracts, property, and family law. It is separate from criminal or public law.

The Legal System

Defendant: The person or group accused in a court action.

Plaintiff: A person who files a lawsuit initiating a civil legal action. In criminal actions, the prosecution is the plaintiff, acting on behalf of the people.

Litigant: A party to a lawsuit.

Litigation: A lawsuit or a contest in court.

Jurisdiction: The power, right, and authority given to a court to hear a case and to make a judgment.

Layperson: An individual who does not have training in a specific profession.

Violations of the Law

Crime: An act that violates a criminal law.

Criminal: A person who has committed a crime or who has been proven guilty of a crime.

Accessory: A person who contributes to or aids in the commission of a crime, by either a direct or an indirect act.

Felony: An offense punishable by death or by imprisonment in a state or federal prison. It is a serious crime, such as murder, kidnapping, assault, or rape. Punishment is usually severe: a prison sentence for more than 1 year or, in some cases, death.

Misdemeanor: A crime that is less serious than a felony and consequently carries a lesser penalty. It is punishable by fine or by imprisonment in a facility other than a prison for less than one year.

Tort: A civil wrong committed against a person or property, excluding a breach of contract. A tort is the most common civil claim in medical law. When one person intentionally harms another, the law allows the injured party to seek remedy in a civil suit. If the conduct is judged to be malicious, punitive damages may also be awarded.

Intentional torts: Assault, battery, defamation of character, false imprisonment, fraud, invasion of privacy, trespass, and infliction of emotional distress. Intentional torts may also be crimes. Therefore, some civil wrongs may also be prosecuted criminal acts in separate court actions.

The four Ds of negligence: Duty, dereliction (breach), damage, and direct causation. The patient must show that the physician–patient relationship existed, in which the physician owed the patient a *duty*. Patients must show that the physician failed to comply with the standards of the profession (which is *dereliction*). The patient must prove that an injury *(damage)* was suffered. The patient must also show that any damages were a direct cause of the physician's breach of duty *(direct causation)*.

Assault: A willful attempt or threat by a person to injure another person with the apparent ability to do so.

Defamation: Spoken or written words about a person that are both false and malicious and that injure that person's reputation or means of livelihood and for which damages can be recovered. Defamation can take the form of libel or slander.

Libel: Defamatory writing, such as published material or pictures.

Slander: Defamatory spoken words.

False imprisonment: The intentional, unlawful restraint or confinement of a person. Refusing to dismiss a patient from a health-care facility upon his or her request or preventing a patient from leaving the facility may be seen as false imprisonment.

Fraud: Dishonest and deceitful practices undertaken in order to induce someone to part with something of value or a legal right.

Invasion of privacy: Intrusion into a person's private affairs and public disclosure of private facts about a person, false publicity about a person, or use of a person's name or likeness without permission. Improper use of or breaching the confidentiality of medical records may be seen as an invasion of privacy.

Abandonment: A situation wherein a patient is provided with insufficient care, or no care at all.

Infliction of emotional distress: Intentionally or recklessly causing emotional or mental suffering to others.

Battery: The unlawful use of force on a person. Also, non-consensual or illegal touching of another person. Any health-care practitioner who fails to receive a formal expression of consent to touch a patient could be charged with battery by the patient.

Trespass: Wrongful injury or interference with the property of another.

Burglary: The act of breaking and entering into a building with intent to commit a felony, especially in order to steal. In a medical building, most burglary attempts are made to steal narcotics.

Misuse of legal procedure: Bringing legal action with malice and without probable cause.

Unintentional torts: The more common torts within the health-care delivery system. Unintentional torts are acts that are not intended to cause harm but are committed unreasonably or with a disregard for the consequences. In legal terms, this constitutes negligence. Negligence is charged when a health-care practitioner fails to exercise ordinary care and a patient is injured as a result.

Tortfeasor: A person who commits a tort either intentionally or unintentionally.

The Court System

Court system: There are both federal and state court systems, and each system has two types of court: lower and higher, or inferior and superior.

Supreme court: There are both state and federal supreme courts. A state supreme court is the highest state court. Its decisions are generally final in matters of state law. The federal Supreme Court is the final court of appeal, the highest court in the United States, sometimes also referred to as the court of last resort.

Appeal: A legal proceeding by which a case is transferred from a lower to a higher court for rehearing.

Motion: An application made to a court or judge to obtain an order, ruling, or direction.

Arbitration: The hearing and determination of a case in controversy, without litigation, by a person chosen by the parties involved or appointed under statutory authority.

Mediation: Intervention between conflicting parties to promote reconciliation, settlement, or compromise.

Summons: An official paper issued by the clerk of the court and delivered with a copy of the complaint to the defendant, directing him or her to respond to the charges.

Subpoena: An official paper ordering a person to appear in court under penalty for failure to do so.

Subpoena *duces tecum:* A legal document requiring the recipient to bring certain records to court to be used as evidence in a lawsuit. Under this court-issued document, an original medical record may be requested for release to and examination by the court.

Witness: A person who can testify under oath to events he or she has heard or observed, such as the signing of a will or a consent form.

Testimony: Statements sworn to under oath by witnesses testifying in court and giving depositions.

Deposition: Sworn pretrial testimony given by a witness in response to written or oral questions and cross-examination. It is made before a public officer for use in a lawsuit, and it may also be presented at the trial if the witness cannot be present.

Perjury: The voluntary violation of an oath to tell the truth; also, a false statement made under oath.

Interrogatory: Formal written questions about a case, addressed to one party by another, that are required to be answered under direction of a court.

Credibility: The quality or power of a witness to inspire belief.

Disposition: The final settlement of a case in criminal law.

Verdict: The finding or decision reached by a jury or judge on the matter submitted to trial.

Bench trial: A trial in which a judge serves without a jury and rules on the law as well as the facts.

Assumption of risk: A legal defense that holds that the defendant is not guilty of a negligent act because the plaintiff knew of and accepted beforehand any risk involved.

Burden of proof: The task of presenting testimony to prove guilt or innocence at a trial.

Statute of limitations: The period of time established by state law during which a lawsuit may be filed.

8.2 The Law and Medicine

Confidentiality: The principle and practice of treating something as a private matter not intended for public knowledge. Confidentiality protects information so that it is not released to anyone unless such release is required by law. Confidentiality is important because it builds trust and maintains patient dignity. Care should also be taken that any information about a patient cannot be overheard by others. Tables 8-1 and 8-2 present principles for preventing the improper release of information.

Releasing medical records: A release permitted only when authorized in writing by the patient or the patient's legal guardian, when ordered by subpoena, or when dictated by statute to protect public health or welfare. The patient or guardian must sign a legal release form before records can be released to another physician or to an insurance company. The unauthorized disclosure of client information can be considered an invasion of privacy.

Maintaining patients' privacy: Keep these considerations in mind when handling sensitive information about patients:

- Do not leave confidential papers anywhere on the copier.
- Do not discard copies in shared trash containers. Always shred them.

- Always verify the telephone number of the receiving location before faxing confidential material.
- Never fax confidential material to an unauthorized person or in a room where others can observe the material. Use a fax cover sheet with a cautionary statement, "Confidential: To addressee only. Please return by mail if received in error."
- Do not leave a computer monitor unattended if confidential material is displayed on it.
- It is recommended that you not send confidential materials via e-mail.
- Do not print confidential material on a printer shared by other departments or in an area where others can see the printed output.
- Do not leave a printer unattended while printing confidential material.

Durable power of attorney: A written document in which one person appoints another to act as his or her agent. This confers authority to the agent to act or function on the behalf of the person making the request.

Privilege: Authority granted to a physician by a hospital governing board to provide patient care in the hospital.

Privileged communication: Information held confidential within a protected relationship, such as attorney-client and physician-patient. Physicians are prohibited from revealing information about clients in court.

Consent: Approval and permission from a patient to allow touching, examination, treatment, or release of medical information by medically authorized personnel. Consent is unnecessary in emergency situations. When more-complex procedures are anticipated, the physician must obtain the patient's informed consent. The patient also must understand that consent may be withdrawn at any time. Types of consent include informed, implied, and expressed consent.

AT A GLANCE — **Principles for Preventing Improper Release of Information from a Medical Office**

It is the patient's right to keep information confidential. If the patient wants to disclose the information, it is unethical for the physician not to do so.

All patients should be treated with the same degree of confidentiality, whatever the health-care professional's personal opinion of the patient might be.

Be aware of all applicable laws, including HIPAA, and of the regulations of agencies such as public health departments.

When it is necessary to break confidentiality, and when there is a conflict between ethics and confidentiality, discuss the matter with the patient. If the law does not dictate what to do in the situation, the attending physician should make the judgment based on the urgency of the situation and any danger that might be posed to the patient or others.

Legally required disclosures include those ordered by subpoena, those dictated by statute to protect public health or welfare, and those considered necessary to protect the welfare of a patient or third party.

Get written approval from the patient before releasing information. For common situations, the patient should sign a standard release of records form.

Table 8-1

Do not disclose information, including whether the person is a patient, to any third party without the patient's signed consent.

Do not decide confidentiality on the basis of whether you approve of or agree with the views or morals of the patient.

Do not reveal financial information about a patient. Be discreet when discussing a patient's account balance so that others in the office waiting room do not overhear.

When talking on the telephone, do not use the caller's name if others in the room might overhear.

Use caution in giving the results of medical tests to patients over the telephone to prevent others in the medical office from overhearing.

When leaving a message at a patient's home or place of employment, simply ask the patient to return a call regarding a recent visit or appointment on a specific date. Do not mention the nature of the call.

It is preferable not to leave a message for a patient to call an oncologist, OB-GYN physician, or other specialist. If test results are abnormal, the physician generally speaks directly to the patient and an appointment is made to discuss the results.

Do not leave medical charts, insurance reports, or patient sign-in sheets where patients or office visitors can see them.

Make sure that the confidentiality protocol is noted in the office procedures manual and that new employees learn it.

Table 8-2

Informed consent: Approval and permission by a mentally competent individual to receive medical services, based on the understanding of all essential information about what will be done, and possible outcomes.

Implied consent: The granting of permission for receiving medical services without a formal agreement between the patient and the provider, such as making an appointment regarding a physical complaint, which implies consent to be treated.

Expressed consent: The granting of permission for medical services via an individual's direct communication with a health-care provider.

Doctrine of informed consent: A legal precept that is usually outlined in a state's medical practice acts. Informed consent implies that the patient understands the proposed modes of treatment, why the treatment is necessary, the risks involved in the proposed treatment, available alternative modes of treatment, the risks of alternative modes of treatment, and the risks involved if treatment is refused. After the patient signs an informed consent form, the medical assistant should document that fact in the patient's chart and note that the patient's questions were answered and that risks and alternative treatments were discussed.

Patient incompetence: A legal term that describes individuals who are unable to properly exercise certain individual rights and options due to mental incapacity.

Mature minor: An individual younger than 18 years of age who has an understanding of the nature and consequences of proposed medical treatment.

Contract: A voluntary agreement between two or more parties in which specific promises are made for a consideration. Health-care delivery occurs under various types of contracts, which must include an agreement, a consideration, legal subject matter, and the contractual capacity of the signing parties to understand the contract.

Good Samaritan Act: A statute that provides immunity from liability to volunteers at the scene of an accident who render emergency care. Today all 50 states have Good Samaritan statutes. They provide a measure of protection to physicians who might otherwise be discouraged by the possibility of a lawsuit from intervening at accident sites.

Mandatory reports: Statutory reports that must be submitted by physicians on a regular basis to various governmental agencies. Certain reports are required from all practicing physicians, including reports of births, deaths, and cases of food poisoning and communicable diseases (AIDS, hepatitis, neonatal herpes, Lyme disease, rabies, and sexually transmitted diseases). Communicable disease information can be released by the physician without written consent from the patient. Physicians also need to report known or suspected abuse of any individual (child, elderly adult, or battered spouse), drug abuse, and criminal acts (indicated by injuries resulting from violence, such as gunshot or stab wounds).

Birth certificate: A legal document that records information about a birth. It is used throughout a person's life to prove age, parentage, and citizenship. It also tells whether a certified midwife was present at birth.

Minor: A person who has not reached the age of majority, or legal age. The age of majority is 18 years in most jurisdictions, 21 in some. Minors usually cannot consent to their own medical treatment unless they are substantially independent of their parents (emancipated minors), are married, or are in other ways self-sufficient. Based on state law, minors may seek medical treatment without parental consent for birth control, pregnancy, and sexually transmitted diseases.

Standard of care: The degree of care that a reasonably prudent person should exercise under the same or similar circumstances.

Medical practice acts: State laws that govern the practice of medicine. Nonlicensed personnel may perform clinical procedures while employed by licensed physicians. These acts (which are classified as *mandates)* differ by state, but are designed to monitor and discipline doctors. They are enforced by state medical boards.

Medical boards: Boards established by each state's medical practice act to protect the health, safety, and welfare of health-care consumers by licensing health-care practitioners.

Protocol: A written plan specifying the procedures to be followed in giving a particular examination. It is also the rules or standards of behavior applicable to one's place of employment.

Patient's Bill of Rights: A statement by the American Hospital Association that guarantees patients certain rights, as shown in Table 8-3.

Defensive medicine: The practice of performing medical tests and procedures in order to protect against future liability and to document the health-care provider's judgment.

Forensic medicine: A division of medicine that involves medical issues or medical proof at trials having to do with malpractice, crimes, and accidents.

Equal Employment Opportunity Commission (EEOC): A body appointed by the president of the United States to administer the Civil Rights Act of 1964, primarily to investigate complaints of discrimination in employment among businesses engaged in interstate commerce.

Public health statutes: Regulations set forth by individual states to promote the health and well-being of a specific population.

Complying with public health statutes: By following these state regulations, there are proven reductions in communicable diseases, abuse, neglect, exploitation, and injuries caused by violence.

Locum tenens: A Latin term meaning "to hold a place." For example, a "locum tenens physician" fills in for other physicians on a temporary basis, typically for a few days to six months.

Malpractice

Medical malpractice: Medical professional misconduct, also called professional negligence. It stems from a lack of the professional knowledge, experience, or skill that is expected from practitioners and results in injury or harm to the patient. The most common malpractice claims against physicians involve negligence. However, it has been shown that the incidence of malpractice claims is directly related to the personal relationship and trust existing between physicians and patients. Incidence is also often directly related to the extent of the patient's injury.

Negligence: Elements necessary to prove negligence: duty, dereliction, direct cause, and damage. These elements are often called the four Ds of negligence.

Malfeasance: The performance of a totally wrongful, unlawful act; example: when a person prescribes medications but is not licensed to do so.

Misfeasance: The performance of a lawful act in a way that is illegal or improper, resulting in harm; example: when sterile technique is not used while preparing an IV, resulting in an infection in the patient.

Nonfeasance: The failure to act when one is required to do so; example: not scanning a barcode on a package when this is a required job function.

Res ipsa loquitur: A Latin phrase meaning "the matter speaks for itself," also known as the doctrine of common knowledge. This doctrine applies if a result could not have occurred without someone's being negligent. Negligence cases chiefly involve acts such as unintentionally leaving foreign bodies inside a patient during surgery, accidentally injuring a patient in surgical procedures, and injuring a portion of the patient's body outside the field of treatment. In these cases, the physician has the burden of proving innocence and non-negligence. If a

---

AT A GLANCE   Patient's Bill of Rights

The patient has a right to

- Receive considerate and respectful care.

- Receive complete, current information concerning his or her diagnosis, treatment, and prognosis.

- Receive information necessary to give informed consent prior to the start of any procedure and/or treatment.

- Refuse treatment to the extent permitted by law.

- Receive every consideration of his or her privacy.

- Be assured of confidentiality.

- Obtain reasonable responses to requests for service.

- Obtain information about his or her health care.

- Know whether treatment is experimental.

- Expect reasonable continuity of care.

- Examine his or her bill and have it explained.

- Know which hospital rules and regulations apply to patient conduct.

Table 8-3

malpractice case is not tried under this doctrine and general law of negligence, the patient has the burden of proving that the physician was at fault and negligent.

Contributing negligence: A legal term defining a situation in which both the plaintiff and the defendant share in the negligence that caused injury to the plaintiff.

Quid pro quo: A Latin phrase that means "something for something"—that is, giving something in return for something else.

Abuse: The improper use of equipment, a substance (such as a drug), or a service (such as a program), either intentionally or unintentionally.

Respondeat superior: A Latin phrase meaning "let the higher-up answer"—that is, that the physician is responsible for employee acts.

Scope of education and training: Laws dictating what medical assistants may or may not do. For example, in some states it is illegal for medical assistants to draw blood. It is illegal in all states for a medical assistant to diagnose a condition, prescribe treatment, and engage in deception about certification, title, or level of education.

Res judicata: A Latin phrase meaning "the matter has been decided." It signifies that a claim cannot be retried between the same parties if it has already been legally resolved.

Statute of limitations: A statute that sets a limit of time during which a suit may be brought, or criminal charges may be made. In a malpractice suit, dispute of limitations begins to run at the time of the injury, or at the time of the discovery of the injury.

Criminal Law

Child abuse: The physical, sexual, or emotional maltreatment of a child.

Child Abuse Prevention and Treatment Act: A law passed by Congress mandating the reporting of cases of child abuse. In all states, teachers, physicians, and other licensed health-care practitioners are responsible for reporting such cases in person or by telephone and for following up with a written report within a specific time frame, such as 72 hours.

Elder abuse: The physical abuse, neglect, intimidation, or cruel punishment of an elderly individual as defined by the Older Americans Act, which created the Administration on Aging and outlined 10 objectives aimed at preserving the rights and dignity of older citizens.

Amendments to the Older Americans Act: A law passed by Congress that defines elder abuse, neglect, and exploitation but that does not deal with enforcement. In 42 states, however, reporting suspected elder abuse is mandatory for physicians; such reporting is voluntary in the other eight states.

Rape: A sexual assault involving intercourse without consent. Rape is a crime of violence, and the victims are treated for medical and psychological trauma. Rapes are criminal acts that should be reported to local law enforcement officials.

Drug Enforcement Administration (DEA): The agency responsible for enforcing the Comprehensive Drug Abuse Prevention and Control Act of 1970. Requirements for physicians include registration (renewed every three years), keeping of records (maintained for two years and specifying the patient, the drug, the dosage, the date, and reason for use), inventory

(taken on the date of registration and every two years following), disposal of drugs (recorded in a log and witnessed), and proper security especially for controlled substances, all of which are major responsibilities of medical assistants.

Business Law

Contracts: Voluntary agreements between two or more parties in which specific promises are made for a consideration. There are three parts to any contract: the offer, the acceptance, and the consideration.

Offer: The beginning of the contract process, when one party makes an offer to another. The offer must be communicated effectively and must be made in good faith and not under duress or as a joke. The offer must also be clear enough to be understood by both parties, and it must define what both parties will do if the offer is accepted.

Acceptance: Agreement to the terms of a contract; a patient indicates acceptance of the physician's offer of practicing medicine by scheduling appointments, submitting to physical examinations, and allowing the physician to prescribe or perform medical treatment.

Consideration: Something of value that is bargained for as part of a contract. It is what each party agrees to provide for the other.

Breach of contract: Failure of a party to comply with the terms of a legally valid contract.

Void: Without legal force or effect.

Implied contract: An unwritten and unspoken agreement, the terms of which result from the actions of the parties involved.

Termination of contract: Generally takes place when all treatment has been completed and all bills have been fully paid.

Premature termination of contract: May occur as a result of failure to pay for services, missed appointments, failure to follow the physician's instructions, or obtaining the services of another physician.

Liable: Accountable under the law.

Bonding: Insurance against embezzlement for employees who handle financial matters in the medical office.

Licensure: The granting of permission by a competent authority to an individual or organization to engage in a practice or activity that would otherwise be illegal. Licensure is a mandatory credential process established by law. It is the strongest form of regulation. It gives legal permission, granted by state statutes, to perform specific acts.

Registration: The recording of professional qualification information relevant to government licensing regulations.

Certification: A voluntary credential process usually made by a nongovernmental agency. The purpose of certification is to ensure that the standards met are those necessary for safe and ethical practice of the profession.

Reciprocity: The policy under which a professional license obtained in one state may be accepted as valid in other states by prior agreement.

Telemedicine: Remote consultation by patients with physicians or other health professionals via telephone, the Internet, or closed-circuit television. Legal concerns over telemedicine involve matters such as state licenses, reimbursement, confidentiality, and informed consent.

Business structures: Legally, business structures include sole proprietorships, partnerships, and corporations.

Sole proprietorship: A type of medical practice management in which a physician practices alone and is responsible for all profits and liabilities of the business. It is the oldest form of business and is the easiest to start, operate, and dissolve. The advantages are simplicity of organization, being one's own boss, being the sole receiver of all profits, and having fewer government regulations to follow.

Partnership: A type of medical practice management involving the association of two or more individuals practicing together under a written agreement specifying the rights, obligations, and responsibilities of each partner. The partnership agreement should be written and reviewed by an attorney. Each partner is responsible or liable for the business.

Corporation: A body formed by a group of people who are authorized by law to act as a single person. Corporations are governed by state law. There are income and tax advantages to incorporating.

Professional corporation: A corporation designed for professionals such as physicians, dentists, lawyers, and accountants.

Group practice: A medical management system in which a group of three or more licensed physicians share their collective income, expenses, facilities, equipment, records, and personnel. There are single-specialty, multi-specialty, and primary care group practices.

Indemnity: A security against loss, hurt, or damage. Indemnity is a traditional form of health insurance that covers the insured against a potential loss of money from medical expenses for an illness or accident.

Managed care: A system in which the financing, administration, and delivery of health care are combined to provide medical services to subscribers for a prepaid fee.

Capitation: A payment method for health-care services in which a fixed amount of money is paid per month or other period to an HMO, medical group, or individual health provider for full medical care of subscribers.

Liability insurance: Contract coverage for potential damages incurred as a result of a negligent act.

Workplace Legalities

Employment-at-will: A concept of employment whereby either the employer or the employee can terminate employment at any time and for any reason.

Wrongful discharge: A concept established by precedent whereby an employer risks litigation if he or she does not have just cause for firing an employee.

Legal protections: Laws against wrongful discharge that prevent employers from firing someone for refusing to commit an illegal act, whistle-blowing, performing a legal duty, or exercising a private right.

Wagner Act of 1935: A statute that makes it illegal to discriminate in hiring or firing because of union membership or organizing activities.

Fair Labor Standards Act of 1938: A statute that prohibits child labor and the firing of employees for exercising their rights under the act's wage and hour standards. It also provides for overtime pay and a minimum wage.

Equal Pay Act of 1963: A statute that requires equal pay for men and women doing equal work.

Title VII of the Civil Rights Act of 1964: A statute that applies to businesses with 15 or more employees working at least 20 weeks of the year. The act prevents employers from discriminating in hiring or firing on the basis of race, color, religion, sex, or national origin. Some states have laws that also prohibit discrimination based on marital status, parenthood, mental health status, mental retardation, other disabilities, sexual orientation, personal appearance, or political affiliation.

Right-to-know laws: State laws that allow employees access to information about toxic or hazardous substances, employer duties, employee rights, and other workplace health and safety issues.

Americans with Disabilities Act: A 1990 act designed to eliminate discrimination against individuals with disabilities. It includes areas such as telecommunications, housing, public transportation, air carrier access, voting accessibility, education, and rehabilitation. Health-care facilities are public accommodations, which must comply with specific requirements for architectural standards and modifications suited to disabled individuals.

Patient Safety and Quality Improvement Act of 2005 Statute and Rule: This legislation established a voluntary reporting system designed to enhance the data available to assess and resolve patient safety and health-care quality issues. It encourages the reporting and analysis of medical errors.

Health Information Technology for Economic and Clinical Health (HITECH) Act: A 2009 law designed to promote the adoption and meaningful use of health information technology. Its Subtitle D addresses privacy and security concerns associated with electronic transmission of health information. For more information, see http://www.hhs.gov.

Documentation and Records Management

POMR: A system of *problem-oriented medical records* based on client problems—conditions or behaviors that result in physical or emotional distress or interfere with functioning. It also includes educational and diagnostic components. The POMR system has four basic parts: database, problem list, plan, and progress notes. The *database* includes patient health history, examination findings, and results of baseline laboratory and diagnostic procedures. The *problem list* identifies health problems and is kept at the front of the patient chart. The written *plan* outlines further studies, treatments, and patient education concerning items on the problem list. Using the first letter of each part of the progress notes spells the acronym *SOAP,* and this portion is called *SOAP notes,* or *SOAPE notes* (when *evaluation* is included).

SOAP: An approach to documentation that is part of the POMR system, which provides an orderly series of steps for dealing with a medical case. SOAP lists (1) the patient's symptoms (*subjective* data), (2) the measurable, observable factors of the patient *objective* data, (3) an *a*ssessment, and (4) a *p*lan of action.

SOMR: Source-oriented medical record, which is the most common form of record keeping used in medical offices by physicians. Charts have divided sections such as History and Physical (H&P), Progress Notes, Laboratory Results, and Consultations. The most recent report or progress note is placed on top.

EMR: Electronic medical record, a type of information collection system used by many different types of care settings. Data is entered directly and downloaded in patient computer files during interviews and assessments, via personal digital assistants (PDAs), laptop computers, or other types of computers.

Ownership of medical records: Patients' medical records are considered the legal property of the owners of the facility where they were created. For example, a physician in private practice owns his or her records; records in a clinic are property of the clinic. This is true even after the deaths of patients. These medical records should not be released unless the patient or legal guardian has signed legal release forms, a court has subpoenaed the records, an act or law mandates that the records be released to protect public welfare and safety, or the physician determines that the release is necessary to protect the patient or a third party.

Transferring medical records: Clients who request that their medical records be transferred to another physician should do so in writing. The original record may be retained in the office. No information should be released from the medical record without the approval of the physician and the written permission of the patient. If the client is incompetent, the court-appointed guardian signs the release form.

Children's medical records: The parent or legal guardian may sign the release forms. If the parents are legally separated or divorced, release forms must be signed by the parent who has legal custody.

HIPAA

Health Insurance Portability and Accountability Act (HIPAA): A law passed by the U.S. Congress in August 1996 to create national guidelines for health privacy protection.

TITLE I, Health-Care Portability: The part of HIPAA that deals with protecting health-care coverage for employees who change jobs. Heath-Care Portability provides the following protection for employees and their families:

- Increases the ability to get health coverage when starting a new job
- Reduces the probability of losing existing health-care coverage
- Helps workers maintain continuous health-care coverage when changing jobs
- Helps workers purchase health insurance on their own if they lose coverage under an employer's group plan and have no other health coverage available

TITLE II, Preventing Health-Care Fraud and Abuse, Administrative Simplification, and Medical Liability Reform: Commonly known as the HIPAA Privacy Rule, the part of HIPAA that provides the first comprehensive federal protection for the privacy of health information. It is designed to provide strong, national privacy protections that do not interfere with patient access to health care or the quality of health-care delivery. The privacy rule is intended to:

- Give patients more control over their health information
- Set boundaries on the use and release of health-care records
- Establish appropriate safeguards that health-care providers and others must achieve to protect the privacy of health information
- Hold violators accountable, with civil and criminal penalties that can be imposed if they violate patients' privacy rights
- Strike a balance when public responsibility supports disclosure of some forms of data (e.g., to protect public health)

Individually identifiable health information: An individual's personal information that is gathered in the process of providing health care. Individually identifiable health information includes:

- Name
- Address
- Phone numbers
- Fax number
- Dates (birth, death, admission, discharge, etc.)
- Social Security number
- E-mail address
- Medical record numbers
- Health plan beneficiary numbers
- Account numbers
- Certificate or license numbers
- Vehicle identifiers and serial numbers, including license plate numbers
- Device identifiers and serial numbers
- Web universal resource locators (URLs)
- Internet protocol (IP) address numbers

Protected health information (PHI): Individually identifiable health information that is transmitted or maintained by electronic or other media, such as computer storage devices. This information is protected by the HIPAA Privacy Rule.

Use: As defined by HIPAA, the act of doing any of the following to individually identifiable health information by employees or other members of an organization's workforce:

- Sharing
- Employing

- Applying
- Utilizing
- Examining
- Analyzing

Disclosure: As defined by HIPAA, the act of doing any of the following by the party holding the information so that the information is outside that party:

- Release
- Transfer
- Providing access to
- Divulging in any manner

Treatment, payment, and operations (TPO): The uses that HIPAA authorizes for sharing patient information:

- Treatment—Providers are allowed to share information in order to provide care to patients.
- Payment—Providers are allowed to share information in order to receive payment for the treatment provided.
- Operations—Providers are allowed to share information to conduct normal business activities, such as quality improvement.

Notice of Privacy Practices (NPP): A document given to patients by health-care providers that informs patients of their rights as outlined by HIPAA.

HIPAA Security Rule: The technical safeguards that protect the confidentiality, integrity, and availability of health information covered by HIPAA. The Security Rule specifies how patient information is protected on computer networks, the Internet, disks, and other storage media. See Chapter 12.

8.3 Ethics

Ethics: The study of values or principles governing personal relationships, including ideals of autonomy, justice, and conduct. The code of ethics for the profession of medical assisting is reproduced in Table 8-4.

Bioethics: A discipline dealing with the ethical and moral implications of biological research and applications, especially as they relate to life and death.

Moral: Conforming to a standard of right behavior or a rule of conduct based on standards of right and wrong. Moral beliefs are usually formed through the influence of family, culture, and society, and they serve as a guide for personal ethical conduct.

Philosophy: A basic viewpoint or system of values, general beliefs, concepts, and attitudes.

Etiquette: Standards of behavior considered appropriate within a profession. Etiquette describes a body of courtesies and manners to be observed in social situations.

Beneficence: Active goodness or kindness.

Nonmaleficence: Abstinence from committing any harm. As human beings, we have an obligation not to harm others.

Fee splitting: An unethical practice in which a physician accepts payment from another physician solely for referral of a patient. In these cases, both physicians are guilty.

Overcharging: An unethical practice of charging excessive or illegal fees.

Professional courtesy: The provision of medical care to physician colleagues or their families in staff free of charge or at a reduced fee.

Ghost surgery: The deceitful, unethical substitution of another surgeon without the patient's consent.

Physician ownership of a health facility: An allowed practice, as long as the physician reveals such ownership to the patient before admitting or referring the patient.

AT A GLANCE | Medical Assisting Code of Ethics

The Code of Ethics of the American Association of Medical Assistants (AAMA) shall set forth principles of ethical and moral conduct as they relate to the medical profession and the particular practice of medical assisting.

Members of the AAMA dedicated to the conscientious pursuit of their profession, and thus desiring to merit the high regard of the entire medical profession and the respect of the general public which they serve, do pledge themselves to strive always to:

A. render service with full respect for the dignity of humanity;

B. respect confidential information obtained through employment unless legally authorized or required by responsible performance of duty to divulge such information;

C. uphold the honor and high principles of the profession and accept its disciplines;

D. seek to continually improve the knowledge and skills of medical assistants for the benefit of patients and professional colleagues;

E. participate in additional service activities aimed toward improving the health and well-being of the community.

Reprinted by permission from The American Medical Association of Medical Assistants.

Table 8-4

Substance abuse: The unethical practice of medicine while under influence of a controlled substance, alcohol, or other chemical agents; this could impair the physician's ability to provide proper care.

Missed appointment charges: An ethical practice of charging for a missed or inappropriately canceled appointment, per the patient's understanding and acceptance that such charges may be incurred.

Duty to improve oneself: As a medical assistant you should always continue your education, learn new competencies and skills, learn from your own mistakes, learn from others you work with, and strive to be a good role model.

Genetics

Genetic: Pertaining to reproduction, birth, or origin or to being produced by genes or attributable to them.

Genetic diseases: Diseases linked to genetic defects. There are as many as 4,000 human genetic diseases. Approximately 500 of them are linked to a defect in a single gene.

Genetic screening: A test for genetic problems that requires a DNA sample from solid tissues, saliva, or blood. Genetic testing is appropriate for prospective parents whose genetic histories indicate an elevated risk for genetic disorders. When a genetic defect is found in the fetus, parents may have to make an ethical decision to request or refuse an abortion. Other ethical concerns include genetic testing by employers and the release of genetic information to insurance companies.

Genetic engineering: Gene splitting, recombinant DNA research, chemical synthesis of DNA, and other technology. It involves numerous ethical issues and requires following stringent ethical guidelines.

Gene therapy: The insertion of a normally functioning gene into cells in which an abnormal or absent element of the gene has caused disease. The goal of gene therapy is to alleviate suffering and disease, not to enhance desirable characteristics or to diminish undesirable characteristics not related to disease.

Cloning: A procedure for producing multiple copies of genetically identical organisms or individual genes.

Eugenics: The study of hereditary improvement achieved by controlling the characteristics of genes.

Pregnancy and Termination of Pregnancy

Artificial insemination: The mechanical injection of viable semen into the vagina. If the donor and the recipient are not married, the recipient will be considered the sole parent of the child except in cases in which both the donor and the recipient agree to recognize a paternity right.

In vitro fertilization (IVF): Fertilization that takes place outside a woman's body, usually in a test tube. Because of ethical concerns, fertilized human eggs should not be subjected to laboratory research.

Gestation: The length of time after conception during which developing offspring are carried in the uterus. In humans, the duration is approximately 280 days, or 40 weeks. Live birth with a gestation time of less than 37 weeks is considered premature. Beyond 42 weeks, the fetus is considered postmature.

Amniocentesis: A small amount of amniotic fluid is aspirated for the purpose of analyzing whether a fetus is developing normally.

Amniotomy: The artificial rupture of the fetal membranes. It is performed to stimulate or accelerate the onset of labor. The procedure is painless.

Anencephaly: A congenital deformity in newborns characterized by absence of the brain and spinal cord.

Stillbirth: The death of a fetus before or during delivery. It is known as fetal death if the weight of the fetus is more than 1,000 g. Stillbirths may require neither birth nor death certificates.

Spontaneous abortion: Also known as a miscarriage, usually before the 20th week of pregnancy.

Abortion: The voluntary termination of pregnancy before gestation is complete and, in most cases, before the fetus is viable. Methods include uterine aspiration, dilation and curettage, saline injection, and cesarean section. Its legality as a medical procedure was affirmed by the U.S. Supreme Court in a 1973 case known as *Roe v. Wade* and in several subsequent cases. People's opinions on the controversial subject are based on their own personal ethical and moral values as well as on the law.

Stem cell: Early embryonic cells that have the potential to become any type of body cell. The debate on the therapeutic use of stem cells remains intense because stem cells have shown promise for treating patients with a wide variety of medical problems.

Organ and Tissue Donation and Transplantation

Uniform Anatomical Gift Act: A law adopted by all states. Its provisions are that (1) any person over 18 years may give all or any part of his or her body after death for research, transplantation, or placement in a tissue bank; (2) physicians who accept organs or tissue, relying in good faith on the documents, are protected from lawsuits; and (3) the time of death must be determined by a physician.

Transplant: The transfer of an organ or tissue from one person to another or from one part of the body to another. Medical transplants are divided into four categories, depending on the source of the tissue used: autograft, heterograft, homograft, and isograft.

Autograft: Surgical transplantation of a person's own tissue from one part of the body to another location. Autografts are used in several kinds of plastic surgery, most commonly to replace skin lost in severe burns. The term can also be applied to transplants between identical twins.

Heterograft: The transplant of animal tissue into a human. It is also called a xenograft.

Homograft: The nonpermanent transplant of tissue from one body to another (in the same species), such as a tissue transplant between two humans who are not identical twins. It is also called an allograft.

Isograft: Surgical transplantation from genetically identical individuals, such as identical twins.

8.4 Death and Dying

Patient Self-Determination Act: A federal law that requires health-care providers to provide written information to patients about their rights under state law to make medical decisions and to execute advance directives. It requires that medical care facilities ask patients whether they have prepared an advance directive for guidance in the event that they are terminally ill.

Advance directives: Documents that make wishes known in the event that individuals are unable to speak for themselves. Examples are living wills, durable powers of attorney, and health-care proxies.

Living will: A document in which an individual expresses his or her wishes regarding medical treatment. It may detail circumstances under which treatment should be discontinued, which treatments to suspend, and which to maintain. A living will is legal only if the person is competent to create such a document and if two witnesses have attested to its accuracy by signing it.

Durable power of attorney: A document that gives a designated person the authority to make legal decisions on behalf of the grantor, usually including health-care decisions.

Health-care proxy: A durable power of attorney issued for purposes of making health-care decisions only.

Do-not-resuscitate (DNR) order: A document written at the request of patients or their authorized representatives stating that cardiopulmonary resuscitation should not be used to sustain life in a medical crisis.

Geriatrics: The branch of medicine pertaining to elderly individuals and the treatment of diseases affecting them.

Termination phase: The period of life of persons who are expected to die within six months. It is the last stage of therapy for patients.

Curative care: Treatment to cure a patient's disease.

Palliative care: Treatment of symptoms to make a dying person more comfortable. It is also called comfort care. Patients should never be abandoned when cure or recovery is impossible. They should continue to receive emotional support, adequate pain control, respect for their autonomy, and effective communication.

Euthanasia: The administration of a lethal agent by another person to a patient with an incurable disease or condition.

Physician-assisted suicide: Euthanasia by a physician at the request of a person who wishes to die. This practice is under intense, ongoing legal and ethical debate.

Brain death: An irreversible cessation of all function in the entire brain. Brain death or irreversible coma is declared when electrical activity is absent on two electroencephalograms performed 12–24 hours apart.

Signs of death: There are six signs for pronouncing a comatose patient dead: no breathing without assistance, no coughing or gagging reflex, no blinking reflex when the cornea is touched, no pupil response to light, no response to pain, and no grimace reflex when the head is rotated or ears are flushed with ice water.

Thanatology: The study of death, dying, and psychological methods of coping with death and dying.

Autopsy: A postmortem examination of a body performed by a specially trained medical person to confirm or determine the cause of death.

Grief: A normal reaction to loss, such as the loss of a job, the loss of a close friend or family member, death, or a diagnosis of a terminal illness.

Stages of grief: A pattern of emotional and physical responses to separation and loss. Elisabeth Kübler-Ross defines five stages or responses of dying patients:

Stage 1	denial and isolation
Stage 2	anger, asking "why me?"
Stage 3	bargaining and guilt
Stage 4	depression
Stage 5	acceptance

STRATEGIES FOR SUCCESS

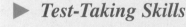 **▶ *Test-Taking Skills***

Don't leave any questions blank!
Make an educated guess for every question even when you don't know the right answer. There is no penalty for guessing, and you might get a few extra points just answering every question.

CHAPTER 8 REVIEW

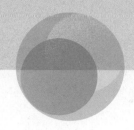

Instructions:

Answer the following questions.

1. *Liable* means
   A. without legal force or effect.
   B. a moral code.
   C. accountable under law.
   D. false, defamatory writing.
   E. a crime that is less serious than a felony and consequently carries a lesser penalty.

2. The power and authority given to a court to hear a case and to make a judgment is called
   A. jurisdiction.
   B. judiciary.
   C. judging.
   D. judicial.
   E. litigation.

3. Professional negligence is also called
   A. malpractice.
   B. malfunction.
   C. malice.
   D. arbitration.
   E. felony.

4. In order to protect the confidentiality and privacy of patients, medical assistants should not
   A. discuss confidential matters such as test results and finances over the telephone.
   B. leave messages with someone other than the patient about test results or finances.
   C. release medical records without the signed consent of the patient or legal guardian.
   D. none of these
   E. all of these

5. A contract
   A. is a voluntary agreement.
   B. is made for a consideration.
   C. involves a specific promise made.
   D. involves two or more parties.
   E. all of these

6. The transplant of animal tissue into a human is known as
   A. a homograft.
   B. an autograft.
   C. a heterograft.
   D. a tissue graft.
   E. cloning.

7. The age of majority in most jurisdictions is _____ years.
   A. 21
   B. 19
   C. 16
   D. 17
   E. 18

8. Good Samaritan laws
   A. encourage physicians to render emergency first aid.
   B. exist in all 50 states.
   C. protect physicians against liability for negligence in certain circumstances.
   D. deal with the treatment of accident victims.
   E. all of these

9. *Res ipsa loquitur* is a Latin phrase that refers to
   A. the responsibility of the physician for employee acts.
   B. something that is common knowledge or that speaks for itself.
   C. the failure to do something that should have been done.
   D. getting something as a result of doing something.
   E. doing something in order to get something in return.

10. When is it also permissible to release information from a patient's records?
   A. when the patient signs a release
   B. when a physician calls to request it
   C. when the insurance company signs a release
   D. when the patient has signed a living will
   E. when the patient is in an accident

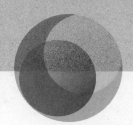
CMA Questions for the End of Section 1 (Chapters 1–8, mixed)

1. The goal of the 1996 AAMA Role Delineation Study was to

   A. revise and update the CMA exam questions.
   B. revise and update the standards used for the accreditation of medical assisting programs.
   C. create a new role and policy of practicing medicine.
   D. establish a new organization that would combine the AAMA and AMT into one organization.
   E. publish all materials needed for medical assisting programs.

2. The first period of menstrual bleeding is called

   A. menses.
   B. menopause.
   C. menstruation.
   D. menarche.
   E. mendacious.

3. All of the following are causative factors for pernicious anemia *except*

   A. vitamin B_{12} deficiency.
   B. folic acid deficiency.
   C. lack of intrinsic factor.
   D. decreased hydrochloric acid in the stomach.
   E. regional enteritis (Crohn's disease).

4. A dying patient refuses to eat, refuses visitors, and refuses further medical treatment. According to Elisabeth Kübler-Ross, this stage of dying most likely represents

   A. denial.
   B. depression.
   C. anger.
   D. acceptance.
   E. bargaining.

5. Vitamin B_9 is also known as

   A. cyanocobalamin.
   B. niacin.
   C. riboflavin.
   D. folic acid.
   E. thiamine.

6. Which of the following behaviors might be displayed by a medical assistant who is behaving unprofessionally?

   A. knocking on the door before entering the examination room
   B. using a term of endearment when talking to a patient
   C. explaining long delays to patients waiting in the reception area
   D. being calm while dealing with an angry patient
   E. thanking a patient for paying for services

7. A translucent band that is present in thick skin is called

   A. stratum corneum.
   B. stratum granulosum.
   C. stratum germinativum.
   D. stratum spongiosum.
   E. stratum lucidum.

8. Which of the following terms means "inflammation of the inner lining and valves of the heart"?

   A. valnulitis
   B. vasculitis
   C. pericarditis
   D. endocarditis
   E. myocarditis

9. An 18-month-old boy temporarily forgets potty training when his parents bring his newborn sister home from the hospital. This is an example of which of the following defense mechanisms?

   A. repression
   B. regression
   C. rationalization
   D. introjection
   E. suppression

10. A physician is required to report all of the following *except*

    A. births.
    B. deaths.
    C. abuse.
    D. communicable diseases.
    E. stroke.

11. The prefix *epi-* means

    A. good.
    B. out.
    C. off.
    D. within.
    E. upon.

12. The most common cyanotic cardiac defect is

    A. patent ductus arteriosus.
    B. angina pectoris.
    C. ventricular septal defect.
    D. coarctation of the aorta.
    E. tetralogy of Fallot.

13. According to Maslow's hierarchy of needs, which of the following is a biological need?

    A. approval

    B. shelter

    C. love

    D. award

    E. self-esteem

14. How many glasses of water a day should people drink on average?

    A. 3–5

    B. 6–8

    C. 10–12

    D. 9–11

    E. 48–64

15. The suffix *gravida* refers to

    A. a pregnancy.

    B. the condition of aging.

    C. a serious condition.

    D. a stomach ache.

    E. a malignancy.

16. Diverticulosis occurs particularly in the

    A. lungs.

    B. cecum.

    C. mouth.

    D. anus.

    E. colon.

17. A 74-year-old man has severe gangrene of the right foot and right lower leg. His physician recommends above-the-knee amputation to prevent further problems. The patient refuses to consider this recommendation and states that he will stop smoking to control the condition, so that amputation will not be necessary. Which of the following defense mechanisms is this patient demonstrating?

    A. denial

    B. repression

    C. rationalization

    D. compensation

    E. sublimation

18. A crime punishable by a fine or imprisonment for less than one year is known as a

    A. misdemeanor.

    B. felony.

    C. mitigation.

    D. mutual assent.

    E. arbitration.

19. The prefix *peri-* means

    A. behind.

    B. underneath.

    C. inside.

    D. half.

    E. surrounding.

20. Which of the following fractures of the bone is common in children?

    A. comminuted

    B. open

    C. incomplete

    D. compound

    E. greenstick

21. An irritable and complaining patient states to you that everyone around him is negative and irritable. You recognize this defense mechanism as

    A. sublimation.

    B. repression.

    C. rationalization.

    D. projection.

22. It is permissible to release private and confidential information about a patient

    A. when you disagree with the patient's choices.

    B. when the patient has signed a release form.

    C. to a friend of the patient who is concerned about the patient's well-being.

    D. over the telephone when others can overhear.

    E. Never; it is always inappropriate to release private or confidential information about a patient.

23. Which of the following contains the central meaning of a word?

    A. prefix

    B. suffix

    C. root

    D. combining vowel

    E. combining form

24. A prolapse of one section of the intestine into the lumen of another segment, causing intestinal blockage, is called

    A. intussusception.

    B. diverticulosis.

    C. volvulus.

    D. Crohn's disease.

    E. luminescence.

25. Psychology is

    A. the scientific study of the mind.

    B. the scientific study of behaviors.

    C. the scientific study of mental processes.

    D. all of these

26. Which of the following items is the most important for medical assistants to keep in mind during their daily work routing in medical offices?

    A. burglary

    B. confidentiality

    C. privilege granted to a physician

    D. consent

    E. Good Samaritan laws

27. The strands of DNA in the nucleus are called

    A. chromatin.

    B. nucleolus.

    C. network.

    D. granules of RNA.

    E. guanine.

28. An organism that obtains its nutrients from dead organic matter is called

    A. diplococcus.

    B. chlamydia.

    C. saprophyte.

    D. mycoplasma.

    E. protozoon.

29. In obesity, body weight exceeds normal by at least

    A. 10%.

    B. 20%.

    C. 30%.

    D. 40%.

    E. 50%.

30. The Uniform Anatomical Gift Act includes the provision that

    A. physicians who accept organs and tissue in good faith, relying on apparently valid documents, are protected from lawsuits.

    B. the time of death must be determined by a physician.

    C. any person over 18 years of age may give all or any part of his or her body up after death for research or transplantation.

    D. none of these

    E. all of these

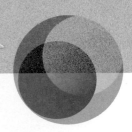

RMA Questions for the End of Section 1 (Chapters 1–8, mixed)

1. The junction between two neurons is known as a(n)

    A. nerve impulse.
    B. axon.
    C. synapse.
    D. microglion.

2. How often must RMA recertification occur?

    A. every year
    B. every two years
    C. every three years
    D. every five years

3. Which of the following terms means "irregular bleeding from the uterus between periods"?

    A. menorrhagia
    B. metrorrhagia
    C. amenorrhea
    D. hemorrhage

4. Which of the following vitamins is an antidote for an overdose of an anticoagulant?

    A. vitamin D
    B. vitamin E
    C. vitamin A
    D. vitamin K

5. A crime that is less serious than a felony and consequently carries a lesser penalty is referred to as

    A. a misdemeanor.
    B. assault.
    C. slander.
    D. battery.

6. The third stage of dying, according to Elisabeth Kübler-Ross, is known as

    A. isolation and denial.
    B. depression.
    C. acceptance.
    D. bargaining and guilt.

7. The prefix *iso-* means

    A. separate.
    B. equal.
    C. recent.
    D. around.

8. The ciliary body of the eye, which changes the shape of the lens, is part of the

    A. vitreous humor.
    B. pupil.
    C. uvea.
    D. cornea.

9. A group of bacteria considered to be the smallest free-living organisms is known as

    A. mycoplasma.
    B. chlamydia.
    C. rickettsia.
    D. viruses.

10. Which of the following means "removal of one or both testes"?

    A. mastectomy
    B. hysterectomy
    C. orchiectomy
    D. vasectomy

11. In the tissues, a basophil is called a

    A. reticulocyte.
    B. granulocyte.
    C. goblet cell.
    D. mast cell.

12. Cyanocobalamin is also known as

    A. vitamin B_{12}.
    B. vitamin B_6.
    C. vitamin B_2.
    D. vitamin C.

13. Approval and permission from a patient to allow touching, examination, treatment, or release of medical information by medically authorized personnel is called

    A. privilege.
    B. consent.
    C. protocol.
    D. contract.

14. The prefix *ambi-* means

    A. before.
    B. around.
    C. against.
    D. both.

15. Dead, keratinized cells located on the outer surface of the epidermis form the

   A. stratum corneum.
   B. stratum lucidum.
   C. stratum spinosum.
   D. stratum granulosum.

16. The most abundant plasma protein is

   A. globulin.
   B. fibrinogen.
   C. albumin.
   D. agglutinin.

17. Which of the following endocrine glands releases epinephrine?

   A. thyroid
   B. adrenal cortex
   C. adrenal medulla
   D. anterior pituitary

18. Cholesterol is continuously synthesized in the body by the

   A. spleen.
   B. liver.
   C. pancreas.
   D. colon.

19. An application made to a court or judge to obtain an order, ruling, or direction is known as a(n)

   A. summons.
   B. subpoena.
   C. motion.
   D. appeal.

20. A condition caused by the lack of melanin pigment in the skin, hair, and eyes is called

   A. keratosis.
   B. albinism.
   C. xerosis.
   D. ankylosis.

21. Calcitonin is released from which of the following endocrine glands?

   A. thymus gland
   B. thyroid gland
   C. parathyroid gland
   D. pancreas

22. Necrophilia means

   A. fear of death.
   B. attraction to dead bodies.
   C. attraction to children.
   D. fear of fire.

23. Which of the following cranial nerves may cause Bell's palsy?

   A. the facial nerve
   B. the vagus nerve
   C. the trigeminal nerve
   D. the trochlear nerve

24. The muscle that flexes the leg and extends the thigh is the

   A. sartorius.
   B. gluteus maximus.
   C. gastrocnemius.
   D. hamstring.

25. The degree of pathogenicity or relative power of a micro-organism to produce a disease is called

   A. infective dose.
   B. virulence.
   C. pathogenicity.
   D. exotoxin.

26. The medical abbreviation meaning "as desired" is

   A. n.p.o.
   B. p.o.
   C. p.r.n.
   D. b.i.d.

27. Which of the following may be described as "let the master answer"?

   A. *res judicata*
   B. *respondeat superior*
   C. *res ipsa loquitur*
   D. informed consent

28. The third cranial nerve is the

   A. optic nerve.
   B. abducens nerve.
   C. accessory nerve.
   D. oculomotor nerve.

29. Which of the following is the term meaning "slow heartbeat"?

   A. tachycardia
   B. tachypnea
   C. bradycardia
   D. bradypnea

30. Nonconsensual or illegal touching of another person is called

   A. battery.
   B. slander.
   C. assault.
   D. libel.

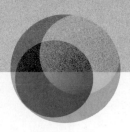

CCMA Questions for the End of Section 1 (Chapters 1–8, mixed)

1. According to the American Hospital Association, which of the following guarantees that the patient has the right to refuse treatment, to the extent permitted by law?

 A. defensive medicine
 B. Patient's Bill of Rights
 C. mandatory report
 D. consent

2. The most common combining vowel is

 A. i.
 B. u.
 C. o.
 D. a.

3. An abnormality of the red blood cells, in which they are of unequal size, is called

 A. poikilocytosis.
 B. hemoptysis.
 C. homeostasis.
 D. anisocytosis.

4. A negatively charged ion is known as a(n)

 A. cation.
 B. ionic bond.
 C. anion.
 D. covalent bond.

5. Corepraxy is a procedure to

 A. centralize a pupil that is abnormally situated.
 B. remove both testes.
 C. widen a bronchus.
 D. remove the uterus.

6. Which of the following terms relates to a male reproductive disorder?

 A. mastoptosis
 B. onychomalacia
 C. ankylosis
 D. cryptorchidism

7. A small, membranous structure found in most cells that forms the carbohydrate side chains of glycoproteins is called the

 A. mitochondrion.
 B. Golgi apparatus.
 C. endoplasmic reticulum.
 D. ribosome.

8. Sebaceous glands are examples of

 A. holocrine glands.
 B. apocrine glands.
 C. merocrine glands.
 D. mammary glands.

9. A tightness and narrowing of the prepuce on the penis that prevents the retraction of the foreskin over the glans penis is referred to as

 A. epididymis.
 B. phimosis.
 C. perineum.
 D. acrosome.

10. Which of the following terms explains the relationship in which both organisms benefit?

 A. commensalism
 B. symbiosis
 C. mutualism
 D. parasitism

11. An element that increases resistance to tooth decay is

 A. iron.
 B. iodine.
 C. zinc.
 D. fluoride.

12. *Ren/o* refers to which of the following?

 A. the bladder
 B. the rectum
 C. the kidney
 D. the spleen

13. The suffix *-oma* means

 A. disease.
 B. tumor.
 C. inflammation.
 D. enlargement.

14. The universal donor blood group is known as type

 A. O.
 B. AB.
 C. A.
 D. B.

15. A disease that causes the bones to enlarge and become deformed and weak is called

 A. kyphosis.
 B. Crohn's disease.
 C. lordosis.
 D. Paget's disease.

16. The torsion of a loop of intestine, causing intestinal obstruction, with or without strangulation, is called

   A. intussusception.
   B. diverticulosis.
   C. volvulus.
   D. regional enteritis.

17. Which of the following words is misspelled?

   A. rickettsia
   B. streptococci
   C. mycoplasma
   D. myecobacteria

18. Which of the following vitamins is called pyridoxine?

   A. vitamin B_2
   B. vitamin B_6
   C. vitamin B_9
   D. vitamin B_{12}

19. Eating a large amount of food in a short time without subsequent purging is referred to as

   A. binge eating.
   B. dumping syndrome.
   C. bulimia.
   D. anorexia nervosa.

20. The CCMA credential is awarded by the

   A. AAMA.
   B. AMT.
   C. NHA.
   D. ARMA.

21. A major somatoform disorder that involves an actual physical disturbance is known as

   A. conversion disorder.
   B. personality disorder.
   C. bipolar disorder.
   D. schizophrenia.

22. Which of the following means "the matter has been decided"?

   A. *respondeat superior*
   B. *quid pro quo*
   C. *res ipsa loquitur*
   D. *res judicata*

23. When an oocyte and sperm fuse together, the result is called a(n)

   A. zygote.
   B. oogonium.
   C. gestation.
   D. cleavage.

24. Balanitis is an inflammation of the

   A. cervix.
   B. epididymis.
   C. glans penis.
   D. vagina.

25. Which of the following conditions is caused by the lack of melanin pigment in the skin, hair, and eyes?

   A. keratosis
   B. albinism
   C. leukoplakia
   D. lithiasis

26. The power plant of the cell that provides energy is called the

   A. ribosome.
   B. lysosome.
   C. Golgi apparatus.
   D. mitochondrion.

27. The process of attributing unwanted feelings to someone else is known as

   A. projection.
   B. regression.
   C. displacement.
   D. repression.

28. Which of the following is the best source of vitamin C?

   A. yogurt and cheese
   B. soybeans
   C. fruits
   D. liver and egg yolk

29. Standards of behavior considered appropriate within a profession are called

   A. morals.
   B. etiquette.
   C. philosophy.
   D. laws.

30. A ridge, wrinkle, or fold, as in the mucous membrane lining the urinary bladder, is known as a

   A. ruga.
   B. trigone.
   C. lobule.
   D. uvula.

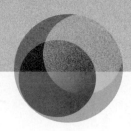

NCMA Questions for the End of Section 1 (Chapters 1–8, mixed)

1. An unethical practice in which a physician accepts payment from another physician solely for referral of a patient is called

    A. professional courtesy.
    B. etiquette.
    C. beneficence.
    D. fee splitting.

2. Which of the following means "let the higher-up answer"?

    A. *novus ordo seclorum*
    B. *respondeat superior*
    C. *res ipsa loquitur*
    D. malfeasance

3. Aseptic hand washing techniques include all of the following *except*

    A. using a nailbrush to scrub under the nails and cuticles.
    B. using liquid soap.
    C. turning off the faucet with the hands.
    D. removing all jewelry.

4. The Uniform Anatomical Gift Act includes the provision that

    A. the time of death must be determined by a physician.
    B. any physician who accepts organs and tissues must pay the donor.
    C. any person, at any age, may donate any part of his or her body for research or transplantation.
    D. none of these

5. Mrs. M. Johnson shares with you that she is very upset when she has to wait in line or sit in a traffic jam. You recognize this stressor as a

    A. personal stressor.
    B. cataclysmic stressor.
    C. background stressor.
    D. post-traumatic stressor.

6. Good Samaritan laws

    A. deal with the treatment of accident victims.
    B. exist in 44 states.
    C. protect only non-health-care professionals against liability for negligence.
    D. all of the above

7. Professional negligence is also referred to as

    A. mutual assent.
    B. felony.
    C. malpractice.
    D. arbitration.

8. According to the Patient's Bill of Rights, which of the following is a patient right?

    A. to be provided with sample medications
    B. to participate in research without informed consent
    C. to expect continuity of care
    D. to waive payment if treatment is unsatisfactory

9. A four-year-old girl with leukemia is brought to the office for a follow-up examination after spending several days in the hospital undergoing many invasive procedures. On arrival at the office, she has a "white-coat-syndrome reaction." Which of the following best describes the child's reaction?

    A. angry
    B. anxious
    C. alert
    D. aggressive

10. The death of a fetus before or during delivery is called

    A. stillbirth.
    B. prematurity.
    C. abortion.
    D. amniotomy.

11. Which of the following makes an individual's wishes known in the event that he or she is unable to speak for any reason?

    A. patient intake form
    B. senior health questionnaire
    C. advance directive
    D. beneficence

12. It is permissible to release private and confidential information about a patient

    A. never. It is always inappropriate to release private or confidential information about a patient.
    B. when the patient has signed a release form.
    C. to a father of a patient who is concerned about the patient's well-being.
    D. when you disagree with the patient's choices.

13. Part of the problem-oriented medical records (POMR) system that identifies health problems, and is kept at the front of the patient chart, is known as the

A. problem list.
B. objective clinical evidence.
C. assessment.
D. subjective impression.

14. In cases of malpractice involving *res ipsa loquitur*, which of the following is true?

A. The physician is not bound by physician–patient confidentiality.
B. The patient has the burden of proving the physician's negligence.
C. The physician has the burden of proving his or her innocence.
D. None of the above is true.

15. Which of the following terms means "standards of behavior considered appropriate within a profession"?

A. beneficence
B. etiquette
C. morals
D. bioethics

16. Individually identifiable health information is protected by

A. the DEA.
B. the CDC.
C. HIPAA.
D. OSHA.

17. The hearing and determination of a case in controversy, without litigation, by a person chosen by the parties involved is called

A. motions.
B. subpoena.
C. appeal.
D. arbitration.

18. Freedom from infection or infectious material is called

A. virulence.
B. asepsis.
C. sterilization.
D. bacteriostatic.

19. When a patient understands why a treatment is necessary, and what related risks are involved, which of the following is the most closely related term?

A. reciprocity
B. disclosure

C. informed consent
D. mature minor

20. A nerve cell process that conducts impulses away from the cell body is known as a(n)

A. dendrite.
B. axon.
C. neuron.
D. neuronal cell body.

21. Which of the following terms means "rupture of the heart"?

A. cardiomegaly
B. cardiorrhexis
C. cardiotomy
D. cardiopexy

22. The hormone that stimulates milk production during pregnancy is referred to as

A. epinephrine.
B. glucagon.
C. insulin.
D. prolactin.

23. Which of the following items is the most important for medical assistants to keep in mind during their daily work routine in medical offices?

A. confidentiality
B. consent
C. burglary
D. Good Samaritan laws

24. Which of the following medical terms means "in order to face stress, an earlier developmental period is sought"?

A. displacement
B. sublimation
C. regression
D. projection

25. Which of the following organisms does not Gram stain well?

A. *Clostridium botulinum*
B. *Haemophilus influenzae*
C. *Staphylococcus aureus*
D. *Mycobacterium tuberculosis*

26. Blood in the pleural cavity caused by trauma is known as

A. hemothorax.
B. pleurisy.
C. pneumothorax.
D. pneumonia.

27. Which of the following medical terms means "prediction about the outcome of a disease"?

A. prophylaxis
B. remission
C. prognosis
D. malaise

28. The transplant of animal tissue into the human body is known as a(n)

A. heterograft.
B. homograft.
C. tissue graft.
D. autograft.

29. Which of the following terms means "cell eating"?

A. exocytosis
B. endocytosis
C. pinocytosis
D. phagocytosis

30. Which of the following terms describes the period beginning at birth and ending at death?

A. neonatal
B. postnatal
C. prenatal
D. antepartum

SECTION 2

ADMINISTRATIVE MEDICAL ASSISTING KNOWLEDGE

SECTION OUTLINE

CHAPTER 9

RECEPTION, CORRESPONDENCE, MAIL, TELEPHONE TECHNIQUES, AND SUPPLIES

LEARNING OUTCOMES

9.1 Describe the duties of the medical receptionist.

9.2 Describe the proper handling of incoming and outgoing mail and correspondence within the medical office.

9.3 Demonstrate proper techniques for handling all types of telephone calls in the medical office.

9.4 Demonstrate proper use of equipment and the maintenance of stock and supplies in the medical office.

9.5 Recall the information needed when making travel arrangements.

9.6 List the different methods and materials that may be utilized when educating patients.

MEDICAL ASSISTING COMPETENCIES

COMPETENCY	CMA	RMA	CCMA	NCMA
Administrative				
Perform basic clerical skills	X	X	X	X
Manage the physician's professional schedule and travel	X	X	X	X
General/Legal/Professional				
Respond to and initiate written communications by using correct grammar, spelling, and formatting techniques	X	X	X	X
Recognize and respond to verbal and nonverbal communications by being attentive and adapting communication to the recipient's level of understanding	X	X	X	X
Demonstrate proper telephone techniques	X	X	X	X
Instruct individuals according to their needs	X	X	X	X

MEDICAL ASSISTING COMPETENCIES (cont.)

General/Legal/Professional

Project a positive attitude	X	X	X	
Be a "team player"	X	X	X	
Exhibit initiative	X	X	X	
Serve as a liaison between the physician and others	X	X		
Interview effectively	X	X	X	
Use appropriate medical terminology	X	X	X	X
Receive, organize, prioritize, and transmit information appropriately	X	X	X	X

STRATEGIES FOR SUCCESS

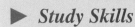 *Study Skills*

Manage your time!

It's easy to develop good study habits if you manage your time effectively. Every day, set aside a time when you can study without interruption. Don't let anything else intrude on this time—not shopping, not paying bills, not running errands, not socializing with friends, not even family (except in the direst emergencies). In this way you will have study time and still be able to get everything else done you want to. Write a daily to-do list and check tasks off as you complete them.

9.1 Reception

Receptionist: The receptionist greets patients, assists with office functions, and is the first person who will have contact with the patient and help the patient form a first impression about the facility and its employees.

Receptionist Duties

Receptionist duties: Receptionists should be professional, confident, and caring. They are responsible for ensuring patient safety and confidentiality at all times. Generally, a receptionist's duties include:

- Opening and closing the office
- Replenishing supplies
- Greeting patients
- Signing in patients
- Registering new patients
- Answering patients' questions
- Assisting with patient forms
- Collating records
- Answering the phone
- Writing charge slips
- Inputting no-shows
- Preparing the office for patients' arrival

- Escorting and instructing patients
- Making sure that the reception area is safe and clean
- Handling patients' complaints

Scheduling: Set up appointments according to the method used by the physician to provide efficient services.

Opening the office: The receptionist responsible for opening the office should arrive 15–20 minutes before office hours begin.

Registering new patients: New patients need to fill out a complete patient registration form containing demographic information. Assist patients who are unable to read or write.

Collating records: Collect all records, test results, and information pertaining to the patient who is scheduled to be seen by the physician. Collation is usually done the day before the patient is seen.

Professionalism: Always be professional. Get to know patients, but only on a professional level, not on a personal level. Call patients by name. Be polite, tactful, and respectful.

9.2 Managing Correspondence and Mail

Classification: Mail can be classified according to type, weight, and destination. The measurement units are the ounce and pound. The U.S. Postal Service (USPS) has recently updated its classification system.

The following classifications of mail are used under the new system:

- First-Class Mail
- Priority Mail
- Periodicals
- Standard Mail
- Express Mail (also called Priority Mail Express)

To get the most current information on classifications and rates or to order supplies, call the USPS (800-ASK-USPS) or visit http://www.usps.com.

Types of Mail

Regular Mail: Includes several classes of mail plus Priority and Express Mail. Each class determines how quickly delivery will occur.

First-Class Mail: Only items that weigh 13 ounces or less may be sent as First-Class Mail. If you mail envelopes larger than the standard No. 10 size, the envelope should have a green diamond border to expedite First-Class delivery. Another way to expedite First-Class Mail is to separate letters according to zip code. If you mail 500 or more items, you can get a discounted bulk rate from the post office. Most medical office correspondence is sent via First-Class Mail.

Second-Class Mail: Designed for newspapers and periodicals only.

Periodicals: Mailed items including newspapers, magazines, journals, newsletters, and so on.

Media Mail: This classification is used for books, manuscript, printed test materials, film, printed music, sound recordings, and printed educational charts. It is also used for videotapes and computer recorded media (CD-ROMs and diskettes). Media Mail cannot weigh over 70 pounds. It is also known as *Third-Class Mail.*

Parcel Post: Formerly called *Fourth-Class Mail,* it is used for items weighing 1–70 pounds that do not require quick delivery. Rates are based on weight and distance. A special rate exists for books, manuscripts, and certain types of medical publications.

Bound Printed Matter: Used for promotional advertising and directories, but not for personal correspondence. Bulk rates are available beginning at 300 pieces.

Priority Mail: Provides First-Class handling for all items that weigh 70 pounds or less. First-Class Mail that weighs more than 13 ounces *must* be sent as Priority Mail. Priority Mail provides second-day service between all major business markets and three-day service everywhere else within the United States.

Express Mail: (Priority Mail Express): The fastest mail service offered by the USPS. It provides guaranteed expedited service for any mailable matter. Express Mail is deliverable seven days a week including holidays. Express Mail packaging supplies are available at no charge from your local post office. Express Mail should be used for urgent business documents, such as contracts and sales orders. A flat rate is charged for anything mailed in the special USPS flat-rate envelope, regardless of weight. Overnight delivery is guaranteed. Federal Express (FedEx) and United Parcel Service (UPS) also offer next-day delivery service.

Online postage: With USPS-approved software, postage can now be purchased online, via the Internet.

International mail: The majority of letters to distant foreign countries, as well as to Mexico and Canada, are sent by air mail at international rates determined by the USPS.

Standard mail: This is mail not required to be mailed as First-Class Mail or periodicals. It includes flyers, circulars, advertising, newsletters, bulletins, catalogs, and small parcels.

Combination mailing: A package with an accompanying letter is called Combination Mail. The letter should be attached to the outside of the package, or the letter should be placed inside the package and the package marked *Letter Enclosed* just below the space for the postage. Separate postage is paid for the parcel and the letter. This method is commonly used to send X-rays with an accompanying report.

Mail Characteristics

Prohibited items: The USPS prohibits the mailing of fraudulent or pornographic materials. The responsibility for mailing any materials, whether or not they are prohibited or hazardous, rests with the mailer.

Hazardous materials: Materials designated by the U.S. Department of Transportation (DOT) as being capable of posing unreasonable risk to health, safety, and property during transportation. Certain drugs and medicines can be classified as hazardous materials.

Minimum size: The post office prescribes minimum sizes for mail to prevent individuals from mailing items so small that they might be lost. If a mail piece is 0.25-inch thick or less, it must be at least 3.5 inches high by 5 inches long. All mailable matter must be at least 0.007-inch thick.

Maximum size: The maximum size for mail pieces is 108 inches in combined length and girth. The maximum mailable weight of any mail piece is 70 pounds. Items mailed as Parcel Post can have a maximum combined length and girth of 130 inches.

Shape: The shape of your mail can determine the rate you pay. The post office separates mail into four size-and-shape categories: cards, letters, flats/nonletters, and parcels.

Cards: Eligible for First-Class services, such as forwarding and return.

Flats: A category for large envelopes, newsletters, and magazines. Flats should not be more than 12 inches high by 15 inches long by 4.75 inches thick.

Special Mail Services

Return Service Requested: Provides no forwarding service, only return with a new address notification. This service is free for First-Class and Priority Mail; Standard Mail is charged First-Class or Priority Mail rates for the return.

Forwarding Service Requested: Provides forwarding and return, but new address notification is provided only for returned items. First-Class, Priority, and Express Mail automatically get this service without any endorsement and free of charge. Periodicals are forwarded without charge for 60 days when postage is fully prepaid by the sender.

Special Delivery: A service that was used to ensure that mail got delivered as soon as it reached the recipient's post office. Special Delivery could be used for regular First-Class, Second-Class, and insured mail. It could not be used for mail addressed to a post office box or military installation. Although Special Delivery is no longer available, please note that questions about this service may still appear on the certification exams.

Special Handling: A method of sending Third- and Parcel Post mail that offers the fastest ground transportation possible, at nearly the speed of First-Class Mail handling. A special handling fee is added, which is determined by the item's weight.

Certified Mail: A special mailing method that uses First-Class rates plus an additional fee; it is used for contracts, other legal documents, financial documents, passports, insurance policies, money orders, and any other documents that would be difficult to replace if lost. A record of certified mail is kept at the post office of delivery for two years. Medical assistants should keep certified mail forms and return receipts in the medical office.

Insurance: Any piece of domestic mail may be insured for damage or loss. Insurance is available for Priority, First-Class, and Standard Mail.

Registered Mail: The most secure service offered by the post office. Registered Mail provides insurance coverage for valuable items and is controlled from the point of mailing to the point of delivery. This service should be reserved for mailing items of tangible value, such as gifts or items that cannot be replaced in case of loss or damage.

Delivery Confirmation: For an added fee, mail is tracked using a tracking number, by its delivery date and signature of the recipient.

Restricted Delivery: Mail is delivered only to a specific addressee or to someone authorized in writing to receive mail for the addressee. Restricted Delivery is available only for Registered Mail, Certified Mail, COD mail, and mail insured for more than $50.

Return Receipt Requested: A receipt that will be returned to the sender to prove that the item was delivered. For a small fee, this signed receipt may be obtained on Express Mail, COD, Registered Mail, Certified Mail, and most insured mail.

Collect on Delivery (COD): Used when the mailer wants to collect payment for merchandise or postage from the recipient when the mail is delivered.

Tracing mail: If a piece of Registered or Certified Mail is lost, you may ask the post office to trace it. You should bring any receipts associated with the item.

Recalling mail: You can recall mail by filling out a written application at the post office and submitting it along with an envelope that is addressed identically to the one you want to recall. A mail carrier is not permitted to simply give mail back to you.

Postal money orders: A convenient way to mail money; each domestic money order may be purchased for an amount as high as $1,000.

Private delivery services: Many private services offer various delivery options and also deliver mail overnight. They include FedEx, UPS, Consolidated Freightways, and DHL Express. These services are well advertised and competitive. Private courier services are also available, though these are usually smaller, local companies who serve a specific area.

U.S. Postal Service state abbreviations: The USPS recommends using the two-letter state abbreviations listed in Table 9-1.

Mail Processing

Opening mail: In general, mail processing involves sorting, opening, recording, annotating, and distributing. Some physicians prefer to open letters from attorneys or accountants. Mail such as routine office expense bills, insurance forms, and checks for deposit may not need to be opened by the physician. In general, when you transmit letters to the physician, place the most important letters on the top and the least important ones on the bottom. Usually something marked *Special Delivery* is considered important mail. After opening the mail, medical assistants usually need to date-stamp the letters, check for enclosures, and in some cases annotate the letter. You should not open mail marked *Personal* or *Confidential* unless you have the addressee's explicit permission.

Recording: Keeping a daily log of all received mail, which also indicates the completion and date of any follow-up correspondence. Recording helps to trace items and track correspondence.

Annotate: To furnish with notes, which are usually critical or explanatory. You must highlight key points of the letter or write reminders and comments in the margins of the letter.

Distributing: Sorting individual mail pieces into batches for distribution to each individual recipient, including physicians, the billing supervisor, and others. Present each batch of mail to recipients organized in file folders, or arranged with most important items on top.

Handling of Drugs and Product Samples: According to procedures required by the physician or office manager, drugs and product samples may be placed in a consultation room for evaluation, in locked storage cabinets, or in patient treatment areas. Samples should be sorted and labeled by category. All distribution to patients must be recorded in patient charts. Outdated samples must be disposed of according to law.

Preparing outgoing mail: To mail a letter that has been edited and proofread, preparation includes having it signed, preparing its envelope, folding and inserting the letter into the envelope, and affixing the proper postage. On an envelope, the right upper corner below the stamp is the most appropriate place to put notations for the postal service.

Multiple delivery addresses: If the envelope has a post office box as well as a street address, it will be delivered to the address that appears directly above the city-state-zip code.

Signatures: The physician may authorize another staff member to sign letters. If you, the medical assistant, are designated by the physician to do this, then sign the physician's name and place your initials after the signature. If instead the physician signs all documents, place all letters to be signed in a file folder marked "For Your Signature."

Postage meter: Most medical offices use a postage meter that automatically stamps large mailings. The meter can print postage directly onto an envelope or a special gummed label. The cost of a postage meter must be weighed against the expense and inconvenience of making trips to the post office and keeping several different denominations of stamps on hand. Remember to change the date daily on the postage meter.

State	Abbreviation	State	Abbreviation
Alabama	AL	Montana	MT
Alaska	AK	Nebraska	NE
Arizona	AZ	Nevada	NV
Arkansas	AR	New Hampshire	NH
California	CA	New Jersey	NJ
Colorado	CO	New Mexico	NM
Connecticut	CT	New York	NY
Delaware	DE	North Carolina	NC
District of Columbia	DC	North Dakota	ND
Florida	FL	Ohio	OH
Georgia	GA	Oklahoma	OK
Hawaii	HI	Oregon	OR
Idaho	ID	Pennsylvania	PA
Illinois	IL	Puerto Rico	PR
Indiana	IN	Rhode Island	RI
Iowa	IA	South Carolina	SC
Kansas	KS	South Dakota	SD
Kentucky	KY	Tennessee	TN
Louisiana	LA	Texas	TX
Maine	ME	Utah	UT
Maryland	MD	Vermont	VT
Massachusetts	MA	Virginia	VA
Michigan	MI	Washington	WA
Minnesota	MN	West Virginia	WV
Mississippi	MS	Wisconsin	WI
Missouri	MO	Wyoming	WY

Table 9-1

Business Letter Components

Components: Business letters consist of letterhead on which are printed a dateline, an inside address, a salutation, a subject line, the body of the letter, a complimentary closing, a signature block, an identification line, and notations. See Figure 9-1.

Dateline: Usually keyed 2.5 inches below the top edge or 0.5 inch below the letterhead. The date should be completely written out, as in *December 15, 2016*.

Inside address: States the title and address of the person for whom the letter is intended. Degree designations should always be abbreviated, and when a professional degree is used, no other title should be placed in front of the name. For a physician, therefore, the title should read either *Dr. John Smith* or *John Smith, M.D.* The form *Dr. John Smith, M.D.* is incorrect.

Use numerals for the building number unless it is a single digit, which should be spelled out: *Three Broadway Place.* Also spell out the words *Street, Drive, Boulevard, Place,* and so on.

Salutation: Keyed flush with the left margin on the second line below the inside address. The formal salutation should refer to the receiver of the letter, using a title and surname (last name): *Dear Mrs. Brown.* If the receiver and sender know each other well, the receiver's given name (first name) may be used. No salutation is necessary in a memorandum.

Subject: A subject line is sometimes used to bring the subject of the letter to the reader's attention. It should be typed two lines below the salutation and two lines above the body of the letter.

Body: Begins two lines below the salutation or subject line. It is single spaced with a blank line between paragraphs.

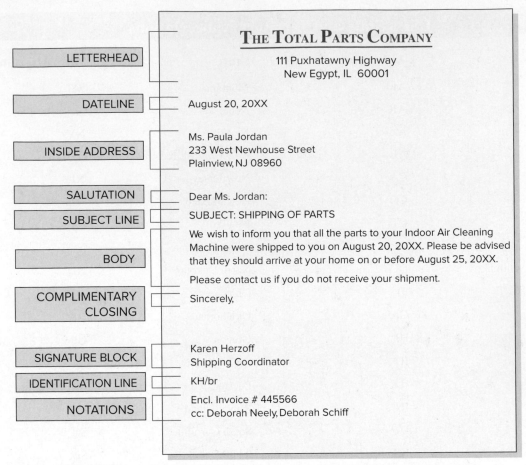

Figure 9-1 *Knowing the parts of a typical business letter enables medical assistants to create written communications that reflect well on the office.*

Complimentary closing: Placed two lines below the last line of the body and consisting of one of the following: *Sincerely, Yours truly,* or *Best regards.* It is followed by a comma.

Signature: The signature block contains the sender's name on the first line and title on the second line.

Identification line: The typist's initials are sometimes included two lines below the signature block. These initials are often preceded by a colon or a slash. The traditional full form includes the initials of the person responsible for creating the letter followed by a colon or a slash and then the typist's initials.

Continuation pages: Pages of a letter that are in addition to the first page. They should begin on the tenth line from the top of the page, or on the third line below the page heading.

Notation: Includes information such as the number and type of enclosures and the names of other people who receive copies of the letter (referred to as carbon copies or courtesy copies, abbreviated *cc*). The word *enclosure(s)* can be abbreviated as *Enc, Encl,* or *Encs*. The notation is typed two lines below the signature block or identification line.

Correspondence Style and Format

Format: The physical presentation of the message is as important as the written content. The guidelines for formatting letters are as follows:

- For most letters, margins should be one-inch wide.
- For shorter letters, use wider margins and start the address farther down the page.
- The body of the letter should be single spaced; use double spacing between paragraphs.
- Use short sentences (fewer than 20 words).
- Use short paragraphs. Most business correspondence should be no more than a page long.
- For multiple-page letters, use letterhead for the first page and blank paper for the other pages. This paper should be of the same bond and quality as the letterhead. On the second and subsequent pages, insert a header that contains the name of the addressee, page number, date, and subject (if needed).
- Sign letters of routine business (such as ordering office supplies). Most other letters should be signed by the physician.
- Letters with misspelled words or errors may give the receiver a negative impression of the staff of the medical practice. Table 9-2 lists frequently misspelled and misused words.

Letter styles: There are four major styles of letters: full block, modified block, indented, and simplified.

Medical Terms

abscess	diluent	larynx	pleurisy
aerobic	dissect	leukemia	pneumonia
anergic	eosinophil	leukocyte	polyp
anesthetic	epididymis	malaise	prescription
aneurysm	epistaxis	menstruation	prophylaxis
anteflexion	erythema	metastasis	prostate
arrhythmia	eustachian	muscle	prosthesis
asepsis	fissure	neuron	pruritus
asthma	flexure	nosocomial	psoriasis
auricle	fomites	occlusion	psychiatrist
benign	glaucoma	ophthalmology	pyrexia
bilirubin	glomerular	oscilloscope	respiration
bronchial	gonorrhea	osseous	rheumatism
calcaneus	hemocytometer	palliative	roentgenology
capillary	hemorrhage	parasite	serous
cervical	hemorrhoids	parenteral	specimen
chancre	homeostasis	parietal	sphincter
choroid	humerus	paroxysm	sphygmomanometer
chromosome	ileum	pericardium	squamous
cirrhosis	ilium	perineum	staphylococcus
clavicle	infarction	peristalsis	surgeon
curettage	inoculate	peritoneum	vaccine
cyanosis	intussusception	pharynx	vein
defibrillator	ischemia	pituitary	venereal
desiccation	ischium	plantar	wheal

Other Words

absence	defendant	irritable	proceed
accept	definite	its	professor
accessible	dependent	it's	pronunciation
accommodate	description	labeled	psychiatry
accumulate	desirable	laboratory	psychology
achieve	development	led	pursue
acquire	dilemma	leisure	questionnaire
adequate	disappear	liable	rearrange
advantageous	disappoint	liaison	recede
affect	disapprove	license	receive
aggravate	disastrous	liquefy	recommend
all right	discreet	maintenance	referral
a lot	discrete	maneuver	relieve

Table 9-2

Other Words

already	discrimination	miscellaneous	repetition
altogether	dissatisfied	misspelled	rescind
analysis	dissipate	necessary	résumé
analyze	earnest	noticeable	rhythm
apparatus	ecstasy	occasion	ridiculous
apparent	effect	occurrence	schedule
appearance	eligible	offense	secretary
appropriate	embarrass	oscillate	seize
approximate	emphasis	paid	separate
argument	entrepreneur	pamphlet	similar
assistance	envelope	panicky	sizable
associate	environment	paradigm	stationary
auxiliary	exceed	parallel	stationery
balloon	except	paralyze	stomach
bankruptcy	exercise	pastime	subpoena
believe	exhibit	persevere	succeed
benefited	exhilaration	persistent	suddenness
brochure	existence	personal	supersede
bulletin	fantasy	personnel	surprise
business	fascinate	persuade	tariff
category	February	phenomenon	technique
changeable	fluorescent	plagiarism	temperament
characteristic	forty	pleasant	temperature
cigarette	grammar	possession	thorough
circumference	grievance	precede	transferred
clientele	guarantee	precedent	truly
committee	handkerchief	predictable	tyrannize
comparative	height	predominant	unnecessary
complement	humorous	prejudice	until
compliment	hygiene	preparation	vacillate
concede	incidentally	prerogative	vacuum
conscientious	indispensable	prevalent	vegetable
conscious	inimitable	principal	vicious
controversy	insistent	principle	warrant
corroborate	irrelevant	privilege	Wednesday
counsel	irresistible	procedure	weird
courtesy			

Table 9-2, concluded

From Booth, Kathryn (et al.) *Medical Assisting, 5/e.* Copyright © McGraw-Hill Education. Reprinted by permission of McGraw-Hill Education.

Full block: Typed with all lines in standard letter format, flush left. It is quick and easy to write. This style is one of the most common formats used in medical practices. See Figure 9-2.

Modified block: All lines begin at the left margin, with the exception of the date line, complimentary closing, and keyed signature, which usually begin at the center position.

Simplified: Omits the salutation and the complimentary closing. All lines are keyed flush with the left margin. It is the most modern letter style. However, in most situations in a medical office, the simplified letter style may be too informal. See Figure 9-3.

Letterhead: Formal business stationery on which the name and address of the office or the physician are printed.

ABC PUBLISHERS, INC.

July 10, 20XX

Ms. Lara Erickson
2594 Hughes Boulevard
Hamilton City, NJ 08999

Dear Ms. Erickson:

SUBJECT: SHIPMENT DELAY

Thank you for contacting us regarding your order for *Smith and Doe's New Medical Dictionary*. Due to an unexpectedly heavy demand for the book, we are experiencing delays in processing and shipping orders.

We expect to ship your book in four weeks, around August 15. Because of this delay, we offer you the option of canceling your order with a full refund. If you would like to cancel at this point, please fill out and return the enclosed postcard. If we do not hear from you, your order will be shipped when ready.

We are sorry for any inconvenience this delay may cause you. Please be assured that ABC Publishers values its customers and always endeavors to fulfill orders in a timely fashion.

Sincerely yours,

Andrew Williams

Andrew Williams
Customer Service Manager

AW/cjc
Enclosure

117 New Avenue New York, NY 10000

Figure 9-2 *The full-block letter style is quicker and easier to type than other styles.*

Standard letterhead: Letterhead that is 8.5 by 11 inches in size and is used in professional correspondence and letters that discuss general business.

Executive letterhead: Letterhead that is 7.25 by 10.5 inches in size and is used for social and informal correspondence.

Baronial letterhead: Letterhead that is 5.5 by 8.5 inches in size and is used for short letters and memos.

Felt side of letterhead: The side from which the watermark is readable and the side on which printing and typing should be done.

ABC PUBLISHERS, INC.

July 10, 20XX

Ms. Lara Erickson
2594 Hughes Boulevard
Hamilton City, NJ 08999

SHIPMENT DELAY

Thank you for contacting us regarding your order for *Smith and Doe's New Medical Dictionary*. Due to an unexpectedly heavy demand for the book, we are experiencing delays in processing and shipping orders.

We expect to ship your book in four weeks, around August 15. Because of this delay, we offer you the option of canceling your order with a full refund. If you would like to cancel at this point, please fill out and return the enclosed postcard. If we do not hear from you, your order will be shipped when ready.

We are sorry for any inconvenience this delay may cause you. Please be assured that ABC Publishers values its customers and always endeavors to fulfill orders in a timely fashion.

Andrew Williams

ANDREW WILLIAMS, CUSTOMER SERVICE MANAGER

AW/cjc
Enclosure

117 New Avenue New York, NY 10000

Figure 9-3 *An example of the simplified letter style.*

Memoranda (memos): Periodically used by medical offices, clinics, and hospitals. Memos generally facilitate informal written communication within an office.

Writing style: Good writing style demands accuracy, clarity, simplicity, and courtesy.

Proofreading: Requires concentration and attention. Common mistakes involve content, punctuation (including the use of apostrophes, hyphens, and parentheses), grammar, spelling, and spacing. Proofread each document twice: once on the screen and then on a hard copy. See Figure 9-4 for common proofreader's marks. For the basic rules of writing, see Table 9-3.

Tools for proofreading and editing: These include the following reference books:

- **Dictionary:** Contains word definitions, correct spellings, ways to divide and pronounce words, and parts of speech (whether each word is a noun, verb, adjective, etc.). Dictionaries are available over the Internet or in printed book form.

- **Medical Dictionary:** Contains medical terms and definitions, correct spellings, prefixes, suffixes, etc. Medical dictionaries are more regularly updated when accessed over the Internet than in printed book form.

- **Thesaurus:** Contains *synonyms,* which are similar words to a specific word you are using. This helps to find other words to express ideas in writing and avoid repetition of words. Thesauruses are available over the Internet, as part of word-processing programs, and in printed form.

Mark	Meaning	Mark	Meaning
stet	Leave as is	|	Align vertically
℈	Delete	wf	Wrong font
ital	Italic type	∨ ∧	Insert here
rom	Roman (regular) type	⊙	Insert period
bf	Bold type	∧	Insert comma
lc.	Lowercase	" " ∨ ∨	Insert quotation marks
caps	All capital letters	=	Insert hyphen
◠	Close up space	(|)	Insert parentheses
fl	Flush left	; |	Insert semicolon
fr	Flush right	: |	Insert colon
] [	Center	#	Insert space
[	Set farther left	¶	Insert a return/ start a new paragraph
]	Set farther right		
tr	Transpose words/ punctuation		

Figure 9-4 *Proofreader's marks.*

AT A GLANCE Basic Rules of Writing

Word Division

Divide:

- According to pronunciation
- Compound words between the two words from which they are derived
- Hyphenated compound words at the hyphen
- After a prefix
- Before a suffix
- Between two consonants that appear between vowels
- Before –*ing* unless the last consonant is doubled, in which case, divide before the second consonant

Do not divide:

- Such suffixes as –*sion,* –*tial,* and –*tion*
- A word so that only one letter is left on a line

Capitalization

Capitalize:

- All proper names
- All titles, positions, or indications of family relation when preceding a proper name or in place of a proper noun (Do not capitalize when the word is used alone or with possessive pronouns or articles.)
- Days of the week, months, and holidays
- Names of organizations and membership designations
- Racial, religious, and political designations
- Adjectives, nouns, and verbs that are derived from proper nouns (including currently copyrighted trade names)
- Specific addresses and geographic locations
- Sums of money written in legal or business documents
- Titles or headings of books, magazines, and newspapers

Table 9-3

Plurals

- Add -*s* or -*es* to most singular nouns. (Plural forms of most medical terms do not follow this rule.)

- With medical terms ending in -*is,* drop the *is* and add *es:* metastasis/metastases.

- With terms ending in -*um,* drop the *um* and add *a:* diverticulum/diverticula.

- With terms ending in -*us,* drop the *us* and add *i:* calculus/calculi.

- Exception: The plural forms of some words, mainly from Latin, involve other changes: corpus/corpora, genus/genera, sinus/sinuses, virus/viruses.

- With most terms ending in -*ma,* add *ta:* stoma/stomata.

- With terms otherwise ending in -*a,* drop the *a* and add *ae:* vertebra/vertebrae.

Possessives

To show ownership or relation to another noun:

- For singular nouns, add an apostrophe and an *s.*

- For plural nouns that do not end in an *s,* add an apostrophe and an *s.*

- For plural nouns that end in an *s,* add just an apostrophe.

Numbers

Use numerals:

- In general writing, when the number is 11 or greater

- With abbreviations and symbols

- When discussing laboratory results or statistics

- When referring to specific sums of money

- When using a series of numbers in a sentence

Tips:

- Use commas when numerals have more than three digits.

- Do not use commas when referring to account numbers, page numbers, or policy numbers.

- Use a hyphen (or an en dash, if possible) with numerals to indicate a range.

Table 9-3, concluded

Spell checking: A function within a word-processing program that scans a document for spelling errors. Higher-level *medical spell-checking programs* are available, which contain medical terminology as well as standard vocabulary terms.

Editing: The editing process ensures that the content of all documents is accurate, clear, complete, and organized logically.

Abbreviations: Abbreviations recommended by the USPS do not use punctuation marks. See Table 9-4. States and U.S. territories are designated by two-letter abbreviations (see Table 9-1).

ZIP plus 4 codes: Nine-digit codes that identify the city, the individual post office, and the zone within the city.

Envelopes: There are three commonly used sizes: Number 6¾, Number 7, and Number 10 (also called business size). Most common in the medical office are Number 6¾ and Number 10. The Number 6¾ size with a window is often used for mailing statements.

Address: Individual First-Class letters must be addressed clearly and legibly. The recipient address must be printed single spaced on the envelope in all capital letters with no punctuation. Put the addressee's name on the first line, the department on the second line, and the company name on the third line. If the letter is being sent to someone's attention at a company, put the company name first and *ATTENTION: [NAME]* on the second line. The last line in the address must include the city, the two-letter state abbreviation, and the zip code. See Figure 9-5.

Return address: A return address for the sender should always be placed in the upper-left corner. This ensures return of the letter if the postage falls off or it is mistakenly mailed without postage. A return address ensures that the letter will be returned in an official envelope with a notice of postage due.

Notations: Terms placed on an envelope, such as *Confidential* or *Personal;* they are typed in all-capital letters immediately below the postage area.

Word	Abbreviation	Word	Abbreviation
Apartment	APT	Lane	LN
Avenue	AVE	North	N
Boulevard	BLVD	Parkway	PKY or PKWY
Center	CTR	Place	PL
Circle	CIR	Plaza	PLZ
Corner	COR	Road	RD
Court	CT	Room	RM
Drive	DR	South	S
East	E	Street	ST
Expressway	EXPY	Suite	STE
Highway	HWY	West	W
Junction	JCT		

Table 9-4

Handling instructions: Instructions, such as the words *Personal* or *Confidential*, should be placed three lines below the return address.

9.3 Telephone Techniques

Telephone calls: Classified as incoming, outgoing, and inter-office. First impressions matter in telephone communications.

Because you are usually the first contact most people have with a medical office, you should convey a professional and positive attitude by what you say and how you sound to the caller. You also need to take care to maintain patient confidentiality.

Volume: Should be the same as when speaking to someone in the same room, just loud enough for them to hear clearly. Bear in mind that some patients may be hard of hearing.

Enunciation: Speak clearly and articulate carefully. Do not slur your speech.

Pronunciation: Adopt a speech pattern that is considered standard. Make sure that you use terminology you are comfortable with so that all of your pronunciation is correct.

Speed: Should be at a normal rate, neither too fast nor too slow.

Answering system: May be an automated voice mail system, an answering machine, or an answering service.

Answering service: Answering services employ people rather than machines to answer the telephone. They take messages and communicate them to the doctor on call. Answering machines sometimes are programmed to refer callers to an answering service in case of emergencies, or the answering service may directly answer the phone after a certain number of rings during specific hours. It is best to set a regular schedule to retrieve messages from the answering service.

Voice mail: A system in which callers can leave recorded messages over the telephone. The recorded message itself is also called voice mail.

Telecom teletype machine: A specially designed telephone that looks like a laptop computer with a cradle for the receiver of a traditional telephone. The receiver is placed in the cradle and the hearing-impaired patient can then type the communication on the keyboard. The message can be received by another telecom teletype machine or relayed through a specialty relay service.

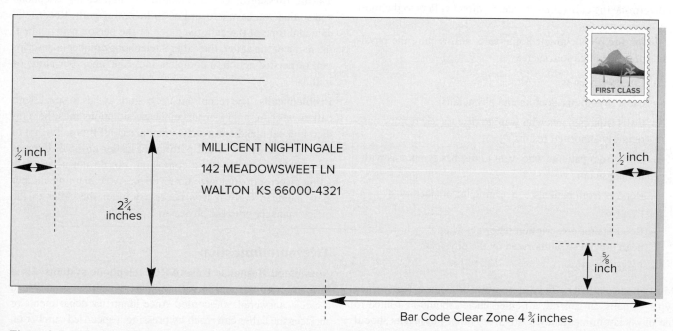

Figure 9-5 *Following this format for typing an envelope ensures that it can be processed by USPS electronic equipment.*

Incoming Calls

Incoming calls: Handle incoming calls as follows:

- Answer telephone calls promptly, by the second or third ring.
- Hold the phone's mouthpiece about an inch away from your mouth, and leave at least one hand free for writing.
- Never eat or chew gum while answering the phone.
- Greet callers first with the name of the office and then with your name. Do not answer the phone by simply giving the number of your office or by saying, "Hello."
- Identify the caller. Demonstrate your willingness to assist the caller by asking, "How may I help you?"
- Be courteous, calm, and pleasant, using phrases such as "please" and "thank you."
- Pay full attention to the caller, and listen carefully. Identify the nature of the call.
- Use words appropriate to the situation, but avoid using technical terms.
- Avoid unnecessarily long conversations. Keep any personal conversations to a minimum.
- If you get interrupted by a second call, excuse yourself to the first caller and answer the second call. Determine the identity of the second caller and the nature of the call. Return to the first call as soon as possible.
- At the end of the call, say "goodbye" and use the caller's name.
- Always ask the caller for permission before putting him or her on hold.

Telephone screening: When receiving incoming telephone calls, the medical assistant should use a screening technique to determine the call's importance, to direct callers to the most appropriate person.

Calls for the physician(s): Some calls will require the physician's personal attention, such as:

- Emergency calls
- Calls from other doctors and physicians
- Calls from patients who want to discuss test results, particularly abnormal results
- Calls from patients who want to discuss symptoms with the physician
- Reports from patients concerning unsatisfactory progress
- Requests for prescription renewals when they have not been previously authorized by the physician
- Personal calls

Most medical offices have a routing procedure for various types of calls. In general, all emergencies should be routed to the physician immediately. Calls from other physicians should also be routed to the doctor immediately, if possible.

Transferring calls: When you transfer calls, identify the person calling to the physician and give a brief description of the nature of the call. If a caller refuses to be identified, you should not put the call through to the physician.

Administrative-issue calls: Common calls to a physician's office that a medical assistant can handle. These calls include:

- Appointment scheduling, rescheduling, and canceling
- Insurance questions
- Inquiries about bills
- X-ray and laboratory reports
- Routine reports from hospitals regarding a patient's progress
- Satisfactory progress reports from patients
- Requests for referrals to other doctors
- Questions concerning office policies, fees, hours, and other such items
- Calls such as complaints about administrative matters
- Prescription refills when they have been previously authorized by the physician

Emergency triage: The screening and sorting of emergency situations, used as a process of evaluating the urgency of a medical condition and deciding what necessary action to take. Depending on the medical facility, some medical assistants may be required to perform triage; therefore, you should be familiar with this concept. See Table 9-5 for information on which symptoms and conditions require immediate medical help.

Documenting calls: Proper documentation protects the physician if the caller takes legal action. This documentation provides an accurate record and helps guard against lawsuits.

Taking messages: Use a standard self-duplicating telephone pad so that you have a record of all incoming calls. Record the date and time of the call, the name of the person being called, the name of the caller, the caller's telephone number, a description of needed action, a complete message, and your name or initials.

Problem calls: The receptionist occasionally has to speak with callers who are angry or upset. These situations must be handled in a calm and constructive manner at all times. Try not to interrupt the caller. Avoid putting the caller on hold. Express regret that the caller has a complaint, but do not necessarily admit an error or apologize for an error. Avoid blaming another staff member. Only if it is necessary, refer the caller to the office manager or to the physician.

Telecommunication

Automated Response Unit (ARU) telephone systems: Used in many hospitals and larger ambulatory care settings. When a call is answered, a recorded voice identifies departments or services the caller can reach by pressing a specified number on the telephone keypad.

Unconsciousness

Lack of breathing or trouble breathing

Severe bleeding

Persistant pressure or pain in the abdomen

Severe vomiting

Bloody stools

Poisoning

Injuries to the head, neck, or back

Choking

Drowning

Electrical shock

Snakebites

Vehicle collisions

Allergic reactions to foods or insect stings

Chemicals or foreign objects in the eye

Fires, severe burns, or injuries from explosion

Human bites or any deep animal bites

Heart attack (Symptoms: chest pain or pressure; pain radiating from the chest to the arm, shoulder, neck, jaw, back, or stomach; nausea or vomiting; weakness; shortness of breath; pale or gray skin color)

Stroke (Symptoms: seizures, severe headache, slurred speech)

Broken bones (Symptoms: inability to move or put weight on the injured body part, misshapen appearance of body part)

Shock (Symptoms: paleness, feeling faint and sweaty, weak and rapid pulse, cold and moist skin, confusion or drowsiness)

Heatstroke (Symptoms: confusion, loss of consciousness, flushed skin that is hot and dry, strong and rapid pulse)

Hypothermia (Symptoms: increasing clumsiness; unreasonable behavior; irritability; confusion; sleepy, slurred speech; slipping into a coma with slow, weak breathing and heartbeat)

Table 9-5

Fax (facsimile) machines: Common in the physician's office, these machines are used to send reports, referrals, insurance approvals, and informal correspondence. A fax is sent over telephone lines from one fax machine (or fax modem) to another. The fax machine must be in a secure location where only authorized personnel have access to it.

Electronic mail (e-mail): The process of sending, receiving, storing, and forwarding messages in digital form through telephone lines or via dedicated Internet connections. Messages are transmitted from computer to computer. The messages are stored until the receiver retrieves them. Both the sender and the receiver may print messages or forward them to another electronic mailbox. E-mail can save time and money.

Intercom: A direct line of an intercommunication system within the facility.

9.4 Supplies and Equipment in the Medical Office

Budgeting: Most medical offices use an annual budget to determine how money will be spent on supplies and equipment. The budget should also take into account salaries, utilities, rent or mortgage, insurance, maintenance, taxes, and laboratory fees. All receipts for purchases should be kept. Expense categories are used to itemize purchases, and are included in the *overhead* expenses of the office.

Price comparisons: Vendor prices should always be compared to guarantee the lowest cost. Also take into account opportunities for bulk purchasing, warranties, product quality, and maintenance agreements.

Ordering supplies: Ideally, only one person should handle ordering of supplies. Printouts of spreadsheets are often posted in storage areas so that stock can easily be checked and noted. Other methods include the use of stickers identifying stock on hand, and bar coding to scan in supplies used, which calculates stock on hand in the computer system. Many supplies are ordered over the Internet. To avoid ordering and purchasing unnecessary medical office supplies, the medical assistant should take an inventory of supplies frequently. Office supplies include stationery, paper clips, staples, pens, pencils, and so on.

Ordering equipment: Equipment ordering is different from supply ordering because equipment is defined as a *capital* purchase. Due to equipment's higher cost, the physician is often involved in these decisions. Office equipment includes photocopiers, computes, scanners, printers, and so on.

Photocopiers: They primarily use dry toner and a heat process to reproduce text and images. The medical assistant must order all supplies needed for photocopiers, including paper and toner.

Computers: Various types of computing devices are used in the medical office for word processing, spreadsheets, scheduling, e-mail, and many other applications.

Scanners: Various devices that scan documents are utilized along with computers.

Printers: Most medical offices utilize all-in-one printers that also fax, copy, and scan laser-quality documents.

Receiving: Open received shipments only when there is sufficient time to verify their contents completely. Never take items out of shipping boxes unless they are checked against the *packing slip.*

Packing slips: Lists of items ordered and actual items shipped.

Warranties: Periods in which a manufacturer protects the purchaser against defects or other problems with a purchased product. The warranty period begins on the date of purchase and usually lasts for one year (or more).

Invoices: Itemized lists of goods shipped that specify prices and terms of sale.

Statements: Summaries of financial accounts showing balances due and transactions that affect the accounts. Invoices precede statements.

Equipment failure: When equipment fails, consult the owner's manual to take steps to troubleshoot the problem. Many manufacturers provide quick, direct access to support personnel over the Internet for equipment failure.

Equipment maintenance: Testing equipment, and other equipment, must be maintained regularly. Controls and calibrations must be performed according to Clinical Laboratory Improvement Act (CLIA) guidelines. Only authorized personnel should perform equipment maintenance.

9.5 Travel Arrangements

Preparations for a trip: In preparing for a trip, the medical assistant should consult with the person traveling, carefully noting the date and time of departure, destinations, length of stay at each destination, and times of arrival at and departure from each destination.

Itinerary: A list that specifies each place the traveler will visit, the name and address of the hotel, the date and time of arrival and departure, and the schedule of the convention if relevant.

Meetings: An *agenda* is a list of topics to be discussed, in a specific order, at a meeting or presentation. The medical assistant must take notes of what is discussed during meetings, which are known as *minutes.*

Duties during the physician's absence: Make sure that adequate arrangements are made with the physician before he or she leaves about how to handle bills, telephone calls, appointments, and mail. If patients have regular appointments scheduled for this time already, they should be notified about the physician's planned absence, and you should make arrangements for new appointments. Also keep a daily log of all telephone calls and what action, if any, was taken. Receipts must be kept for all expenditures that occur during business travel. Also, the office may provide *advance money* to the person traveling; this must be reconciled with all collected receipts.

Substitute physician: In larger practices and more urban areas, physicians in the same or a nearby practice often provide coverage while the physician is away. If a local physician is not readily available, a *locum tenens* (substitute physician), may be hired to see patients while the regular physician is unavailable.

9.6 Patient Education

Forms of patient education: Materials can be as simple as a single sheet of paper, or longer and more complex. Among the formats are brochures, booklets, fact sheets, educational newsletters, and community directories.

Visual materials: May be easier than written material for many patients to understand. DVDs are common, as are seminars and classes.

Patient information packet: Material specific to the practice to help patients feel more comfortable with it. The packet normally contains the following information:

- Introduction to the office
- Physicians' qualifications
- Description of the practice
- Introduction to the office staff
- Office hours
- Appointment scheduling policy and procedure
- Telephone policy
- Payment policy
- Insurance policies
- Patient confidentiality statement

Preoperative education: Instruction given to patients before surgery. It informs them about the details of the procedure and about diet and activity restrictions, among other things.

Promoting patient health and preventing injury: One of the goals of patient education is to promote good health behaviors and to teach patients how to prevent common injuries. As a medical assistant, you can help patients develop healthy practices and habits.

Instructions:

Answer the following questions.

1. Which of the following terms means the act of articulating and speaking clearly?

    A. communication
    B. conversation
    C. telecommunication
    D. pronunciation
    E. enunciation

2. Account statements for a medical practice should be sent as

    A. First-Class Mail.
    B. Standard Mail.
    C. Priority Mail.
    D. Special Standard Mail.
    E. Express Mail (Priority Mail Express).

3. If a patient calls about insurance coverage, the call should be handled by

    A. the physician who performed the test or procedure in question.
    B. the medical assistant.
    C. the next available physician.
    D. the insurance company.
    E. an insurance specialist only.

4. According to U.S. Postal Service guidelines, which of the following is the correct state abbreviation for an envelope addressed to Key West?

    A. MS
    B. MA
    C. MT
    D. FL
    E. TX

5. The physician should handle calls from patients about which of the following?

    A. insurance questions
    B. X-ray and laboratory reports
    C. unsatisfactory progress
    D. prescription refills previously authorized
    E. scheduling appointments

6. Which of the following is an introductory form that provides demographic data about patients?

    A. physical examination form
    B. patient referral form
    C. patient encounter form
    D. patient information form
    E. patient health questionnaire

7. When a patient does not respond to past-due billing statements and does not return telephone calls, which of the following types of mail should be used to determine if the patient is receiving mail?

    A. Insured
    B. Priority
    C. Express
    D. Registered
    E. Certified, return receipt

8. Which proofreader's mark means "close up space"?

    A. [
    B. ◠
    C.][
    D.]
    E. ⊙

9. A medical assistant is asked by the physician to make travel arrangements for a seminar that the physician will be attending. The detailed outline that the medical assistant prepares for the physician is called which of the following?

    A. minutes
    B. a synopsis
    C. an itinerary
    D. an abstract
    E. an agenda

10. Which of the following refers to the practice of underlining or highlighting important words and phrases when opening the mail?

    A. indexing
    B. prioritizing
    C. annotating
    D. conditioning
    E. coding

CHAPTER 10

APPOINTMENTS, SCHEDULING, MEDICAL RECORDS, FILING, POLICIES, AND PROCEDURES

LEARNING OUTCOMES

10.1 Recall the different types of appointments and scheduling methods used in the medical office.

10.2 Demonstrate proper filing methods and the correct techniques for the handling of medical records.

10.3 Describe the importance of the policy and procedures manual.

MEDICAL ASSISTING COMPETENCIES

COMPETENCY	CMA	RMA	CCMA	NCMA
Administrative				
Schedule and oversee appointments	X	X	X	X
Schedule inpatient and outpatient admissions and procedures	X	X	X	X
Prepare, organize, and maintain medical records	X	X	X	X
File medical records	X	X	X	X
General/Legal/Professional				
Identify and respond to issues of confidentiality by maintaining confidentiality at all times and following appropriate guidelines when releasing records or information	X	X	X	X
Determine the needs for documentation and reporting, and document accurately and appropriately	X	X	X	X

MEDICAL ASSISTING COMPETENCIES (cont.)

General/Legal/Professional

Explain general office policies and procedures	X	X	X	X
Perform an inventory of supplies and equipment	X	X	X	
Maintain the physical plant or facility	X	X	X	
Evaluate and recommend equipment and supplies for practice	X	X	X	
Exercise efficient time management	X	X	X	
Adapt to change	X	X	X	X
Have a responsible attitude	X	X	X	
Be impartial and show empathy when dealing with patients	X	X	X	

STRATEGIES FOR SUCCESS

▶ Study Skills

Medical assistants must always concentrate on medical records and filing. They must follow the policies and procedures of their medical office, because medical records are the most important documents that are handled. Misfiling will cause difficulty in locating patient information, which can impact patient care.

10.1 Appointments and Schedules

Appointment scheduling: The process that determines which patients will be seen by the physician, how soon they will be seen, and how much time will be allotted to each patient—based on the patient's complaint and the physician's availability.

Appointment book: The basic format of appointment books is the matrix, which requires blocking off times on the schedule during which the doctor is not available to see patients. An appointment matrix provides an accurate record of available patient scheduling times. Time slots are blocked off with an "X" on a paper schedule, or specified time periods are automatically blocked out on a computer schedule. These times include:

- Lunch
- Consultations
- Visits with drug company representatives
- Catch-up time
- Emergencies
- Hospital rounds
- Surgery
- Days off
- Holidays

See Figure 10-1 for a sample page from an appointment book.

Legal record: The appointment book is a legal record. Some experts advise holding on to old appointment books for at least three years.

Scheduling abbreviations: The receptionist who maintains the appointment book should be familiar with the abbreviations in Table 10-1 to save space and time when entering information.

Types of Appointments

Types of appointments: A medical assistant may schedule appointments for any one of the following purposes:

- New patients
- Follow-up
- Admissions
- Laboratory tests
- Surgery
- Physician referrals
- Salespersons, including pharmaceutical sales representatives
- Returning patients
- Specialists
- Buffer time

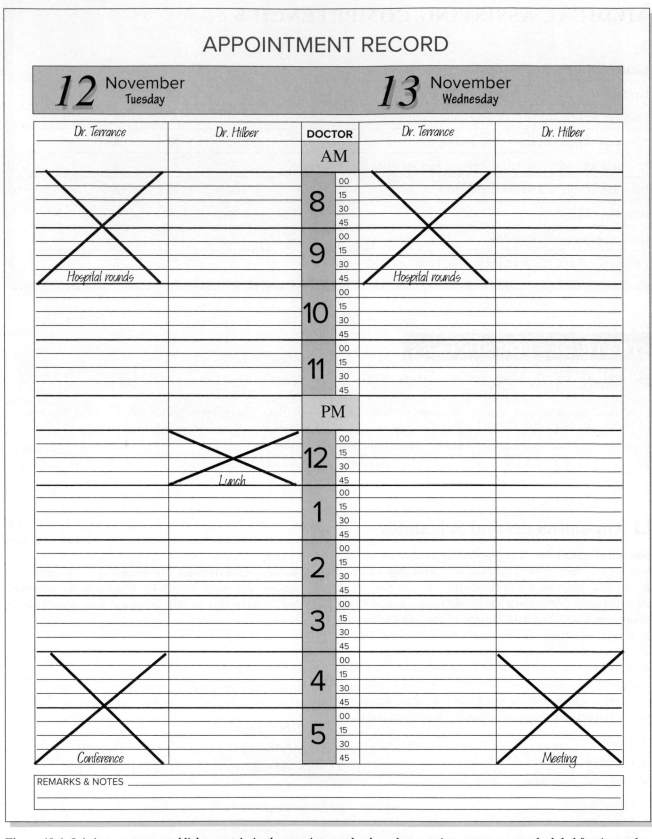

APPOINTMENT RECORD

		DOCTOR		
12 November Tuesday			**13** November Wednesday	
Dr. Terrance	Dr. Hilber		Dr. Terrance	Dr. Hilber
		AM		
✕ Hospital rounds		8 / 9	✕ Hospital rounds	
		10		
		11		
		PM		
	✕ Lunch	12		
		1		
		2		
		3		
✕ Conference		4 / 5		✕ Meeting

REMARKS & NOTES _____

Figure 10-1 *It is important to establish a matrix in the appointment book so that appointments are not scheduled for times when the doctor will be out of the office.*

Abbreviation	Meaning
cx	Cancellation
cons	Consultation
CPE	Complete physical examination
FU	Follow-up appointment
NP	New patient
NS	No-show patient
PT	Physical therapy
re✓	Recheck
ref	Referral
RS	Reschedule
surg	Surgery

Table 10-1

New patient: A patient who is not established at the medical practice and is scheduling the first visit, or has not been seen by the physician for more than three years. The most important information to give these patients is office hours and the fee schedule. When you schedule appointments for new patients, make sure to allow enough time for filling out forms and making files.

Pharmaceutical sales representatives: Some doctors may be willing to schedule a short appointment with sales reps to take a look at products that might be useful in their medical practice.

Buffer time: Appointment slots held open in case of emergencies. Every medical practice should have at least one or two slots open for buffer time each day.

Fasting or diabetic patients: It is advisable to schedule fasting patients as early in the day as possible, to minimize blood sugar deficiencies. For diabetic patients, avoid scheduling them late in the morning, prior to lunch. The medical office should have some type of snacks on hand for diabetic patients.

Emergencies: For certain emergency situations, the patient may be required to see the physician immediately, but not need to go to the emergency department of a hospital. These patients must take precedence over all other scheduled patients. The screening and sorting of emergency situations is called emergency triage. The medical assistant must be aware of any patients that have potentially life-threatening conditions and make sure they are seen first by the physician.

Repeat visits: It is advisable to schedule appointments on the same days and times, for patients who must be seen regularly; this will balance the schedule and help avoid missed appointments.

Referrals: Patients referred by other physicians to your medical office should be scheduled with the next available appointment. If the physician in your office needs to refer a patient to another physician, give the patient at least two referral names, with complete contact information. Verify that the referred physicians' offices accept the patient's insurance.

Scheduling Process

Matrix: The schedule matrix contains the times already allotted, which therefore are not available for scheduling patients. The first step in preparing an appointment book is to block off these times and establish a matrix.

Scheduling guidelines: Once the matrix has been established, you can schedule patient appointments based on:

- Patient needs and preferences
- Physician preferences and habits
- Degree of illness and/or contagion
- Available facilities

Considerations: When scheduling appointments, you should consider:

- Legal issues
- Tailoring the scheduling system
- Analyzing patient flow
- Waiting time
- Flexibility

Appointment cards: On reminders given to patients, the medical assistant should write the date and time when they are scheduled to return to the office for another appointment. The card is sent through the mail or handed to the patient if the appointment is made in person. Appointment cards should contain the physician's name, address, and telephone number.

Phone: You may call patients one–two days before an appointment to remind them of and to confirm the scheduled time.

Special problems: There will be times when you will have to deal with patients who are late for appointments or do not show up at all. For legal purposes, you must have careful and accurate documentation of these incidents. The best way to manage a patient who is chronically late is to schedule the patient for the last appointment of the day.

Cancellations: When a patient calls to cancel an appointment, offer to reschedule the appointment immediately, or make a note to remind yourself to call the patient later to reschedule. Also note the canceled appointment in the appointment book as well as the patient's medical record.

Rescheduling: Appointments are often rescheduled because of emergencies or other unforeseen problems.

Types of Scheduling Systems

Open hours: Some providers do not schedule appointments; instead they conduct their practices with open office hours. This system is the least structured of all the scheduling systems. Patients come in during given hours of the day, sign in, and are seen on a first-come, first-served basis—unless there is an extreme emergency. One of the main disadvantages of this system is the inefficient use of the staff's time that results from uneven patient flow.

Time-specified scheduling: Also known as *stream scheduling,* it assumes there will be a steady flow of patients all day, at regular intervals. Minor problems such as sore throats usually require 15 minutes (or less), new patient visits usually require 30 minutes, and more extensive procedures, such as physical exams, usually require 60 minutes.

Double booking: The scheduling of two or more patients in the same time slot. This method is limited to practices in which more than one patient can be attended to at a time. In all other practices, you should not schedule multiple patients in the same time slot unless they can be seen in a fairly short amount of time (about five minutes). Patients may become impatient and upset with long waits.

Wave scheduling: A method that can be used effectively in medical facilities that have several procedure rooms and adequate personnel to staff them. This method provides built-in flexibility to accommodate unforeseen situations, such as a patient who requires more time with the physician, a patient who arrives late, or a patient who fails to keep an appointment.

Modified wave scheduling: Wave scheduling can be modified to prevent long waits by patients. In the modified wave method, appointments for two or more patients are scheduled at the beginning of each hour, followed by single appointments every 10–20 minutes for the remainder of the hour.

Cluster scheduling: This groups similar appointments together, and is also called *categorization scheduling.* For example, all physical exams may be clustered on certain days, between certain hours.

Advance scheduling: In some specialties, appointments may be made weeks or even months in advance.

Grouping: Reserving certain times, such as a day of the week or time of the day to perform a number of similar procedures.

Exceptions: A few types of patients cannot be fit neatly into a regular schedule:

- Emergency patients
- Acutely ill patients
- Patients who have a physician referral
- Walk-ins

Streaming: The scheduling of appointments for a certain amount of time, based on patient need.

Computerized scheduling: Becoming more common in medical offices because it has several advantages over handwritten systems. One of the main advantages of a computerized system is that the scheduling information can be accessed from all terminals. It is still important to print the computer schedule daily for the physician to review.

Online scheduling: This allows patients to schedule themselves over the Internet. It requires the office staff to undergo additional training to manage the process and to ensure adequate patient privacy and security of information.

10.2 Medical Records and Filing

Medical records: Accurate medical records are essential to proper patient care. Medical records provide a continuous story of a patient's progress from the first visit to the last with all the important information, observations, illnesses, treatments, and outcomes carefully documented. These records are important communication and research tools as well as legal documents. Electronic medical record (EMR) usage is becoming more prevalent in practice today. The Federal EMR Electronic Medical Records Mandate 2014/2015 Deadline established the goal of converting all medical records in the United States into the electronic format. From 2015 onward, penalties may be levied against health-care entities who have not upgraded to electronic records.

Reasons for medical records: Good reasons for careful recording of medical information include:

- To provide the best medical care to patients. Good medical records help a physician provide continuity in a patient's medical care.
- To supply statistical information. Properly conducted studies based on objective measurements can lead to revised techniques and treatments.
- To be used in lawsuits and malpractice cases either to support a patient's claim or to support the physician's defense against such a claim.
- To evaluate the quality of treatment a doctor's office provides.
- To facilitate reimbursement. Medical records provide documentation for insurance billing and the basis for defending audits by managed care and government (Medicare and Medicaid) regulatory agencies.

Documentation: The recording of information in a patient's medical record. The term also refers to information recorded.

Standard information to include in medical records: Each new patient who comes to the office will need a medical record. Each medical facility has its own forms and charts, but all records must contain certain standard information. For adequate legal protection, a patient's medical record should include the following items:

- Patient registration form
- Patient medical history
- Physical examination results
- Results of laboratory tests
- Copies of prescriptions and notes on refill authorizations
- Diagnosis and treatment plan
- Patient progress reports, documentation of follow-up visits, and notes on telephone calls

- Informed consent forms
- Discharge summary
- Correspondence with and about the patient

Make sure that you date and initial all entries. Always record all signs, symptoms, and other information the patient wishes to share with you. Use the patient's own words, not your interpretation of them. Make sure that any interviews are conducted in a private room where others cannot hear. The main reason for documenting patient education efforts in writing is to make recommendations for patient care and compliance.

Six *Cs* of charting: In order to maintain accurate patient records, keep these six concepts in mind:

- *C*lient's words—Do not interpret the patient's words.
- *C*larity—Use precise and accurate medical terminology. Write legibly and neatly.
- *C*ompleteness—Fill out all forms. All information should be complete and accurate.
- *C*onciseness—Use abbreviations where appropriate.
- *C*hronological order—Date all entries, and keep medical records up to date by entering all current reports and information.
- *C*onfidentiality—Protect the patient's privacy. Only the patient, the attending physician, and the medical assistant are allowed to see the charts without the patient's written consent or a court order.

Items to exclude: The following items should not be included in a patient's medical records:

- Reports from consulting physicians should not be placed in the record until carefully reviewed.
- Financial information is not included.
- Transferred records from the patient's previous physician are never added to the patient's record.
- Prejudicial, personal, or flippant comments are never entered into the record.

Records management: Assembling the medical record for each patient and having an efficient filing system for retrieval, transfer, protection, retention, storage, and destruction of these files. Some of the objectives of good records management include:

- Saving space
- Reducing filing equipment expenditures
- Preventing the creation of unnecessary records
- Retrieving information faster
- Reducing misfiles
- Complying with legal safeguards
- Saving the physician's and patient's time

SOAP: This is an acronym for *subjective* impressions, *objective* clinical evidence, *assessment,* and *plans* for more studies, treatment, or management. The letter "E" may be added to represent patient *evaluation* or *education,* and an "R" may be added to represent patient *response* and compliance.

Subjective information: Chief complaint, history of present illness, pertinent symptoms, pertinent medical history, surgical history, family history, social history, current medications, smoking status, drug/alcohol/caffeine use, level of physical activity, and allergies.

Objective information: Vital signs, body measurements, findings from physical examinations, laboratory and test results, medication list obtained from pharmacy or medical records.

POMR or **POR:** Also known as the *Weed system,* it is a record of clinical practice that utilizes *problem-oriented medical records,* including a database, problem list, treatment plan, and progress notes.

Retaining files: The length of time to retain patient files differs for each medical office; usually the physician makes the decision. The medical assistant will help prepare a *retention schedule* that specifies which files will be kept, for how long, after being closed or inactivated. This schedule will also detail how and when files will be moved to storage, and for how long they will be stored there prior to being destroyed. Legal requirements for storage vary, between 2–10 years; however, immunization records should be kept in the medical office *permanently,* and not put into storage.

Meaningful use: The use of electronic medical records by providers to achieve significant improvements in care. Today, payments are tied to the achievement of advances in health-care processes and outcomes.

Transcription and Dictation

Medical transcription: The transformation of spoken words into accurate written form. These written notes are then entered into the patient's record. Transcribed material must be accurate and complete, with correct grammar, spelling, medical abbreviations, medical codes, and terminology. Dictated materials are confidential and should be regarded as potential legal documents.

Ensuring accurate transcription: Fast, accurate transcription is achieved by following these recommendations:

- Have needed materials at hand.
- Adjust the transcribing equipment's speed, tone, and volume.
- Listen all the way through before starting to transcribe.
- If problems with the recorded material arise, write down the time on the digital counter so that you can find them quickly when requesting clarification.
- Listen carefully.

Dictation: Medical assistants may be required to take dictation directly from the physician. In order to take dictation properly, follow these guidelines:

- Use a writing pad with a stiff back or a clipboard.
- Use incomplete sentences to keep up with the speed of speech.

- Use abbreviations when you can.
- When something is unclear, ask for clarification right away.
- Read the dictation back to the physician to verify accuracy.

Machine transcription: This involves dictation, listening back to the dictation, and keying the dictation as text in a printed document, with correct formatting and punctuation.

Dictation machine: The unit into which the physician dictates; it may be handheld or desktop.

Transcription machine: The unit used by the transcriber, which may use digital disks or various magnetic tapes. Offers rewind, fast-forward, speed-volume-tone controls, and indicators for finding special instructions as well as determining length of the dictation.

Transcription computer: The unit used to produce the printed text of the dictation; it utilizes foot pedals and headphones for direct transcribing, as well as transcription software.

Voice recognition software: A new technology being used more frequently for transcription; it uses *artificial intelligence* to "learn" the speaker's voice patterns. It offers all of the advantages of traditional transcription, with more speed and less cost.

Confidentiality: The principle of treating something as a private matter not intended for public knowledge. Confidentiality protects information so that it is not released to anyone unless required by law. When children reach the age of 18, most states consider them adults with the right to privacy. No one, not even their parents, may see their medical records without their written consent or a court order. The Health Insurance Portability and Accountability Act (HIPAA) Privacy Rule protects patient confidentiality.

Filing Methods

Alphabetical filing: Strict alphabetical filing is one of the simplest filing methods. It involves alphabetizing the files from A to Z. Files are labeled with the patient's surname (last name) first, followed by the given name (first name), and the middle initial. It is a *direct filing system,* and is one of the most common filing systems for maintaining patient files in sequential order.

Alphanumerical filing: A filing system based on combinations of letters and numbers.

Subject filing: Arranging records alphabetically by names of topics or things rather than by names of individuals. It can be either alphabetical or alphanumerical, such as A1–5, B1–2. It is a widely used filing system for medical practices. It offers the most appropriate order for adding new progress notes to source-oriented medical records.

Chronological filing: A filing system based on time.

Numerical filing: The filing of records, correspondence, or cards by number. Such a system is often used when patient information is highly confidential. Numerical filing is used by practically every large clinic or hospital serving more than 5,000 patients. It is an *indirect filing system.*

Color coding: A filing system based on color. One commonly used system breaks the alphabet up into five different colors: red, yellow, green, blue, and purple. Red is for A through D, yellow for E through H, green for I through N, blue for O through Q, and purple for R through Z. This is the easiest system for locating a misfiled record.

Alphabetic color coding: This system may use 5–13 different colors of folders, each representing different segments of the alphabet. Often, names beginning with A to M are placed in one set of 13 colors, with names beginning with N to Z placed in a second set.

Numeric color coding: Numbers 0–9 are assigned different colors, often based on the last digit of the number.

Outguides: Stiff markers placed on medical files when they are removed, serving as placeholders in file cabinets so that any removed files are traceable within an office. They either have a list to sign out the file, or a clear pocket in which a piece of paper is inserted listing the location of the file, and which individual has signed it out. Outguides are removed when files are returned to file drawers.

Filing guidelines: When pulling a file or filing a chart, look at it to make sure the papers are in the proper order. Keep files neat at all times; they should not be too full of papers. Multiple files for a single patient may be required so that each is not overfull. File drawers should also not be overcrowded. Uppercase and lowercase letters should be used on file labels so that the first letters of names are easier to read. Different tab positions should be used to make folders easier to find and pull out.

Computer records: Some medical practices use computer software to create and store patient records. One of the main advantages to computerization is that a physician can call up the record whenever it is needed, review or update the file, and save it to the central computer again.

Tickler file: A chronological file used as a reminder that something needs to be done on a certain date. An example of its use would be for patients' annual physical exams.

Filing Procedures

Filing procedures: There are five steps involved in filing:

- Conditioning
- Releasing
- Indexing and coding
- Sorting
- Storing and filing

Conditioning: Removing paper clips and other fasteners, stapling related papers together, attaching smaller pieces of paper to full-size sheets of paper with tape or rubber cement, and fixing damaged records.

Releasing: Placing a mark on the paper to indicate it is ready for filing; this is usually the MA's initials, or a stamp with the word FILE, onto the upper-left corner.

Indexing and coding: An organized method of identifying and separating items to be filed, such as letters or papers, by assigning essential pieces of information to numbered units (sometimes called fields). The key unit, unit 1, is generally the surname (last name). Unit 2 is the given name (first name). Unit 3 is the middle initial. Unit 4 is a title or special designation (Ms., Dr., Jr., Sr., etc.). Some files can be placed in more than one location, such as the file of a recently married female who has changed her last name. The MA can cross-reference files that are under both her maiden name and her married name.

Place some indication of the index on the material to be filed. Coding may be done by underlining the name or the subject. Every paper placed in a patient's medical record should have the date and the name of the patient on it, usually in the upper-right corner.

Sorting: Arranging items to be filed in a sequence by removing loose pieces of tape or paper clips before going to the file cabinet or shelf.

Storing and filing: Place items face up, top edge to the left, with the most recent date at the front of the folder. Lift folders a few inches out of the drawer before inserting new material, or preferably, attach items to the file folder permanently. Arrange completed folders in indexing order before refiling.

Active files: Files that you use frequently.

Inactive files: Files that you use infrequently. Each practice develops guidelines for determining the point at which a file becomes inactive. In some practices, the file of a patient who has not been seen for a year may be considered inactive, whereas in others the amount of time may be two–three years.

Closed files: Files of patients who have died or moved away.

Transfer: Removing inactive records from the active files.

Retention period: The amount of time to keep different types of patient records in the office after files have become inactive or closed. Some legal requirements for retaining certain types of information are listed in Table 10-2.

Identical names: When filing identical names, use date of birth, patient identification number, or some other form of identification in order to distinguish between the two patients.

Business and organization records: File business and organization records according to subject and topic.

Misplaced files: Always replace files promptly after use. If a file cannot be found, check through its folder, the surrounding folders, between folders, under all folders, in a similarly named file, and in the sorter.

Filing Equipment

File shelves: An advantage of keeping files on shelves is that it allows several people to retrieve and return files at one time.

File cabinets: Three types of file cabinets are used in the medical office: vertical, lateral, and movable.

Vertical file cabinets: Have two–six drawers. They are the least efficient type of cabinet because half of the filing time goes into opening and closing drawers. Also, bending, squatting, and stretching to reach files makes these cabinets that much more inefficient.

Open-shelf file cabinets: Take up 50% less space, permit quick access, and have no drawers to open or close. They have the disadvantage of collecting dust.

Movable file units: Allow easy access to large record systems and require less space than vertical or lateral files.

Filing supplies:

- Divider guides are heavy card stock or plastic dividers that separate approximately every 10 folders; they have a protruding tab. Divider guides support folders and aid in searching files.

- Labels are used to identify shelves, drawers, divider guides, and folders.

- File folders designed for the type of cabinet in use.

AT A GLANCE	Requirements for Retaining Records	
Source	**Type of Record**	**Retention Period**
National Childhood Vaccine Injury Act of 1986	Immunization records	Permanently
Labor Standards Act	Employee health records	3 years
Statute of limitations	Records needed for civil suits	Varies by state, most commonly 2 years
Legal consultants	Patient records	At least 7 years
Internal Revenue Service	Financial records	10 years
State laws	Records of minors	From 2 to 7 years after the child reaches legal age, depending on the state
American Medical Association, American Hospital Association, other medical groups	Patient records	10 years after patient's final visit or contact

Table 10-2

- Identification labels, affixed either along the top of the file folder or along the side of the file folder in open-shelf file cabinets.
- Guides and captions: Guides are used to separate the file folders. Captions are used to identify major sections of file folders by more manageable subunits.

10.3 Policies and Procedures

Policy and procedures manual: A written document that covers all office policies and clinical procedures, developed by the physicians and the staff (particularly the medical assistant) for use by permanent and temporary employees. This manual should begin with a *mission statement*.

Policies: Rules or guidelines that dictate the day-to-day workings of an office. Most manuals cover the following policy areas:

- Office purposes, objectives, and goals
- Rules and regulations
- Job descriptions and duties
- Office hours

- Dress code
- Insurance and other benefits
- Vacation, sick leave, and other time away from the office
- Performance evaluations and salary
- Maintenance of equipment and supplies
- Mailings
- Bookkeeping
- Scheduling appointments
- Maintaining patient records
- Health and safety guidelines
- Organizational chart

Procedures: Detailed instructions for maintaining clinical and quality assurance.

Developing a manual: Begins with planning the format and outline, which should be approved by the office manager and physicians. Sources for developing and updating material include journals, product literature, textbooks, and standards publications, among others.

Manual format: Many offices prefer a loose-leaf binder in which pages can be replaced when necessary.

STRATEGIES FOR SUCCESS

▶ Test-Taking Skills

Eliminate wrong answers!

When answering multiple-choice questions, you can increase your chances of answering correctly by eliminating answers that you know are wrong. As you read the possible answers, put an X next to ones you know are incorrect, or cross them out completely. If you are taking an exam on a computer, ask for scratch paper and write down the question number and the answer choices that you know are incorrect. Once you have narrowed down your possible choices, you have a better chance of making an educated guess about the correct answer.

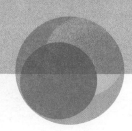

Instructions:

Answer the following questions.

1. Which of the following is a widely used filing system for medical practices, and may utilize letters or numbers as identifiers?

   A. numeric
   B. subject
   C. alphabetical
   D. chronological
   E. alphanumeric

2. In appointment scheduling, the matrix indicates

   A. time available for scheduling vacations.
   B. time not available to schedule patients.
   C. time open for pharmaceutical representatives.
   D. time open for surgery.
   E. time not available for surgery.

3. A chronological file used as a reminder is called a(n)

   A. index file.
   B. tickler file.
   C. active file.
   D. closed file.
   E. timer file.

4. Scheduling patients so that two come in at the beginning of each hour and the others are scheduled every 10–20 minutes is called

   A. wave scheduling.
   B. appointment time pattern.
   C. modified wave scheduling.
   D. double booking.
   E. advance scheduling.

5. SOAP pertains to

   A. malpractice.
   B. computer code.
   C. dictation equipment.
   D. asepsis.
   E. patient records.

6. An appointment book is considered

   A. an interpersonal skill.
   B. a patient analysis.
   C. a legal document.
   D. a scheduling system.
   E. both a legal document *and* a scheduling system.

7. Which of the following scheduling methods allows short-term flexibility within an hour to account for variables in appointments?

   A. wave
   B. open hours
   C. stream
   D. cluster
   E. double booking

8. In the SOAP method of medical record documentation, the "P" stands for which of the following?

   A. prescription
   B. prognosis
   C. patient
   D. plan
   E. physical examination

9. Which of the following is substituted in the place of a patient's official file when the file is removed?

   A. outguide
   B. index guide
   C. divider guide
   D. hanging folder
   E. cross-reference notation

10. Arranging items to be filed in a sequence before going to the file cabinet is called

    A. indexing.
    B. coding.
    C. sorting.
    D. storing.
    E. filing.

CHAPTER 11

COMMUNICATION IN THE MEDICAL OFFICE

LEARNING OUTCOMES

11.1 Recall the five Cs of communication.

11.2 Recall the elements of the communication cycle.

11.3 Describe positive and negative communication, including verbal, nonverbal, and written.

11.4 Recognize the importance of possessing strong listening, interpersonal, and therapeutic communication skills, as well as the ability to be assertive.

11.5 Demonstrate the ability to remain diplomatic and professional during all types of communication.

11.6 Recognize the importance of remaining supportive, loyal, and professional when communicating with coworkers and superiors.

11.7 Recall methods used to minimize stress and prevent burnout.

11.8 Explain the importance of utilizing the policy and procedures manual.

MEDICAL ASSISTING COMPETENCIES

COMPETENCY	CMA	RMA	CCMA	NCMA
General/Legal/Professional				
Respond to and initiate written communications by using correct grammar, spelling, and formatting techniques	X	X	X	X
Recognize and respond to verbal and nonverbal communications by being attentive and adapting communication to the recipient's level of understanding	X	X	X	X
Demonstrate proper telephone techniques	X	X	X	X
Identify and respond to issues of confidentiality by maintaining confidentiality at all times and following appropriate guidelines when releasing records or information	X	X	X	X
Explain general office policies and procedures	X	X	X	X
Instruct individuals according to their needs	X	X	X	X
Project a positive attitude	X	X	X	X
Be a "team player"	X	X	X	X

MEDICAL ASSISTING COMPETENCIES (cont.)

General/Legal/Professional

Adapt to change	X	X	X	X
Have a responsible attitude	X	X	X	X
Be courteous and diplomatic	X	X	X	
Be impartial and show empathy when dealing with patients	X	X	X	
Serve as a liaison between the physician and others	X	X	X	
Interview effectively	X	X	X	
Use appropriate medical terminology	X	X	X	X
Receive, organize, prioritize, and transmit information appropriately	X	X	X	X

STRATEGIES FOR SUCCESS

▶ *Study Skills*

Study the things you don't know, not what you do know. As you test yourself, you will find areas that you know very well and those with which you are not as comfortable. Even though it feels good to study those things you know, you should put those subjects aside and spend time with the material you do not know as well. If you study with note cards, make two piles, an "I know that" pile and an "I don't know that" pile. Soon your "I know that" pile will grow larger than your "I don't know that" pile.

11.1 Communicating with Patients and Families

The way that you interact with patients significantly influences how comfortable they feel with being in your medical office, as well as setting the overall tone for their visit.

The Five Cs of communication:

- Completeness—The message must contain all necessary information.
- Clarity—The message must be free from obscurity and ambiguity.
- Conciseness—The message must not include any unnecessary information.
- Courtesy—The message must be respectful and considerate of others.
- Cohesiveness—The message must be organized and logical.

Developing Good Communication Skills

Attitude: Your confidence and self-esteem can positively affect your success in the medical field. The way you represent yourself is the way others will see you. Communicating a positive attitude begins by doing the following:

- Smiling instead of frowning
- Saying something pleasant instead of complaining
- Using positive statements instead of negative statements

11.2 The Communication Cycle

The communication cycle consists of giving and receiving information. You also will be responsible for receiving information from the patient.

Elements of the Communication Cycle

The communication cycle is formed as the sender, or source, sends the message to the receiver and the receiver responds with

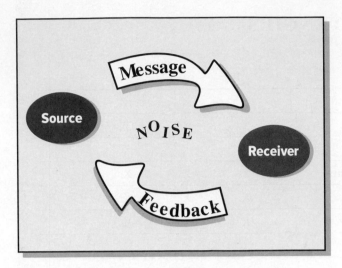

Figure 11-1 *The process of communication involves an exchange of messages through verbal and nonverbal means.*

feedback. The message may be verbal or nonverbal. This circle of communication also may include noise, which is anything that distorts the message in any way or interferes with the communication process. Noise includes sounds, such as a siren or alarm, and also can include physical discomfort (e.g., pain) or personal worries or concerns that may interfere with what is being communicated. Figure 11-1 illustrates the communication cycle.

11.3 Types of Communication

Communication can be verbal, nonverbal, or written. It also can be positive or negative.

Positive Communication

Positive communication: Promotes patients' comfort and well-being. Positive communication is essential in the medical office. Some examples of positive communication include:

- Being friendly, warm, and attentive
- Verbalizing your concern for patients
- Encouraging patients to ask questions
- Asking patients to repeat your instructions in order to make sure they understand
- Looking directly at patients when you speak to them
- Smiling naturally
- Speaking slowly and clearly
- Listening carefully

Negative Communication

Negative communication: Most people do not intend to communicate negatively; however, some communication practices have a negative effect on others. Negative communication includes:

- Mumbling
- Speaking sharply or too intensely

- Avoiding eye contact
- Interrupting patients as they are speaking
- Rushing through explanations or instructions
- Treating patients impersonally
- Forgetting common courtesies such as "please" and "thank you"
- Using negative body language, such as frowning, slouching, and crossing one's arms
- Showing boredom

Nonverbal Communication

Body language: Nonverbal communication is also known as body language. In many cases, body language conveys a person's true feelings when words may not. Be aware of your body language, and note the body language of others. Examples of nonverbal communication include the following:

- Facial expressions—These should be nonjudgmental and correspond to your words.
- Hand gestures—This type of body language can emphasize your words.
- Eye contact—Establishing eye contact with others shows interest, attention, and sensitivity.
- Nodding—This gesture acknowledges information and encourages the patient to continue speaking.
- Posture—Turning and leaning your body toward a person helps to communicate your interest in what he or she is saying. Posture may be *open* or *closed*.
- Attention to personal space—This aspect shows respect for the person's privacy and comfort.
- Touch—This type of body language can communicate sensitivity and empathy. In general, a touch on the shoulder, back, or hand is acceptable. However, not everyone is comfortable being touched. Be aware of cultural and personal differences and adjust your style to the preferences of others.

11.4 Improving Your Communication Skills

Listening Skills

Listening is the act of receiving a message. Three different listening patterns are used in a medical office: active, passive, and evaluative.

Active listening: Requires two-way communication, positive body language, asking questions, and offering feedback.

Passive listening: Involves listening without answering and offering feedback.

Evaluative listening: Provides an immediate response and opinion. It is very important to listen to everything a patient says; avoid "selective hearing."

Leading Questions

You should avoid asking *leading questions,* which give hints as to the answer you hope the patient will give. An example is, "You don't drink alcohol, do you?" This makes the patient feel like you don't approve of drinking, leading to an answer that will please you but may not be the truth. You must keep all of your questions positive. The way to do this, for this example, would be to ask, "Have you ever consumed alcoholic beverages?" or "Do you drink alcoholic beverages?"

Talking Too Much

Always remember that you should listen more to what the patient says than to talk excessively. Often, to avoid explaining what he or she is experiencing, the patient will allow you to talk. You should pay attention to his or her body language in order to decide whether you are allowing enough opportunity for the patient to discuss the health problem.

Giving Advice

You must avoid giving advice to patients. Often patients will ask you what you would do if you were in their situation. Patients must make their own decisions about what to do concerning their health. You can ask the patient, "Following along with what the doctor told you, what do you think you should do?" If the patient still is not sure, you can ask, "Do you need more information before you can make a decision?" You should always encourage patients to talk to the physician some more if they have additional questions about a health-care decision.

Using Medical Terminology

Each patient has a different level of understanding concerning various medical terms. You must adjust the words you use in order to fit each patient. Each patient needs to understand, as fully as possible, all of the information concerning his or her condition. The most common error in patient care is *misinterpreted communication.* Medical terminology can be partially or totally confusing to people who have never studied medicine. Watch patients' body language to gauge whether they understand your words, or if they appear to be uncomfortable with them. Ask patients to repeat back what you said in their own words. This is known as the *demonstration-return* method of providing feedback. It gives you a chance to clarify anything a patient has misunderstood.

Interpersonal Skills

Interpersonal skills are used when you interact with people. You demonstrate good interpersonal skills when you make a patient feel at ease with your warmth and friendliness. Other valuable interpersonal skills include the following:

- Empathy
- Respect
- Genuineness
- Openness
- Consideration and sensitivity

Therapeutic Communication Skills

Patients in the medical office will come from a variety of backgrounds and will have their own perceptions of the medical office and its staff. It is important to be able to interact with all patients, addressing each of their individual needs and circumstances. Therapeutic communication is the ability to communicate in terms that patients can understand while making them feel at ease and comfortable with what is being said. Therapeutic communication is also the ability to communicate with other health-care professionals by using technical terms appropriate in the health-care setting. Table 11-1 summarizes techniques for therapeutic communication.

AT A GLANCE **Techniques for Therapeutic Communication**

Technique	Therapeutic Value
Rapport / Acknowledgment	Use good communication skills to build a positive and harmonious relationship. / Acknowledgment shows that you respect the patient's autonomy as well as the importance of his or her role.
Focusing / Establishing guidelines	You should use direct questions to ask for specific information, with (usually) a yes or no answer. / Guidelines help the patient understand how the interview will be conducted.
Open-ended questions and statements	These are used to encourage the patient to reply with greater detail.
Reflecting / Summarizing	This shows that you acknowledge the patient's feelings. / This keeps the interview clear, and helps the patient to sort out relevant material from nonrelevant material.
Restating	This verifies and validates your interpretation of what the patient has told you.
Silence / Listening	The patient can see your acceptance, and that you are willing to wait until a response is ready to be given to your question(s). / Listening communicates your interest in the patient without saying so.

Table 11-1

Silence: Periods in which there is no verbal communication. Silence can allow the patient to think without pressure to speak.

Restating: Repeating to a patient what you believe is the main thought or idea expressed. It helps to paraphrase ideas rather than just repeat statements verbatim. In this way you can make sure that you understand what is being communicated.

Reflecting: Encouraging patients to think through and answer their own questions and concerns.

Open-ended questions: General questions that allow patients to elaborate on their answers, providing as much information as they wish to. Open-ended questions lead to better communication.

Focusing: Helping the patient stay on a particular topic with directing questions and statements.

Rapport: Involves a positive and harmonious relationship between a patient and a medical assistant, or between patients and other members of the medical staff. You can build rapport with good communication skills.

Ineffective Therapeutic Communication Methods

Ineffective therapeutic communication includes roadblocks that can interfere with your communication style.

Reassuring: Indicates to the patient that there is no need for anxiety or worry. By doing this, you devalue the patient's feelings and give false hope if the outcome is not positive.

Giving approval: Usually done by overtly approving of a patient's behavior. Giving approval may lead the patient to strive for praise rather than progress.

Disapproving: Done by overtly disapproving of the patient's behavior. This may cause a patient to discontinue communication.

Agreeing/disagreeing: Either one of these is an ineffective way to communicate with patients. When you agree with patients, they will have the perception that they are right because you agree with them. Conversely, when you disagree with patients, you become the opposition to them instead of their caregiver.

Advising: Telling the patient what you think should be done places you outside your scope of practice. You cannot advise patients.

Probing: Discussing a topic that the patient has no desire to discuss.

Defending: Protecting yourself, the medical office, and others from verbal attack. Doing so may make the patient feel the need to discontinue communication.

Requesting an explanation: Involves asking patients to provide reasons for their behavior. "Why" questions may have an intimidating effect on some patients.

Minimizing feelings: Judging or making light of a patient's discomfort or concerns. It is important for you to perceive what is taking place from the patient's point of view, not your own.

Making stereotyped comments: Involves using meaningless clichés when communicating with patients, such as "It's for your own good." Comments of this type are given in an automatic, mechanical way as a substitute for a more reasonable and thoughtful explanation.

Prejudice: Holding a negative opinion of an individual because of his or her beliefs or culture.

Defense Mechanisms

Patients will often develop defense mechanisms, which they are usually not conscious of, to protect themselves from anxiety, guilt, shame, or other uncomfortable situations. It is important for you to observe defense mechanisms when working with patients in order to better understand what they are trying to communicate. The following are common defense mechanisms that patients may display.

Compensation: Overemphasizing a trait to make up for either a perceived or actual failing.

Denial: An unconscious attempt to reject unacceptable wishes, thoughts, needs, feelings, or external reality factors.

Displacement: The unconscious transfer of unacceptable desires, feelings, or thoughts from the self to a more acceptable external substitute.

Dissociation: Disconnecting emotional significance from specific events or ideas.

Identification: Mimicking the behavior of another person in order to cope with feelings of inadequacy.

Introjection: Adopting the unacceptable feelings or thoughts of others.

Projection: Projecting onto another person one's own feelings, as if they were originally the other person's feelings.

Rationalization: Justifying unacceptable feelings, thoughts, and behaviors into tolerable behaviors.

Regression: Unconsciously returning to more infantile thoughts or behaviors.

Repression: Putting unpleasant events, feelings, or thoughts out of one's mind.

Substitution: Unconsciously replacing an unacceptable or unreachable goal with another more acceptable goal.

Assertiveness Skills

As a professional, you need to be assertive. This means being firm and standing by your principles while still showing respect for others. Being assertive is not the same as being aggressive. Aggressive actions make others feel that the aggressive person is trying to impose his or her position on others or is trying to manipulate others.

11.5 Communicating in Special Circumstances

Part of the medical assistant's role includes setting the tone for communications. Medical assistants must therefore be aware of all obstacles that affect communication between human beings. As you interact with patients and their families, you will encounter many different kinds of patients—including those from different cultures, different socioeconomic backgrounds, and different educational levels. Normal personal space in most cultures is approximately two feet, but this varies. For example, many people from a Latino/a background are comfortable with much smaller distances concerning personal space. In addition, patients' ages will range widely, and some patients may have lifestyles that are very different from your own. Medical assistants must be able to remain professional and diplomatic with all of the patients with whom they communicate.

Communicating with Patients as Individuals

If you make an effort to develop good interpersonal skills, communicating with most patients will be easy. However, some situations can cause difficulties in communication. Sometimes communication problems occur in special circumstances, such as with anxious or angry patients, patients from different cultures, or patients with visual or hearing impairments. Additional problems may be encountered in communicating with patients who are mentally or emotionally disabled, have AIDS or are HIV-positive, are terminally ill, or are elderly or young.

Anxious patients: It is common for patients to become anxious in a health-care setting such as a doctor's office. This reaction is commonly known as "white-coat syndrome" and can have many different reasons. Some patients, particularly children, may not be able to express in words their feelings of fear or anxiety. You should be alert to signs of anxiety, which include the following:

- Tense appearance
- Increased blood pressure, pulse rate, and rate of breathing
- Sweaty palms
- Reported problems with sleep or appetite
- Irritability
- Agitation

Angry patients: Anger may occur in a medical setting for many different reasons. It may be a way to hide the patient's fear about an illness or a surgical outcome. Anger may come from feelings of being treated unfairly or without compassion. It may be a reaction to an invasion of privacy, feelings of loss of control or self-esteem, disappointment, rejection, or frustration. The medical assistant should help angry patients refocus their emotional energy on solving the problem. The following are some tips for communicating with an angry patient.

1. Learn to recognize anger and its causes.
2. Remain calm and continue to demonstrate respect and genuineness.
3. Focus on the patient's medical and physical needs.
4. Maintain adequate personal space to help the patient feel comfortable.
5. Avoid the feeling of needing to defend yourself or giving reasons that the patient should not be angry.
6. Encourage patients to be specific in describing their feelings, including the cause of their anger and their thoughts about it. Avoid agreeing or disagreeing with the patient. Instead, state what you can and cannot do for the patient.
7. Present your point of view firmly but calmly to help the patient better understand the situation.
8. Avoid a communication breakdown with the patient.
9. If you feel threatened by a patient's anger—or if you have concerns about the patient becoming violent—leave the room and seek assistance from other members of the office staff.

Patients from other cultures: Our cultural background shapes our views of the world, as well as our values, attitudes, beliefs, and use of language. Each culture and ethnic group has its own values, traditions, and behaviors. These differences among cultures should not be viewed as barriers to communication. Remember that these beliefs are neither superior nor inferior to your own beliefs—they are just different. For example, people from some Asian countries believe that direct eye contact is considered rude, whereas Americans consider this a sign of trust. Also, *personal space* differs among cultures. As mentioned, people from many Latino/a cultures have a much closer sense of personal space than most Americans.

Patients with visual impairments: Visually impaired patients cannot usually rely on nonverbal clues; therefore, your tone of voice, inflection, and speech volume take on a greater importance when you are communicating with them. Be aware of what you say and how you say it. Use large-print materials whenever possible. Make sure there is adequate lighting in all patient areas. Use a normal speaking voice, talk directly and honestly, and avoid talking down to the patient. The patient's dignity must be preserved in order for effective communication to occur.

Patients with hearing impairments: Communicating effectively with a hearing-impaired patient depends on the degree of impairment and on whether the patient has effective use of a hearing aid. Hearing loss can range from mild to severe. Find a quiet area to talk, and try to minimize background noise. Position yourself close to the patient and face him and her at all times. Speak slowly, and use body language. Note: In some situations, the physician may need to hire an interpreter for a patient with hearing impairments.

Patients who are mentally or emotionally disabled: Sometimes you will need to communicate with patients who are mentally or emotionally disabled. When communicating with such patients, first determine the level of communication they can understand. The following are some suggestions that can help improve communication with these patients.

- Remain calm if the patient becomes confused or agitated.
- Do not raise your voice or appear to be impatient.
- Ask the patient to repeat what you do not understand.

Elderly patients: Medical assistants now spend 50% or more of their time caring for older patients. Elderly patients should not be stereotyped as frail or confused, as most of them are not. Each patient deserves to be treated according to his or her individual abilities. Always treat elderly patients with respect. Use the title "Mr." or "Mrs." to address older patients unless they ask you to call them by their first name.

Terminally ill patients: Because they are often under extreme stress, terminally ill patients can be difficult to treat. Health-care professionals must respect the rights of terminally ill patients and always treat them with dignity. It is also important that medical assistants communicate with the families of terminally ill patients, offering support and empathy as these patients accept their conditions. Empathy differs from sympathy, in that empathy involves understanding other people's feelings based on your own experience. Sympathy involves acknowledging another person's problems and providing comfort and assurance.

Young patients: Children are more receptive to the requests and suggestions made by a medical assistant once they realize that you take their feelings seriously. Explain any procedure in very simple terms, no matter how basic it is. Let the child examine the instruments you will need to use. Use praise for his or her good behavior, and always be truthful.

Parents: Because parents are naturally concerned about their children, reassuring parents and keeping them calm also can help children relax.

Patients with AIDS and patients who are HIV-positive: Patients with AIDS and patients who are HIV-positive have a serious illness to deal with. These patients often feel depressed, angry, and guilty about their condition. In communicating effectively with them, you need accurate information about the disease and the risks involved. These patients will have many questions, and part of your role as an effective communicator will be to answer as many questions as you can.

11.6 Communicating with Coworkers and Superiors

Communicating with Coworkers

As a medical assistant, you are part of a larger health-care team. The quality of communication that you have with your coworkers is vitally important and influences the development of positive or negative work environments, as well as a team approach to patient care.

Communicating with Superiors

Positive or negative communication affects the quality of your relationship with superiors. Problems arise when communication about your job responsibilities is unclear or when you do not have an open line of communication with your superior. The following are some suggestions for good communications with superiors.

- Keep superiors informed.
- Ask questions.

- Minimize interruptions.
- Show initiative.

Dealing with Conflict

Conflict can arise when the lines of communication break down or when a misunderstanding between staff members or between a medical assistant and a superior occurs. A lack of mutual respect or trust can also cause conflicts among office staff. The following suggestions can help improve communication among coworkers.

- Do not participate in other people's negative attitudes.
- Try your best at all times to be personable and supportive of coworkers.
- Refrain from passing judgment on others or stereotyping them.
- Do not gossip. Act professionally at all times.
- Do not jump to conclusions. You do not know until you ask.

11.7 Managing Stress and Preventing Burnout

Stress is a communication barrier. Health-care professionals may experience high levels of stress in their daily work environment. Stress can result from feelings of being under pressure, or it can be a reaction to frustration, anger, or a change of routine. You can minimize stress by maintaining a balance between work, family, and leisure activities, as well as by exercising and eating a healthy diet. It is important to learn how to manage stress in order to prevent burnout. Burnout is an energy-depleting condition that will affect your health and career. Table 11-2 provides tips for reducing stress.

11.8 The Policy and Procedures Manual

In the medical office setting, the policy and procedures manual is a key written communication tool. These important documents should be reviewed by all employees for a thorough understanding of their office's rules, standards, and ways of operating.

Policies: Rules or guidelines that determine the daily working of an office. They include:

- Office purposes, objectives, and goals as established by the physician(s)
- Rules and regulations
- Job descriptions and duties of staff personnel
- Office hours
- Dress code
- Insurance and other benefits
- Vacation, sick leave, and other time away from the office

- Maintain a healthy balance in your life among work, family, and leisure activities.

- Exercise regularly.

- Eat balanced, nutritious meals and healthful snacks. Avoid foods high in caffeine, salt, sugar, and fat.

- Get enough sleep.

- Allow time for yourself, and plan time to relax.

- Rely on the support that family, friends, and coworkers have to offer. Don't be afraid to share your feelings.

- Try to be realistic about what you can and cannot do. Do not be afraid to admit that you cannot take on another responsibility.

- Try to set realistic goals for yourself.

- Remember that there are always choices, even when there appear to be none.

- Be organized. Good planning can help you manage your workload.

- Redirect excess energy constructively—clean your closet, work in the garden, do volunteer work, have friends over for dinner, exercise.

- Change some of the things you have control over.

- Keep yourself focused. Focus your full energy on one thing at a time, and finish one project before starting another.

- Identify sources of conflict, and try to resolve them.

- Learn and use relaxation techniques, such as deep breathing, meditation, or imagining yourself in a quiet, peaceful place. Choose what works for you.

- Maintain a healthy sense of humor. Laughter can help relieve stress. Joke with friends after work. Go see a funny movie.

- Try not to overreact. Ask yourself if a situation is really worth getting upset or worried about.

- Seek help from social or professional support groups, if necessary.

Table 11-2

- Salary and performance evaluations
- Maintenance of equipment and supplies
- Mailing
- Bookkeeping
- Scheduling of appointments and maintenance of patient records

- Occupational Safety and Health Administration (OSHA) and HIPAA guidelines

Procedures: Detailed instructions for specific procedures. The instructions include clinical procedures and quality assurance programs.

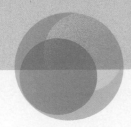

Instructions:

Answer the following questions.

1. Which of the following is *not* part of the communication cycle?

   A. message
   B. sender
   C. witness
   D. receiver
   E. feedback

2. Which of the following terms describes the verbal and nonverbal evidence that a message was received and understood?

   A. affirmation
   B. feedback
   C. medical records
   D. communication
   E. noise

3. Rapport involves

   A. a positive and harmonious relationship.
   B. silence.
   C. close-ended questions.
   D. repeating.
   E. a direct, confrontational relationship.

4. When in the medical office, anxious patients may exhibit

   A. decreased blood pressure.
   B. white-coat syndrome.
   C. nervous coughing.
   D. blue-coat syndrome.
   E. a tired appearance.

5. Which of the following types of materials should you use when dealing with visually impaired patients?

   A. large print
   B. braille
   C. nonverbal
   D. brightly colored
   E. infrared

6. Open-ended questions

   A. should never be asked of patients.
   B. should be asked of children but not of adults.
   C. should be asked of adults but not of children.
   D. should be asked of all patients.
   E. should help communication with patients who have hearing impairments.

7. Patients with AIDS

   A. often feel depressed, angry, and guilty.
   B. often feel hateful toward others.
   C. will not want to ask questions about their disease.
   D. will often deny that they have the disease.
   E. require a patient confidentiality statement.

8. Which one of the following defense mechanisms is defined as putting unpleasant events, feelings, or thoughts out of one's mind?

   A. substitution
   B. compensation
   C. displacement
   D. dissociation
   E. repression

9. The five Cs of communication include

   A. cyclic communication.
   B. cohesiveness.
   C. channeling.
   D. contact.
   E. closing.

10. Which therapeutic communication technique keeps the interview clear, and helps the patient to sort out relevant material?

    A. reflecting
    B. silence
    C. rapport
    D. restating

KEYBOARDING AND COMPUTER APPLICATIONS

LEARNING OUTCOMES

12.1 Demonstrate the ability to perform basic computer functions.

12.2 Describe the three basic types of computers.

12.3 Demonstrate the ability to operate the physical components of the computer, including input, output, processing, and storage devices.

12.4 Recognize the computer programs and operating systems used in the medical office.

12.5 Explain the HIPAA Privacy Rule.

12.6 Identify the uses of surge protectors and screen savers.

12.7 Explain telemedicine and speech recognition technology.

MEDICAL ASSISTING COMPETENCIES

COMPETENCY	CMA	RMA	CCMA	NCMA
General/Legal/Professional				
Operate and maintain facilities, and perform routine maintenance of administrative and clinical equipment safely	X	X	X	X
Utilize computer software and electronic technology to maintain office systems	X	X	X	X
Evaluate and recommend equipment and supplies for practice	X	X	X	X

12.1 The Computer Revolution

In today's world, computer skills are essential for most career choices, including medical assisting. Today's computers are faster and more accurate than ever before. Understanding the fundamentals of computers is essential to being able to perform all the duties of a medical assistant.

12.2 Types of Computers

The three basic types of computers used today are the personal computer, the minicomputer, and mainframe computers.

Personal computers: Also called microcomputers, personal computers are small, self-contained units that come in several different types.

- Desktop—The desktop computer is the most common type, and is found in large and small medical offices.

- Notebook—Notebook computers are also called *laptops*. They use batteries as an alternate power source. Because of their portability, they allow users to travel with them.

- Tablet—Tablets generally cannot do everything that the other types of computers can do, but they can be extremely useful for tasks such as entering patient data from remote locations.

Personal digital assistant (PDA): A handheld computer that functions similarly to cellular (cell) phones, including data storage and transfer, Web browsing, and scheduling functions. Though still used, they are widely being replaced by newer devices such as smartphones.

Mainframes and minicomputers: Essentially used by larger companies and institutions, mainframes and minicomputers are not often used directly by small medical offices.

Supercomputers: As the name indicates, these computers are the biggest, fastest, and most complex computers in use today. Supercomputers are primarily used in medical research applications. They are used for genetic coding and DNA and cancer research.

12.3 Computer Systems

Computer systems consist of hardware and software. As a medical assistant, you should be familiar with the components and uses of a computer. See Figure 12-1.

Computer Hardware

Hardware: Consists of the physical components of a computer system, including the monitor, keyboard, and printer. Figure 12-2 illustrates some types of hardware devices.

Ergonomics: The design of work stations to maximize the user's safety, comfort, and effectiveness. For optimal ergonomics, the computer monitor, keyboard, and mouse should be positioned at the proper heights in order to avoid straining the wrists, back, neck, and eyes. Ergonomics helps to avoid repetitive strain injuries (RSIs), such as carpal tunnel syndrome, and other strains upon muscles, tendons, and nerves.

Input Devices

Input is defined as information entered into and used by the computer. Several types of input devices may be used to enter data into the computer. Keyboards, pointing devices, modems, and scanners are input devices.

Keyboards: The most common type of input device. The keyboard resembles a typewriter. Many specialized functions can be controlled by computer keyboards. Text can be inserted, programs can be accessed, and certain commands can be made easier by accessing specific keys. The calculator section of the keyboard, which specifically controls mathematical functions, is known as the *keypad*.

Tab key: Used to advance the cursor to the next "tab stop," which is a preset location moving horizontally from left to right across the page, as in a word-processing program.

Pointing devices: A device used to enter information into the computer. When you move the pointing device, an arrow appears. You can point and click the arrow on various buttons that appear on the screen. The three types of pointing devices are the mouse, the trackball, and the touch pad.

- Mouse—The most common pointing device. The user moves the mouse across a pad to direct the cursor to the desired place on the computer screen.

- Trackball—Similar to a mouse, but the ball is at the top of the device rather than encased in the body of the mouse unit.

- Touch pad—A small and flat device that is very sensitive to touch. It allows the user to simply slide his or her finger across it in order to move the cursor on the screen.

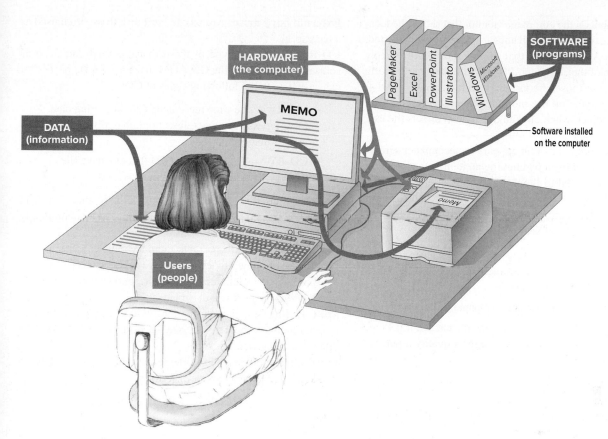

Figure 12-1 *The computer system.*

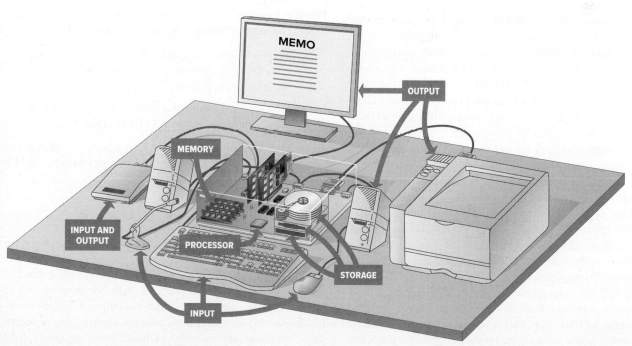

Figure 12-2 *Types of hardware devices.*

Cursor: A symbol on the computer monitor that shows the location where the next character will appear when typed or inserted.

Touch screen: A technology that allows the user to simply touch the screen of the computer, PDA, or cell phone to perform functions similar to those of a mouse, trackball, or touch pad.

Icon: A small graphic on the monitor screen that represents a program or an object; when clicked on, an icon directs the user to the program or object.

Menu: A list of commands that appears on a computer screen, which can be selected from by clicking an item in the list.

Scanners: Devices used to input printed matter and convert it into a format that can be read by the computer. The scanners can convert nonelectronic graphics and text into a computerized format. Three types of scanners are available:

- Handheld—The least expensive type of scanner, it is more difficult to use and produces lower-quality input than other types of scanners.
- Single-sheet—Feeds one sheet of paper through at a time.
- Flatbed—The most expensive type of scanner, it is the easiest to use and produces the highest-quality input.

Processing Devices

Motherboard: The main circuit board that controls components within the computer system.

Central processing unit (CPU): A microprocessor, it is the primary computer chip responsible for interpreting and executing programs. The CPU allows the computer to perform all of its operations; it is also called the "brain" of the computer.

Storage Devices

Storage devices include memory and different types of external computer drives.

Random-access memory (RAM): Temporary memory that functions while you are using a computer's software.

Read-only memory (ROM): Permanent memory that the computer can access but that the user cannot change. It provides the basic operating instructions the computer needs to function.

Cache: Special high-speed storage that is part of the main computer memory or a separate storage device, often used to store previously visited websites for faster recall.

Bits: The smallest units of information inside a computer, each represented by the digit 0 or the digit 1.

Byte: A unit of data containing eight binary digits (bits).

Kilobyte: Approximately 1,024 bytes of information.

Megabyte: Approximately one million bytes of information.

Gigabyte: Approximately one billion bytes of information.

Terabyte: Approximately one trillion bytes of information.

Megahertz: Abbreviated "MHz"; a unit of measure for the clock speed of a microprocessor.

Hard disk drive: A magnetic disk inside the computer used to permanently store data. It offers large amounts of memory and quick access to files. Application software is normally saved to the hard disk and stored there on the computer for use when needed. This is commonly called the C drive.

External hard drive: A separate hard disk drive often used as a backup.

CD-ROM drive: A type of drive that can read data such as software programs. If the CD-ROM drive has a CD "burner," it can save data to the following types of CDs:

- **CD-R**—A one-time recordable CD for storing data. Most types of compact discs hold up to 600 megabytes of information.
- **CD-RW**—A re-recordable CD that can have files rewritten onto it numerous times.

Digital video disk (DVD): An optical disk that can hold approximately 4.7 gigabytes of information, and is commonly used for movies and other forms of video files.

Flash drive: A small, portable memory device. Capacities of flash drives range up to 256 gigabytes of information. A flash drive plugs into a computer's USB port, and is also known as a *thumb, jump,* or *portable* drive.

Multimedia: Graphics, animation, video, sound, and text, as presented on a computer, that may be stored on a CD, DVD, or other storage device.

Purging: The process of removing data that is outdated or no longer needed from a disk or disk drive.

Output Devices

Output is defined as information processed by the computer and transmitted to the monitor, printer, or other output device. Output devices are used to display data after it has been processed. Monitors and printers are the two primary types of output devices.

Monitor: Consists of a screen that looks similar to a television screen. A monitor displays the information that is currently active, such as word processing, spreadsheet, and e-mail files.

Printer: Produces a hard copy or printout of information onto paper. The most commonly used printers are ink jet and laser.

- Ink jet—Offers high-quality printing at an affordable price. This type of printer is commonly used in the home and in small businesses.
- Laser—Offers the highest resolution and therefore the highest-quality output of all printer types.

Default printer: More than one printer may be attached to the same computer; when this occurs, the primary printer used by the computer is considered the default printer.

Transfer Devices

Modems: Devices that transfer information from one computer to another over telephone lines. Modems function by converting data into signals that are transmitted and then converted back into data at the receiving end. With the development of digital subscriber lines (DSLs) and other direct lines, the transfer rates of information have increased significantly in recent years. Modems are essential in transferring electronic files such as insurance claim forms.

Router: A device used to connect any number of local area networks, communicating with other routers to determine the best signal transmission between two or more computers.

Hub: A common connection point for networked devices with multiple ports, often used as part of a local area network (LAN).

Computer Software

Software: Consists of the programs or operating instructions that the computer needs to function. There are two types of software: systems software and applications software.

Systems software: Serves as the operating system of the computer and allows it to run and carry out the functions that the computer performs.

Operating systems: The most popular computer operating systems include Microsoft Windows, Apple (Macintosh, or Mac), and Linux.

Applications software: Refers to the programs loaded onto the computer that carry out the work for the actual users of the computer. Application programs are designed to perform specific tasks, such as word processing, billing, accounting, payroll, insurance form preparation, appointment scheduling, and database management. Popular *practice management* software programs used in the medical office include *Allscripts Professional PM, AthenaHealth, eClinicalWorks, McKesson Practice Choice,* and *NextGen.*

Optical character recognition (OCR): Allows images to be converted to text so that they can be used and edited similarly to any word-processing document. It utilizes optical scanners and special software that is compatible with word-processing software programs.

Driver: Also called a *device driver,* it is the software program or series of commands that enable a computer-connected device to function.

12.4 Using Computer Software

Software includes applications (computer programs) and the operating system.

Word Processing

Word processing can include writing correspondence and reports, transcription, addressing envelopes, and creating form letters. In the medical office, word-processing software is used to produce doctors' notes, transcripts, reports, memos, and letters. The tasks associated with word processing include text editing and proofreading.

Desktop publishing: A type of software used to design a large variety of materials that can be printed or used electronically, including office brochures, letters, memos, reports, and others.

Fonts: Computer *typefaces,* also referred to as "the size and style of type," used in word-processing programs. Two of the most common fonts are Times New Roman and Arial.

Proofreading: The process of checking transcribed materials or text for accuracy and clarity; it helps to reduce errors.

Horizontal centering: Typing text midway between the left and right margins, as used in word-processing or other types of software.

Computer crash: A software or hardware error that causes the computer to malfunction or break down.

Database Management

A database is a collection of related files that serve as a foundation for retrieving information. Accessing patient records is one of the most important uses of computers in the medical office. Databases are forms of software that store patient records, including insurance information, medical charts, and billing records. Information stored in medical databases includes the names of providers, addresses, phone numbers, tax and medical identifier numbers, patient chart numbers, personal patient records, data about insurance carriers and types of plans, electronic insurance claim submission records, diagnosis codes, procedure codes, drug libraries, and all transaction information.

Data hierarchy: An organization of data within a database, from simple to more complex. It includes fields, records, and files.

Fields: Basic data, usually arranged in columns. The data may be alphanumeric (combining letters, numbers, or symbols), numeric, logical (yes/no, true/false, etc.), or in "memo" form (providing additional information or explanation).

Records: Collections of related fields, usually organized in rows. Every record within a file will have the same types of fields.

Files: Collections of related records.

Entry operations: Additions, deletions, or modifications of information within a database.

Addition: Adding fields, records, or files to a database by either appending or inserting it.

Appending: Adding data at the end of a set of other data.

Inserting: Adding data between sets of other data.

Deleting: Removing fields, records, or files from a database.

Modification: Changing existing fields, records, or files.

Database operations: The sorting or indexing of information in a database.

Sorting: Arranging data in a specific sequence or order, such as ascending or descending numerical or alphabetical order.

Indexing: Creating new files by using existing fields and records without altering the original database files.

Database reports: Information from a database organized into summary, exception, or detail reports.

Summary reports: Those that provide counts, subtotals, or totals of specific fields within a database.

Exception reports: Those that identify fields or records having unique characteristics, usually that are outside of predetermined or normal data.

Detail reports: Those that list the records within each file.

Medical practice software: Specially designed software used for all types of data manipulation required by a medical practice. It offers the following:

- Billing, collection, scheduling
- Databases of demographic, financial, and insurance information
- Adding of each new patient to the database

- Coding of services in order to generate claims for payers or patients
- Electronic mailing of claims to payers or payment clearinghouses
- Posting of paid claims into the system
- Creation of financial reports
- Code checking to prevent improper coding of claims
- Rules for submitting claims, which help to avoid denials of payment
- Sorting and "triage" of tasks to alert staff of most important items
- Interfacing with tablets, handheld devices, and voice recognition
- Accessing of data on individual patients or groups of patients
- E-prescribing, which integrates electronic health records, websites used to collect patient information, appointment requests, prescription renewals, test result requests, and online bill payment

Accounting and Billing

This type of software can track patient accounts, create statements and invoices, prepare financial reports, and maintain tax records.

Spreadsheet Software

Spreadsheet software simulates business or scientific worksheets, as well as performs calculations when certain pieces of data are changed. It is most popularly used for bookkeeping and accounting. In the medical office, computer spreadsheet programs are most commonly used for tracking accounts payable.

Appointment Scheduling

Scheduling software can allow patient preferences, such as day of the week and time, to be stored. Available appointments are then listed on the basis of these preferences.

Electronic Health Records

Electronic health records (EHRs) coordinate hardware, software, individuals, policies, and processes with the goal of improving patient care. Data is captured from many sources and used at the point of care (POC) to assist in making clinical decisions. Information is exchanged easily between all levels of health-care professionals. Evidence-based medicine is supported. Documentation is simplified by using embedded medical terminology.

Benefits of EHRs: Interaction with POC while treating patients, documentation of findings and procedures, medication administration reminders, alerts about less expensive drugs, procedure protocols, alerts about duplicate services,

scheduling, patient registration, billing, exchange of data with other providers' systems, and establishing a Continuity of Care Record.

Continuity of Care Record: Standard content that physicians agree should be included in a referral. Abbreviated as "CCR."

Technology used in EHRs: Databases, data exchange, electronic clinical imaging storage, workflow systems that allow multiple users to access information at the same time, flexible data retrieval; data capture technology that includes speech/handwriting recognition, patient devices, and wireless/handheld devices; ability to communicate with a variety of computer network types; real-time data storage and retrieval, and workstations that facilitate easy use of data.

Health care data sets: Single facts or measurements called *data elements*; analyzed meaningful information collection; aggregate data about groups of patients; data sets of information with uniform definitions; identification of elements needed to be collected for each patient; uniform definitions used for commonly used terms; comparison of data from different facilities; and defined uses of comparison data, including accreditation, research, and performance improvement.

Common data sets: Collections of data for a variety of health-care systems, as follows:

- Uniform Hospital Discharge Data Set (UHDDS)—inpatient hospital care
- Uniform Ambulatory Care Data Set (UACDS)—for patients who return home on the day of service
- Minimum Data Set for Long-Term Care (MDS)—nursing home patients
- Outcome and Assessment Information Set (OASIS)—Medicare beneficiaries receiving home health agency care
- Data Elements for Emergency Department Systems (DEEDS)
- Essential Medical Data Set (EMDS)—works with DEEDS to provide concise medical histories on all patients
- Health Plan Employer Data and Information Set (HEDIS)—gives consumers information with which to compare managed care plans

Electronic Transactions

By utilizing modems and special software, transaction information in the form of electronic data interchanges can be sent and received quickly, avoiding the use of ground mail services. Common electronic transactions include sending insurance claims and communicating with other computer users. The date of service is important, to ensure that insurance forms will be sequential.

Sending insurance claims: Insurance claims can be sent directly from medical offices to insurance carriers; claims processed in this way take much less time and are usually processed more efficiently. The electronic claim transaction is the HIPAA Health Care Claim or Equivalent Encounter Information; its official name is the X12 837 Health Care Claim. The HIPAA Electronic Health Care Transactions and Code Sets (TCS) mandate means that health plans are required to accept the standard claim submitted electronically. HIPAA stands for the Health Insurance Portability and Accountability Act of 1996.

Communications

Electronic mail and the Internet help users in different locations save time and money in their communications.

Electronic mail: Also known as e-mail, a method of communication that allows messages to be sent through a computer network. Information sent electronically moves quickly, regardless of the distance it is sent.

Internet: A global computer network that allows communication among computer users worldwide. Large sources of information, including medical information, may be accessed on the Internet. An advantage of the Internet is that information can be updated frequently.

E-commerce: The sale and purchase of goods and services over the Internet.

Browser: A software program that allows Internet sites (Web pages) to be viewed on a computer.

HTML: Hypertext markup language, which is used to create Internet documents.

HTTP: Hypertext transfer protocol, which is used to instruct a Web server where to retrieve a desired Web page.

HTTPS: Hypertext transfer protocol secure, which allows for secure communication while instructing a Web server where to retrieve a desired Web page. It combines HTTP with the secure sockets layer (SSL) / transport layer security (TLS) protocol, adding security to standard communications.

Search engine: A program that searches Internet documents for keywords, returning a list of documents containing those words.

Server: A computer or other networked device that manages shared resources.

URL: Uniform resource locator, which is the global address of a Web page or other Internet information.

12.5 Security in the Computerized Office

Much of the information used in a medical office is confidential and should be accessible only to authorized personnel.

Passwords: Passwords are often used so that the computer system administrator can keep track of who is accessing information at any given time. Each employee is given a distinct password that should not be shared with anyone.

Activity-monitoring systems: Some health-care facilities use activity-monitoring systems that keep track of user names and the files they have viewed or changed.

Data backup: Any type of storage that prevents loss of files due to hard-disk failure. To protect against data loss from any

cause, the MA should make backup copies of all files nightly. These copies should be stored at a secure location that is off the premises.

Batch processing: A procedure in which accumulated similar programs and input data are processed simultaneously.

HIPAA Privacy Rule

The HIPAA Standards for Privacy of Individually Identifiable Health Information provides the first comprehensive federal protection for the privacy of health information. It creates national standards to protect individuals' medical records and other personal health information. The core of the HIPAA Privacy Rule is the protection, use, and disclosure of protected health information (PHI). PHI refers to individually identifiable health information that is transmitted or maintained by electronic or other media, such as computer storage devices. The privacy rule protects all PHI held or transmitted by a covered entity, which includes health-care providers, health plans, and health-care clearinghouses.

12.6 Computer System Care and Maintenance

The first step in computer care and maintenance is to keep the area near each computer free from dirt, food, liquids, and similar substances that could enter and cause damage to the system components and devices. In addition, computer components should be located in well-ventilated locations. A computer maintenance agreement should include software upgrades.

Surge protector: An electrical power strip that helps keep a computer system's delicate circuits from being damaged by the increased voltage of an electrical power surge.

Screen saver: Protects computer monitors from screen burn-in by automatically changing the monitor display at short intervals or by showing constantly moving images.

Printer supplies: Printers should be regularly maintained with fresh ribbons, ink cartridges, and toner cartridges. Most printers alert the user when one of these items needs to be replaced.

Disk and tape maintenance: Disks should be kept away from magnetic fields, direct sunlight, and extreme temperatures. They should be handled carefully as dirt and dust can cause them to not operate properly. CD-ROMs should be handled only by their edges and by the hole in the center; they should be stored in their plastic cases. Smudges, fingerprints, and dust can cause a CD-ROM to be misread by the CD drive. Magnetic tapes should be stored in cool, dry places. It is especially important to store these tapes away from magnetic fields as they can be erased by magnetism.

12.7 Computers of the Future

Computers are constantly being improved and upgraded. This includes both their hardware and the software that is used to operate them. Examples of new computer technologies include telemedicine and speech recognition technology.

Telemedicine: Refers to using telecommunications to transmit video images. Physicians in rural areas can easily send patient information via these images to physicians with more expertise in the patient's type of condition, which can aid in the patient's treatment and diagnosis.

Speech recognition technology: Enables computers to comprehend and interpret spoken words. Instead of using a keyboard, mouse, scanner, or other input device, the user inputs information by speaking into a microphone connected to the computer. As this technology becomes more advanced, it may largely eliminate the need for the physician's notes to be transcribed by medical assistants.

CHAPTER 12 REVIEW

Instructions:

Answer the following questions.

1. Which of the following is a type of temporary memory?

   A. ergonomics
   B. cache
   C. random-access memory
   D. read-only memory
   E. megabytes

2. Which of the following helps to avoid repetitive strain injuries when working with a computer system?

   A. touchscreens
   B. routers
   C. megahertz
   D. hubs
   E. ergonomics

3. Spreadsheets are most commonly used for which of the following tasks?

   A. word processing
   B. desktop publishing
   C. accounting and billing
   D. appointment scheduling
   E. electronic mailing

4. Which of the following devices is able to interpret printed text, illustrations, or photos and put them into a format that can be used by the computer?

   A. cache
   B. motherboard
   C. modem
   D. mouse
   E. scanner

5. The process of removing data that is outdated or no longer needed from a disk or disk drive is

   A. scanning.
   B. printing.
   C. backing up.
   D. purging.
   E. saving.

6. Which one of the following devices helps protect a computer system's delicate circuits from damage?

   A. motherboard
   B. mainframe
   C. surge protector
   D. activity-monitoring system
   E. scanner

7. Any individually identifiable health information that is transmitted or maintained by electronic or other media is known as

   A. PHI.
   B. HIPAA.
   C. CPU.
   D. CD-RW.
   E. data.

8. Which of the following is often called the "brains" of the computer?

   A. read-only memory (ROM)
   B. random-access memory (RAM)
   C. video display terminal (VDT)
   D. cathode ray tube (CRT)
   E. central processing unit (CPU)

9. Which of the following terms refers to programs loaded on to a computer that carry out the work for the users of the computer?

   A. systems software
   B. applications software
   C. spreadsheet software
   D. password
   E. icon

10. The primary printer used by a computer is considered to be the

    A. accessory printer.
    B. default printer.
    C. laser printer.
    D. inkjet printer.
    E. dot matrix printer.

CHAPTER 13

FINANCIAL MANAGEMENT

LEARNING OUTCOMES

13.1 Describe the process of taking inventory, ordering, receiving, storing, and paying for supplies.

13.2 Recognize terminology used when recording, classifying, and analyzing financial transactions.

13.3 Identify the types of bank accounts and banking transactions utilized by the medical office.

13.4 Describe the billing and collections process.

13.5 Identify financial obligations the physician has to others for equipment and services.

MEDICAL ASSISTING COMPETENCIES

COMPETENCY	CMA	RMA	CCMA	NCMA
Administrative				
Prepare a bank deposit record	X	X		
Post entries on a daysheet	X	X		
Maintain accounts payable and receivable	X	X		X
Perform billing and collection procedures	X	X		X
Post adjustments	X	X		X
Process a credit balance	X	X		X
Process refunds	X	X		
Post NSF checks	X	X		
Post collection agency payments	X	X		X
Reconcile a bank statement	X	X		
Prepare a check	X	X		
Establish and maintain a petty cash fund	X	X		X
Use manual and computerized bookkeeping systems	X	X		X
Maintain records for accounting and banking purposes	X	X		X
Process employee payroll	X	X		

▶ *Study Skills*

Use your energy!
Know your daily cycle of high and low energy. Are you a morning person or a night person? Try to use your high-energy times to study and tackle difficult subject matter. Arrange your daily schedule so that you can study when you feel most refreshed and energized.

13.1 Purchasing

Medical office supplies: Purchasing and maintaining supplies for medical practices is essential. The medical assistant is usually responsible for taking inventory of equipment and supplies and for ordering anything that is needed.

Types of Supplies

The types of supplies used in the medical office include administrative, clinical, and general. Table 13-1 lists the most commonly used supplies.

Administrative supplies: Items used to keep the office running, such as stationery, typing paper, photocopy paper, medical record forms, appointment books, pens, colored highlighters, correcting tape, and toner.

Clinical supplies: Medically related items, such as towels, drapes, gowns, table paper, instruments, lubricants, tongue blades, syringes, suture material, laboratory reagents, and elastic bandages.

General supplies: Items used by both patients and staff, such as paper towels, soap, and toilet tissue.

Vital supplies: Can be both clinical and administrative in nature. These items are absolutely essential to ensure the smooth running of the practice. Examples include prescription pads and paper for examinations. To help keep track of supplies, categorize them according to the urgency of need, making sure that vital supplies are readily available.

Incidental supplies: Can be clinical, administrative, or general in nature. The efficiency of the office is not threatened if these supplies run low. Incidental supplies include rubber bands and staples.

Durable items: Pieces of equipment that are used indefinitely, such as telephones or computers, that are not considered supplies.

Expendable items: Items that are used and then must be restocked, also known as consumables. Expendable items are used up within a short period of time, and they are relatively inexpensive.

Capital equipment: Items that are considered major and involve expenditures above a predetermined dollar value. Capital equipment includes general, large lab, administrative, and clinical equipment. Table 13-2 lists some examples of capital equipment.

Ordering and Receiving Supplies

Vendors: The medical assistant should obtain recommendations from other medical offices, gather competitive prices, and compare vendors on the basis of price, quality, service, and payment policies. It takes multiple vendors to provide all the supplies for a medical practice. Many medical vendors provide their services and supplies only over the Internet.

Local vendors: It is a good idea to establish good credit and business relationships with local vendors, even if they cost a little more. Local vendors may offer special discounts, emergency service, information about sales and specials, and personal assistance.

Catalog services: Can provide ease of availability, competitive pricing, and fast delivery. Many vendors accept telephone, fax, and e-mail orders as well as traditional order forms.

Ordering supplies: Expendable supplies and equipment must be replaced and reordered in time. A copy of the order form should be retained to check against the order when it arrives.

Purchase requisitions: Some practices require approval of a formal request before supplies can be ordered.

Receiving supplies: Orders should be checked for completeness. One person should be responsible for receiving and signing for deliveries. This person must check invoices and/or packing slips against the items delivered, initial and date the invoices as items are received, and distribute goods to the storage room.

Packing slip: A list of supplies packed and shipped, supplied by the vendor in the package with the supplies. It is used to verify that ordered supplies were received.

Statement: The monthly bill summarizing invoices. It is a request for payment.

Supply budget: The average medical practice spends from 4–6% of its annual gross income on supplies. If costs exceed 6%, you might be required to reevaluate the office's spending practices.

Storage of Supplies

Storage room: Should be arranged with the most commonly used items within easiest reach. Place new stock in the back of the storage area, and move the old supplies up front for first use. This practice is referred to as rotating stock. You must know the storage requirements for various kinds of supplies. You must maintain an adequate quantity of supplies in a well-organized storage space to run the office smoothly.

Inventory: A list of articles in stock, with the description and quantity of each. Inventory control requires constant supervision because a medical office cannot afford to run out of supplies. Most offices maintain an ongoing inventory system, which helps determine when to reorder supplies.

AT A GLANCE Typical Supplies in a Medical Office

Administrative Supplies

Appointment books, daybooks	Local welfare department forms
Back-to-school/back-to-work slips	Patient education materials
Clipboards	Pens, pencils, erasers
Computer supplies	Rubber bands, paper clips
Copy and facsimile (fax) machine paper	Social Security forms
File folders, coding tabs	Stamps
History and physical examination sheets / cards	Stationery: appointment cards, bookkeeping supplies (ledgers, statements, billing forms), letterhead, second sheets, envelopes, business cards, prescription pads, notebooks, notepads, telephone memo pads
Insurance forms: disability, HMO and other third-party payers, life insurance examinations, Veterans Administration, workers' compensation	
Insurance manuals	

Clinical Supplies

Alcohol swabs	Microscopic slides and fixative
Applicators	Needles, syringes
Bandaging materials: adhesive tape, gauze pads, gauze sponges, elastic bandages, adhesive bandages, roller bandages (gauze and elastic)	Safety pins
	Silver nitrate sticks
	Suture removal kits
Cloth or paper gowns	Sutures
Cotton, cotton swabs	Thermometer covers
Culture tubes	Tongue depressors
I.V. solutions	Topical skin freeze
Disposable sheaths for thermometers	Urinalysis test sticks
Disposable tips for otoscopes	Urine containers
Gloves: sterile, examination	Medications, chemicals, solutions, ointments, lotions, and disinfectants
Hemoccult test kits	
Iodine or Betadine pads	
Lancets	
Lubricating jelly	

General Supplies

Liquid hypoallergenic soap
Paper cups
Paper towels
Feminine hygiene products
Tissues: facial, toilet

Table 13-1

AT A GLANCE Examples of Capital Equipment

General	Administrative	Clinical
Office furnishings	Computers	Examination room furnishings
Carpeting	Copy machines	Examination equipment such as microscopes, autoclaves, and ultrasound machines

Table 13-2

Reminder cards: Many offices develop color-coded reorder reminder cards, which are inserted into the stack of inventory items. When the card comes to the top of the stack, it is time to reorder.

Payment

Invoice: A paper describing a purchase and the amount due. Check the invoice against the original order and the packing slip, mark it to confirm that the order was received, and pay it. The check number, date, and payment amount should then be recorded on the invoice. Invoices should be placed in a special folder until paid.

Payment terms: Many vendors do not charge a handling fee if an order is prepaid. Others offer a discount for enclosing a check with an order. Some delay billing for 30 to 90 days. The vendor's invoice usually describes payment terms.

Records: Copies of all bills and order forms for supplies should be kept on file for at least 7 years in case the practice is audited by the IRS.

Disbursement: Payment of funds, whether in cash or by check. Usually, you will write a check to the vendor and have the physician sign it. At the time of payment, write the date and check number on the statement, and place it in the paid file. Disbursements can be entered into the accounting records in several ways, depending on the accounting system used.

Purchasing procedure: The purchasing procedure should follow certain standard practices:

- An authorized person should be in charge of purchasing.

- High-quality goods and services should be ordered at the lowest possible prices.

- Receipts of goods should be recorded.

- Shipments received should be checked against packing slips to verify that all goods have been received.

- Invoices should be paid in a timely manner.

- Paid invoices should be kept on file.

13.2 Accounting

Accounting: A system of recording, classifying, summarizing, and interpreting financial statements.

Accounting bases: Methods of accounting, which include the *cash basis* and the *accrual basis*. In the cash basis (used by most physicians), charges for services are entered as income when payment is collected, and expenses are recorded when they are paid. In the accrual basis, revenues are recognized on an income statement when they are earned, rather than when payment is received.

Account: In bookkeeping terms, a single financial record category or division. It is used to track debit and credit changes, by date, in reference to a specific matter. For example, when a practice accepts a new patient, the patient is assigned an account. As the patient is charged for services and the patient (or third-party payer, such as an insurance company) pays those charges, entries are made in the patient's account.

Account balance: The debit or credit balance remaining in an account.

Accounts payable: Records of the amounts charged with suppliers or creditors that remain unpaid.

Accounts receivable: Records of all outstanding accounts and the amounts that are due.

Record of office disbursements: A list of the amounts paid for medical supplies, rent, utilities, wages, postage, and equipment over a certain time period. The person receiving the payment is called the *payee*.

Assets: Possessions of value, which in a medical office are inventory, equipment, prepaid rent, and the amounts due from patients.

Liabilities: Amounts owed to creditors, such as a mortgage on the medical building and the accounts payable.

Balance sheet: A financial statement for a specific date or period that indicates the total assets, liabilities, and capital of the business.

Auditing: The review of financial data to verify accuracy and completeness. Medical assistants responsible for bookkeeping must provide required financial records and answer questions about accounting systems used. According to the Internal Revenue Service, financial records must be retained for at least seven years.

Bookkeeping Systems

Bookkeeping: The recording part of the accounting process. Bookkeeping records income, charges, and disbursements. There are two types of bookkeeping: electronic and manual. There are three types of manual bookkeeping systems: single entry, double entry, and pegboard.

Electronic bookkeeping: Computerized bookkeeping that often utilizes the *double-entry system*. Spreadsheet programs are used to handle all tasks that can be performed in manual bookkeeping, but with the advantages of increased speed and the ability to back up data. Various software programs are also available that combine accounting, bookkeeping, scheduling, records, and billing.

Single-entry system: The oldest bookkeeping system, requiring only one entry for each transaction. This straightforwardness makes it the easiest system to learn and use. Because it is not self-balancing, however, it is the hardest system in which to spot errors. It includes several basic records, such as:

- Daily log to record charges and payments (see Figure 13-1)

- Patient ledger cards

- Payroll records

- Cash payment journal

- Petty cash records

Double-entry system: Based on the accounting equation *assets = liabilities + owner equity*. The materials required for a double-entry bookkeeping system are inexpensive, but the system requires more skill and knowledge of accounting procedures than the single-entry system. It is also more time consuming to use. After each financial transaction, the medical office using a double-entry system must debit one account and credit another

Dr. _____		Date _____		
Hour	**Patient**	**Service Provided**	**Charge**	**Paid**
1				
2				
3				
4				
5				
6				
7				
8				
9				
10				
11				
12				
13				
14				
15				
16				
		Totals		

Figure 13-1 *A daily log is used to record charges and payments.*

account. For example, when the practice charges for a medical service, the patient's account is debited and the appropriate account for the practice is credited.

Pegboard system: A system consisting of daysheets, ledger cards, patient charge slips, and receipt forms or superbills. A pegboard system usually includes a lightweight board with pegs on the left or right edges and is sometimes called a write-it-once system. It is the most commonly used manual medical accounts receivable system and the most expensive to maintain. It was once the most widely used bookkeeping system in medical practices, but is now less common.

A pegboard system has several main advantages:

- The system is efficient and saves time.
- The daysheet provides complete and up-to-date information about accounts receivable status at a glance.
- The system is easy to learn.

Charge slip: The original record of the doctor's services and the charge for those services.

Posting to Records

General journal: A record of the physician's practice. It includes records of services rendered, charges made, and monies received. The general journal is also known by the names *daily log, daybook, daysheet, daily journal,* and *charge journal.* This journal is also called the *book of original entry* because it is where all transactions are first recorded.

Patient ledger card: A card that contains the patient's name, address, home and work telephone numbers, and the name of the person who is responsible for the charges (if different from the patient). It also contains a record of charges, payment, and adjustments for individual patients or families. See Figure 13-2.

Accounts receivable: Amounts owed to the physician or the medical office.

Accounts receivable ledger: A record of the charges and payments posted on patient accounts. It includes all the individual patients' financial accounts on which there are balances.

Posting: The process of copying or recording an amount from one record, such as a journal, onto another record, such as a ledger—or from a daysheet onto a ledger card.

Manual posting: Facilitated by a section at the bottom of each daysheet and a check register page at the end of each month, plus monthly and annual summaries. Accounting records must show every amount paid out, date and check number, and purpose of payment.

Computer posting: Using a computer to keep track of and print accounts receivable and accounts payable. Computers are also used to print checks, as well as payment information.

Accrual basis accounting: Recording income when it is earned and expenses when they are incurred.

Trial balance: A method of checking the accuracy of accounts. It should be done once a month after all posting has been completed and before preparing the monthly statements. The purpose of a trial balance is to disclose any discrepancies between the journal and the ledger.

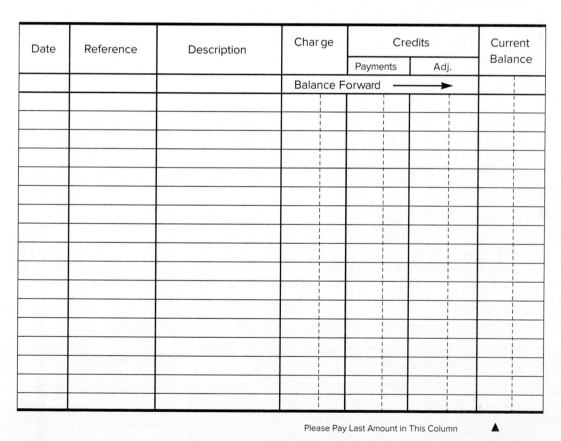

Patient's Name   Jonathan Jackson

Home Phone   (612) 555-9921   Work Phone   (612) 555-1000

Patient's ID No.   111-21-4114

Employer   Ashton School District

Insurance   National Insurance Co.

Policy #   123-4-56-788

Person Responsible for Charges (If Different from Patient) _____

JONATHAN JACKSON
123 Fourth Avenue
Ashton, MN 70809-1222

Date	Reference	Description	Charge	Credits		Current Balance
				Payments	Adj.	
		Balance Forward ⟶				

Please Pay Last Amount in This Column ▲

OV— Office Visit   C—Consultation   EX—Examination
X—X-ray   NC—No Charge   INS—Insurance
ROA—Received on Account   MA—Missed Appointment

Figure 13-2 *Patient ledger cards are used to show how much each patient owes.*

Daily journal: A chronological record of the medical practice, also known as its *financial diary*. Practices using a manual pegboard system refer to this as their *daysheet*. All transactions should be recorded.
Disbursement journal: A summary of accounts paid out.

Account Balances

Equity: The net worth of the medical office. Equity equals the practice's total assets minus the total liabilities.
Balance: The difference between the debit and credit totals.
Adjustment column: An account column, sometimes included to the left of the balance column, used for entering discounts, debits, credits, refunds, and write-offs.
Balance column: The account column on the far right that is used for recording the difference between the debit and credit columns.
Debit: An amount usually representing things acquired for the intended use or benefit of a business. It is recorded in the column to the left of the credit column. In each journal entry, the dollar amount of the debit must be equal to the dollar amount of the credit. A debit is also called a charge. Debits are incurred when the practice pays for something, such as medical supplies.
Credit: An amount constituting an addition to a revenue, net worth, or liability account. It is recorded in the column to the right of the debit column. Credits constitute payments received by the practice, such as from patients or third-party insurance providers.
Credit balance: Money owed to the patient that results when a patient has paid in advance and there has been an overpayment. The medical assistant should circle the payment on the daysheet and ledger. A credit balance may occur when a partial payment is made and then the patient's insurance allows a higher payment than the remaining balance.
Refunds: Debit adjustments. If a patient wishes to have an overpayment refunded, write a check for the amount due and enter the transaction on the daysheet.
Credit bureau: A company that provides information about the creditworthiness of a person seeking credit. If a patient's credit history is in question, you may request a report from a credit bureau. A sample credit bureau report is shown in Figure 13-3.
Equal Credit Opportunity Act: An act that states that credit arrangements may not be denied on the basis of a patient's sex, race, religion, national origin, marital status, or age. Also, credit cannot be denied because the patient receives public assistance or has exercised rights under the Consumer Credit Protection Act, such as disputing a credit card bill or a credit bureau report. Under the Equal Credit Opportunity Act, the patient has a right to know the specific reason that credit was denied.
In balance: Accounts are in balance when the total ending balances of patient ledgers equals the total of accounts receivable.
Receipts: Money received.

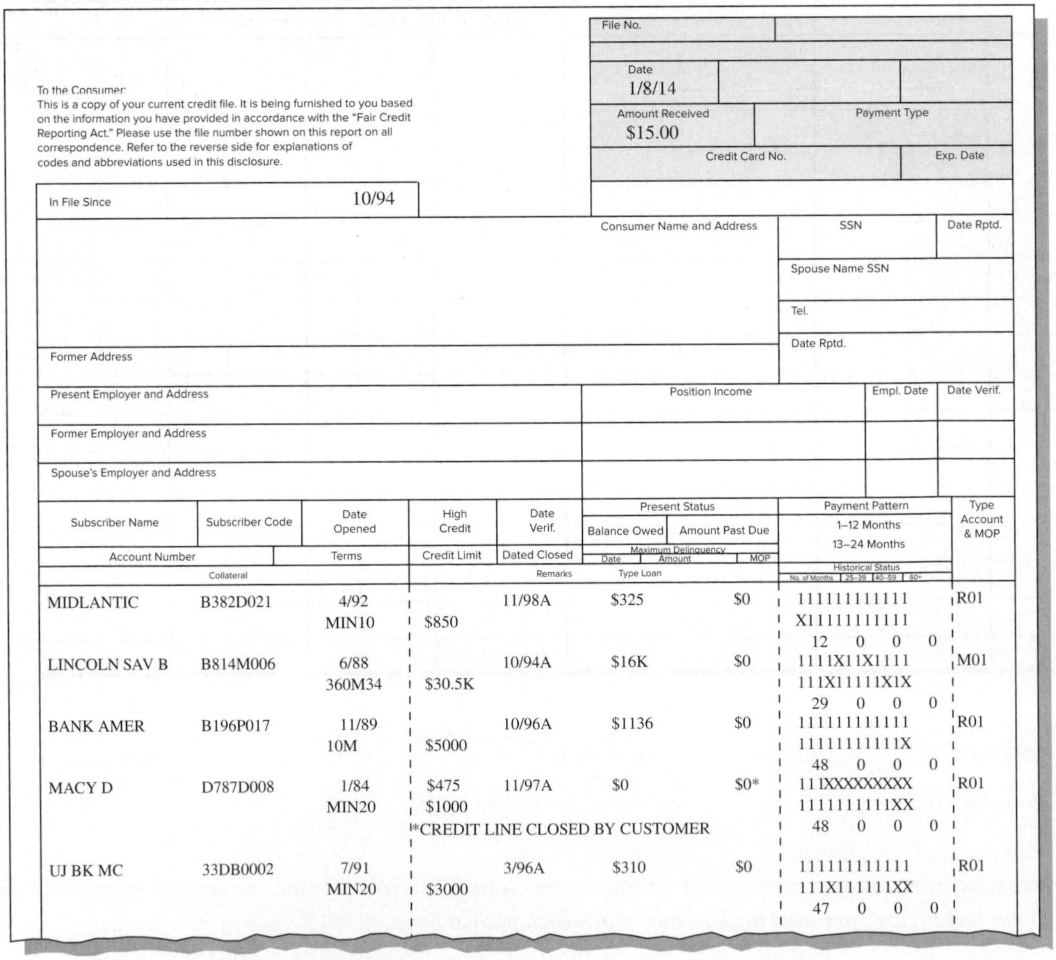
File No.

Date 1/8/14

Amount Received $15.00 | Payment Type

Credit Card No. | Exp. Date

To the Consumer:
This is a copy of your current credit file. It is being furnished to you based on the information you have provided in accordance with the "Fair Credit Reporting Act." Please use the file number shown on this report on all correspondence. Refer to the reverse side for explanations of codes and abbreviations used in this disclosure.

In File Since 10/94

Consumer Name and Address | SSN | Date Rptd.

Spouse Name SSN

Tel.

Former Address | Date Rptd.

Present Employer and Address | Position Income | Empl. Date | Date Verif.

Former Employer and Address

Spouse's Employer and Address

Subscriber Name / Account Number / Collateral	Subscriber Code	Date Opened / Terms	High Credit / Credit Limit	Date Verif. / Dated Closed / Remarks	Present Status: Balance Owed / Maximum Delinquency Date, Amount / Type Loan	Amount Past Due / MOP	Payment Pattern: 1–12 Months / 13–24 Months / Historical Status (No. of Months, 25–39, 40–59, 60+)	Type Account & MOP
MIDLANTIC	B382D021	4/92 MIN10	$850	11/98A	$325	$0	111111111111 X11111111111 12 0 0 0	R01
LINCOLN SAV B	B814M006	6/88 360M34	$30.5K	10/94A	$16K	$0	1111X11X1111 111X11111X1X 29 0 0 0	M01
BANK AMER	B196P017	11/89 10M	$5000	10/96A	$1136	$0	111111111111 11111111111X 48 0 0 0	R01
MACY D	D787D008	1/84 MIN20	$475 $1000	11/97A	$0	$0*	11XXXXXXXXXX 1111111111XX 48 0 0 0	R01
*CREDIT LINE CLOSED BY CUSTOMER								
UJ BK MC	33DB0002	7/91 MIN20	$3000	3/96A	$310	$0	111111111111 111X111111XX 47 0 0 0	R01

Figure 13-3 ***Credit reports are generated by credit bureaus.***

Petty cash fund: A fund used to pay for small or unpredictable expenditures. These include parking fees, postage due, emergency supplies, small contributions, and miscellaneous items. This fund is usually no more than $50.

Petty cash log: A financial record that shows payments for minor office expenses.

Reconciliation of bank statement: The process of verifying that the bank statement and the checkbook balances are in agreement. As you reconcile the bank statement with your accounts, be aware of outstanding checks, outstanding deposits, and any service fees the bank may have charged. The bank statement may have an entry for service charges, which must be deducted from the checkbook balance. When reconciling a bank statement for the medical practice, daily deposits should be added to the bank statement balance.

Superbill: A combination charge slip, statement, and insurance reporting form. A superbill includes the charges for services rendered on a day, an invoice for payment or insurance copayment, and all the information for submitting an insurance claim. It is also called an encounter form. See Figure 13-4.

13.3 Banking for the Medical Office

Medical business: A medical practice is a business that must produce a profit—that is, its income must exceed its expenses. Bookkeeping and banking are essential and must be 100% accurate.

Absolute accuracy: Necessary when working with bank deposits, reconciliation of statements, and all bookkeeping activities. The medical assistant acts as the agent for the physician.

Banks: Maintain checking and savings accounts for their customers.

Banking functions: Basic bank-related activities carried out by a medical practice include:

- Depositing funds
- Withdrawing funds
- Reconciling statements
- Using auxiliary services

Types of Bank Accounts

Types of bank accounts: Medical practices typically use three types of bank account:

- Regular checking account
- Interest-earning, or interest-bearing, checking account
- Savings account

Regular checking account: Most medical practices have a regular checking account for office expenses. This account does not pay interest but offers availability and flexibility.

Interest: Money paid to a depositor by a bank or other financial institution for the use of the depositor's money.

Electronic banking: Banking with the use of computers. Electronic banking has several advantages over traditional banking: It can improve productivity, cash flow, and accuracy. The computer screen can display all checks and deposits that were logged into the register in the order they were posted.

In electronic banking, someone must still be responsible for recording and physically depositing checks.

Bank statements: All contain certain basic information, including:

- Closing date
- Caption
- List of checks processed
- List of deposits

Caption: A summary of the account activity that has taken place during the month up to the closing date. It includes the beginning balance, total value of checks processed, total amount of deposits made, service charges, and ending balance.

Checks

Check: A written order to a bank to pay or transfer money. It is payable on demand and is considered a negotiable instrument. The person who writes the check is called the payer or drawer.

Types of checks: Cashier's checks, certified checks, money orders, limited checks, traveler's checks, voucher checks, bank drafts, and warrants.

Cashier's check: Written using the bank's own check form and signed by a bank representative. The funds for payment of the check are debited from the payer's account at the time the check is written. A service charge is usually added. Another term for a cashier's check is treasurer's check.

Certified check: Written on the payer's own check form and verified by the bank with an official stamp. The bank withdraws the money from the payer's account when it certifies the check. The stamp indicates that the bank certifies the availability of the funds.

Money order: A certificate of guaranteed payment. It is purchased for the cash value printed on the certificate plus a nominal handling fee. Money orders may be purchased from banks, post offices, and some convenience stores. International money orders can be acquired in U.S. dollars to be cashed in foreign countries. Money orders are often used by people without checking accounts who want to have a receipt of payment for record keeping.

Limited check: Issued on a special check form that displays a preprinted maximum dollar amount for which the check can be written. This type of check often is used for payroll or insurance payments.

Traveler's check: A check purchased for a small fee for a specified amount of money. It is designed for people who are traveling where personal checks may not be accepted and for people who do not want to carry large amounts of cash. Traveler's checks are also available in foreign currencies. They can be purchased at a bank. A traveler's check is available in many denominations. It requires a signature when purchased and when used.

Counter check: A special bank-issued check that allows the depositor to withdraw funds from his or her account only.

Voucher check: Contains a detachable voucher form. It is frequently used for payroll checks because additional information about the transaction can be supplied to the payee. The voucher portion is used to itemize the purpose of the check, deductions, or other information.

Lakeridge Medical Group
262 East Pine Street, Suite 100
Lakeridge, NJ 07500

☐ PRIVATE ☐ BLUECROSS ☐ IND. ☐ MEDICARE ☐ MEDI-CAL ☐ HMO ☐ PPO

PATIENT'S LAST NAME		FIRST	ACCOUNT #	BIRTHDATE / /	SEX ☐ MALE ☐ FEMALE	TODAY'S DATE / /
INSURANCE COMPANY		SUBSCRIBER		PLAN #	SUB. #	GROUP

ASSIGNMENT: I hereby assign my insurance benefits to be paid directly to the undersigned physician. I am financially responsible for non-covered services.
SIGNED: (Patient, or Parent, if Minor)   DATE: / /

RELEASE: I hereby authorize the physician to release to my insurance carrers any information required to process this claim.
SIGNED: (Patient, or Parent, if Minor)   DATE: / /

✔	DESCRIPTION	M/Care	CPT/Mod	DxRe	FEE	✔	DESCRIPTION	M/Care	CPT/Mod	DxRe	FEE	✔	DESCRIPTION	M/Care	CPT/Mod	DxRe	FEE
	OFFICE CARE						PROCEDURES						INJECTIONS/IMMUNIZATIONS				
	NEW PATIENT						Tread Mill (In Office)		93015				Tetanus		90718		
	Brief		99201				24 Hour Holter		93224				Hypertet	J1670	90782		
	Limited		99202				If Medicare (Set up Fec)		93225				Pneumococcal		90732		
	Intermediate		99203				Physician Interpret		93227				Influenza		90724		
	Extended		99204				EKG w/Interpretation		93000				TB Skin Test (PPD)		86585		
	Comprehensive		99205				EKG (Medicare)		93005				Antigen Injection-Single		95115		
							Sigmoidoscopy		45300				Multiple		95117		
	ESTABLISHED PATIENT						Sigmoidoscopy, Flexible		45330				B12 Injection	J3420	90782		
	Minimal		99211				Sigmoidos., Flex. w/Bx.		45331				Injection, IM		90782		
	Brief		99212				Spirometry, FEV/FVC		94010				Compazine	J0780	90782		
	Limited		99213				Spirometry, Post-Dilator		94060				Demerol	J2175	90782		
	Intermediate		99214										Vistaril	J3410	90782		
	Extended		99215										Susphrine	J0170	90782		
	Comprehensive		99215				LABORATORY						Decadron	J0890	90782		
							Blood Draw Fee		36415				Estradiol	J1000	90782		
	CONSULTATION-OFFICE						Urinalysis, Chemical		81005				Testosterone	J1080	90782		
	Focused		99241				Throat Culture		87081				Lidocaine	J2000	90782		
	Expanded		99242				Occult Blood		82270				Solumedrol	J2920	90782		
	Detailed		99243				Pap Handling Charge		99000				Solucortef	J1720	90782		
	Comprehensive 1		99244				Pap Life Guard		88150-90				Hydeltra	J1690	90782		
	Comprehensive 2		99245				Gram Stain		87205				Pen Procaine	J2510	90788		
	Dr.						Hanging Drop		87210								
	Case Management		98900				Urine Drug Screen		99000				INJECTIONS - JOINT/BURSA				
													Small Joints		20600		
	Post-op Exam		99024										Intermediate		20605		
							SUPPLIES						Large Joints		20610		
													Trigger Point		20550		
													MISCELLANEOUS				

	DIAGNOSIS:	ICD-9									
	Abdominal Pain	789.0	Gout	274.0	C.V.A. - Acute	436.	Electrolyte Dis.	276.9	Herpes Simplex	054.9
	Abscess (Site)	682.9	Asthma	493.90	Cere. Vas. Accid. (Old)	438	Fatigue	780.7	Herpes Zoster	053.9
	Adverse Drug Rx	995.2	Asthmatic Bronchitis	493.90	Cerumen	380.4	Fibrocys. Br. Dis	610.1	Hydrocele	603.9
	Alcohol Detox	291.8	Atrial Fib.	427.31	Chestwall Pain	786.59	Fracture (Site)	829.0	Hyperlipidemia	272.4
	Alcoholism	303.90	Atrial Tachi.	427.0	Cholecystitis	575.0	Open/Close		Hypertension	401.9
	Allergic Rhinitis	477	Bowel Obstruct.	560.9	Cholelithiasis	574.00	Fungal Infect. (Site)	110.8	Hyperthyroidism	242.9
	Allergy	995.3	Breast Mass	611.72	COPD	492.8	Gastric Ulcer	531.90	Hypothyroidism	244.9
	Alzheimer's Dis.	290.1	Bronchitis	490	Cirrhosis	571.5	Gastritis	535.0	Labyrinthitis	386.30
	Anemia	285.9	Bursitis	727.3	Cong. Heart Fail.	428.9	Gastroenteritis	558.9	Lipoma (Site)	214.9
	Anemia - Pernicious	281.0	Cancer, Breast (Site)	174.9	Conjunctivitis	372.30	G.I. Bleeding	578.9	Lymphoma	202.8
	Angina	413.9	Metastatic (Site)	199.1	Contusion (Site)	924.9	Glomerulonephritis	583.9	Mit. Valve Prolapse	424.0
	Anxiety Synd.	300.00	Colon	153.9	Costochondritis	733.99	Headache	784.0	Myocard. Infarction (Area)	410.9
	Appendicitis	541	Cancer, Rectal	154.1	Depression	311.	Headache, Tension	307.81	M.I., Old	412
	Arterioscl. H.D.	414.0	Lung (Site)	162.9	Dermatitis	692.9	Migraine (Type)	346.9	Myositis	729.1
	Arthritis, Osteo.	715.90	Skin (Site)	173.9	Diabetes Mellitus	250.00	Hemorrhoids	455.6	Nausea/Vomiting	787.0
	Rheumatoid	714.0	Card. Arrhythmia (Type)	427.9	Diabetic Ketosis	250.1	Hernia, Hiatal	553.3	Neuralgia	729.2
	Lupus	710.0	Cardiomyopathy	425.4	Diverticulitis	562.11	Inguinal	550.9	Nevus (Site)	216.9
			Cellulitis (Site)	682.9	Diverticulosis	562.10	Hepatitis	573.3	Obesity	278.0

DIAGNOSIS: (IF NOT CHECKED ABOVE)

SERVICES PERFORMED AT: ☐ Office ☐ E.R. ☐	☐ ☐ CLAIM CONTAINS NO ORDERED REFERRING SERVICE	REFERRING PHYSICIAN & I.D. NUMBER

RETURN APPOINTMENT INFORMATION: 5 - 10 - 15 - 20 - 30 - 40 - 60	NEXT APPOINTMENT M - T - W - TH - F - S	ACCEPT ASSIGNMENT?	DOCTOR'S SIGNATURE
[DAYS] [WKS.] [MOS.] [PRN]	DATE / / TIME: AM PM	☐ YES ☐ NO	

INSTRUCTIONS TO PATIENT FOR FILING INSURANCE CLAIMS:	☐ CASH	TOTAL TODAY'S FEE	
1. Complete upper portion of this form, sign and date. 2. Attach this form to your own insurance company's form for direct reimbursement. **MEDICARE PATIENTS - DO NOT SEND THIS TO MEDICARE. WE WILL SUBMIT THE CLAIM FOR YOU.**	☐ CHECK # _____ ☐ VISA ☐ MC ☐ CO-PAY	OLD BALANCE	
		TOTAL DUE	
		AMOUNT REC'D. TODAY	

INSUR-A-BILL ® BIBBERO SYSTEMS, INC. • PETALUMA, CA • UP. SUPER. © 6/94 (BIBB/STOCK)

Figure 13-4 *A superbill is a form that can also be used as a charge slip and invoice and can be submitted with insurance claims.*

Bank draft: A check written by a bank against its funds in another bank.

Warrant: A nonnegotiable check. It is a statement issued to indicate that a debt should be paid, for example, by an insurance company.

ABA number: Part of a coding system originated by the American Bankers Association (ABA). It is always located in the upper-right corner of a printed check to identify the location of the bank at which the check is to be redeemed.

MICR code: Stands for magnetic ink character recognition code, which appears along the bottom of a check and consists of numbers and characters printed in magnetic ink.

Accepting checks: The majority of bills are paid by personal checks drawn on patients' bank accounts. Some checks may be considered risky, such as third-party checks, postdated checks, checks drawn on an out-of-town bank, and checks marked "paid in full" that do not represent the total due. Avoid accepting such checks.

Power of attorney: A directive that grants a person the legal right to handle financial matters for another person who is unable to do so.

Postdated check: A check that bears a date in the future and cannot be cashed until then.

Predated or **backdated check:** A check made out with a date in the past. Predated checks can be accepted as long as the date shown is no more than six months before the date on which it is cashed.

Third-party check: A check written by an unknown party to a payee (e.g., your patient) who wishes to release the check to you for payment of an outstanding balance. Government and payroll checks used in this way are also third-party checks.

Canceled check: A check that has been cashed and thus cannot be issued again.

Deposits

Deposits: Cash or checks placed into a bank account. They can be made to either checking or savings accounts. Checks should be deposited promptly for the following reasons:

- They may be lost, misplaced, or stolen.
- There is the possibility of a stop-payment order.
- They may have a restricted time for cashing.

Endorsement: A check must be endorsed to transfer the funds from one person to another. Endorsement is accomplished by signing or rubber-stamping the back of the check, in ink, at the left end. When you accept a check, immediately endorse it and write the words "for deposit only" on the back.

Types of endorsements: There are four principal kinds of endorsements: blank, restrictive, special, and qualified. Blank and restrictive endorsements are the most commonly used.

Blank endorsement: A signature only. Also known as an open endorsement, it is the simplest and most common type of endorsement on personal checks.

Restrictive endorsement: The words "for deposit only" followed by the account number and signature.

Limited endorsement: The words "pay to the order of" and the name, followed by a signature. A check with a limited endorsement functions as a third-party check. For example, a patient might give you a check that was originally made out to someone else, who used a limited endorsement to sign the check over to the patient. This original payee would become a third-party payer if the practice were to accept the check from the patient.

Qualified endorsement: Used to disclaim future liability of the endorser, generally consisting of the words "without recourse" above the signature. It is most commonly used by lawyers who accept checks on behalf of clients.

Deposit slip: After endorsing the check, fill out a deposit slip.

Methods of deposit: There are three different ways to deposit funds: in person, by mail, or at commercial night depositories. Making deposits in person is the most direct method, and banks immediately provide a receipt to verify transactions. Avoid sending cash through the mail, but if it is absolutely necessary to do so, use registered mail.

Returned checks: Occasionally, the bank returns a deposited check because of problems such as a missing signature or missing endorsement. A check is also returned if the payer has insufficient funds on deposit to cover it. The patient's account should be adjusted.

NSF: Abbreviation for not sufficient funds, meaning that there is not enough money in the account on which a check has been drawn to cover the amount of the check.

Handling returned checks: If a check is returned, begin by contacting the person who gave you the check. If payment is not made, or if you cannot track down the person, turn the account over to a collection agency.

Bill Payment

Bills: All bills should be paid by check for documentation and control purposes. For small payments, such as public transportation costs, petty cash may be used.

Office banking policy: Should indicate who is responsible for writing and signing all checks. For good control, one person should write the checks, and another person should be authorized to sign them. Sometimes two authorized signatures are required in order to transfer funds from one account to another or to write checks over a certain amount, such as $1,000.

Check writing: Checks are printed on sensitized paper so that erasures are easily noticeable. The bank has the right to refuse payment on any check that has been altered. You must not cross out, erase, or change any part of a check.

Check stub: The part of a check that remains in the checkbook after the check has been written and removed.

Payee: The person to whom the check is payable.

Payer: The person who signs the check to release the funds to the payee.

Lost and stolen checks: Occasionally, an outgoing check may be lost or stolen after it has been issued. You must report this situation to the bank promptly. The bank will place a warning on the account, and signatures on cashed checks will be carefully inspected to detect possible forgeries.

Coordination of benefits: Preventing duplication of payment for the same service.

Reimbursement allowance: A fixed amount paid monthly for medical bills, regardless of whether the patient submitted the supporting bills. This is part of coordination of benefits in regard to nonduplication of payment.

Federal reimbursement allowance: A reimbursement allowance related to federal medical insurance programs. Some insurance companies use coordination of benefits in practice, and some use the federal reimbursement allowance.

13.4 Billing and Collections

Medical Billing

Billing duties of a medical assistant: To be an effective account manager, follow these rules:

- Do not be embarrassed to ask for payment for services. The physician or facility has the right to charge for the care and services provided.
- Practice good judgment.
- Give personal attention and consideration to each patient.
- Show a desire to help patients with financial difficulties.

Payment at the time of service: Every practice should encourage time-of-service collection. There will be no further billing and bookkeeping expenses if patients get into the habit of paying their current charges before they leave the office. The most appropriate time to discuss payment arrangements with a new patient is at the time of the first scheduled appointment.

Payment plans and extensions of credit: For procedures and services involving large fees, such as surgery and long-term care, inform patients of:

- What the charges will be
- What services these charges cover
- Credit policies of the facility
  - When payment is due
  - Circumstances in which the practice requires payment at the time of service
  - When or whether assignment of insurance benefits is accepted
  - Whether insurance forms will be completed by the office staff
  - Collection procedures, including circumstances in which accounts will be sent to a collection agency

It is a good idea to have credit policies in writing, for example, included in a new patient brochure.

Balance billing: Billing the patient for the difference between the fee and the amount the insurance company allows. Whether balance billing is acceptable depends on the contract with the insurance company.

Exceptions and rules: Although there will be exceptions, there must be rules, which should be conveyed in writing to the patient at the outset of the relationship. Any patient who needs special consideration can be counseled individually.

Internal billing: In a practice with only a moderate number of accounts, the medical assistant handles the preparation and mailing of statements. A printed statement may be computer generated, based on a superbill, typewritten, or photocopied from the ledger card.

Statement: Should show the service rendered on each date, the charge for each service, the date on which a claim was submitted to the insurance company, the date of payment, and the balance due from the patient. A regular system of mailing statements should be put into operation. Time limits also must be observed in billing third-party payers. Bills for minors must be addressed to parents or legal guardians.

Cycle billing: A common billing system that bills each patient once a month but spreads the work of billing over the month. In this system, invoices are sent to patients whose names begin with A–D on one day, those whose names begin with E–H on another day, and so on.

Fair Credit Billing Act: A federal law mandating that billing for a balance due or reporting a credit balance of $1 or more must occur every 30 days.

Collection Policies and Procedures

Standard payment period: Normally, people are expected to pay bills within 30 days. When a bill is 30 days overdue, the MA should send a letter or a reminder statement to the patient.

Open-book account: The most typical account for patients of a medical practice, in which the account is open to charges made occasionally. It uses the last date of payment or charge for each illness as the starting date for determining the time limit on that debt.

Written-contract account: An account in which the physician and patient sign an agreement stating that the patient will pay the bill in more than four installments.

Single-entry account: An account with only one charge, as is created, for example, when an out-of-town vacationer consults a local physician for an illness.

Delinquent accounts: Accounts in which payment is overdue. Payment is the most difficult to collect from two groups of patients: those with hardship cases and those who have moved and have not received an invoice.

Hardship cases: Accounts of patients who are poor, uninsured, underinsured, or elderly and on a limited income. Physicians may decide to treat such patients at a deep discount or for free.

Payment collection: Evaluation of the success of collections is based on (1) the collection ratio and (2) the accounts receivable ratio.

Collection ratio: Measures the effectiveness of the billing system. The basic formula for figuring the collection ratio is to divide the total collections by the net charges (gross charges minus any discounts) to reach the percentage figure.

Accounts receivable ratio: Measures how fast outstanding accounts are being paid. The formula for figuring the accounts receivable ratio is to divide the current accounts receivable balance by the average gross monthly charges.

Age analysis: The process of classifying and reviewing delinquent accounts by age from the first date of billing. It should list all patient account balances, when charges were incurred, the most recent payment date, and any notes regarding the account. The age analysis is a tool to show, at a glance, the status of each account. See Figure 13-5.

Reasons for collecting delinquent accounts: The main reasons to attempt collection of all delinquent accounts are:

- Physicians must be paid for services so that they can pay expenses and continue to treat patients.
- Although a patient cannot be "fired" for nonpayment (in the sense that necessary treatment cannot be withheld

ACCOUNTS RECEIVABLE–AGE ANALYSIS

Date: October 1, 2014

Patient	Balance	Date of Charges	Most Recent Payment	30 days	60 days	90 days	120 days	Remarks
Black, K.	120.00	5/24	5/24			75.00	45.00	3rd Notice
Brown, R.	65.00	8/30	8/30	65.00				
Green, C.	340.00	8/25						Medicare filed
Jones, T.	500.00	6/1	6/30		125.00	125.00	250.00	3rd Notice
Perry, S.	150.00	7/28	7/28	75.00	75.00			1st Notice
Smith, J.	375.00	6/15	7/1			375.00		2nd Notice
White, L.	200.00	6/24	7/5	20.00	30.00	150.00		2nd Notice

Figure 13-5 *An age analysis organizes delinquent accounts by age.*

because of an inability to pay), failure to collect payment can result in the termination of the established patient–physician relationship.

- Noncollection of medical bills may imply guilt, and a malpractice suit may result.
- Abandoning accounts without collection follow-up encourages nonpayment; as a result, the paying patients indirectly subsidize the cost of medical care for those who can pay but do not.

Collection techniques: Include telephone collection calls, collection letters or statements, and personal interviews. Send the first letter or statement when the account is 30 days past due, then follow up at 60 days, at 90 days, and again at 120 days. Table 13-3 lists laws governing credit and collections. If you call the patient, make sure that you do so in private and during reasonable hours. Always be respectful and professional, and demonstrate your willingness to help the patient meet his or her financial obligation. Get a definite answer from the patient if you can, and follow up later if the payment has not been received. Do not call the patient's place of work, especially if you do not know whether the patient can take personal calls at work. When writing collection letters, make sure that the first few letters simply remind the patient about a possible oversight of debt, and make sure that each letter is specific to the individual situation.

Illegal collection techniques: It is illegal to harass a debtor. Harassment includes making threats or calls late at night (after 9 p.m.). It is also illegal to threaten action that cannot be legally taken or that is not intended to be taken.

Statute of limitations: A statute that limits the time in which rights can be enforced by action. After the statute of limitations expires, no legal collection suit may be brought against a debtor. This time limit depends on the state in which the debt was incurred.

Outside collection assistance: When you have done everything possible internally to follow up on an outstanding account and have not received payment, there are still steps you can take.

- Use a collection agency. If the patient has failed to respond to your final letter or has failed to fulfill a second promise on payment, send the account to the collector without delay. After an account has been released to a collection agency, your office makes no further collection attempts.
- Collect through the court system. Most physicians believe that it is unwise to resort to the courts to collect medical bills unless there are extraordinary circumstances.

Collection agencies: Medical practices should be careful to avoid collection agencies that use harsh collection practices. Once an account has been turned over to an agency, do not

Law	Requirements	Penalties for Breaking the Law
Equal Credit Opportunity Act (ECOA)	• Creditors may not discriminate against applicants on the basis of sex, marital status, race, national origin, religion, or age. • Creditors may not discriminate because an applicant receives public assistance income or has exercised rights under the Consumer Credit Protection Act.	• If an applicant sues the practice for violating the ECOA, the practice may have to pay damages, penalties, lawyers' fees, and court costs. • If an applicant joins a class action lawsuit against the practice, the practice may have to pay damages of up to $500,000 or 1% of the practice's net worth, whichever is less. (In a class action lawsuit, one or more people sue a company that wronged all of them in the same way.) • If the Federal Trade Commission (FTC) receives many complaints from applicants stating that the practice violated the ECOA, the FTC may investigate and take action against the practice.
Fair Credit Reporting Act (FCRA)	Credit bureaus are required to supply correct and complete information to businesses to use in evaluating a person's application for credit, insurance, or a job.	• If one applicant sues the practice in federal court for violating the FCRA, the practice may have to pay actual damages, punitive damages (punishment for intentionally breaking the law), court costs, and lawyer fees. • The FTC may investigate and take action against the practice if it receives too many complaints.
Fair Debt Collection Practices Act (FDCPA)	Debt collectors are required to treat debtors fairly. Certain collection tactics are also prohibited, such as harassment, false statements, threats, and unfair practices.	• If it is sued by a debtor, the practice may have to pay damages, court costs, and lawyer fees. • In a class action lawsuit, the practice might have to pay damages of up to $500,000 or 1% of the practice's net worth, whichever is less. • The FTC may investigate and take action.
Truth in Lending Act (TLA)	Creditors are required to provide applicants with accurate and complete credit costs and terms, in clear and understandable language.	• If it is sued by a debtor, the practice may have to pay damages, court costs, and lawyer fees. • The FTC may investigate and take action against the practice if it receives too many complaints.

Table 13-3

send bills or discuss the account with the patient. If the agency is unable to collect the money, the physician should decide whether to write off the debt or take the matter to court.

Write-offs: Charges considered noncollectable by a business. An example would be if a patient owing $150 were to unexpectedly die. There are many types of write-offs, which should be identified as *bad debts, contractual discounts, professional courtesy discounts,* etc. Write-offs must be approved by the physician or office manager.

13.5 Accounts Payable

Accounts payable: Amounts the physician owes to others for equipment and services, including:

- Office supplies
- Medical supplies and equipment
- Equipment repair and maintenance
- Utilities
- Taxes
- Payroll
- Rent

Accounts payable records: Include purchase orders, packing slips, and invoices.

Payroll

Payroll: The total direct and indirect earning of all employees. Federal, state, and local laws require records to be kept of all salaries and wages paid to employees. All records of employment taxes must be kept for at least four years.

Payroll tasks: Include calculating the amount of wages or salaries paid and amounts deducted from employees' earnings.

Other payroll tasks involve writing checks, tracking data for payroll taxes, and filling out payroll tax forms.

Retention of payroll records: The physician is required by law to keep payroll data for four years. The records should include the following information.

- Employee's social security number
- Number of withholding allowances claimed
- Gross salary
- Deductions for social security tax; Medicare tax; federal, state, and other tax withholding; state disability insurance; and state unemployment tax

Employer tax identification number (EIN): Every employer, no matter how small, must have an EIN for reporting federal taxes. It is obtained by completing Form SS-4, Application for Employer Identification Number.

Employee identification: Employees are identified for tax purposes by their social security numbers.

Payroll register: A list of all employees and their earnings, deductions, and other information. See Figure 13-6.

Payroll accounting: Involves payroll records being sent to an accountant or bookkeeper, entered in the journal, and posted to the ledgers. Timely, accurate financial statements and tax returns can then be prepared.

State disability benefit laws: Those that provide disability insurance to employees absent from work due to nonwork-related injury or illness. Participating states include California, Hawaii, New Jersey, New York, Rhode Island, and the territory of Puerto Rico.

Gross earnings: Total earnings before any deductions are made.

Net earnings: Gross earnings minus total deductions.

Employee earnings: Either salaries or wages, plus indirect forms of payment, such as paid time off and employee benefit and service programs.

Salary: A fixed amount paid to an employee on a regular basis regardless of the number of hours worked.

Wages: Pay based on a specific rate per hour, day, or week.

Payroll deductions: Amounts regularly withheld from a paycheck, such as those for federal, state, and local taxes, as well as those for such options as a 401(k) plan, life insurance, or savings bonds. These deductions include income taxes, court-ordered deductions (garnishments), IRS-ordered tax levies, union fees, and miscellaneous other deductions.

Payroll records: Complete records of pay for every employee that are frequently reported to the government. Taxes are withheld from employees, and certain taxes are paid by both employers and employees. Payroll records include the employee's social security number, amount of withholding allowances claimed, amount of gross salary, social security and Medicare deductions, withholding taxes for various jurisdictions, state disability insurance, and (if applicable) state unemployment tax.

Methods for calculating payroll checks: Include the manual, the pegboard, and the computer system. Regardless of the accounting system used, attention to accuracy in bookkeeping is necessary. In addition, it is necessary to maintain confidentiality in matters related to employees' wages and salaries.

Payroll services: Some offices hire an outside payroll service to process all payroll checks and withholding payments, as well as to keep records.

Tax

Types of tax: The federal government mandates payment of the following taxes through withholding:

- Social security
- Medicare
- Federal income tax

These taxes are based on a percentage of the employee's total gross income.

Income tax withholding: Taxes withheld from employees' earnings that are reported and forwarded to the IRS, and applied toward payment of income tax. It is based on total earnings, the claimed withholding allowances, marital status, and length of the pay period.

Form W-4: In order to determine the amount of money to be withheld from each paycheck, each new employee must complete a Form W-4, and each employee should update the W-4 regularly. Figure 13-7 shows a Form W-4, which asks for the

Pay Period 6/1–6/14

Emp. No.	Name	Earnings to date	Hrly. Rate	Reg. Hrs.	OT Hrs.	OT Earnings	TOTAL GROSS	Earnings Subject to Unemp.	Earnings Subject to FICA	Social Security (FICA)	Medicare	Federal W/H	State W/H	Health Ins.	Net Pay	Check No.
0010	Scott, B.	9,823.14	14.00	70.00			980.00	980.00	980.00	60.50	14.10	147.92	15.10	25.00	717.38	11747
0020	Wilson, J.	14,290.38	17.00	70.00	6.50	153.00	1343.00	1343.00	1343.00	83.26	19.47	160.45	15.85	67.50	996.47	11748
0030	Diaz, J.	2,750.26	5.50	46.25			254.37	254.37	254.37	15.77	3.68	38.20	3.75		192.97	11749
0040	Ling, W.	2,240.57	6.80	30.00			204.00	204.00	204.00	12.66	2.96	26.02	3.12		159.54	11750
0050	Harris, E.	2,600.98	10.00	23.50			235.00	235.00	235.00	14.57	3.41	33.52	3.36		180.14	11751

Figure 13-6 *A payroll register is designed to summarize information about all employees and their earnings.*

Form W-4 (2013)

Purpose. Complete Form W-4 so that your employer can withhold the correct federal income tax from your pay. Consider completing a new Form W-4 each year and when your personal or financial situation changes.

Exemption from withholding. If you are exempt, complete **only** lines 1, 2, 3, 4, and 7 and sign the form to validate it. Your exemption for 2013 expires February 17, 2014. See Pub. 505, Tax Withholding and Estimated Tax.

Note. If another person can claim you as a dependent on his or her tax return, you cannot claim exemption from withholding if your income exceeds $1,000 and includes more than $350 of unearned income (for example, interest and dividends).

Basic instructions. If you are not exempt, complete the **Personal Allowances Worksheet** below. The worksheets on page 2 further adjust your withholding allowances based on itemized deductions, certain credits, adjustments to income, or two-earners/multiple jobs situations.

Complete all worksheets that apply. However, you may claim fewer (or zero) allowances. For regular wages, withholding must be based on allowances you claimed and may not be a flat amount or percentage of wages.

Head of household. Generally, you can claim head of household filing status on your tax return only if you are unmarried and pay more than 50% of the costs of keeping up a home for yourself and your dependent(s) or other qualifying individuals. See Pub. 501, Exemptions, Standard Deduction, and Filing Information, for information.

Tax credits. You can take projected tax credits into account in figuring your allowable number of withholding allowances. Credits for child or dependent care expenses and the child tax credit may be claimed using the **Personal Allowances Worksheet** below. See Pub. 505 for information on converting your other credits into withholding allowances.

Nonwage income. If you have a large amount of nonwage income, such as interest or dividends, consider making estimated tax payments using Form 1040-ES, Estimated Tax for Individuals. Otherwise, you may owe additional tax. If you have pension or annuity income, see Pub. 505 to find out if you should adjust your withholding on Form W-4 or W-4P.

Two earners or multiple jobs. If you have a working spouse or more than one job, figure the total number of allowances you are entitled to claim on all jobs using worksheets from only one Form W-4. Your withholding usually will be most accurate when all allowances are claimed on the Form W-4 for the highest paying job and zero allowances are claimed on the others. See Pub. 505 for details.

Nonresident alien. If you are a nonresident alien, see Notice 1392, Supplemental Form W-4 Instructions for Nonresident Aliens, before completing this form.

Check your withholding. After your Form W-4 takes effect, use Pub. 505 to see how the amount you are having withheld compares to your projected total tax for 2013. See Pub. 505, especially if your earnings exceed $130,000 (Single) or $180,000 (Married).

Future developments. Information about any future developments affecting Form W-4 (such as legislation enacted after we release it) will be posted at *www.irs.gov/w4*.

Personal Allowances Worksheet (Keep for your records.)

A Enter "1" for **yourself** if no one else can claim you as a dependent . . . . **A** _____

B Enter "1" if:
- You are single and have only one job; or
- You are married, have only one job, and your spouse does not work; or
- Your wages from a second job or your spouse's wages (or the total of both) are $1,500 or less.

. . . **B** _____

C Enter "1" for your **spouse.** But, you may choose to enter "-0-" if you are married and have either a working spouse or more than one job. (Entering "-0-" may help you avoid having too little tax withheld.) . . . . **C** _____

D Enter number of **dependents** (other than your spouse or yourself) you will claim on your tax return . . . . **D** _____

E Enter "1" if you will file as **head of household** on your tax return (see conditions under **Head of household** above) . . **E** _____

F Enter "1" if you have at least $1,900 of **child or dependent care expenses** for which you plan to claim a credit . . . **F** _____
(**Note.** Do **not** include child support payments. See Pub. 503, Child and Dependent Care Expenses, for details.)

G **Child Tax Credit** (including additional child tax credit). See Pub. 972, Child Tax Credit, for more information.
- If your total income will be less than $65,000 ($95,000 if married), enter "2" for each eligible child; then **less** "1" if you have three to six eligible children or **less** "2" if you have seven or more eligible children.
- If your total income will be between $65,000 and $84,000 ($95,000 and $119,000 if married), enter "1" for each eligible child . . . **G** _____

H Add lines A through G and enter total here. (**Note.** This may be different from the number of exemptions you claim on your tax return.) ▶ **H** _____

For accuracy, complete all worksheets that apply.	• If you plan to **itemize** or **claim adjustments to income** and want to reduce your withholding, see the **Deductions and Adjustments Worksheet** on page 2.
	• If you are **single and have more than one job** or are **married and you and your spouse both work** and the combined earnings from all jobs exceed $40,000 ($10,000 if married), see the **Two-Earners/Multiple Jobs Worksheet** on page 2 to avoid having too little tax withheld.
	• If **neither** of the above situations applies, **stop here** and enter the number from line H on line 5 of Form W-4 below.

- - - - - - - - - - **Separate here and give Form W-4 to your employer. Keep the top part for your records.** - - - - - - - - - -

---

Form W-4

Department of the Treasury
Internal Revenue Service

Employee's Withholding Allowance Certificate

▶ **Whether you are entitled to claim a certain number of allowances or exemption from withholding is subject to review by the IRS. Your employer may be required to send a copy of this form to the IRS.**

OMB No. 1545-0074

2013

1 Your first name and middle initial	Last name	2 Your social security number

Home address (number and street or rural route)

3 ☐ Single ☐ Married ☐ Married, but withhold at higher Single rate.
Note. If married, but legally separated, or spouse is a nonresident alien, check the "Single" box.

City or town, state, and ZIP code

4 If your last name differs from that shown on your social security card, check here. You must call 1-800-772-1213 for a replacement card. ▶ ☐

5 Total number of allowances you are claiming (from line **H** above **or** from the applicable worksheet on page 2) | **5** |

6 Additional amount, if any, you want withheld from each paycheck . . . . | **6** $ |

7 I claim exemption from withholding for 2013, and I certify that I meet **both** of the following conditions for exemption.
- Last year I had a right to a refund of **all** federal income tax withheld because I had **no** tax liability, **and**
- This year I expect a refund of **all** federal income tax withheld because I expect to have **no** tax liability.

If you meet both conditions, write "Exempt" here . . . . ▶ | **7** |

Under penalties of perjury, I declare that I have examined this certificate and, to the best of my knowledge and belief, it is true, correct, and complete.

Employee's signature
(This form is not valid unless you sign it.) ▶ _____ Date ▶ _____

8 Employer's name and address (Employer: Complete lines 8 and 10 only if sending to the IRS.)	9 Office code (optional)	10 Employer identification number (EIN)

For Privacy Act and Paperwork Reduction Act Notice, see page 2.   Cat. No. 10220Q   Form **W-4** (2013)

Figure 13-7 *Update all Employee's Withholding Allowance Certificates (Form W-4) at least once a year.*
I9 Form. United States Citizenship and Immigration Services

(1) employee's name and current address, (2) social security number, (3) marital status, and (4) number of allowances the employee claims that should be used in calculating withholding.

Employers income tax: A physician in individual practice is expected to make an estimated tax payment four times per year, instead of being subjected to withholding tax.

Social security (FICA): The Federal Insurance Contribution Act governs the social security system. The employee pays half of the contribution, and the employer pays the other half. IRS Circular E lists the FICA tax percentages that should be applied, based on the level of taxable earnings, length of the payroll period, marital status, and number of withholding allowances claimed.

Payroll taxes: These include income tax, FICA, Medicare (if applicable), and unemployment compensation tax.

Payroll tax returns: Related forms are known as W-2, W-3, and W-4, as well as the following:

- Form SS-4: Application for Employer Identification Number
- Form SS-5: Application for Social Security number

- Form 940: Employer's Annual Federal Unemployment Tax Return
- Form 941: Employer's Quarterly Federal Tax Return
- Form 8109: Federal Tax Deposit Coupon Book

Federal Unemployment Tax Act (FUTA): Requires employers to pay a percentage of each employee's income, up to a specified dollar amount, to fund an account used to pay employees who have been laid off for a specified time while they are seeking new employment. Although FUTA is based on employees' gross income, it must not be deducted from employees' wages. Payments into a state unemployment fund can generally be applied as credit against the FUTA tax amount. FUTA deposits are calculated quarterly. See Figure 13-8.

State unemployment tax: All states have unemployment compensation laws. Most states require only the employer to make payments to the unemployment insurance fund. However, a few states require both the employer and employee to make a payment. In some states, the employer does not have to make

Figure 13-8 *Taxes submitted with the FUTA tax return (Form 940) provide money to workers who are unemployed.*
Form 940. United States Citizenship and Immigration Services

unemployment compensation payments if there are very few employees (four or fewer).

State disability insurance: Some states require a certain amount of money to be withheld from the employee's check to cover a disability insurance plan. This plan covers employees in the event of injury or disability.

Insurance withholding: Money also may be withheld, as requested by the employee, for health insurance, life insurance, and disability insurance that are available from the employer as employee benefits.

Form W-2: Must be completed at the end of each year and given to each employee, with copies to the federal and state governments. The W-2 lists the total gross income; total federal, state, and local taxes withheld; taxable fringe benefits; tips; and the employee's total net income. The amount of wages taxable under social security and Medicare must be listed separately on the W-2. See Figure 13-9.

Form W-3: This is the Transmittal of Wage and Tax Statements form, which is submitted along with a W-2 form. See Figure 13-10.

Immigration and Nationality Act: Requires employers to verify that all employees are authorized to work, regardless of their citizenship status.

Form I-9: This is the Employment Eligibility Verification form, which employees are required to complete by the Department of Justice, Immigration, and Naturalization Service. It is designed to ensure that all employed persons are U.S. citizens.

Employment eligibility: This must be proven and recorded on the I-9 form once the employee presents a social security card, a government-issued identification card, or other items proving authorization for employment.

Deposit requirements: Federal tax withholding and FICA payments must be made to a federal deposit account in a federal reserve bank or authorized banking institution at regular intervals, at least monthly. The IRS imposes a severe penalty for failure to deposit this money.

Employer's quarterly federal tax return: Form 941 must be filed quarterly to report federal income and FICA taxes withheld from employees' paychecks. It is due before the last day of the first month after the end of a quarter: April 30, July 31, October 31, and January 31. If deposits equaling full payment of taxes due have been made, the due date for the return will be extended for 10 days.

Fair Labor Standards Act (FLSA): Also called the federal wage and hour law, it affects organizations doing business in more than one state. It sets the minimum wage required to be paid to employees, and requires employers to pay one and one-half times the regular wage for work in excess of 40 hours per week.

Civil Rights Act of 1964: Title VII of this act prohibits discrimination in hiring, firing, or the promotion of employees due to race, color, religion, national origin, or gender.

Age Discrimination in Employment Act (ADEA): Prohibits unfair employment practices regarding people over the age of 40 years.

Figure 13-9 *Each employee's Wage and Tax Statement (Form W-2) records the total amount of taxes withheld during the previous year.* W2 Form. United States Citizenship and Immigration Services

Americans with Disabilities Act of 1990: Prohibits unfair employment practices regarding people with disabilities, who are otherwise qualified for employment. Employers must make reasonable accommodations for these employees.

Employee Retirement Income Security Act (ERISA): Protects and regulates pension funds and their operation.

Immigration Reform Act of 1985: Requires employers to certify that new hires are authorized to work in the United States regardless of citizenship.

State minimum wage law: For states that set their own minimum wage rate, this rate must be higher than the federal rate.

Workers' compensation laws: In most states, these laws exist and require employers to provide workers' compensation insurance for employees, to compensate for work-related injuries, illnesses, or death. Employers must purchase this insurance or contribute to a state fund.

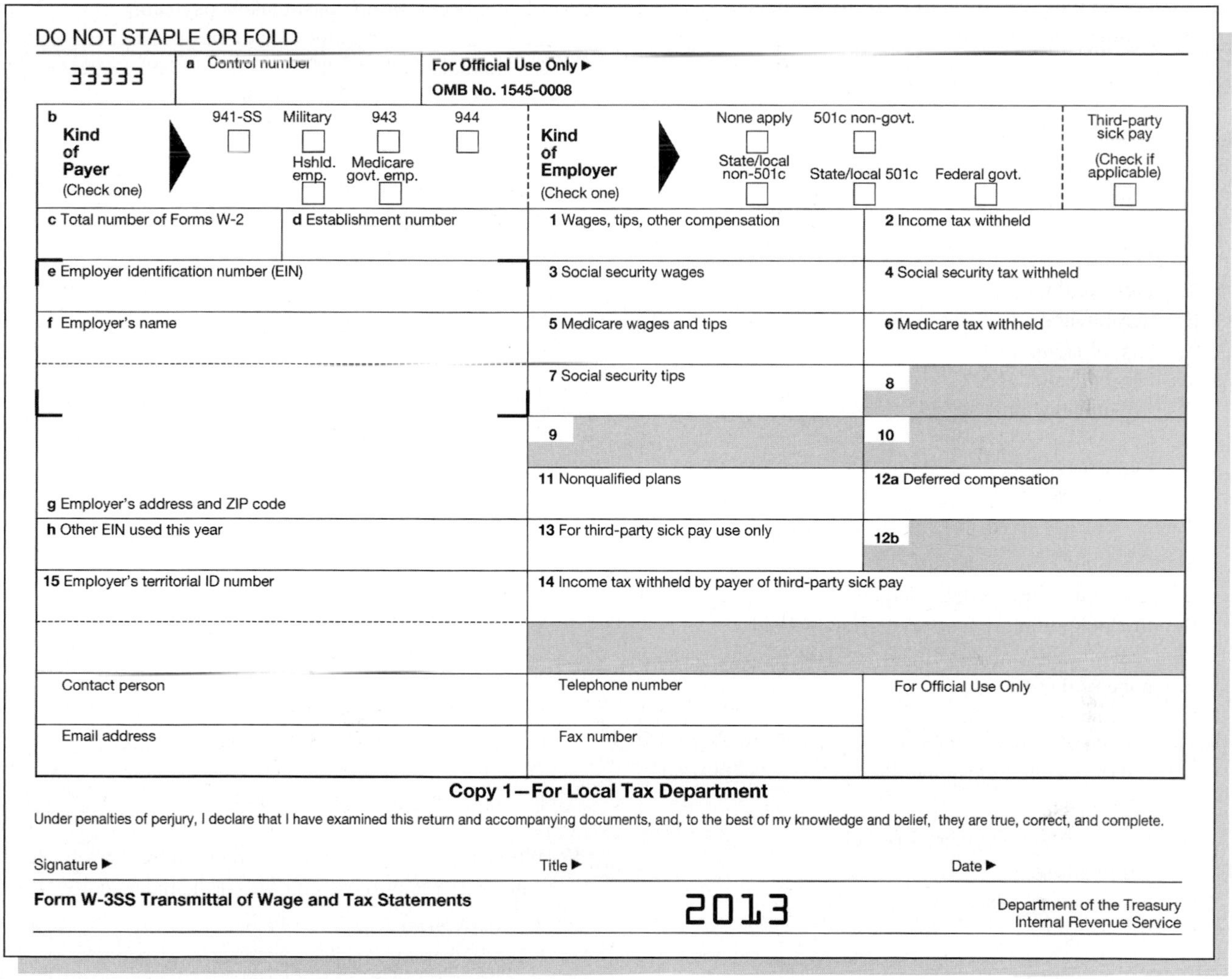

DO NOT STAPLE OR FOLD

| 33333 | a Control number | For Official Use Only ▶ OMB No. 1545-0008 |

| b Kind of Payer (Check one) | 941-SS ☐ Military ☐ 943 ☐ 944 ☐ Hshld. emp. ☐ Medicare govt. emp. ☐ | Kind of Employer (Check one) | None apply ☐ 501c non-govt. ☐ State/local non-501c ☐ State/local 501c ☐ Federal govt. ☐ | Third-party sick pay (Check if applicable) ☐ |

c Total number of Forms W-2	d Establishment number	1 Wages, tips, other compensation	2 Income tax withheld
e Employer identification number (EIN)		3 Social security wages	4 Social security tax withheld
f Employer's name		5 Medicare wages and tips	6 Medicare tax withheld
		7 Social security tips	8
		9	10
		11 Nonqualified plans	12a Deferred compensation
g Employer's address and ZIP code			
h Other EIN used this year		13 For third-party sick pay use only	12b
15 Employer's territorial ID number		14 Income tax withheld by payer of third-party sick pay	
Contact person		Telephone number	For Official Use Only
Email address		Fax number	

Copy 1—For Local Tax Department

Under penalties of perjury, I declare that I have examined this return and accompanying documents, and, to the best of my knowledge and belief, they are true, correct, and complete.

Signature ▶ _____ Title ▶ _____ Date ▶ _____

Form W-3SS Transmittal of Wage and Tax Statements   **2013**   Department of the Treasury Internal Revenue Service

Figure 13-10 *Submit a Transmittal of Wages and Tax Statements (Form W-3) with the W-2 forms.*
W4 Form. United States Citizenship and Immigration Services.

STRATEGIES FOR SUCCESS

▶ *Test-Taking Skills*

Dress in layers!

On the day of the exam, you should dress in layers, especially if you are sensitive to the temperature of the environment. Adding or removing layers will allow you to adjust to the room temperature, whether it's hot or cold, and the temperature won't become a distracting factor in taking the exam.

Instructions:

Answer the following questions.

1. A list of all employees and their earnings, deductions, and other information is called

   A. employee earnings.
   B. payroll tasks.
   C. accounts payable.
   D. payroll register.
   E. employee financial listing.

2. Paper towels are considered

   A. incidental items.
   B. durable items.
   C. capital equipment.
   D. clinical supplies.
   E. expendable items.

3. A collection ratio is

   A. the amount of money collected this year divided by the amount of money collected last year.
   B. the total collections divided by net charges.
   C. the total collections divided by gross charges.
   D. the total amount of money collected divided by any discounts.
   E. none of these

4. The portion of salary held back from payroll checks for the purpose of paying government income taxes is known as

   A. W-4 forms.
   B. Federal Unemployment Tax Act.
   C. withholding.
   D. annual tax returns.
   E. FICA.

5. Accounts receivable age analysis

   A. means that the physician must collect the receivables on time.
   B. is not necessary in a single-physician office.
   C. is a tool to show the status of each account.
   D. involves writing off accounts that are more than one year past due.
   E. involves writing off accounts that are more than five years past due.

6. Which of the following statements regarding state unemployment tax is correct?

   A. Only employees must make a payment.
   B. Only employers must make a payment.
   C. A few states require both employees and employers to make a payment.
   D. A few states do not make it available.
   E. none of these

7. Amounts that are paid by cash or check are called

   A. disbursements.
   B. statements.
   C. receivables.
   D. payables.
   E. none of these.

8. The reviewing of financial data to verify accuracy and completeness is called

   A. withholding taxes.
   B. auditing.
   C. annual tax returns.
   D. accounts payable.
   E. taking a trial balance.

9. A bank draft is a check drawn by a bank

   A. that is not limited.
   B. that can be used as a third-party check.
   C. that is less reliable than a cashier's check.
   D. on the guaranteed funds of a depositor.
   E. on its funds in another bank.

10. Which type of check is frequently used for payroll because it itemizes the purposes for the check and deductions?

    A. bank draft
    B. voucher check
    C. limited check
    D. certified check
    E. cashier's check

CHAPTER 14

MEDICAL INSURANCE

LEARNING OUTCOMES

14.1 Define terminology used in association with medical insurance.

14.2 Identify the different types of health insurance.

14.3 Identify the different types of health plans.

14.4 Describe how benefits are determined.

14.5 Explain the process of submitting claims for reimbursement.

MEDICAL ASSISTING COMPETENCIES

COMPETENCY	CMA	RMA	CCMA	NCMA
Administrative				
Apply managed care policies and procedures	X	X	X	
Analyze and apply third-party guidelines	X	X	X	
Perform procedural and diagnostic coding	X	X	X	X
Complete insurance claim forms	X	X	X	
Use the physician fee schedule	X	X		
General/Legal/Professional				
Be aware of and perform within legal and ethical boundaries	X	X	X	X
Receive, organize, prioritize, and transmit information appropriately	X	X	X	X

14.1 Medical Insurance Terminology

Insurance: Economic protection against financial loss caused by possible but unplanned events affecting an individual or business.

Coinsurance: A fixed percentage of covered charges paid by the insured person after a deductible has been met.

Premium: The amount charged for a medical insurance policy. The insurer agrees to provide certain benefits in return for the premium. It is also called coverage cost.

Insurance benefits: Payments for medical services that can be submitted by an insurance company under a predefined policy issued to an individual or group of individuals.

Lifetime maximum benefit: The total sum that the health plan will pay out over the patient's life.

Determination: A payer's decision about the benefits due for a claim.

Rider: A special provision or provisions that may be added to a policy to expand or limit benefits that would otherwise be payable. It may increase or decrease benefits or coverage, waive a condition, or amend the original contract in other ways.

UCR: The *u*sual, *c*ustomary, and *r*easonable fee. It is determined by payers comparing the actual fee charged by a physician, the fee charged by most physicians in a community, and the amount determined to be appropriate for the service.

Usual fee: The fee an individual physician most frequently charges for a service to private patients.

Customary fee: The range of fees charged by most physicians in the community for a particular service.

Reasonable fee: The generally accepted fee a physician charges for an exceptionally difficult or complicated service. A charge is considered reasonable if it is deemed acceptable after peer review even if it does not meet the criteria for a customary fee or prevailing charges.

Fee schedule: A list of charges for services performed.

Prevailing charges: The most frequently charged fees in an area by a specialty group of physicians.

Medical billing cycle: A series of steps that lead to maximum, appropriate, timely payments for patients' medical services.

Payment: Cash, a check, a credit card payment, an insurance payment, or a money order received for professional services rendered.

Payment plan: A patient's agreement to pay medical bills over time according to an established schedule.

Truth in Lending Act: Federal law requiring disclosure of finance charges and late fees for payment plans.

Collections: The process of following up on overdue accounts.

Third-party payer: A health plan or other party that agrees to carry the risk of paying for a patient's medical services.

Assignment of benefits: An authorization to an insurance company to make payment directly to the physician.

Acceptance of assignment: An agreement by a physician to accept the amount established by Medicare, Medicaid, or a private insurer as full payment for covered services. The patient is not billed for the difference because it is illegal to bill the patient for the balance.

Carrier (insurer): An insurance company, payer, or third-party payer.

Allowed charge: The maximum charge an insurance carrier or government program will cover for specific services. The allowed charges are detailed in an insurance carrier's explanation of benefits. In managed care, a participating provider agrees to accept allowed charges in return for various incentives, such as fast payment. If a participating provider normally charges more for a service than the allowed charge, the physician must write off the difference, and the patient may not be billed for this amount. However, nonparticipating providers may bill patients for this difference.

Disallowed charge: The difference between what has been billed by the health-care provider, and what the insurance company has paid. This is not billed to the patient, but written off by the provider.

Limiting charge: The highest amount that an insured person can be charged for a covered service by providers who do not accept assignment. This only applies to certain services, and not to supplies or equipment.

Coordination of benefits: Prevents duplicate payment for the same service. For example, if a child is covered by both parents' insurance policies, a primary carrier is designated to pay benefits according to the terms of its policy, and the secondary plan may cover whatever charges are still left. If the primary carrier pays $105 of a $150 charge, the most the secondary carrier will pay is $45.

Adjudication: The process followed by health plans to examine claims and determine benefits.

Remittance: The statement of the results of the health plan's adjudication of a claim.

Clean claim: A claim that is accepted by a health plan for adjudication.

Suspended: Claim status during adjudication when the payer is developing the claim.

Medical provider: A licensed professional who performs medical procedures.

Participating (PAR) provider: A physician or other health-care provider who participates in an insurance carrier's plan. The physician must keep a list of valid plans, because benefits vary for participating and nonparticipating providers. Claims will be denied or have reduced reimbursement if the physician is not a participating provider. Disallowed charges and charges not eligible for payment must be written off.

Nonparticipating (nonPAR) provider: A physician or other health-care provider who has not joined a particular insurance plan. Patients who obtain services from nonPAR providers generally must pay more of the cost than those who obtain services from PAR providers.

Referral: Transfer of patient care from one physician to another.

Subscriber: The person named as the principal in an insurance contract, also called the *insured*.

Guarantor: A person who is financially responsible for a bill from a health-care practice.

Tertiary insurance: The third insurance policy responsible for paying a claim.

Beneficiary: The person named in an insurance policy to receive the benefits.

Overpayment: Payment by the insurer or by the patient of more than the amount due.

Schedule of benefits: The list of services that are paid for and the amounts that are paid by the insurance carrier. For example, the schedule of benefits may say that the insurance carrier will pay only 80% of all medical fees for surgeries, making the subscriber responsible for payment of coinsurance, the remaining 20% of the medical fees. Such a plan is often referred to as an 80:20 plan.

Deductible: The fixed dollar amount that must be paid out of pocket, by the insured, before an insurer will pay any additional expenses.

Provider fee profile: Also called a *provider profile;* an examination of services provided, claims filed, and benefits allocated by various providers, to access quality of care and cost management.

Advance Beneficiary Notice (ABN): A document signed by the patient, accepting responsibility for paying for certain services that the primary care provider thinks are appropriate but Medicare does not.

Explanation of Benefits (EOB): A document from an insurance carrier that shows how the amount of the benefit was determined.

Waiting period: The initial period of time when a newly insured individual is not eligible to receive benefits.

Copayment (copay): The amount of money due from the subscriber to cover a portion of a bill. For most health maintenance organizations (HMOs), this amount is usually a small fixed fee, such as $10, per office visit.

Exclusions: Expenses that may not be covered under the insured's contract. The insured is required to pay for services not covered by the health plan.

Utilization: A pattern of usage for a medical service or procedure.

Utilization review: Examination of services by an outside group. A utilization review committee reviews individual cases to ensure that the medical care services are medically necessary.

Peer review organizations: Groups of practicing physicians paid by insurance companies to review medical records with respect to effectiveness and efficiency. The purpose of reviewing is to monitor the validity of diagnoses and the quality of care and to evaluate the appropriateness of hospital admissions and discharges.

Balance billing: A usually illegal practice, in which providers bill patients for the balance between what they wish to charge and what the insurance company has already reimbursed.

Health information management (HIM): The hospital department that organizes and maintains patient medical records.

14.2 Types of Health Insurance

Basic medical: Covers some or all nonsurgical services provided by a physician, whether in the office, the patient's home, or a hospital. Each time service is received, there is usually a copayment or coinsurance charge as well as a deductible amount payable by the patient. Some insurance plans cover pathology, X-ray, and diagnostic lab fees.

Major medical: A policy designed to offset heavy medical expenses resulting from catastrophic or prolonged illness or injury.

Hospital coverage: Pays for a hospital room, board, and special services in total or in part. Often a maximum number of days in the hospital or a maximum amount payable per day is set by hospitalization policies.

Surgical coverage: Covers suturing, fracture reduction, aspiration, removal of foreign bodies, excisions, and incisions performed in a doctor's office, a hospital, or elsewhere. Part or all of a surgeon's and possibly an assistant surgeon's fees are paid for by surgical coverage.

Disability protection: Covers loss of income that results from illness. It is not to be used for payment of specific medical bills, and it is paid directly to the patient.

Dental care: Employers' benefit packages often include dental coverage, usually based on an incentive and copayment program. Often a company's portion of a copayment increases by the year, until 100% coverage is achieved.

Vision care: Reimburses for all or some costs for frames, lenses, and eye exams.

Liability insurance: Covers people injured in their homes or cars. The many types include homeowner, business, and automobile policies.

Life insurance: A plan that pays benefits to a beneficiary in case of loss of life.

14.3 Types of Health Plans

Indemnity plans: The insurer pays the subscriber a set amount for each service or procedure performed because of illness or injury. These fees are usually paid directly to the insured unless previous arrangements have been made for them to go straight to the provider. This type of plan does not pay for complete services rendered, and there is often a difference between the physician's fee and the amount the insurance company pays out. A fee schedule is given to the purchaser at the beginning of the contract, and benefits are determined on a fee-for-service basis.

Group policies: Cover groups of people under a master contract, which is generally issued to an employer for the benefit of the employees. Such a plan usually provides greater benefits at lower premiums than an individual plan. Every person in a group contract has identical coverage. Physical examinations are not required in order to receive coverage.

Individual policies: Individuals who do not qualify for group policies may apply for individual policies. Premiums will probably be greater and the benefits less than in group policies. Individual policies usually require applicants to pass physical examinations in order to receive coverage.

Service benefit plans: Cover certain medical or surgical services without any additional cost to the insured. There are no scheduled set fees.

Government Plans

Government policies: Government-sponsored insurance coverage for eligible individuals. The federal government provides coverage under Medicare, Medicaid, TRICARE or CHAMPUS, and CHAMPVA.

Medicare Plans

Original Medicare plan: Provides health insurance to citizens aged 65 and older and to younger patients who are blind or widowed or who have serious long-term disabilities, such as kidney failure. **Medicare Part A** covers hospital, nursing facility, home health, hospice, and inpatient care. Those who are eligible for social security benefits are automatically enrolled in Medicare Part A. **Medicare Part B** covers outpatient services, services by physicians, durable medical equipment, and other services and supplies. Medicare Part B coverage is optional. Everyone eligible for Part A can choose to enroll in Part B by paying monthly premiums. Deductibles must be met in Parts A and B before payment benefits begin. **Part C** is not a separate benefit. It allows private health insurance companies to provide Medicare benefits. These Medicare *private health plans* (such as HMOs and PPOs) are sometimes known as *Medicare Advantage* plans. It is possible to obtain Medicare coverage through a Medicare private health plan instead of "original" Medicare. These private plans must offer "at least the same" coverage as original Medicare, but may have different costs attached. **Medicare Part D** provides outpatient prescription drug coverage, only through private insurers with no connection to the government.

Bundled payment: An experimental Medicare payment method by which an entire episode of care is paid for by a predetermined single payment.

Diagnosis-related groups (DRGs): Groups of procedures or tests related directly to a diagnosis. The fixed fees paid by Medicare Part A are based on DRGs. In other words, Medicare uses DRGs to determine appropriate reimbursement for medical diagnoses and procedures, as do many private insurers. DRGs are assigned in the hospital when a patient is discharged.

Three-day payment window: A rule under which Medicare bundles all outpatient services provided by a hospital to a patient within three days before admission into the DRG payments for the patient.

Medicare fee schedule (MFS): Providers participating in Medicare must accept the charges listed in this schedule as payment for covered services. The MFS is developed by using the Resource-Based Relative Value Scale. The participating physician may bill the patient for coinsurance and deductibles but may not collect excess charges.

Medicare supplements (Medigap policies): Private insurance contracts that supplement regular Medicare coverage. They are kept uniform in their benefits so as not to be confusing to purchasers. These supplemental plans pay for a beneficiary's deductibles, for coinsurance, and in some cases for services not covered by Medicare. If the subscriber has Medigap insurance, Medicare is still the primary payer, which means that claims must be filed with Medicare first. If a patient has both Medicare and Medicaid, charges must be filed with Medicare first, and Medicaid is the secondary payer.

Medicare + Choice Plans

Medicare also offers a group of plans called the Medicare + Choice Plans. Beneficiaries can choose to enroll in one of three major types of plans instead of the original Medicare plan:

1. Medicare managed care plans
2. Medicare preferred provider organization plans
3. Medicare private fee-for-service plans

Medicare managed care plans: These plans charge a monthly premium and a small copayment for each office visit, but not a deductible. Like private payer managed care plans, Medicare managed care plans often require patients to use a specific network of physicians, hospitals, and facilities. Some plans offer the option of receiving services from providers outside the network for a higher fee. All plans offer coverage for services not reimbursed in the original Medicare plan, such as physical examinations and inoculations. Participants are generally required to select a primary care provider (PCP) from within the network. The PCP provides treatment and manages the patient's medical care through referrals.

Medicare preferred provider organization plans (PPOs): In these plans, physicians, hospitals, and other health-care providers join together and agree to offer services to members of a group (subscribers) at a lower cost or discount. Patients pay less to use doctors within a network, but they may choose to go outside the network for additional costs, such as a higher copayment or higher coinsurance. Patients do not need a PCP, and referrals are not required. This can give the individual more control over his or her health care.

Medicare private fee-for-service plans: Patients in these plans receive services from the provider they choose, as long as Medicare has approved the provider or facility. The plan is operated by a private insurance company that contracts with Medicare to provide services to beneficiaries. The plan sets its own rates for services, and physicians are allowed to bill patients the amount of the charge not covered by the plan. A copayment may or may not be required.

Accountable care organizations (ACOs): Groups of physicians, hospitals, and other health-care organizations that voluntarily work together to coordinate care for Medicare patients.

Medicaid Plans

Medicaid: A health benefit program designed for low-income people (people receiving welfare payments or other forms of public assistance) who cannot pay their medical bills. People covered under Medicaid are medically indigent. Eligibility for coverage might vary from month to month based on the recipient's income. Medicaid is a health-cost assistance program, not an insurance program, and physicians may choose to accept or not to accept Medicaid patients. By treating Medicaid patients, physicians accept Medicaid reimbursement for covered services and cannot charge patients for any difference. In some states, Medicaid is known by a different name. For example, in California Medicaid is called MediCal. Always ask for a Medicaid card from patients who state that they are entitled to Medicaid coverage (see Figure 14-1). Medicaid is always last to be billed when there is another form of existing health coverage.

Medicaid fee-for-service: Patients are treated by the provider of their choice as long as the provider accepts Medicaid. The provider submits the claim and Medicaid pays it directly.

Medicaid managed care: As used by many states, about 70% of Medicaid recipients are in managed care plans. Enrollment is mandatory or voluntary, based on state regulations. Patients are restricted to a network of providers, and must obtain all services and referrals through their PCP, who is responsible for coordinating and monitoring all care. The PCP must provide referrals to specialists if needed, or the plan will not pay for their services. It is usually easier for patients to find providers who will accept managed care plans under Medicaid, instead of the fee-for-service plans. Managed care also offers immunizations and health screenings. Claims are sent to the managed care organization instead of to the state Medicaid department.

Medicaid payment for services: Participating providers sign contracts with the Department of Health and Human Services (HHS), and managed care plans also contract with HHS. Providers agree to accept Medicaid payments as "payments in full" for services, and cannot bill for additional amounts. The differences are entered as "write-offs." Certain states require selected Medicaid recipients to make small payments of deductibles, coinsurance, or copayments, which are referred to as *cost-share payments.* Emergency services and family planning services are exempted from copayments. If Medicaid will not cover a certain service, the patient must be informed and given a form to sign acknowledging his or her understanding.

Third-party liability: An obligation of a governmental program or insurance plan to pay all or part of a patient's medical costs. Eligibility for Medicaid does not relieve Medicare of its responsibility to cover health-care costs. In other words, Medicaid is always a secondary carrier or a payer of last resort.

Medi/Medi: Older or disabled patients who have Medicare and who cannot pay the difference between the bill and the Medicare payment may qualify for Medicare and Medicaid. This type of coverage is known as Medi/Medi. In such cases, Medicare is the primary payer, and Medicaid is the secondary payer.

State guidelines: Medicaid benefits can vary from state to state. It is important to understand the Medicaid guidelines in your state so that your office's Medicaid reimbursement is prompt and without complications. Here are some suggestions:

- Always ask for a Medicaid card from patients who state that they are entitled to Medicaid.
- Check the patient's Medicaid card, which is issued monthly and shows the patient's eligibility for services or procedures.
- Ensure that the physician signs all claims. Then send them to the state's Medicaid-approved contactor (which pays on behalf of the state) or to the state department that administers Medicaid (e.g., the state department of social services or public health).
- Unless the patient has a medical emergency, Medicaid often requires authorization before services are performed.
- Check the time limit on claim submissions. It can be as short as two months or as long as one year.
- Meet the deadlines. If a Medicaid claim is submitted after the time limit, the claim may be rejected.
- Treat Medicaid patients with the same professionalism and courtesy as you extend to other patients. Simply because a patient qualifies for Medicaid assistance does not mean that the patient is in any way inferior to those with private insurance.

INDIANA MEDICAID

AND OTHER MEDICAL ASSISTANCE PROGRAMS

100341842799   001

Danny L Owens
07/19/62

Figure 14-1 *A Medicaid card gives the patient's name and identification (or social security) number.*

TRICARE and CHAMPVA

TRICARE: The U.S. government provides health-care benefits to families of current military personnel, retired military personnel, and veterans through the TRICARE and CHAMPVA programs. They are run by the Defense Department. TRICARE is a health-care benefit for families of uniformed personnel and retirees from the uniformed services, including the Army, Navy, Marines, Air Force, Coast Guard, Public Health Service, and National Oceanic and Atmospheric Administration. TRICARE offers families three choices of health-care benefits:

1. TRICARE Prime, a health maintenance organization
2. TRICARE Extra, a managed care network of health-care providers that families can use on a case-by-case basis without a required enrollment
3. TRICARE Standard, a fee-for-service plan

TRICARE for Life: A program aimed at Medicare-eligible military retirees and Medicare-eligible family members. This program offers the opportunity to receive health care at a military treatment facility to individuals aged 65 and older who are eligible for both Medicare and TRICARE.

TRICARE participating providers: Those who agree to accept the allowable charge as payment in full for services. Providers may participate on a case-by-case basis, and are required to file claims on behalf of patients.

TRICARE nonparticipating providers: Those who do not wish to participate may not charge more than 115% of the allowable charge. If they do, the patient may refuse to pay the excess amount.

CHAMPVA: Stands for Civilian Health and Medical Program of the Veterans Administration. It covers the expenses of the families of veterans with total, permanent, service-connected disabilities. It also covers surviving spouses and dependent children of veterans who died in the line of duty. CHAMPVA is a service benefit plan rather than an insurance plan.

Sponsor: The uniformed service member in a family who is qualified for TRICARE or CHAMPVA.

DEERS: Stands for Defense Enrollment Eligibility Reporting System, maintained by the Department of Defense. DEERS is a worldwide database of people covered by TRICARE.

Payments under TRICARE and CHAMPVA: Payments on assigned claims are made directly to the physician. As with Medicaid, the physician who does not participate has the option to accept assignment on a case-by-case basis.

Cost-share: The term TRICARE and CHAMPVA use for coinsurance.

Catastrophic cap: The maximum amount a beneficiary might need to pay out as coinsurance within a span of a year. When the cap is reached, TRICARE and CHAMPVA pay all allowed charges for the rest of the year.

Avoiding duplication: TRICARE and CHAMPVA are primary payers when an insured individual also has Medicaid. If the insured is also covered under Medicare, claims must be filed with Medicare first. TRICARE and CHAMPVA also do not pay for illnesses or injuries covered by workers' compensation unless compensation benefits have been exhausted. Claims must be filed within one year from date of service.

Private Plans

Coverage with private insurance companies: Physicians and medical societies control neither the premiums paid nor the benefits received from such policies. Insurance payments may be made to the subscriber and not to the physician.

Blue Cross and Blue Shield (BCBS) Association: A nationwide federation of local nonprofit service organizations that offer prepaid health-care services to subscribers. Under a prepaid health coverage plan, the carrier will pay for specified medical expenses if premiums are paid in advance. The Blue Cross part of BCBS covers hospital services, outpatient and home care services, and other institutional care. Blue Shield covers physician services and dental, vision, and other outpatient benefits. Some local BCBS organizations help the government administer Medicare, Medicaid, and TRICARE programs.

Local BCBS organizations: Operate under the laws of the states in which they are located. There are 86 local BCBS plans in the United States, each with its own claim form. Plans make direct payments to member physicians, but payments may be made to the subscriber (patient) if the physician is a nonmember. Many small groups and individuals who may not be able to get coverage elsewhere can join a BCBS plan. Some plans offer coverage regardless of medical condition during special periods of time. Plans also must get permission from the state to raise their rates.

Blue Card Program: The Blue Card Program is a nationwide program that makes it easy for patients to receive treatment when outside their local service area, and also makes it easy for providers to receive payment when treating patients enrolled in plans outside the provider's service area.

Customary maximum: The term BCBS plans use to describe the fee based on actual fees charged by most physicians in the community.

Fixed-fee schedule: A list used by BCBS plans of maximum fees allowed for specific services.

Blue card: An agreement among BCBS plans through which a local plan may provide benefits for any out-of-town BCBS plan subscriber.

Kaiser Foundation Health Plan: A type of prepaid group practice (HMO). The Kaiser Foundation was a pioneer of nonprofit prepaid group practice beginning in California in 1933. The plan owns the medical facilities and directly employs the physicians and other providers.

Workers' compensation: A contract carried by the employer that insures a person against on-the-job injury or illness. The employer is responsible for the premium payment. See Table 14-1 on managing workers' compensation cases. Generally, a workers' compensation plan covers only specific medical bills, such as laboratory bills, physicians' fees, medical treatment, physical therapy, disability income, and income replacement. This type of plan recommends any private medical records for an individual patient be kept separate from any workers' compensation records for the same individual.

Short-term disability: Insurance coverage that provides 40–70% of the individual's predisability base salary. It covers temporary disability in which a person cannot work for a short

If your medical practice accepts workers' compensation cases, you should follow this procedure when contacted by a patient:

- Call the patient's employer to verify that the accident occurred on the employer's premises.

- Obtain the employer's approval to provide treatment.

- Ask the employer for the name of the workers' compensation insurance company.

- Remind the employer to report the accident or injury to the state labor department.

- Contact the insurance company to verify that the employer has a policy in good standing.

- Obtain a claim number from the insurance company.

- Create a patient record.

Table 14-1

period of time, usually less than three months, due to sickness or injury not related to his or her job.

Long-term disability: Insurance coverage that usually begins after a short-term disability policy has run out. These policies usually pay 75% of the predisability base salary, or 50% of the base salary until the employee turns 65.

Self-insured plans: These exist when a company's employee base is large enough to allow self-funding. Though not technically *true insurance*, self-insured plans often use a *fiscal intermediary* or *third-party administrator* to handle paperwork and claim payments. The employer pays employee health-care costs from the company's own funds.

Medical savings accounts: Tax-free accounts, which are a type of self-insurance. Companies of 50 employees or fewer, self-employed people, and uninsured people can buy health insurance and make tax-free deposits to an MSA. This money is then used to pay small, routine health expenses. Interest earned from money in the account is tax free.

Managed Care

Managed care organizations: Organizations that manage, negotiate, and contract for health care with the goal of keeping costs down. Managed care organizations sign up health-care providers who agree to charge a fixed fee for services. These fixed fees are set by the managed care organization or by the governmental agency responsible for managed care.

Cost-containment practices: Developed by insurance carriers such as managed care organizations to keep premiums as low as possible. Such practices may include, for example, requiring fewer overnight stays after certain surgeries or requiring preauthorization of a service before the procedure is performed.

Health maintenance organization (HMO): A type of managed care program that provides specific services to enrollees. Enrollees are expected to receive treatment only from participating providers, and they may see specialists only when referred by their primary care physicians, who act as gatekeepers.

Group model HMO: Physicians in this type of an arrangement see both members of the HMO and nonmember patients, and

they remain self-employed. Physicians receive fixed payments from the HMO for each member patient, rather than reimbursement for the services provided. This fixed fee is paid to the physician monthly regardless of the number of times the patient visits the physician. This type of reimbursement is called capitation. Examples of a group model HMO include independent practice associations (IPAs) and network model HMOs.

Staff model HMO: Under this arrangement, the physicians are employees of the HMO and work full time seeing member patients. In this type of HMO, a primary care physician is assigned as the gatekeeper for patients.

Preferred provider organization (PPO): A type of managed care plan in which enrollees receive the highest level of benefits when they obtain services from a physician, hospital, or other health provider designated by their program as a preferred provider. Enrollees receive reduced benefits when they obtain care from a provider who is not designated as a preferred provider by their program. PPO patients may see specialists without prior authorization from their primary care physicians. HMOs offering point-of-service options are more like PPOs.

Point-of-service: An option added to some HMO plans that allows patients to choose a physician outside the HMO network and to pay increased deductibles and coinsurance.

Physician-hospital organization (PHO): An approach to coordinating services for patients in which physicians join hospitals to create an integrated medical care delivery system. This union then makes arrangements for insurance with a commercial carrier or an HMO.

Patient-centered medical home (PCMH): A model of primary care that is comprehensive, team based, coordinated, accessible, and focused on quality and safety in health care while remaining based on the patient's direct needs.

Fee-for-service: A system of retroactive reimbursement in which the physician or other provider bills for each service that is provided. BCBS is a fee-for-service plan.

Capitation: A system of payment used by managed care plans in which physicians and hospitals are paid a fixed, per capita amount for each patient enrolled over a stated period of time, regardless of the type and number of services provided.

Withhold: A portion of the monthly capitation payment to physicians retained by an HMO until the end of the year to create an incentive for efficient care. If the physician exceeds utilization norms, he or she will not receive this portion.

Relative value scale (RVS): A system of assigning values to medical services on the basis of an analysis of the skill and time required to provide them. Both indemnity plans and many managed care plans are moving to this approach for assigning allowed charges. The RVS assigns numerical values to medical services, which then have to be multiplied by a dollar conversion factor to calculate fees.

Precertification: A call to the patient's insurance carrier to find out whether the treatment, surgery, tests, or hospitalization is covered under the patient's health insurance policy.

Preauthorization: Permission by the insurance carrier that must be obtained before giving a certain treatment to a patient.

Utilization management: A process, based on established criteria, of reviewing and controlling the medical necessity for services and providers' use of medical care resources. In managed care systems such as HMOs, reviews are done to establish medical necessity.

Referrals: In managed care, the primary care physician needs to refer a patient to a specialist before that patient can make an appointment with the specialist. A referral form must be completed showing the following information:

- Referring physician
- Specialist to whom the patient is being referred
- Diagnosis
- Treatment (past and present, including medications)
- Chart notes
- Minor surgical procedures

Types of referrals: There are three types of referrals:
- Regular referral, which usually takes 3–10 days
- Urgent referral, which usually takes 24 hours
- STAT referral, which can be done on the phone immediately

Authorization: A referral that is approved.

Processing authorizations: Follow these guidelines in processing authorizations:
- Always review the authorization before providing services.
- Deny unauthorized procedures.
- Unauthorized services provided cannot be billed to the patient, and the practice will eventually have to write off the charges.
- Obtain the patient's signature on an agreement to pay for services not covered by insurance.

Formulary: A list of medications that are covered by a health plan.

Member services: A department designed to assist patients with inquiries and/or concerns that may arise.

Provider relations: This department is designed to assist the physician's office with inquiries about capitation, contracts, credentialing, physician appeals, formularies, and so forth.

HIPAA: Health Insurance Portability and Accountability Act created to improve continuity of health insurance coverage and the administration of health-care services. HIPAA provides federal income tax advantages to people who purchase certain long-term-care insurance policies.

HIPAA's Privacy Rule: Protects patient information so that it is available to those who need to see it but unavailable to those who should not.

Pay-to provider: The person or organization that is to receive a payment for services reported on a HIPAA claim, which may be the same as or different from the billing provider.

14.4 Determination of Benefits

Benefits are determined via indemnity schedules, service benefit plans, usual/customary/reasonable fees, and the resource-based relative value scale. The first three are defined here; the fourth is defined later in this chapter.

Indemnity schedules: Traditional health insurance plans that pay for some or all of the cost of covered services, regardless of the licensed health-care provider that is used. Indemnity schedules often are called *fee-for-service plans*.

Service benefit plans: The insurance company pays for certain medical or surgical services with no additional cost to the insured person. There is no set fee schedule, but premiums and payments may be higher. The provider may accept a certain amount for a procedure even if it is less than he or she would otherwise charge.

Usual, Customary, and Reasonable Fee: The insurer may pay all of, or a percentage of, this fee to a provider. These fees are based on a database of charges for the same service to other patients by the same type of provider.

14.5 Claims Processing

HIPAA claims: The electronic claim transaction is the HIPAA Health-Care Claim or Equivalent Encounter Information, commonly referred to as the HIPAA claim. Its official name is X12 837 Health-Care Claim. Medicare mandates the X12 837 transaction for all Medicare claims except for those from very small practices. Third-party payers may continue to accept paper transactions.

Follow these tips when entering data in medical billing programs:
- Enter data in all capital letters.
- Do not use prefixes for people's names, such as Mr., Ms., or Dr.
- Unless required by a particular insurance carrier, do not use special characters such as hyphens, commas, or apostrophes.
- Use only valid data in all fields; avoid words such as *same*.

The X12 837 transaction requires many data elements on correct claims. Most billing programs or claim transmission programs automatically reformat data, such as dates, in the correct formats. These data elements are reported in five major sections.

1. Provider
2. Subscriber (the insured or policyholder)
3. Patient (who may be the subscriber or another person) and payer
4. Claim details
5. Services

Paper claim: The paper claim is the "universal claim" known as the CMS-1500 claim form (or the CMS-1500), which is the most commonly used insurance claim form. The CMS-1500 form is required by law to be filed for all eligible Medicare patients. Practices that elect to use paper claims must have two versions of their medical billing software: one to capture the necessary data elements for HIPAA-compliant electronic Medicare claims and an older version to generate CMS-1500 claims. Also, under HIPAA regulations, only medical offices that do not handle any other HIPAA-related transactions can still use paper claims. It is anticipated that eventually, for cost reasons, all payers will require electronic submissions and add this provision to their contracts with providers. See Figure 14-2. After completing the form, the medical assistant acting as the medical insurance specialist should:

- Proofread the form.
- Photocopy the form and place a copy in the patient's medical records.
- Enter the date sent, the patient's name, and the name of insurance carrier in the insurance log (if any).
- Enter the date and the words "insurance filed" in the patient ledger.
- Transmit the form.

Claim attachment: Documentation that a provider sends to a payer in support of a health-care claim.
Electronic filing: The electronic filing of claims utilizes Electronic Data Interchange (EDI), in which they are sent from one computer to another, avoiding expensive paperwork. It is also much quicker and safer to use.
Data format: An arrangement of electronic data for transaction.
Violating HIPAA's Privacy Rule: Any individual who discovers that his or her privacy has been misused or disclosed without permission can file a complaint with the Department of Health and Human Services (DHHS) that his or her health-care provider, his or her health plan, or a clearinghouse has not followed HIPAA's regulations. The penalties for this violation include fines that may be imposed for civil wrongdoing, as well as up to $250,000 and up to 10 years in prison for criminal breach.
File acknowledgment: Immediate feedback that lets the physician's office know that the file has arrived at the insurance carrier's claims department.
Format rejection: Immediate feedback that the file has details missing or incorrect information, such as a required field left blank.

National Standard Format (NSF): The most widely accepted format for transmitting CMS forms electronically.
Advantages of electronic claim submission:
- Immediate transmission and feedback about errors
- Faster payment and electronic funds transfer
- Faster explanation of benefits and appeal resolution
- Easier tracking of claim status

Insurance claim reimbursement criteria: There are four bases for determining payment.

1. UCR charges
2. The Medicare Resource-Based Relative Value Scale (RBRVS)
3. Fee schedules
4. DRGs

The most common reason for the return of insurance claim forms is missing or mistyped information. To minimize the chance of errors, it is extremely important always to proofread all claims before submitting them.
RBRVS: Used to determine physician fees, utilizing a fee-for-service system for Medicare Part B, based on customary, prevailing, and reasonable charges.
Steps in claims processing: Following are the general steps in processing a claim:

1. Gather health insurance information from the patient and verify insurance coverage.
2. Complete the CMS-1500 claim form.
3. Base the claim on the superbill, which lists the name and address of the patient, the name of the insurance carrier, the insurance identification number, a brief description of each service by code number, the fee for the service, the place and date of service, the diagnosis, the physician's name and address, and the physician's signature. You also should have the current editions of the *ICD-9-CM* and the *Current Procedural Terminology* (CPT) for diagnostic and procedural coding.
4. If possible, use electronic claims submission. Prepare claims on a computer and submit them via modem to the insurance carrier's computer system. Such claims are also called electronic media claims (EMCs).
5. Track insurance claims. Follow up with the insurance company until the claim is paid in a timely manner.
6. Remember that if a claim form is not sufficiently detailed, complete, and accurate, it will be rejected by the insurance company.

Prospective audit: Internal audit of particular claims conducted before they are transmitted to payers.
Tracing: If after 30 days the insurance company has not paid the claim or responded to a claim, the choices are to bill again or to call the carrier. Because second billings are sometimes rejected as duplicates, the medical office can send a tracer, a letter to the insurance company containing the basic billing information.

DRAFT - NOT FOR OFFICIAL USE

HEALTH INSURANCE CLAIM FORM

APPROVED BY NATIONAL UNIFORM CLAIM COMMITTEE (NUCC) 02/12

| | PICA | | | | | | | | PICA | |

1. MEDICARE MEDICAID TRICARE CHAMPVA GROUP HEALTH PLAN FECA BLK LUNG OTHER
(Medicare#) (Medicaid#) (ID#/DoD#) (Member ID#) (ID#) (ID#) (ID#)

1a. INSURED'S I.D. NUMBER (For Program in Item 1)

2. PATIENT'S NAME (Last Name, First Name, Middle Initial)

3. PATIENT'S BIRTH DATE MM DD YY SEX M F

4. INSURED'S NAME (Last Name, First Name, Middle Initial)

5. PATIENT'S ADDRESS (No., Street)

6. PATIENT RELATIONSHIP TO INSURED Self Spouse Child Other

7. INSURED'S ADDRESS (No., Street)

CITY STATE

8. RESERVED FOR NUCC USE

CITY STATE

ZIP CODE TELEPHONE (Include Area Code) (   )

ZIP CODE TELEPHONE (Include Area Code) (   )

9. OTHER INSURED'S NAME (Last Name, First Name, Middle Initial)

10. IS PATIENT'S CONDITION RELATED TO:

11. INSURED'S POLICY GROUP OR FECA NUMBER

a. OTHER INSURED'S POLICY OR GROUP NUMBER

a. EMPLOYMENT? (Current or Previous) YES NO

a. INSURED'S DATE OF BIRTH MM DD YY SEX M F

b. RESERVED FOR NUCC USE

b. AUTO ACCIDENT? PLACE (State) YES NO

b. OTHER CLAIM ID (Designated by NUCC)

c. RESERVED FOR NUCC USE

c. OTHER ACCIDENT? YES NO

c. INSURANCE PLAN NAME OR PROGRAM NAME

d. INSURANCE PLAN NAME OR PROGRAM NAME

10d. CLAIM CODES (Designated by NUCC)

d. IS THERE ANOTHER HEALTH BENEFIT PLAN? YES NO If yes, complete items 9, 9a, and 9d.

READ BACK OF FORM BEFORE COMPLETING & SIGNING THIS FORM.
12. PATIENT'S OR AUTHORIZED PERSON'S SIGNATURE I authorize the release of any medical or other information necessary to process this claim. I also request payment of government benefits either to myself or to the party who accepts assignment below.

SIGNED _____ DATE _____

13. INSURED'S OR AUTHORIZED PERSON'S SIGNATURE I authorize payment of medical benefits to the undersigned physician or supplier for services described below.

SIGNED _____

14. DATE OF CURRENT ILLNESS, INJURY, or PREGNANCY (LMP) MM DD YY QUAL.

15. OTHER DATE QUAL. MM DD YY

16. DATES PATIENT UNABLE TO WORK IN CURRENT OCCUPATION FROM MM DD YY TO MM DD YY

17. NAME OF REFERRING PROVIDER OR OTHER SOURCE

17a.
17b. NPI

18. HOSPITALIZATION DATES RELATED TO CURRENT SERVICES FROM MM DD YY TO MM DD YY

19. ADDITIONAL CLAIM INFORMATION (Designated by NUCC)

20. OUTSIDE LAB? $ CHARGES YES NO

21. DIAGNOSIS OR NATURE OF ILLNESS OR INJURY Relate A-L to service line below (24E) ICD Ind.
A. ____ B. ____ C. ____ D. ____
E. ____ F. ____ G. ____ H. ____
I. ____ J. ____ K. ____ L. ____

22. RESUBMISSION CODE ORIGINAL REF. NO.

23. PRIOR AUTHORIZATION NUMBER

24. A. DATE(S) OF SERVICE From MM DD YY To MM DD YY	B. PLACE OF SERVICE	C. EMG	D. PROCEDURES, SERVICES, OR SUPPLIES (Explain Unusual Circumstances) CPT/HCPCS MODIFIER	E. DIAGNOSIS POINTER	F. $ CHARGES	G. DAYS OR UNITS	H. EPSDT Family Plan	I. ID. QUAL.	J. RENDERING PROVIDER ID. #
1									NPI
2									NPI
3									NPI
4									NPI
5									NPI
6									NPI

25. FEDERAL TAX I.D. NUMBER SSN EIN

26. PATIENT'S ACCOUNT NO.

27. ACCEPT ASSIGNMENT? (For govt. claims, see back) YES NO

28. TOTAL CHARGE $

29. AMOUNT PAID $

30. Rsvd for NUCC Use

31. SIGNATURE OF PHYSICIAN OR SUPPLIER INCLUDING DEGREES OR CREDENTIALS (I certify that the statements on the reverse apply to this bill and are made a part thereof.)

SIGNED _____ DATE _____

32. SERVICE FACILITY LOCATION INFORMATION

a. NPI b.

33. BILLING PROVIDER INFO & PH # (   )

a. NPI b.

NUCC Instruction Manual available at: www.nucc.org PLEASE PRINT OR TYPE OMB APPROVAL PENDING

CARRIER PATIENT AND INSURED INFORMATION PHYSICIAN OR SUPPLIER INFORMATION

Figure 14-2 *The CMS-1500 is the universal health insurance claim form accepted by most insurers, even if they have their own forms.*

Universal health insurance claim form.

Rebilling: Make a copy of the original claim form submitted and write "SECOND BILLING" in red letters at the top. Reasons to rebill include:

- The insurance company is delinquent in responding to a claim.
- A mistake has been made in billing.
- Charges must be detailed to receive maximum reimbursement.
- A claim was overlooked by the physician's office.
- The carrier asked for rebilling because the wrong diagnosis or procedure codes were submitted, some information was incomplete or missing, or the charges did not total properly.

Reasons claims are denied or payments are delayed:

- The claim is not for a covered contract benefit. Bill the patient.
- The patient's preexisting condition is not covered. Bill the patient.
- The patient's coverage has been canceled. Bill the patient.
- Workers' compensation is involved, and the case is under consideration. Check on the claim's progress every 30 days.
- The insurance company considers the physician's procedure to be experimental. Call the carrier to discuss options. Peer review may be requested.
- No preauthorization was obtained. Review the patient's contract and what the sanctions are. Write a letter of appeal if appropriate.
- The physician provided services before the patient's health insurance contract went into effect. Bill the patient.
- The carrier asks for additional information. Send the carrier the requested information and follow up in 30 days.

Claim appeal: A written request to the insurance carrier to review reimbursement. It is usually filed if the preauthorization was not obtained because unusual circumstances exist; the reimbursement was inadequate for a complicated procedure; the physician disagrees that the patient's condition was preexisting; or the patient has unusual circumstances that affect medical treatment.

Medicare claims processing: Guidelines for processing Medicare claims are:

- Providers are required by law to file the CMS-1500 for all eligible patients.
- Providers may be participating or nonparticipating.
- PAR providers accept assignment on Medicare claims and receive the allowed fee.
- NonPAR providers are not required to accept assignment; therefore, the patient is responsible for the balance after Medicare makes its payment. See Table 14-2.
- The allowable payment to nonPAR providers is less than the payment to PAR providers.
- Medicare forms must be signed by both the patient and the physician.
- Claims for Medicare must be filed by December 31 of the year following that in which the services were rendered.

The website address for Medicare regulations is http://www.cms.gov/Regulations-and-Guidance/Regulations-and-Guidance.html.

Medicaid claims processing: Guidelines for processing Medicaid claims are:

- A physician is free to accept or refuse to treat a patient under Medicaid.
- A patient's eligibility should be verified before the delivery of medical service.
- Preauthorization may be required for the service.
- Claims should be filed on the CMS-1500.
- There is always a time limit for filing claims, according to state regulations.
- Medicaid is a secondary carrier for patients who have Medicare, and is a type of Medigap insurance policy.

AT A GLANCE Understanding Medicare Payments

Participating Provider		Nonparticipating Provider	
Physician's standard fee:	$120.00	Physician's standard fee:	$120.00
Medicare PAR fee:	$ 60.00	Medicare nonPAR fee:	$ 57.00
Medicare pays 80% of PAR fee:	$ 48.00	Medicare pays 80% of nonPAR fee:	$ 45.60
Patient or supplemental plan pays:	$ 12.00	Patient or supplemental plan pays:	$ 11.40
Provider writes off:	$ 60.00	Provider writes off:	$ 63.00

Table 14-2

Note: These charges do not represent realistic or accurate medical service fees. They are used here merely as an example.

Medi/Medi claims processing: Guidelines for processing Medi/Medi claims are:

- A physician must always accept assignment.
- A claim form is first processed through Medicare and is then automatically forwarded to Medicaid.
- It is not necessary to prepare two claim forms. The combined claim is sometimes referred to as a crossover claim.

BCBS claims processing: Guidelines for processing Blue card claims are:

- Claims should be submitted as soon as possible after the service is provided.
- Like Medicare, the Blue plans have arrangements with PAR and nonPAR providers. Usually a PAR provider is paid directly for covered services and agrees not to bill the patient for any difference.
- Blue plans have provider manuals that describe coverage and coding features of the plan.
- BCBS offers prepaid health services *and* follows a fee-for-service reimbursement plan.

TRICARE claims processing: Guidelines for processing a TRICARE claim are:

- Use the CMS-1500 claim form.
- If the physician accepts assignment (i.e., the physician is a PAR provider), the medical office files the insurance claim and the patient can be billed for the entire deductible and the coinsurance portion of the allowed charge.
- If the physician does not accept assignment, the patient must submit claim forms to the insurance company and is responsible for all charges.
- The claims must be filed no later than December 31 of the year following that in which services were provided.
- PAR providers are paid within 21 days after submitting a claim, and only PAR providers may appeal a claims decision.

CHAMPVA claims processing: CHAMPVA claims follow the same guidelines as TRICARE claims.

Workers' compensation claims processing: Follow these guidelines:

- Records of the workers' compensation case should be kept separate from the patient's regular history.
- The insurance carrier is entitled to receive copies of all records pertaining to the industrial injury.
- The injured person's records must be personally signed by the physician.
- The insurance carrier may supply its own billing forms.
- Payment is usually made on the basis of a fee schedule.
- At the termination of the treatment, a final report and bill are sent to the insurance carrier.
- Do not bill the patient.

Verification of Insurance Benefits

Insurance must be verified prior to providing service to patients. Insurance coverage protects the physician and patient against unplanned costs. Verification includes eight steps:

1. Identify insurance or managed-care organization coverage when the patient calls.
2. Photocopy or scan both sides of the patient's insurance ID card when the patient arrives.
3. Verify with the insurer that the patient is eligible for benefits, and whether preauthorization is needed for referrals to specialists or for certain services and procedures.
4. Write down the name, title, and phone number of the contact person.
5. Document all information in the patient's medical record and on a Verification of Benefits form.
6. Have the patient sign a letter that outlines insurance requirements, restrictions, and noncovered items. The letter may also outline patient responsibilities.
7. Explain any needed referrals to the patient, and tell the patient that without the referral, he or she would need to pay for the physician's services.
8. Collect any deductibles or copayments.

Legal Considerations

Legal and ethical issues: There are a variety of legal and ethical issues associated with processing claims:

- Stay current on the laws that affect medicine.
- It is the physician's responsibility to identify the procedures that have been performed. Code only for procedures that appear in the medical records. If you think that a certain procedure has been left out by accident, tell the physician to update the medical records before you file a claim.
- An incorrect code used for billing a service can be considered fraud.
- Obtain patient signatures permitting insurance billing.
- Obtain proper authorization from the insurance carrier whenever required.

Fraud: Occurs when someone intentionally misrepresents facts to receive a benefit illegally. A person who cooperates in a fraudulent situation becomes personally liable, or legally responsible. Some fraudulent actions include:

- Altering a patient's chart to increase the amount reimbursed
- Upgrading or falsifying medical procedures to increase the amount reimbursed
- Billing primary or secondary insurance carriers while at the same time collecting payment from the patient
- Under Medicare law, not attempting to collect a required payment from a Medicare patient

Because an incorrect code can seem like fraud, it is very important to code accurately and keep good records of the coordination of benefits.

Fee Schedules

The health-care worker must estimate the value of his or her time, expertise, and services. Based on the type of practice, fee schedules differ widely. Today, government and managed health organizations (third-party payers) have strongly influenced fee schedules of health-care providers. These organizations have established *allowable charges*, which are maximum amounts they will pay for certain services or procedures.

Resource-Based Relative Value Scale

Though Medicare Part B previously used a fee-for-service system that was based on usual, customary, and reasonable fees, today a fee scale has been implemented. It consists of the physician's work, charge-based professional liability expenses, and charge-based overhead. The physician's work includes the effort required for the service or procedure, and the time it took. The Centers for Medicare and Medicaid Services compute professional liability and overhead. The Resource-Based Relative Value Scale's fee schedule provides country-wide uniform, adjusted payments reflecting differences in practice costs over geographic areas. A conversion factor is used, which is a single number applied nationally to all services paid under the fee schedule. These factors are usually changed every year by Congress, upon request by the CMS. There is great variance of contracts between service providers and insurers. The MA must understand the contract terms for each third-party payer. After payment is received, the MA must examine the *explanation of benefits (EOB)* to ensure that all benefits have been appropriately and correctly reimbursed. Medicare also utilizes *remittance advice (RA)*, which is communication that provides information about what has been paid for.

Deductibles and Coinsurance

Deductibles and coinsurance are required by many types of health insurance plans. There is usually an annual deductible amount paid by the patient prior to the plan paying any amount. Members must usually pay a percentage of each charge (coinsurance). In most indemnity plans, there is a yearly out-of-pocket limit that is paid for coinsurance. Indemnity plans reduce major expenses of medical bills while keeping premium costs lower. The amount due from a patient for covered services (from a participating provider) is the difference between the allowed charge and the patient's deductible (and/or coinsurance).

STRATEGIES FOR SUCCESS

▶ Test-Taking Skills

Circle key words?
Do not get a question wrong just because you misread what it was asking you. Notice key words in the question such as *best, not, except, always, never, all*, and any other words that relate to the main point in the question. Doing so will force you to focus on the central point so that you can untangle even more complicated questions.

Instructions:

Answer the following questions.

1. The range of fees charged by most physicians in a community is called the

   A. customary fee.
   B. reasonable fee.
   C. usual fee.
   D. premium.
   E. average fee.

2. If a child is covered by both of her parents' insurances and the total medical charges come to $365—$280 of which is covered by the primary insurance—how are the rest of the charges handled?

   A. The parents are billed for $85.
   B. A claim is submitted to secondary insurance for $85.
   C. A claim is submitted to secondary insurance for $365.
   D. The doctor writes off $85, and no one is charged.
   E. A claim is submitted to secondary insurance for $280.

3. Which of the following is an example of fraud?

   A. miscoding a diagnosis unintentionally
   B. leaving a field blank on the CMS-1500 by mistake
   C. altering a patient's chart to increase the amount reimbursed
   D. releasing patient's medical records without the patient's consent to the patient's wife because you feel morally obligated to do so
   E. all of these

4. Which of the following Medicare programs covers hospital charges?

   A. Part A
   B. Part B
   C. Part C
   D. both Parts A and B
   E. none of these

5. Assume that John Smith got an X-ray through Dr. Jones, a participating provider in Mr. Smith's HMO. The allowed charge for such an X-ray is $75, but Dr. Jones's usual fee is $100. John Smith's copayment due for each office visit is $15. How much can Dr. Jones collect from Mr. Smith?

   A. $25
   B. $10
   C. $15
   D. $0
   E. $75

6. Which of the following types of medical insurance is designed to offset medical expenses resulting from catastrophic or prolonged injury or illness?

   A. basic medical
   B. hospital coverage
   C. disability protection
   D. liability insurance
   E. major medical

7. Capitation is

   A. payment at the time of service.
   B. fixed prospective payment for services provided.
   C. fixed payment made for each enrolled patient rather than reimbursement based on the type and number of services provided.
   D. various payments for specific services provided during a specified time period.
   E. a reduction in payment if services are not provided to a minimum number of enrolled patients.

8. Providers are required by law to file which of the following for all eligible Medicare patients?

   A. CMS
   B. HCPCS
   C. ICD-9
   D. RBRVS
   E. CMS-1500

9. A patient's medical fees come to a total of $600 from a participating provider, and the EOB lists the following information.

Charges:	$78
Not Eligible for Payment:	List item
Allowed Charge:	$63
Applied to Deductible:	$ 7
Coinsurance:	$ 5
Amount Due from Carrier:	$51

   What amount is the patient required to pay?

   A. $7
   B. $5
   C. $27
   D. $12
   E. nothing

10. In the staff model HMO

  A. providers are employees of the HMO.
  B. the HMO has capitation contracts with provider groups.
  C. contracts exist with an administrative group of physicians that in turn contracts with members.
  D. plan members can see out-of-network providers for additional fees.
  E. providers are paid on a fee-for-service basis.

MEDICAL CODING

LEARNING OUTCOMES

15.1 Recognize terminology commonly used in association with medical billing.

15.2 Identify the two types of coding systems and what they are used for.

15.3 Demonstrate the proper procedures for use of the ICD-10-CM.

15.4 Demonstrate the proper procedures for using the CPT.

15.5 Recognize the code range differences between ICD-9-CM and ICD-10-CM.

15.6 Identify Level I, II, and III codes.

15.7 Demonstrate proper coding techniques to avoid fraudulent claims.

MEDICAL ASSISTING COMPETENCIES

COMPETENCY	CMA	RMA	CCMA	NCMA
Administrative				
Apply managed care policies and procedures	X	X	X	
Analyze and apply third-party guidelines	X	X	X	
Perform procedural and diagnostic coding	X	X	X	X
Complete insurance claim forms	X	X	X	
General/Legal/Professional				
Be aware of and perform within legal and ethical boundaries	X	X	X	X
Use appropriate medical terminology	X	X	X	X

15.1 Data and Billing Basics

Coding applies to *prospective payment systems* that apply to various health-care providers. Prospective payment systems exist for inpatient rehabilitation facilities, long-term-care hospitalization, skilled nursing facilities, and others. See Table 15-1.

Inpatient prospective payment system (IPPS): A prospective system with the payment rate set in advance based on the *Medicare severity-diagnosis-related group (MS-DRG)* that is reported.

Medicare severity-diagnosis-related group (MS-DRG): A Medicare system of identification for fixed payment amounts, based on average costs for specified groupings of diagnoses and procedures.

Uniform hospital discharge data set (UHDDS): A standard data set adopted by the federal government for collection of data for Medicare and Medicaid.

Outpatient prospective payment system (OPPS): A system that uses CTP and HCPCS codes, instead of ICD-related codes.

AT A GLANCE | Prospective Payment Systems

Setting	Payment System	Reimbursement	Year Implemented	Data Set
Inpatient acute care hospital	Inpatient prospective payment system (IPPS)	Medicare severity-diagnosis-related groups (MS-DRGs)	DRG—1983 MS-DRG—2007	Uniform Hospital Discharge Data Set (UHDDS)
Physician office	Resource-Based Relative Value Scale (RBRVS)	Medicare fee schedule	1992	None
Skilled nursing facility	Skilled nursing facility prospective payment system (SNF PPS)	Resource utilization groups, Version III (RUG-III)	1998	Minimum Data Set 2.0 (MDS 2.0) Collected using resident assessment instrument (RAI) submitted using data entry software Resident Assessment Validation and Entry (RAVEN)
Outpatient	Outpatient prospective payment system (OPPS)	Ambulatory payment classification (APC)	2000	
Home health	Home health prospective payment system (HH PPS)	Home health resource groups (HHRGs)	2000	Outcome and Assessment Information System (OASIS) submitted using data entry software, Home Assessment Validation and Entry (HAVEN)
Inpatient rehabilitation facility	Inpatient rehabilitation facility prospective payment system (IRF PPS)	Case-mix groups (CMGs)	2002	Inpatient rehabilitation facility patient assessment instrument (IRF-PAI) submitted via Inpatient Rehabilitation Validation and Entry system
Long-term-care hospital	Long-term-care hospital prospective payment system (LTCH PPS)	Medicare severity long-term-care diagnosis-related groups (MS-LTC-DRGs)	2002	None

Table 15-1

Source: Data from ICD-10-CM, Centers for Medicare and Medicaid Services and the National Center for Health Statistics.

However, ICD-related codes are utilized, but must be linked to CPS and HCPCS coding, which completely regulates required payments.

Ambulatory payment classifications (APCs): Categories into which hospital outpatient services are classified for reimbursement.

Outcome and assessment information set (OASIS): An instrument used to document assessment of the home health-care patient's condition.

Home health resource groups (HHRGs): A total of 80 case-mix groups based on clinical presentation, functional factors, and service utilization.

Other data sets: These include the *Data Elements for Emergency Department Systems (DEEDS), National Hospital Ambulatory Medical Care Survey (NHAMCS), National Electronic Disease Surveillance System (NEDSS),* and *Uniform Ambulatory Care Data Set (UACDS).*

15.2 Basic Coding

The two basic types of coding systems are diagnostic and procedural. They are used to keep track of the many thousands of possible diagnoses, procedures, and services rendered by physicians, as well as to simplify the process of verifying the medical necessity of each procedure.

Coding: Converting verbal or written descriptions into numerical and alphanumerical designations. The most important factor in coding is the accuracy of the codes.

Medical coding: The translation of medical terms for diagnoses and procedures into code numbers selected from standardized code sets.

Ancillary diagnostic services: Services that support patient diagnoses, such as radiology or laboratory services.

Ancillary therapeutic services: Services that support patient treatment, such as surgery and visits to specialists.

15.3 Diagnosis Codes: The ICD-10-CM

Like its predecessor, the ICD-9-CM, the new ICD-10-CM contains an alphabetic index and a tabular list (index) with 21 chapters organized by etiology or body system. It consists of three volumes. Its purposes include the compilation of statistical data, indexing of medical records for data storage and retrieval, and facilitating collection of uniform and comparable health information. ICD-10-CM codes may contain as many as seven digits. The first three digits are called the *category,* and are followed by a decimal point. There may be a fourth, fifth, sixth, or seventh digit added for subcategory level coding. Sometimes a *placeholder* character, such as an X, is used after the fourth character. Although the layouts of the ICD-10-CM and ICD-9-CM are similar, the codes are very different.

The ICD-10-CM includes a completely new procedural coding system called the ICD-10-PCS, which is much more detailed and specific than the contents of the ICD-9-CM. The ICD-10-PCS replaced the original "third volume" of the ICD-9-CM. The PCS system is used only for hospital inpatients, and relates to ICD-9-CM procedure codes. All other entities continue to use CPT and HCPCS codes. The ICD-10-CM contains more than 68,000 diagnosis codes and 87,000 procedure codes. Basic terminology is still in use, but coding has become much more extensive.

The three volumes of the ICD-9-CM manual:

- **Volume I:** A tabular list, with 17 chapters; conditions are listed by body systems as well as by causes. This volume also includes:

  - V-codes: Factors that influence health status and contact with health services
  - E-codes: External causes of poisoning and injury
  - M-codes: Morphology of neoplasms
  - American Hospital Formulary drug classifications
  - Industrial accidents, classified by specific agencies
  - Three-digit category list

- **Volume II:** An alphabetic index, organized as follows:

  - Section 1: Diseases and Injuries
  - Section 2: Drugs and Chemicals (in tabular format)
  - Section 3: External Causes of Poisonings and Injuries (to assign E-codes)

- **Volume III:** Procedural codes for hospitals; this is not used in standard medical offices. This volume is titled "Section 3 of Volume II" in some references.

Chief complaint: A description of a patient's medical problem that the patient reports to the physician.

Etiology: The cause of a disorder. A claim is sometimes classified according to its etiology.

Principal diagnosis: The primary condition for which a patient is receiving care.

Preexisting condition: A physical condition that existed before the issuance of a patient's health plan.

Coexisting condition: An additional condition or symptom that is related to a patient's current illness.

Diagnosis: The determination of the nature of a disease, injury, or congenital defect. The diagnosis is communicated to the third-party payer through a diagnosis code on the health-care claim. The abbreviation for diagnosis is Dx.

Medical necessity: In regard to procedural and diagnostic coding, this means something that is reasonable and necessary to diagnosis, or to treat a patient's condition. Coding tells the payer why something was necessary.

Using the ICD-10-CM

New features that you must understand in order to use the ICD-10-CM include:

- *Combination codes:* For external causes of disease and poisonings, information is combined into one code. This means that former complicated sequencing rules are no longer required. For poisonings, alpha extensions are added (the letter *a* stands for *initial encounter,* the letter *d* stands for *subsequent encounter,* and the letter *q* stands for *sequela*).

- *Codes for laterality,* at the fifth or sixth character level, have been added. An example would be C50.511, which stands for malignant neoplasm, lower-outer quadrant, right female breast.

- *Expanded codes* are used for greater detail. An example would be E11.610, which stands for type 2 diabetes mellitus with diabetic neuropathic arthopathy.

- *Flexibility and expandability:* In ICD-10-CM, this allows for much more specificity. An example would be S72.324A, which stands for nondisplaced transverse fracture, shaft of right femur, initial encounter for closed fracture.

- *Requirement for providers to give more detailed diagnoses:* Greater detail in diagnostic information makes it possible to assign the most accurate coding. Most experienced ICD-9-CM coders will easily adapt to ICD-10-CM.

Locating the Correct Codes

In ICD-10-CM, the following basic steps should be performed to locate the correct codes after you review the patient's record and identify the existing conditions.

- Search the *main term* in the alphabetic index, then check for any *subterms* indented below it. Also check for any *cross-reference notes* or *instructional notations.* Sometimes, codes are listed directly next to main terms. Table 15-2 lists basic codes for primary types of conditions. Codes for other specific types of conditions are shown in Tables 15-3 through 15-5. Cross-reference the tabular list and verify that the code selection is the most appropriate. This helps to identify extra characters that must be reported.

AT A GLANCE ICD-10-CM Chapter Structure

Chapter	Code Range	Title
1	A00–B99	Certain infectious and parasitic diseases
2	C00–D49	Neoplasms
3	D50–D89	Diseases of the blood and blood-forming organs and certain disorders involving the immune mechanism
4	E00–E89	Endocrine, nutritional, and metabolic diseases
5	F01–F99	Mental, behavioral, and neurodevelopmental disorders
6	G00–G99	Diseases of the nervous system
7	H00–H59	Diseases of the eye and adnexa
8	H60–H95	Diseases of the ear and mastoid process
9	I00–I99	Diseases of the circulatory system
10	J00–J99	Diseases of the respiratory system
11	K00–K95	Diseases of the digestive system
12	L00–L99	Diseases of the skin and subcutaneous tissue
13	M00–M99	Diseases of the musculoskeletal system and connective tissue
14	N00–N99	Diseases of the genitourinary system
15	O00–O9A	Pregnancy, childbirth, and the puerperium
16	P00–P96	Certain conditions originating in the perinatal period
17	Q00–Q99	Congenital malformations, deformations, and chromosomal abnormalities
18	R00–R99	Symptoms, signs, and abnormal clinical and laboratory findings, not elsewhere classified
19	S00–T88	Injury, poisoning, and certain other consequences of external causes
20	V01–Y99	External causes of morbidity
21	Z00–Z99	Factors influencing health status and contact with health services

Table 15-2
Source: Data from ICD-10-CM, Centers for Medicare and Medicaid Services and the National Center for Health Statistics.

C00–C14	Malignant neoplasms of lip, oral cavity, and pharynx
C15–C26	Malignant neoplasms of digestive organs
C30–C39	Malignant neoplasms of respiratory and intrathoracic organs
C40–C41	Malignant neoplasms of bone and articular cartilage
C43–C44	Melanoma and other malignant neoplasms of skin
C45–C49	Malignant neoplasms of mesothelial and soft tissue
C50–C50	Malignant neoplasms of breast
C51–C58	Malignant neoplasms of female genital organs
C60–C63	Malignant neoplasms of male genital organs
C64–C68	Malignant neoplasms of urinary tract
C69–C72	Malignant neoplasms of eye, brain, and other parts of central nervous system
C73–C75	Malignant neoplasms of thyroid and other endocrine glands
C7A–C7A	Malignant neuroendocrine tumors
C7B–C7B	Secondary neuroendocrine tumors
C76–C80	Malignant neoplasms of ill-defined, other secondary, and unspecified sites
C81–C96	Malignant neoplasms of lymphoid, hematopoietic, and related tissue
D00–D09	In situ neoplasms
D10–D36	Benign neoplasms, except benign neuroendocrine tumors
D3A–D3A	Benign neuroendocrine tumors
D37–D48	Neoplasms of uncertain behavior, polycythemia vera, and myelodysplastic syndromes
D49–D49	Neoplasms of unspecified behavior

Table 15-3

Source: Data from ICD-10-CM, Centers for Medicare and Medicaid Services and the National Center for Health Statistics.

S00–S09	Injuries to the head
S10–S19	Injuries to the neck
S20–S29	Injuries to the thorax
S30–S39	Injuries to the abdomen, lower back, lumbar spine, pelvis, and external genitals
S40–S49	Injuries to the shoulder and upper arm
S50–S59	Injuries to the elbow and forearm
S60–S69	Injuries to the wrist, hand, and fingers
S70–S79	Injuries to the hip and thigh
S80–S89	Injuries to the knee and lower leg
S90–S99	Injuries to the ankle and foot
T07–T07	Injuries involving multiple body regions
T14–T14	Injury of unspecified body region
T15–T19	Effects of foreign body entering through natural orifice
T20–T25	Burns and corrosions of external body surface, specified by site

Table 15-4

T26–T28	Burns and corrosions confined to eye and internal organs
T30–T32	Burns and corrosions of multiple and unspecified body regions
T33–T34	Frostbite
T36–T50	Poisoning by, adverse effect of, and underdosing of drugs, medicaments, and biological substances
T51–T65	Toxic effects of substances chiefly nonmedicinal as to source
T66–T78	Other and unspecified effects of external causes
T79–T79	Certain early complications of trauma
T80–T88	Complications of surgical and medical care, not elsewhere classified

Table 15-4

Source: Data from ICD-10-CM, Centers for Medicare and Medicaid Services and the National Center for Health Statistics.

AT A GLANCE ICD-10-CM Codes for External Causes of Morbidity (V00–Y99)

V00–V09	Pedestrian injured in transport accident
V10–V19	Pedal cycle rider injured in transport accident
V20–V29	Motorcycle rider injured in transport accident
V30–V39	Occupant of three-wheeled motor vehicle injured in transport accident
V40–V49	Car occupant injured in transport accident
V50 V59	Occupant of pickup truck or van injured in transport accident
V60–V69	Occupant of heavy transport vehicle injured in transport accident
V70–V79	Bus occupant injured in transport accident
V80–V89	Other land transport accidents
V90–V94	Water transport accidents
V95–V97	Air and space transport accidents
V98–V99	Other and unspecified transport accidents
W00–W19	Slipping, tripping, stumbling, and falls
W20–W49	Exposure to inanimate mechanical forces
W50–W64	Exposure to animate mechanical forces
W65–W74	Accidental nontransport drowning and submersion
W85–W99	Exposure to electric current, radiation, and extreme ambient air temperature and pressure
X00–X08	Exposure to smoke, fire, and flames
X10–X19	Contact with heat and hot substances
X30–X39	Exposure to forces of nature
X52–X58	Accidental exposure to other specified factors
X71–X83	Intentional self-harm
X92–Y09	Assault
Y21–Y33	Event of undetermined intent
Y35–Y38	Legal intervention, operations of war, military operations, and terrorism
Y62–Y69	Misadventures to patients during surgical and medical care
Y70–Y82	Medical devices associated with adverse incidents in diagnostic and therapeutic use
Y83–Y84	Surgical and other medical procedures as the cause of abnormal reaction of the patient, or of later complication, without mention of misadventure at the time of the procedure
Y90–Y99	Supplementary factors related to causes of morbidity classified elsewhere

Table 15-5

Source: Data from ICD-10-CM, Centers for Medicare and Medicaid Services and the National Center for Health Statistics.

- Look for instructional terms (at the beginnings of chapters, section ranges, or categories). If a condition is described as a *syndrome,* look up the term *syndrome* in the alphabetic index. If there are no additional instructions in the index, the code next to it should be assigned. If there is an additional instruction, you must follow what it says. This continues until all codes are found and no additional instructions remain.

- If there are entries for both *acute* and *chronic,* at the same indentation level, both codes are assigned, usually with the acute code appearing first.

- *Combination codes* must be looked for and used if there are additional details about the patient's condition.

- *Sequela codes* are used if a condition or injury has *late effects,* which may occur anytime in life. Coding depends on whether the condition was confirmed, or is impending or threatening to occur.

Diagnosis codes cannot be reported multiple times for a single encounter—for example, for the same condition occurring bilaterally.

15.4 Procedure Codes

After an office visit, each procedure and service performed for a patient is reported on the health-care claim by using a procedure code. The procedure codes are primarily used in hospitals and other facilities to code the procedures performed in those settings. In ICD-10-CM, procedure codes mostly relate to surgery, but also include patient evaluation, physician management of treatments, medication administration, dental procedures, radiology, laboratory services, and more.

Evolution of CPT Coding

The CPT coding system was developed after the American Medical Association realized that standard descriptions of services were needed for use by all health-care professionals. It originated as a four-digit code, but evolved into the current five-digit format in the 1970s. Its fourth edition introduced periodic annual updating because of rapid advancements in diagnoses and procedures. The fifth edition is the most current edition.

Content of the CPT Manual

Based on which published edition is used, the CPT manual generally contains (1) comprehensive instructions and steps for coding; (2) an alphabetic index; (3) main text ("Tabular List") with six sections, guidelines and notes, and conventions; and (4) 13 appendices.

The Indices

The two primary divisions of the CPT manual are the Alphabetic Index and the Tabular List. The Alphabetic Index is a guide to locating data in the manual; it lists codes or code ranges, which are found in numeric order in each section.

Main Text

The Main Text (Tabular List) has six sections, as follows: (1) evaluation and management, (2) anesthesia, (3) surgery for all body systems, (4) radiology, (5) pathology and laboratory, and (6) medicine. Codes are listed in numeric or alphanumeric order within each section. Each section is divided into general types of service. Further subdivisions include subsections, categories, and subcategories.

Evaluation and Management Section

This section (also referred to as the E&M section) contains codes for various types of visits (encounters) that patients may have with various types of providers. Codes in this section range from 99201 to 99499. Subsections include office/hospital/nursing home visits, consultations, and skilled nursing facility encounters.

Using the CPT

Current Procedural Terminology, commonly known as the CPT, is the most commonly used system of procedure codes. The CPT is published by the American Medical Association (AMA) and is the HIPAA-required code set for physicians' procedures. The CPT is published every year to reflect changes in medical practice. These changes are also available electronically for medical offices that use a computer-based version of the CPT. The medical assistant responsible for coding should attend at least one class each year on ICD-10-CM and CPT.

Locating the Correct Codes

CPT codes are five-digit numbers, organized into six sections (see Table 15-6). Medical offices should have the current year's CPT available for reference. Previous editions of this book also should be kept in case there is a question about previously submitted insurance claims.

Add-on codes: Used for procedures that are usually carried out in addition to another procedure. A plus sign (+) is used to symbolize these codes. Add-on codes are never reported alone. They are used together with the primary code.

Modifiers: Indicate that a procedure was different from the standard description, but not in a way that changed the definition or required a different code. Modifiers are codes that may consist of two digits, two letters, or a combination of both. They help to further describe or clarify the procedure, service, or supply referred to by the primary code. For the modifier section used in CPT coding, there is Appendix A at the end of the book, which explains modifiers that are used. Modifiers are used primarily in the following instances:

- A service or procedure was performed more than once, or by more than one physician.

- A service or procedure has been increased or reduced.

- Unusual difficulties occurred during the procedure.

- Only part of a procedure was performed.

- A service or procedure was altered in some way.

Section	Range of Codes
Evaluation and Management	99201–99499
Anesthesia	00100–01999; 99100–99150
Surgery	10021–69990
Radiology	70010–79999
Pathology and Laboratory	80047–89398
Medicine	90281–99099; 99151–99199; 99500–99607
Category II Codes	0001F–7025F

Table 15-6

Source: Data from ICD-10-CM, Centers for Medicare and Medicaid Services and the National Center for Health Statistics.

Symbols: Commonly used CPT symbols include the following:

- A bullet point (•) indicates a new procedure code.
- A triangle (▲) indicates a change in the code's description.
- Facing triangles (▶◀) are placed at the beginning and end of new or revised information.
- A plus sign (+) is used for add-on codes, indicating procedures that are usually carried out in addition to another procedure.
- An arrow (→) with a circle around it refers to the CPT assistant.
- An asterisk (*) indicates a surgical procedure only.
- A semicolon (;) denotes that everything to its left is applicable to indented shorter descriptions that follow.
- A circle with a line (⊘) through it means modifier-51 is not assigned to the code and the procedures are not add-on procedures.
- A lightning bolt (⚡) indicates the product is pending FDA approval.
- A dot (⊙) surrounded by a circle denotes moderate sedation. It is known as a b*ull's-eye*.

15.5 Comparison of ICD-9-CM and ICD-10-CM

Although many of the chapters in these books have identical or similar titles, the codes themselves are very different. See Table 15-7.

15.6 HCPCS

The Health Care Financing Administration (HCFA) Common Procedure Coding System, commonly referred to as HCPCS, is used to report procedures and services for Medicare patients. This system is also used to report most Medicaid services. HCPCS has three code levels, referred to as Level I, Level II, and Level III.

Level I codes: These codes repeat the CPT's five-number codes for physician procedures and services.

Level II codes: These codes consist of more than 2400 five-digit alphanumerical codes for items that are not listed in CPT-4. Most of these items are supplies, materials, or injections that are covered by Medicare. Level II codes start with a letter followed by four digits, such as J7630. There are 18 sections, each covering a related group of items. See Table 15-8.

Level III codes: Commonly called local carrier codes, these codes are created and used only by the insurance companies that process Medicare for HCFA in the various geographical regions they are assigned.

15.7 Avoiding Fraud

Physicians have the ultimate responsibility for proper documentation and correct coding, as well as for compliance with regulations. Medical assistants help ensure maximum appropriate reimbursement for reported services by submitting correct health-care claims. Ensuring that the proper steps are taken to avoid incorrect coding, false claims, and data entry errors helps to ensure that no fraud takes place in the coding and claims submission process.

Fraud: An act of deception used to take advantage of another person or entity. Claims fraud occurs when physicians or others falsely represent services or charges to payers. Examples of fraud include the following:

- A provider who bills for services that were not performed, overcharges for services, or fails to provide complete services under a contract
- A patient who exaggerates an injury to get a settlement from an insurance company, or one who asks a medical assistant to change a date on the patient's chart so that a service is covered by a health plan

Code linkage: The connection between the diagnostic and procedural information on a health-care claim. Insurance company representatives analyze this connection to evaluate the medical necessity of the reported charges.

ICD-10-CM Chapter Title	ICD-10-CM	ICD-9-CM
Certain Infectious and Parasitic Diseases	A00–B99	001–139
Neoplasms	C00–D49	140–239
Diseases of the Blood and Blood-Forming Organs and Certain Disorders Involving the Immune Mechanism	D50–D89	280–289 (only includes diseases of blood and blood-forming organs)
Endocrine, Nutritional, and Metabolic Diseases	E00–E89	240–279 (also includes immunity disorders)
Mental and Behavioral Disorders	F01–F99	290–319
Diseases of the Nervous System	G00–G99	320–389 (Diseases of the Nervous System and Sense Organs)
Diseases of the Eye and Adnexa	H00–H59	
Diseases of the Ear and Mastoid Process	H60–H95	
Diseases of the Circulatory System	100–199	390–459
Diseases of the Respiratory System	J00–J99	460–519
Diseases of the Digestive System	K00–K94	520–579
Diseases of the Skin and Subcutaneous Tissue	L00–L99	680–709
Diseases of the Musculoskeletal System and Connective Tissue	M00–M99	710–739
Diseases of the Genitourinary System	N00–N99	580–629
Pregnancy, Childbirth, and the Puerperium	O00–O9a	630–677 (Complications of Pregnancy, Childbirth, and the Puerperium)
Certain Conditions Originating in the Perinatal Period	P00–P96	760–779
Congenital Malformations, Deformations, and Chromosomal Abnormalities	Q00–Q99	740–759 (Congenital Anomalies)
Symptoms, Signs, and Abnormal Clinical Laboratory Findings, Not Elsewhere Classified	R00–R99	780–799 (Symptoms, Signs, and Ill-Defined Conditions)
Injury Poisoning and Certain Other Consequences of External Causes	S00–T88	800–999 (Injury and Poisoning)
External Causes of Morbidity	V00–Y98	E800–E999 Supplementary Classification of External Causes of Injury and Poisoning
Factors Influencing Health Status and Contact with Health Services	Z00–Z99	V01–V83 Supplementary Classification of Factors Influencing Health Status and Contact with Health Services

Table 15-7

Source: Data from ICD-10-CM, Centers for Medicare and Medicaid Services and the National Center for Health Statistics.

AT A GLANCE HCPCS (Level II Codes)

Sections	Codes
Transportation	A0000–A0999
Medical and surgical supplies	A4000–A4999
Miscellaneous and experimental	A9000–A9999
Enteral and parenteral therapy	B4000–B9999
Temporary Hospital Outpatient Prospective Payment System	C0000–C9999
Dental procedures	D0000 D9999
Durable medical equipment (DME)	E0000–E9999
Temporary Procedures and Professional Services	G0000–G9999
Rehabilitative Services	H0000–H9999
Drugs administered other than by oral method	J0000–J8999
Chemotherapy drugs	J9000–J9999
Temporary codes for durable medical equipment regional carriers	K0000–K9999
Orthotic procedures	L0000–L4999
Prosthetic procedures	L5000–L9999
Medical services	M0000–M9999
Pathology and laboratory	P0000–P9999
Temporary codes	Q0000–Q0099
Diagnostic radiology services	R0000–R5999
Private Payer Codes	S0000–S9999
State Medicaid Agency Codes	T0000–T9999
Vision services	V0000–V2999
Hearing services	V5000–V5999

Table 15-8

Source: Data from ICD-10-CM, Centers for Medicare and Medicaid Services and the National Center for Health Statistics.

Coding for coverage: Changing a code to match what the insurance company will pay for, rather than to accurately reflect the procedure that was performed.
Upcoding: Using a code on a claim form that indicates a higher level of service than that which was actually performed.
Double billing: Submitting two claims for one encounter.

Correct Coding Initiative (CCI): A computerized system used by Medicare to prevent overpayment for procedures.
Mutually exclusive codes: Codes that are identified in the coding book as not permitted to be used on the same claim form with other specified codes.

CHAPTER 15 REVIEW

Instructions:
Answer the following questions.

1. How many volumes are in ICD-10-CM?

   A. There are two volumes in ICD-10-CM.
   B. There are three volumes in ICD-10-CM.
   C. There are five volumes in ICD-10 CM.
   D. There are 17 volumes in ICD-10-CM.

2. Because coding information is revised annually, medical assistants responsible for coding should

   A. attend at least one CPT class each year.
   B. attend at least one ICD-10 class every two years.
   C. attend at least one ICD-10 and one CPT class every two years.
   D. attend at least one CPT and one ICD-10 class each year.
   E. review codes in their spare time; there is no need to attend classes.

3. How many digits are assigned to the primary code in the CPT coding system?

   A. two
   B. three
   C. four
   D. five
   E. six

4. To locate the correct codes in the ICD-10-CM, you should begin with

   A. the main term and indented subterms below it.
   B. the CPT code.
   C. the HCPCS code.
   D. the sequela codes.
   E. the expanded codes.

5. Which of the following ICD-10-CM codes indicates cancer?

   A. S00–T88
   B. D50–D89
   C. C00–D49
   D. N00–N99
   E. O00–O9a

6. Which of the following is the most important factor in coding?

   A. level of codes
   B. quantity of codes
   C. accuracy of codes
   D. speed of coding process
   E. knowledge and understanding of medical terms

7. Which of the following is indicated by two "facing triangles" (▶ ◀) placed at the beginning and end of a new CPT code?

   A. new procedure code
   B. add-on codes
   C. surgical procedure only
   D. new or revised information

8. Level III of the HCPCS codes are commonly called

   A. international codes.
   B. local carrier codes.
   C. diagnosis-related groups.
   D. G codes.

9. CPT codes are organized into how many sections?

   A. two
   B. three
   C. five
   D. six
   E. nine

10. How many chapters of disease descriptions and codes are included in the *Tabular List* of the ICD-10-CM?

    A. 5
    B. 12
    C. 17
    D. 19
    E. 21

SECTION 2 CMA REVIEW

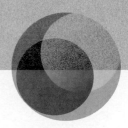

CMA Questions for the End of Section 2 (Chapters 9–15, mixed)

1. When an incoming call is received, the telephone should be answered
   A. within one minute.
   B. by the second or third ring.
   C. by the fourth or fifth ring.
   D. when there is no patient nearby.
   E. after the doctor has been helped.

2. Which of the following word-processing functions is most appropriate for the medical assistant to use when verifying the accuracy of words in a business letter?
   A. word count
   B. spell check
   C. sort
   D. find and replace
   E. autocorrect

3. Which of the following scheduling systems is most likely to decrease the patient's waiting time?
   A. wave
   B. stream
   C. open hours
   D. clustering
   E. modified wave

4. For mentally disabled patients, you should always
   A. spend 50% less time with them than with normal patients.
   B. remain calm if they become confused.
   C. treat them the same as everyone else.
   D. treat them as you would treat an infant.
   E. call them by their first name.

5. Which of the following computer technologies is likely to become further advanced?
   A. telemedicine
   B. software
   C. speech recognition technology
   D. hardware
   E. all of these

6. When new supplies are received, you should
   A. throw out the old ones.
   B. place them in the front of the storage area.
   C. place them in the back of the storage area.
   D. inventory all supplies.
   E. none of these

7. According to the CPT, when a health-care claim for the removal of a melanoma is coded, the code should be listed under which of the following body systems?
   A. respiratory
   B. integumentary
   C. digestive
   D. endocrine
   E. cardiovascular

8. Which of the following parts of a business letter is keyed on the second line below the salutation?
   A. complimentary close
   B. enclosure notation
   C. subject line
   D. reference initials
   E. date line

9. When communicating with very young patients, you should
   A. treat them the same as adults.
   B. bargain with them.
   C. explain any procedure in very simple terms.
   D. mimic their behaviors.
   E. show them videotapes of procedures.

10. What is the trial balance?
    A. a daily summary
    B. a way of checking the accuracy of accounts
    C. an accounting system
    D. accrual accounting
    E. bookkeeping

11. A two-digit modified attached to the five-digit CPT code indicates
    A. the severity of the patient's illness.
    B. the time services were performed.
    C. a service or procedure has been altered.
    D. a surgical procedure was performed.
    E. where services were performed.

12. Two patients are scheduled for an appointment at the same time on the same day. This is an example of which of the following scheduling systems?
    A. stream
    B. modified wave
    C. double booking
    D. cluster
    E. categorization

13. The goal of a medical assistant to treat patients so that they become comfortable and at ease is achieved by

    A. good appointment scheduling.
    B. policy and procedure.
    C. patient confidentiality statement.
    D. good attitude.
    E. therapeutic communication.

14. Copying an amount from a journal onto a ledger is an example of

    A. deducting.
    B. superbilling.
    C. posting.
    D. trial balancing.
    E. crediting.

15. Which of the following is true about Blue Cross and Blue Shield?

    A. It offers prepaid health services.
    B. It helps Medicare to determine covered health services.
    C. It follows a fee-for-service reimbursement plan.
    D. It offers prepaid health services *and* follows a fee-for-service reimbursement plan.
    E. all of these

16. Which of the following is a coding system used to document the procedure for suturing a laceration?

    A. relative value studies (RVS)
    B. resource-based relative value scale (RBRVS)
    C. diagnostic-related groups (DRGs)
    D. International Classification of Diseases, Clinical Modification (ICD-CM)
    E. Current Procedural Terminology (CPT)

17. Financial information

    A. should always be included in the patient's medical records.
    B. should be included in the patient's medical record if the patient has been delinquent in payments.
    C. should not be included in the patient's medical records.
    D. should be included in the patient's medical record if the patient requests it.
    E. should be included in the patient's medical record if the patient's insurance provider requires it.

18. The three types of listening are evaluative, active, and

    A. two-way.
    B. responsive.
    C. selective.
    D. passive.
    E. circumstantial.

19. When similar programs are functioning simultaneously in a computer system, what is this known as?

    A. batch processing
    B. database management
    C. HTML
    D. cache storage
    E. purging

20. The amount due from the patient for covered services from a participating provider is the difference between

    A. the allowed charge and the physician's fee.
    B. the allowed charge and the patient's deductible and/or coinsurance.
    C. the physician's fee and the coinsurance.
    D. the physician's fee and the deductible.
    E. the physician's fee and the capitation.

21. Changing a code to one you know the insurance company will pay for is called

    A. double billing.
    B. unbundling.
    C. coding for packaging.
    D. coding for coverage.
    E. supporting documentation.

22. The screening and sorting of emergency situations is called

    A. emergency reception.
    B. documenting emergencies.
    C. telephone emergencies.
    D. incoming emergencies.
    E. emergency triage.

23. Elderly patients

    A. are often frail or confused.
    B. should be allowed to examine all instruments.
    C. should be praised for good behavior.
    D. are usually in denial.
    E. should be addressed as "Mr." or "Mrs." unless they tell you otherwise.

24. Amounts charged with suppliers or creditors that remain unpaid are referred to as

A. bookkeeping.
B. accounts receivable.
C. account balances.
D. accounts payable.
E. assets.

25. If a policyholder of an 80:20 plan had foot surgery that cost $3,600, then how much of this bill is the subscriber responsible to pay?

A. $450
B. $720
C. $180
D. $2,880
E. $3,600

26. Which of the following is the main purpose of the ICD-10-CM?

A. to compile statistical data
B. to index medical records for data storage and retrieval
C. to facilitate the collection of uniform and comparable health information
D. none of these
E. all of these

27. Which of the following is not one of the five steps involved in filing?

A. conditioning
B. releasing
C. subjecting
D. storing and filing
E. indexing and coding

28. Which of the following pointing devices manipulates the cursor on the monitor screen?

A. mouse
B. trackball
C. touch pad
D. all of these
E. none of these

29. What does "debit" mean?

A. total
B. credit
C. charge
D. subtotal
E. balance

30. The ICD-10-CM codes for classifying injury, poisoning, and certain other consequences of external causes are coded between

A. S00 and T88.
B. D50 and D89.
C. V00 and Y98.
D. R00 and R99.
E. P00 and P96.

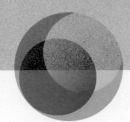
RMA Questions for the End of Section 2 (Chapters 9–15, mixed)

1. When processing incoming mail, adding explanatory notes is known as
   A. indexing.
   B. sorting.
   C. annotating.
   D. postmarking.

2. When a proofreader adds a period with a circle around it, you should
   A. insert a period into the text.
   B. underline the text.
   C. stop the text here and create a new paragraph.
   D. omit all the text before the period.

3. Which of the following methods of preparing outgoing First-Class Mail is most appropriate to expedite delivery?
   A. sorting letters alphabetically by addressee
   B. separating letters according to zip code
   C. verifying all addresses
   D. weighing each piece of mail

4. Interoffice memorandums do not contain which of the following?
   A. the date
   B. written information
   C. the names of any intended recipients
   D. a salutation

5. When reconciling a bank statement for the medical practice, daily deposits should be
   A. subtracted from the bank statement balance.
   B. subtracted from the checkbook balance.
   C. added to the bank statement balance.
   D. added to the checkbook balance.

6. Which of the following forms is the wage and tax statement that identifies an employee's earnings and taxes withheld?
   A. W-2
   B. W-3
   C. W-4
   D. SS-4

7. Which of the following word-processing functions is activated when the "Enter" key is pressed?
   A. indent
   B. word wrap
   C. bold
   D. hard return

8. Which of the following components of a patient's medical record is objective information?
   A. treatment prescribed
   B. medical history
   C. marital status
   D. chief complaint

9. Which of the following tax forms should be completed by new employees, and is referred to as an "employee withholding allowance certificate"?
   A. 1040
   B. W-2
   C. W-3
   D. W-4

10. Traveler's checks can be purchased at which of the following?
    A. United States Post Office
    B. convenience store
    C. bank
    D. airport

11. Which of the following contains detailed instructions for completing tasks in the medical office?
    A. risk management plan
    B. procedure manual
    C. exposure control plan
    D. patient information brochure

12. In addition to the patient's name, which of the following is the most important information to record when scheduling an appointment for a new patient?
    A. home address
    B. insurance company
    C. daytime telephone number
    D. date of birth

13. How many digits are contained in an International Classification of Diseases, Tenth Revision, Clinical Modification (ICD-10-CM) code that is listed at the highest level of specificity?
    A. two
    B. three
    C. four
    D. five

14. In which order should a tickler file be kept?

    A. numeric
    B. subject
    C. alphabetical
    D. chronological

15. Nonverbal communication is also known as

    A. touching.
    B. conciseness.
    C. body language.
    D. nodding.

16. Copies of all bills and order forms for supplies should be kept on file for at least

    A. three years.
    B. five years.
    C. seven years.
    D. 10 years.

17. The most common insurance claim form is the

    A. CMS-1500.
    B. ICD-10.
    C. superbill.
    D. charge sheet.

18. TRICARE is a health-care benefit program for all of the following *except*

    A. families of uniformed personnel.
    B. veterans with service-related disabilities.
    C. the National Oceanic and Atmospheric Administration.
    D. the Coast Guard.

19. The federal law requiring disclosure of finance charges and late fees for payment plans is referred to as the

    A. Truth in Lending Act.
    B. Fair Credit Billing Act.
    C. Equal Credit Opportunity Act.
    D. Wagner Act of 1935.

20. Scheduling obstetric appointments in the morning and gynecologic appointments in the afternoon is an example of which of the following scheduling methods?

    A. wave
    B. stream
    C. modified wave
    D. clustering

21. Which of the following is a financial record that shows payments for minor office expenses?

    A. invoice
    B. petty cash log
    C. purchase order
    D. accounts payable

22. Which of the following terms means "typing text midway between the left and right margins"?

    A. spread heading
    B. formatting
    C. vertical centering
    D. horizontal centering

23. Which of the following is a mail service that provides the sender proof of delivery?

    A. Certificate of Mailing
    B. Express Mail
    C. Registered Mail
    D. Priority Mail

24. Which of the following exists when payments exceed charges?

    A. credit balance
    B. disbursement
    C. payable
    D. adjustment

25. Which of the following medical record filing systems best provides confidentiality of patient information and ease of expansion?

    A. tickler
    B. numeric
    C. alphabetic
    D. subject

26. Which of the following categories of diagnoses is coded on insurance claim forms?

    A. probable
    B. possible
    C. suspected
    D. established

27. A breakdown resulting from software or hardware malfunction is called a

    A. bug.
    B. crash.
    C. syntax error.
    D. backup.

28. Which of the following information included in a patient's medical record is subjective information?

    A. radiology reports

    B. treatment prescribed

    C. patient's family history

    D. laboratory results

29. Which of the following federal statutes protects debtors from harassment?

    A. Fair Debt Collection Practices Act

    B. Equal Credit Opportunity Act

    C. Truth in Lending Act

    D. Fair Credit Reporting Act

30. On an envelope, which of the following is the most appropriate placement of notations for the postal service?

    A. right upper corner, below the stamp

    B. left upper corner, above the return address

    C. left lower corner

    D. below the delivery address

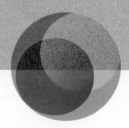

CCMA Questions for the End of Section 2 (Chapters 9–15, mixed)

1. The simplest direct filing system for maintaining patient files is
   A. numeric filing.
   B. chronological filing.
   C. subject filing.
   D. alphabetic filing.

2. The patient record is considered to be the property of the
   A. patient.
   B. physician.
   C. attorney.
   D. court.

3. Which of the following ICD-10-CM codes indicates mental disorders?
   A. F01–F99
   B. G00–G99
   C. H00–H59
   D. J00–J99

4. In most insurance plans, the primary care physician is reimbursed using which of the following methods?
   A. fee-for-service
   B. dual coverage
   C. copayment
   D. capitation

5. A claim that is accepted by a health plan for adjudication is called a
   A. determination.
   B. clean claim.
   C. guarantor.
   D. bundled payment.

6. How long should immunization records be kept in the medical office?
   A. two years
   B. five years
   C. 10 years
   D. permanently

7. Which of the following columns is located on the left side of the accounts receivable ledger, and is used for entering charges?
   A. balance
   B. debit
   C. adjustment
   D. credit

8. Which of the following scheduling systems is limited to practices in which more than one patient can be attended to at a time?
   A. double-booking
   B. wave scheduling
   C. cluster scheduling
   D. grouping

9. Which of the following is another name for the general journal?
   A. cash payment journal
   B. accounts receivable ledger
   C. daysheet
   D. professional income record

10. Which of the following is the correct format for the name in the inside address, in a letter to a physician?
    A. Dr. Smith
    B. Doctor Smith
    C. Doctor David Smith, M.D.
    D. David Smith, M.D.

11. According to current law, employers are responsible for paying which of the following for each employee without matching funds from the employee?
    A. state disability insurance
    B. Medicare assessment
    C. Federal Unemployment Tax Act (FUTA)
    D. Federal Insurance Contribution Act (FICA)

12. Leaving two appointment times open in the daily schedule is known as
    A. offering flexible office hours.
    B. adding buffer time.
    C. using modified-wave scheduling.
    D. performing triage.

13. When is the most appropriate time to discuss payment arrangements with a new patient?
    A. when mailing month-end billing statements
    B. when the patient calls for an appointment
    C. when the patient's insurance form is processed
    D. at the time of the first scheduled appointment

14. The office policy manual should begin with which of the following?
    A. physician's credentials
    B. mission statement
    C. office hours
    D. hierarchy chart

15. Which of the following mail services guarantees overnight delivery?

    A. Express

    B. Insured

    C. Registered

    D. Certified

16. A physician plans to attend a seminar in another state. Which of the following is the most appropriate first step for the medical assistant who is making his or her travel arrangements?

    A. delegate the task to the receptionist

    B. research the city where the seminar is being held

    C. obtain the pertinent details and preferences from the physician

    D. contact a travel agency to make the arrangements

17. Which of the following computer keys is used to remove characters to the right of the cursor?

    A. Escape

    B. Delete

    C. Backspace

    D. Control

18. The insurance program that provides for medically indigent people is

    A. BlueShield.

    B. CHAMPVA.

    C. Medicaid.

    D. Medicare.

19. The proofreader's mark "#" means to insert a

    A. hyphen.

    B. semicolon.

    C. period.

    D. space.

20. Patients who require more examination time are scheduled at the beginning of each hour. Patients who require less examination time are scheduled 20 minutes after the hour. Patients who call at the last minute are scheduled at the end of each hour. This is an example of which of the following types of appointment scheduling?

    A. wave

    B. advance

    C. grouping

    D. clustering

21. Which of the following is a scheduling system in which the office hours are posted and the patients are seen in the order that they arrive?

    A. double-booking

    B. modified wave

    C. open hours

    D. clustering

22. The amount of income tax withheld from an employee's salary is based on which of the following criteria?

    A. number of exemptions

    B. number of years employed

    C. number of employees

    D. gender

23. When using the modified-block letter style (standard), the date line, complimentary close, and typewritten signature should start at which of the following locations?

    A. flush with the right margin

    B. flush with the left margin

    C. five spaces from the left margin

    D. at the center of the page

24. Which of the following forms is used to verify that supplies ordered were received?

    A. supply list

    B. packing slip

    C. purchase order

    D. routing form

25. A computer maintenance agreement should include which of the following stipulations?

    A. replacement of outdated equipment

    B. instructions for minor repairs

    C. timely service

    D. software upgrades

26. An unscheduled patient comes to a primary care physician's office because he has an eye injury. The schedule is full. The most appropriate course of action is to

    A. give him an appointment at the end of the next day.

    B. examine the eye to determine if an appointment is necessary.

    C. take him to an examination room immediately.

    D. ask him to wait and work him into the schedule.

27. Which of the following is often called the "brains" of the computer?

 A. read-only memory (ROM)
 B. central processing unit (CPU)
 C. random-access memory (RAM)
 D. cathode ray tube (CRT)

28. When making arrangements for a meeting, the first logical step is to determine the

 A. number attending.
 B. date and time.
 C. budget allowed.
 D. type of meeting.

29. Which of the following devices transfers information from one computer to another over telephone lines?

 A. modem
 B. printer
 C. flash drive
 D. router

30. Premiums are greater in which of the following types of health plans?

 A. indemnity plans
 B. individual plans
 C. service benefit plans
 D. group policies

SECTION 2 NCMA REVIEW

NCMA Questions for the End of Section 2 (Chapters 9–15, mixed)

1. Which of the following terms is misspelled?

   A. fascinate
   B. entrepreneur
   C. guarante
   D. inimitable

2. A person who cooperates in a fraudulent situation becomes

   A. compliant.
   B. liable.
   C. negligent.
   D. malfeasant.

3. The new ICD-10-CM contains an alphabetic index and a tabular list with how many chapters organized by body system?

   A. 7
   B. 10
   C. 13
   D. 17

4. A physician will most likely terminate a physician–patient relationship for which of the following reasons?

   A. The patient lacks insurance coverage.
   B. The patient has moved to another state.
   C. The patient has been cured.
   D. The patient has been noncompliant.

5. Which of the following is accomplished by using the therapeutic communication technique of restating information obtained from the patient?

   A. showing the importance of the patient's feelings
   B. validating the medical assistant's interpretation of the patient's information
   C. helping the patient understand what information is required before the examination
   D. encouraging a response from the patient

6. Which of the following types of listening behaviors is most effective when questioning a patient about history and symptoms?

   A. passive
   B. selective
   C. active
   D. evaluative

7. The contents of a patient's medical record can be disclosed after written consent has been given by which of the following persons?

   A. the patient
   B. the referred physician
   C. the patient's spouse
   D. the patient's insurance company

8. Which of the following types of mail is most appropriate for sending a letter of dismissal?

   A. First-Class
   B. Priority
   C. Overnight
   D. Certified, returned receipt

9. When an insurance payment is posted to the daysheet, the Medicare nonallowable amount should be posted in which of the following columns?

   A. balance
   B. adjustments
   C. description
   D. credit

10. Which of the following types of filing systems is designed to reduce misfiling of patient folders?

    A. subject
    B. color coded
    C. numeric
    D. cross-reference

11. Which of the following is the primary benefit of numeric filing?

    A. Less storage space is required.
    B. Patient confidentiality is preserved.
    C. Files may be stored either vertically or horizontally.
    D. Color coding is not necessary.

12. Which of the following parts of a business letter is keyed on the second line below the salutation?

    A. subject line
    B. enclosure notation
    C. reference initials
    D. date

13. Which of the following should be placed on top of a stack of incoming mail for the physician's attention?

    A. patient payment
    B. seminar brochure
    C. medical journal
    D. consultant's report

14. Which of the following is the function of the tab key on the computer keyboard?

   A. moving the cursor to a predetermined number of spaces to the right
   B. moving the cursor to the left margin
   C. setting the margins
   D. centering the cursor

15. Which of the following terms refers to assets?

   A. bank debts
   B. notes payable
   C. accounts payable
   D. supplier/vendor inventory

16. Which of the following endocrine glands secretes glucagon?

   A. thyroid gland
   B. thymus gland
   C. kidneys
   D. pancreas

17. Scheduling based on the reality that some patients will arrive late and others will require more or less time is known as which of the following?

   A. wave
   B. time-specified
   C. advance booking
   D. combination

18. Which of the following types of computer software is most appropriate to use when designing an office brochure?

   A. spreadsheet
   B. presentation
   C. desktop publishing
   D. communications

19. How often do employers pay amounts due per the Federal Unemployment Tax Act (FUTA), which are referred to as the FUTA tax?

   A. weekly
   B. monthly
   C. quarterly
   D. yearly

20. Toxemia of pregnancy that results in convulsions and coma is called

   A. eclampsia.
   B. preeclampsia.
   C. endometriosis.
   D. malignant hypertension.

21. A 62-year-old woman with coronary artery disease, hypertension, and stable type 2 diabetes mellitus is seen for evaluation because of dysuria. Which of the following is the most likely primary diagnosis?

   A. hypertension
   B. type 2 diabetes mellitus
   C. coronary artery disease
   D. urinary tract infection

22. Which of the following proofreader's symbols means "move text to the left"?

   A. [
   B.]
   C. ^
   D. lc

23. Which of the following filing systems identifies the patient by primary name and creates a file for all medical records relative to the name?

   A. color-coded
   B. numeric
   C. tickler
   D. subject

24. Which of these steps must be followed to ensure coverage by a patient's insurance company before the patient undergoes surgery to repair a rotator cuff?

   A. verifying the amount of the patient's copayment and deductible
   B. precertifying the surgical procedure
   C. estimating the cost of the surgery
   D. completing a "certificate of need" application

25. Which of the following items is part of a single-entry bookkeeping system?

   A. receipt
   B. calculator
   C. pegboard
   D. computer software

26. Which of the following expenses is most likely to be paid with petty cash?

    A. repair of a photocopier
    B. employee holiday party
    C. laboratory supplies
    D. postage due

27. Which of the following computer terms refers to the size and style of type?

    A. font
    B. format
    C. byte
    D. edit

28. Which of the following documents is most appropriate for verifying a supply order when supplies are received?

    A. packing slip
    B. purchase order
    C. requisition form
    D. billing invoice

29. Which of the following should replace a medical record if it has been temporarily removed from a filing cabinet?

    A. Post-it note
    B. empty folder
    C. outguide
    D. 3 x 5 index card

30. Spreadsheets are used most commonly for which of the following tasks?

    A. word processing
    B. desktop publishing
    C. appointment scheduling
    D. accounting

CLINICAL MEDICAL ASSISTING KNOWLEDGE

SECTION 3

CHAPTER 16

BLOOD-BORNE PATHOGENS AND PRINCIPLES OF ASEPSIS

LEARNING OUTCOMES

16.1 Identify blood-borne pathogens and related terminology.

16.2 Demonstrate proper techniques for performing medical and surgical asepsis.

16.3 Explain the workplace standards set by OSHA and the penalties for failure to comply.

MEDICAL ASSISTING COMPETENCIES

COMPETENCY	CMA	RMA	CCMA	NCMA
Clinical				
Apply principles of aseptic techniques and infection control, including hand washing	X	X	X	X
Wrap items for autoclaving	X	X	X	X
Perform sterilization techniques	X	X	X	X
Dispose of biohazardous materials	X	X	X	X
Practice Standard Precautions	X	X	X	X
Screen and follow up on patient test results	X	X	X	X
General/Legal/Professional				
Identify and respond to issues of confidentiality by maintaining confidentiality at all times and following appropriate guidelines when releasing records or information	X	X	X	X
Be aware of and perform within legal and ethical boundaries	X	X	X	X
Determine the needs for documentation and reporting, and document accurately and appropriately	X	X	X	X

MEDICAL ASSISTING COMPETENCIES (cont.)

General/Legal/Professional

Demonstrate knowledge of and monitor current federal and state health-care legislation and regulation; maintain licenses and accreditation	X	X		X
Perform risk management procedures		X		
Instruct individuals according to their needs	X	X	X	X
Provide patients with methods of health promotion and disease prevention	X	X	X	
Identify community resources and information for patients and employers	X	X	X	
Be courteous and diplomatic		X	X	
Be impartial and show empathy when dealing with patients		X	X	

STRATEGIES FOR SUCCESS

▶ *Study Skills*

Prepare for class!

You can understand a lecture better and retain more information if you take time before class to read the material that is going to be covered. If your instructor tells you which chapters will be discussed on a certain date, you should have plenty of time to review the information beforehand. Even if you don't have time to read a whole chapter, you should scan it for key concepts and headings. This background information will make the lecture material more comprehensible and perhaps even provide an outline for your notes in class.

16.1 Blood-Borne Pathogens

Pathogen: Any microorganism that causes a disease.

Blood-borne pathogens: Disease-causing microorganisms that spread from one person to another via blood. The most common blood-borne pathogens are the hepatitis B virus (HBV) and human immunodeficiency virus (HIV), but blood-borne pathogens are not limited to these two pathogens.

Potentially infectious body fluids: Body fluid visibly contaminated with blood; seminal and vaginal secretions; cerebrospinal, amniotic, and other body fluids; mucus, and tissue cultures.

Contaminated: Exhibiting the presence of blood or other potentially infectious materials. No longer clean or sterile.

Biohazard: Anything that poses a risk to the human body or other living organism, such as blood (which can cause the spread of infections), chemical materials, or ionizing radiation.

Biohazard container: A leakproof, puncture-resistant container that is color-coded red or labeled with a biohazard symbol and is used to store and dispose of contaminated supplies and equipment. When a biohazard container is filled to the three-quarter mark, it should be placed in a locked storage area until pickup. All biohazard containers must have a fluorescent orange or orange-red label with the biohazard symbol and the word *BIOHAZARD* in a contrasting color. Every container must have a lid that is replaced after use. These containers are used for disposable gowns, table covers, items contaminated with blood and body fluids, dressings, gloves, needles, and sharp objects. Biohazard waste must be disposed of in accordance with all federal, state, and local regulations. Disposal methods include treatment by heat, incineration, chemical treatment, steam sterilization, and other safe, equivalent methods that inactivate the waste before it is placed in a landfill. All biohazard containers must have a displayed address in case they get separated on the way to disposal.

Sharps: Needles, scalpels, scissors, or other objects that could cause wounds or punctures to individuals handling them. Sharps should be disposed of into a biohazardous waste container designed to contain them.

Needlestick injuries: Accidental skin punctures resulting from contact with hypodermic syringe needles. These injuries can be dangerous, particularly if the needle has been used in a patient with a severe blood-borne infection. Needles should never be recapped or broken. They must be discarded immediately into a sharps container. If an injury occurs, wash your hands, cover the injury, report and document the injury, and get the injury treated.

Exposure potential: The possibility of bodily contact with a safety hazard, a hazardous chemical, or blood or other potentially infectious material.

Hazardous chemical: A chemical that is explosive, unstable, flammable, carcinogenic, irritating, or that contains toxic agents.

Occupational exposure: Contact with blood or other potentially infected body fluids that occurs as a result of the normal duties of an employee at work.

Disease Profiles
Hepatitis

Hepatitis: Inflammation and infection of the liver that may be caused by several factors, such as drugs, toxins, and microorganisms. The most common cause of hepatitis is a virus. There are six known hepatitis viruses, designated A, B, C, D, E, and G.

Hepatitis A: Inflammation of the liver caused by the hepatitis A virus (HAV), which is transmitted by fecal-oral contamination. Hepatitis A is not generally considered to be an important risk to health-care workers. It is also called acute infective hepatitis.

Hepatitis B: Inflammation of the liver caused by the hepatitis B virus (HBV). It is the main blood-borne hazard for health-care workers. HBV can be transmitted through contaminated serum and plasma; contaminated needles (involved in needle-stick injuries or IV drug use); cuts caused by contaminated sharps; sexual contact with an infected person; and splashes of contaminated material onto the eyes, mouth, nose, or broken skin. HBV is also transmitted from infected mothers to newborns. It is a severe infection that may cause a prolonged illness and become a chronic disease resulting in destruction of liver tissues, cirrhosis, or death. It is also known as serum hepatitis. The virus is capable of surviving for at least a week in a dried state on environmental surfaces.

Acute hepatitis B: Approximately one-third of all patients are asymptomatic. The initial symptoms, if present, last from 2–14 days. No specific treatment or drug kills the hepatitis virus. Approximately 90% of patients recover fully after the acute phase.

Chronic hepatitis B: Approximately 10% of patients who do not recover from the acute phase go on to develop chronic hepatitis. These patients face an increased risk of liver damage, cirrhosis of the liver, liver cancer, or liver failure.

Hepatitis B vaccine: Approximately 90% effective in providing immunity for at least seven years. The vaccine is recommended as a series of three intramuscular doses in infants, children, adolescents, and adults. Employers must offer this vaccine within 10 days of employment if there is a reasonable expectation of exposure to the virus. At the present time, a routine booster dose is not recommended. The hepatitis B vaccine is recommended for the following individuals:

- Health-care workers in high-risk occupations, such as physicians, dentists, dental hygienists, medical assistants, nurses, and laboratory personnel
- Staff members of residential institutions
- Sexually active homosexual men
- Intravenous drug users
- Persons with hemophilia
- Hemodialysis patients
- Household members or sexual contacts of hepatitis B carriers

Hepatitis C (non-A, non-B hepatitis): A chronic disease transmitted largely by a blood transfusion or intravenous drug use (sharing needles). Diagnosis is made by detecting HCV antibodies. There is no cure.

Hepatitis D: Also called delta hepatitis, a form of viral hepatitis that occurs only in patients infected with hepatitis B; consequently, it can be prevented by hepatitis B vaccination. The hepatitis D virus (HDV) is transmitted through needle-sharing and sex. Diagnosis is made by detecting HDV serum antibodies. It is not common in the United States.

Hepatitis E: A common acute infection of the liver, similar to hepatitis A, seen mainly in Southeast Asia, South America, and Africa. Hepatitis E is frequently seen in the rainy season or after natural disasters because of fecally contaminated water or food. There is no serological test available for the detection of the hepatitis E virus (HEV). The disease is most dangerous in pregnant women and increases the mortality rate among them.

Hepatitis G: Inflammation of the liver caused by the single-stranded RNA flavivirus. Mode of spread is usually blood and possibly semen. Incubation period for hepatitis G may be weeks. There is no vaccine, and the symptoms are usually mild. Viremia may be persistent for months or years.

HIV and AIDS

HIV: The human immunodeficiency virus that causes AIDS. It is passed from one person to another through blood-to-blood and sexual contact. Infected pregnant women can pass the virus to their babies during pregnancy or delivery or by breast-feeding. It is not spread through casual contact. HIV infects and destroys T lymphocytes (T cells) of the immune system.

HIV transmission: HIV has been isolated in blood, semen, saliva, tears, breast milk, cerebrospinal fluid (CSF), amniotic fluid, urine, and vaginal secretions. No cases of AIDS have been reported as a result of exposure to saliva or tears. However, definite means of transmission of HIV are through the blood, semen, vaginal secretions, or any body fluid that contains blood.

AIDS: Acquired immunodeficiency syndrome, caused by HIV. It is a fatal disease that attacks the immune system and is characterized by severe opportunistic infections and rare cancers. Approximately 70% of HIV-infected people develop AIDS within 10 years. An HIV-infected person is diagnosed as having AIDS after development of one of the indicator illnesses or on the basis of certain blood tests. AIDS is officially diagnosed when there are 200 or fewer helper T cells in 1 mL of blood.

Risk factors for HIV transmission: The risk factors for HIV transmission are generally the same as the risk factors associated with HBV. People at risk include:

- Those with multiple sexual partners
- Those who have had unprotected anal, vaginal, or oral sex
- Intravenous drug users who share needles
- Sexual partners of an infected person
- Infants born to HIV positive women

Stages of AIDS: A person who is HIV-positive without any symptoms for months or even years is known as a carrier of HIV. The AIDS virus infection cycle has four stages: acute HIV infection, asymptomatic latency period, AIDS-related complex (ARC), and full-blown AIDS.

Acute HIV infection: An infection that lasts from three days to one month. Symptoms are often mistaken for those of other viral infections and include fever, sweats, fatigue, loss of appetite, diarrhea, pharyngitis, myalgia, arthralgia, and adenopathy.

Asymptomatic latency period: A long incubation period, sometimes lasting for years. During this period, the infected individual is asymptomatic. The only evidence of infection during this phase is the body's production of HIV antibodies. These HIV antibodies, however, are unable to destroy the virus. This period is a confounding factor in tests for the presence of HIV infection because testing may fail to detect HIV for as long as three–six months after an individual has been infected.

AIDS-related complex (ARC): A syndrome resulting from HIV infection but lacking an opportunistic infection or Kaposi's sarcoma. Patients with ARC often have chronic systemic symptoms, including enlarged lymph nodes, fever, diarrhea, weight loss, fatigue, and dementia. Most people with ARC progress to having full-blown AIDS.

Final stage of AIDS: Full-blown AIDS is characterized by the presence of opportunistic infections and unusual cancers. A severe pneumonia caused by *Pneumocystis carinii* is commonly seen in AIDS patients, and Kaposi's sarcoma, a rare type of cancer, frequently occurs.

Opportunistic infections: Infections that occur when normal immunity is altered. If the immune system cannot respond to a microbe that it would normally eliminate, the infection that results is termed opportunistic. These infections cause most of the morbidity and mortality in AIDS because they attack many different organs of the body. The lungs are the most commonly affected organs in AIDS since they are the principal target for *Pneumocystis carinii* and atypical tuberculous bacteria.

Kaposi's sarcoma: A malignancy of the skin and lymph nodes that often occurs in AIDS patients. It is the most common HIV-related cancer and usually appears as painless nodules and reddish purple to dark blue colors on the body.

Pneumocystis carinii **pneumonia:** A type of pneumonia caused by the parasite *Pneumocystis carinii*, usually seen in patients with HIV infection. Its symptoms include fever, tachypnea, cough, and cyanosis. The diagnosis is not easy to make. The mortality rate in untreated patients is almost 100%.

Tuberculosis: A disease that is often curable when treatment regimens are followed exactly and completely. However, there has been a rise in the number of cases in recent years as a result of HIV infection and antibiotic resistance. HIV infection is the single largest risk factor for the development of tuberculosis infection into the active form of the disease.

HIV antibody testing: Since 1992, recommendations issued by the Centers for Disease Control and Prevention (CDC) have called for the voluntary testing of people who are at high risk for HIV infection. HIV antibody testing is federally mandated for all military applicants and is also required for those who donate organs, tissue, sperm, or blood.

Inactivation of HIV: HIV is readily destroyed by heat treatment and exposure to disinfectants. The most common disinfectant is 10% NaOCl (sodium hypochlorite, the active ingredient in household bleach).

Other Blood-Borne Pathogens

Toxoplasmosis: An infection caused by *Toxoplasma gondii*, transmitted in cat feces. Pregnant women and AIDS patients should not handle cat litter boxes.

Cytomegalovirus: One of the most common infections. As many as 80% of adults have been exposed to it. In AIDS patients, it may cause severe lung disease. Pregnant women may transmit this infection to the fetus through the placenta, which results in brain damage, mental retardation, blindness, deafness, or death.

16.2 Medical and Surgical Asepsis

Asepsis: The condition in which pathogens are absent or controlled.

Medical asepsis: Also referred to as *clean technique*. It is used for the destruction of organisms after they leave the body, to maintain cleanliness in order to prevent the spread of microorganisms. It ensures that there are as few microorganisms in the medical environment as possible.

Surgical asepsis: Also referred to as *sterile technique*, it is used to create a completely sterile environment without the presence of any microorganisms, or their spores. This procedure is used for invasive or surgical techniques. When you are performing the sterile technique, it is important that nothing interrupts this process and that things are done in the correct order. If there is any question that an area might be contaminated, consider it contaminated and sterilize again. Surgical asepsis is used to destroy pathogenic organisms before they enter the body.

Microbial control: The prevention of infectious diseases by using heat, steam, fire, and chemicals to control the growth of microbes.

Bactericidal or **bacteriocidal:** Destructive to or destroying bacteria.

Bacteriostatic: Inhibiting the growth of bacteria.

Antisepsis: Inhibition, usually through a topical application, of the growth and multiplication of microorganisms.

Aseptic Precautions

Office procedures: The following procedures help promote asepsis.

- Offer separate areas in the waiting room for well and sick patients.
- Maintain a well-lit, well-ventilated, draft-free office with a room temperature of approximately 72°F.
- Prohibit eating and drinking in the office.
- Dispose of trash as often as needed.
- Eliminate insects from the office.
- Post signs asking patients to use tissues, put waste in the trash cans, report safety or health hazards, and tell the receptionist if they are nauseated or need to use the restroom.
- Keep hand sanitizing agents in all (administrative and clerical) areas.

Cross-contamination: Perform procedures in a way that avoids cross-contamination. For example, do not place the lid of a sterile container face down on a surface, and do not pour tablets or capsules into your hand.

Hand washing: One of the most important methods of medical asepsis. Wash your hands:

- At the beginning of the day
- After breaks
- Before and after using the restroom
- Before and after lunch
- Before and after any patient contact, including taking vital signs
- Before and after using gloves

- Before and after handling specimens or waste
- Before and after handling clean or sterile supplies
- Before and after performing any procedure
- After blowing your nose or coughing
- Before leaving for the day

Aseptic hand washing: Removes accumulated dirt and microorganisms that could cause infection. Table 16-1 describes how to perform aseptic hand washing.

Hand hygiene: The CDC has released new recommendations for hand hygiene in health-care settings. *Hand hygiene* is a term that applies to either hand washing or using an antiseptic hand rub (surgical hand antisepsis). Hand antisepsis with an antiseptic hand rub is more effective in reducing nosocomial infections than plain hand washing.

Surgical scrub: Similar to aseptic hand washing, with the following differences:

- A sterile scrub brush is used instead of a nail brush.
- Hands and forearms are washed.
- Hands are held above the elbows so that water cannot run from the arms onto washed areas.
- Sterile towels are used instead of paper towels.
- Sterile gloves are put on immediately after the hands are dried.

Infection Control

Sanitization: A cleansing process that reduces the number of microorganisms to a safe level, via washing and scrubbing equipment to remove body tissue, blood, and other body fluids.

Ultrasonic cleaning: Used to sanitize delicate instruments and those with moving parts. It involves placing the instruments in a special bath that generates sound waves through a cleaning solution.

Disinfection: The process of destroying infectious agents by chemical or physical means. It is used for instruments that do

---

AT A GLANCE | **Aseptic Hand-Washing Method**

Remove all jewelry, except plain gold wedding bands.

Use a paper towel to turn on faucets, and adjust the temperature to moderately warm.

Wet your hands and apply liquid soap. Liquid soap in a foot pump dispenser is less likely to accumulate dirt.

Work the soap into a lather, and make sure that both of your hands are covered in lather. Rub vigorously in circular motions for at least 2 minutes. Keep your hands lower than your forearms so that the dirty water flows into the sink instead of back onto your arms. Interlace your fingers, and clean the palms and between the fingers. Wash the wrists as well.

Use a nailbrush or orange stick to dislodge dirt from the cuticles and nails.

Rinse your hands well, keeping them lower than your forearms and not touching the sink or faucets.

With the water still running, dry your hands with clean, dry paper towels, and then use a clean, dry paper towel to turn off the faucets. Discard the paper towels.

Table 16-1

not penetrate a patient's skin or that come in contact only with a patient's mucous membranes or other surfaces not considered sterile.

Disinfectants: Cleaning products that reduce or eliminate infectious organisms on instruments or equipment. Common disinfectants are chemical germicides, household bleach, boiling water, and steam. A 10% bleach solution reduces or eliminates infectious agents for 24 hours. Hydrogen peroxide is a disinfectant and sterilizing agent without antiseptic properties because it is rapidly inactivated by enzymes in skin. However, the frothing that occurs is beneficial since it loosens debris in wounds. It has a short shelf life.

Antiseptics: Cleaning products used on human tissues as anti-infection agents.

Germicides: Germ-killing additives. The use of soap in the process of disinfection is less important than the scrubbing and rinsing steps, but germicides may increase the effectiveness of soap.

Sterilization: A destruction of all living microorganisms and spores. It is required for all instruments and supplies that penetrate a patient's skin or come in contact with any normally sterile areas of the body. It also is required for instruments that will be used in a sterile field. Examples of items that need to be sterilized are:

- Curettes
- Needle drivers/holders
- Forceps
- Hemostats

Autoclave: A device that forces the temperature of steam above the boiling point of water in order to sterilize instruments and equipment. Distilled water is used for autoclaving. The most common and effective method for sterilizing articles in the medical office is steam under pressure using an autoclave. Most microorganisms are killed in a few minutes at temperatures ranging from 130°F to 150°F. No organism can survive direct exposure to saturated steam at 250°F for 15 minutes or longer.

Autoclave procedures: Take the following steps when using the autoclave:

1. Wrap sanitized and disinfected instruments and equipment, and label each pack.
2. Clean and preheat the autoclave.
3. Perform quality control procedures.
4. Load the instruments and equipment, allowing adequate space around the items.
5. Set the autoclave for the correct time.
6. Run the autoclave through the cycle, including drying time.
7. Remove the instruments and equipment.
8. Store the instruments and equipment for the next use.
9. Clean the autoclave and the surrounding work area.

Sterilization indicators: Tags, inserts, tapes, tubes, or strips that confirm that the items in the autoclave have been exposed to the correct volume of steam at the correct temperature for the correct length of time.

Chemical sterilization: Used on instruments that would be damaged by prolonged exposure to the high temperatures in a steam autoclave.

Dry heat sterilization: Used on items that would be damaged by immersion in chemical solution or by exposure to steam.

Gas sterilization: Uses ethylene oxide, a hazardous gas. It may be performed only in hospital and manufacturing environments.

Microwave sterilization: The fastest method, using low-pressure steam with radiation.

16.3 OSHA Requirements

OSHA: The U.S. Department of Labor's Occupational Safety and Health Administration requires basic safety practices, including infection control. OSHA develops federal regulations that aim to protect health-care workers from health hazards on the job, particularly from accidentally acquired infections.

OSHA Blood-Borne Pathogens Standard of 1991: A set of regulations to protect health-care workers, patients, and other visitors from health hazards. It:

- Requires employers to identify, in writing, tasks, procedures, and job classifications that involve occupational exposure to blood.
- Mandates universal precautions, emphasizing engineering and work practice controls.
- Requires employers to provide and employees to use personal protective equipment.
- Requires a written schedule for cleaning, identifying the method of decontamination to be used, and specifies methods of disposing of regulated waste.
- Specifies procedures to be made available to all employees who have had an exposure incident, including a confidential medical evaluation.
- Requires warning labels, including the biohazard symbol, to be affixed to containers of regulated waste and other containers used to store or transport blood or other potentially infectious materials.
- Mandates training within 90 days of the effective date of assignment and annually thereafter.
- Calls for confidential medical records of employees to be kept for the duration of employment plus 30 years.

Exposure Control Plan: A part of the safety plan used by a medical facility, or a stand-alone document, that must cover all OSHA-required elements. The plan must detail which tasks employees perform that involve a risk of exposure to blood, and classify jobs according to their potential for blood exposure. A *hazardous materials communication* must be included, which explains how to handle spills or exposures involving hazardous substances.

OSHA record-keeping regulations: In 2002, OSHA revised the rules concerning record-keeping in the workplace. Three forms are now primarily used to document accidents, injuries, and illnesses related to the workplace.

- Form 300 is the "Log of Work-Related Injuries and Illnesses" (which also covers deaths).
- Form 301 is the "Injury and Illness Incident Report," which must also be completed for each entry in Form 300.
- Form 300A is the "Summary of Work-Related Injuries and Illnesses." It must be posted in the facility where all employees can view it, and must document all accidents, illnesses, and injuries in the facility for the previous year.

Needlestick Safety and Prevention Act: OSHA revised its Bloodborne Pathogens Standard (in 2001) to comply with the 2000 Needlestick Safety and Prevention Act. Employers must involve employees when selecting needle safety devices. In the medical facility, a needlestick and sharps injury log must be kept, and must include the description of the incident, the type (and brand) of the device involved, the location of the incident, and any other pertinent information. All needlestick and sharps injuries must be reported and documented, not only those that cause severe injury or illness.

OSHA training requirements: All employees, regardless of their work schedule, must receive training about occupational exposures when they are hired, and then every year that they are employed. Training sessions must be documented in each employee's file.

Failure to comply with OSHA standards: Could result in a maximum penalty of $7,000 for the first violation, and up to $70,000 for repeated violations. See Table 16-2.

Universal precautions: An approach to infection control, in which all human blood and certain other human body fluids are treated as if they were known to be infectious for HIV, HBV, and other blood-borne pathogens. Universal precautions apply to blood and blood products; human tissue; semen and vaginal secretions; saliva from dental procedures; cerebrospinal, synovial, pleural, peritoneal, pericardial, and amniotic fluids; and other body fluids if visibly contaminated with blood or of questionable origin in the body.

Standard precautions: The means by which transmission of pathogens in infected materials is prevented. Standard precautions apply to blood, other body fluids, secretions, excretions (except sweat), nonintact skin, and mucous membranes. Standard precautions are used in hospitals for the care of all patients. In medical offices, use universal precautions when dealing with patients.

Work practice controls: Controls that reduce the likelihood of exposure by altering the manner in which a task is performed, such as prohibiting the recapping of needles by using two hands.

Category I tasks: Tasks that expose a worker to blood, body fluids, or tissues, such as assisting with the removal of a cyst, and tasks that have a chance of spills or splashes. These tasks always require special protective measures.

Category II tasks: Tasks that usually do not involve a risk of exposure but that may involve exposure in certain situations. An example is giving mouth-to-mouth resuscitation. These tasks require precautions to be taken.

Category III tasks: Tasks that involve no exposure to blood, body fluids, or tissues and therefore do not require special protection. An example is giving a patient nose drops.

Material Safety Data Sheet (MSDS): Manufacturer-provided paperwork that gives detailed information regarding a chemical,

AT A GLANCE	Infectious Waste Disposal: Penalties for Not Following OSHA Regulations	
Type of Violation	**Characteristics of Violation**	**Penalties for Violation**
Other than serious violation	Direct relationship to job safety and health but would probably not result in death or serious injury	Fine of up to $7,000 (discretionary)
Serious violation	Substantial probability that death or serious physical harm could result and employer knew or should have known of the hazard	Fine of up to $7,000 (mandatory)
Willful violation	Violation committed intentionally and knowingly	Fine of up to $70,000, with a $5,000 minimum; in the event of the death of an employee, possible additional penalties, including a six-month imprisonment
Repeated violation	Substantially similar violation found upon reinspection (not applicable if initial citation is under contest)	Fine of up to $70,000
Failure to correct	Initial violation not corrected	Fine of up to $7,000 for each day the violation continues after the date it was supposed to stop

Table 16-2

its hazards, and steps to take to prevent injury or illness while handling the chemical. A current MSDS must be kept on file for each hazardous chemical stored or used in the workplace. Medical assistants must review the MSDS for any hazardous chemical they will work with.

Postprocedure cleanup: OSHA requires the following steps:

- Decontaminate all exposed work surfaces with bleach or a germ-killing solution.
- Replace protective coverings on surfaces and equipment that have been exposed.
- Decontaminate receptacles.
- Pick up broken glass with tongs.
- Discard all potentially infectious waste materials in appropriate biohazardous waste containers.

Engineering controls: Controls, such as sharps disposal containers and self-sheathing needles, that isolate or remove the hazard of blood-borne pathogens.

Hand-washing facility: A facility providing an adequate supply of running potable water, soap, and single-use towels or hot-air drying machines.

Personal protective equipment: Specialized clothing or equipment worn by an employee for protection against a hazard. It includes gloves, lab coats, protective eyewear, face shields, surgical gowns, and shoe covers.

Filter mask for tuberculosis: Health-care providers working with patients who have tuberculosis must wear a filter mask, which is also called a *filtering face-piece respirator*. This is a nonpowered, air-purifying mask that covers half of the face, and may or may not be disposable. In high-risk situations, additional protection may be required.

Hazard warning label: Each hazardous chemical should be identified by a hazard warning label that displays the following information:

- A stated requirement that the chemical be kept in its original container
- A color code (blue for health hazards, red for flammability, yellow for reactivity, and white for specific hazards, such as radioactivity); these are designated by the National Fire Protection Association (NFPA)
- A numerical rating superimposed on each colored area of the label indicating a level of hazard from 0 (no hazard) to 4 (extreme hazard); also designated by the NFPA

Decontamination: A term used by OSHA to describe the use of physical or chemical means to remove, inactivate, or destroy blood-borne pathogens on a surface or item to the point at which they are no longer capable of transmitting infection and the surface or item is rendered safe for handling, use, or disposal.

Regulated waste: Liquid or semiliquid blood or other potentially infectious materials; contaminated items that would release blood or other potentially infectious materials in a liquid or semiliquid state if compressed; items that are caked with blood or other potentially infectious materials and are capable of releasing these materials during handling; contaminated sharps; and pathological and microbiological wastes containing blood or other potentially infectious materials.

Storing biohazardous materials: OSHA regulations prohibit medical personnel from performing any of the following activities in a room where potentially infectious materials are present.

- Eating
- Drinking
- Smoking
- Chewing gum
- Applying cosmetics
- Handling contact lenses
- Chewing pencils or pens
- Rubbing eyes

You should have separate refrigerators in separate rooms for food and for biohazardous materials. Refrigerators used for specimens should be clearly labeled with biohazard stickers.

Refrigerators: To prevent spoilage or deterioration of testing kits and specimens, the temperature of the laboratory refrigerator should be maintained between 36° and 46°F (2° and 8°C).

STRATEGIES FOR SUCCESS

▶ *Test-Taking Skills*

Choose the best answer!
When taking a multiple-choice test such as the CMA, RMA, or CCMA exam, you may find that the choices do not always include the perfect answer or what you think the answer should be. Remember, you must choose the best answer possible. When you return to a difficult question, you should try not to look at any of the given answers. Instead, supply your own answer and then look for the option that is the closest to your response.

Instructions:

Answer the following questions.

1. Potentially infectious body fluids include all of the following *except*

   A. blood.
   B. vaginal secretions.
   C. sweat.
   D. cerebrospinal fluid.
   E. semen.

2. Clean technique is another term for

   A. medical asepsis.
   B. surgical asepsis.
   C. hand washing.
   D. sterilization.
   E. sanitization.

3. Instruments that penetrate a patient's skin should be

   A. sanitized.
   B. disinfected.
   C. sterilized.
   D. treated with antiseptics.
   E. cleaned ultrasonically.

4. A cleansing process that reduces the number of microorganisms to a safe level is called

   A. sanitization.
   B. disinfection.
   C. sterilization.
   D. autoclaving.
   E. cleaning.

5. Treating all human blood as if it were infectious is known as

   A. engineering controls.
   B. work practice controls.
   C. asepsis.
   D. universal precautions.
   E. isolation methods.

6. After you have rinsed your hands as part of the aseptic hand-washing method, what step should you take next?

   A. Using a nailbrush or orange stick, dislodge the dirt from your nails.
   B. Turn off the faucets using your hands.
   C. Hold your hands above the elbows to prevent water from running onto washed areas.
   D. Put on sterile gloves.
   E. Dry your hands with clean paper towels and turn off faucets by using a clean paper towel.

7. To dispose of a contaminated needle,

   A. recap it and drop it into the nearest biohazardous waste container.
   B. drop it into the biohazardous waste container for sharps.
   C. wash it, recap it, and drop it into the biohazardous waste container for sharps.
   D. sterilize it and put it into the biohazardous waste container.
   E. drop it in the nearest trash can.

8. The autoclave

   A. is used for instruments that would be damaged by prolonged exposure to high temperatures and steam.
   B. involves the use of soap and scrubbing to disinfect instruments.
   C. forces the temperature of steam above the boiling point of water in order to sterilize equipment.
   D. uses ethylene oxide and may be operated only in the hospital or a manufacturing environment.
   E. is used for items that would be damaged by immersion in a chemical solution or by exposure to steam.

9. Standard precautions are

   A. focused on dried body substances.
   B. used to prevent pathogen transmission via infected materials.
   C. used only in medical offices.
   D. never used because they are outdated.
   E. the same as universal precautions.

10. Which of the following liquids is used in an autoclave to sterilize instruments and supplies?

   A. tap water
   B. distilled water
   C. sterile water
   D. alcohol
   E. bleach

CHAPTER 17

PREPARING THE PATIENT

LEARNING OUTCOMES

17.1 Describe the medical assistant's role in maintaining the rights, responsibilities, and privacy of the patient.

17.2 Demonstrate how to conduct a successful medical interview.

17.3 Describe the responsibilities of the medical assistant when assisting the physician with the physical examination of a patient.

17.4 Describe the medical assistant's role when assisting the physician with performing minor surgery.

MEDICAL ASSISTING COMPETENCIES

COMPETENCY	CMA	RMA	CCMA	NCMA
Clinical				
Apply principles of aseptic techniques and infection control, including hand washing	X	X	X	X
Perform sterilization techniques	X	X	X	X
Dispose of biohazardous materials	X	X	X	X
Practice standard precautions	X	X	X	X
Obtain specimens for microbiological testing, including throat specimens and wound cultures	X	X	X	X
Interview the patient to obtain and record the patient's history	X	X	X	X
Prepare and maintain examination and treatment areas	X	X	X	X
Prepare the patient for and assist the physician with routine and specialty examinations, treatments, and minor office surgeries	X	X	X	X
Screen and follow up on patient test results	X	X	X	X

MEDICAL ASSISTING COMPETENCIES (cont.)

General/Legal/Professional

Recognize and respond to verbal and nonverbal communications by being attentive and adapting communication to the recipient's level of understanding	X	X	X	X
Identify and respond to issues of confidentiality by maintaining confidentiality at all times and following appropriate guidelines when releasing records or information	X	X	X	X
Be aware of and perform within legal and ethical boundaries	X	X	X	X
Determine the needs for documentation and reporting, and document accurately and appropriately	X	X	X	X
Instruct individuals according to their needs	X	X	X	X
Provide patients with methods of health promotion and disease prevention	X	X	X	X
Perform an inventory of supplies and equipment	X	X	X	
Operate and maintain facilities, and perform routine maintenance of administrative and clinical equipment safely	X	X	X	X
Maintain the physical plant	X	X	X	
Evaluate and recommend equipment and supplies for practice	X	X	X	
Conduct work within scope of education, training, and ability	X	X	X	X
Be impartial and show empathy when dealing with patients	X	X	X	
Serve as a liaison between the physician and others		X	X	
Interview effectively	X	X	X	
Use appropriate medical terminology	X	X	X	X

STRATEGIES FOR SUCCESS

▶ Study Skills

Review frequently!

As soon as possible after a lecture, it's important to spend some quiet time organizing and clarifying your notes. Doing so will help you retain and understand material much better than waiting until the night before the exam to take out your notes. Also review by rereading your notes throughout the course of your study. Test yourself on the material you should already know. If your instructor does not give midterm exams, give yourself one to check your progress. As you learn new information, try to link it to things you've already learned. For example, before reading the section on conducting medical interviews, you should go back and review the section on patient communication.

17.1 Patient Rights, Responsibilities, and Privacy

All the data you obtain are subject to legal and ethical considerations. The *Patient's Bill of Rights* was written in 1973 and revised in 1992. The *Patient Care Partnership* is a brochure often used in place of the *Patient's Bill of Rights* that informs patients about what they should expect during hospitalization, regarding their rights and responsibilities. Each state encourages health-care workers to be aware of and follow this document when caring for patients. The statement guarantees the patient's rights to:

- Receive considerate and respectful care
- Receive complete and current information concerning his or her diagnosis, treatment, and prognosis
- Know the identity of physicians, nurses, and others involved with his or her care, as well as when those involved are students, residents, or trainees
- Know the immediate and long-term costs of treatment choices
- Receive information necessary to give informed consent before the start of any procedure or treatment
- Have an advance directive concerning treatment or be able to choose a representative to make decisions
- Refuse treatment to the extent permitted by law
- Receive every consideration of his or her privacy
- Be assured of confidentiality
- Obtain reasonable responses to requests for services
- Obtain information about his or her health care, be allowed to review his or her medical record, and have any information explained or interpreted
- Know whether treatment is experimental and be able to consent or decline to participate in proposed research studies or human experimentation
- Expect reasonable continuity of care
- Ask about and be informed of the existence of business relationships between the hospital and others that may influence the patient's treatment and care
- Know which hospital policies and practices relate to patient care, treatment, and responsibilities
- Be informed of available resources for resolving disputes, grievances, and conflicts, such as ethics committees or patient representatives
- Examine his or her bill and have it explained and be informed of available payment methods

Medical assistants also should know that patients have certain responsibilities when they seek medical care. Patients are responsible for:

- Providing information about past illnesses, hospitalizations, medications, and other matters related to their health status. If an incorrect diagnosis is made because a patient fails to give the physician the proper information, the physician is not liable.
- Participating in decision making by asking for additional information about their health status or treatment when they do not fully understand information and instructions.
- Providing health-care agencies with a copy of their written advance directive if they have one.
- Informing physicians and other caregivers if they anticipate problems in following a prescribed treatment.
- Following the physician's orders for treatment. If a patient willfully or negligently fails to follow the physician's instructions, that patient has little legal recourse.
- Providing health-care agencies with necessary information for insurance claims and working with the health-care facility to make arrangements to pay fees when necessary.

Additionally, in April 2003, the enforcement of the Health Insurance Portability and Accountability Act (HIPAA) began. If this act is not followed, individual health-care workers can be subject to fines up to $250,000 and 10 years in jail. The privacy standards of this act ensure the following:

- Health-care facilities must provide patients with a written notice of their practices regarding the use and disclosure of all individually identifiable health information.
- Health-care facilities may not use or disclose protected health information for any purpose that is not in the privacy notice.
- Patient consent is required when protected information is used or disclosed for purposes of treatment, payment, or health operations.
- Written authorization is required for other types of disclosures.
- Hospitals must make the privacy notice available either before or at the time of the delivery of care.
- A privacy notice must be posted in a clear and prominent location within the hospital facility.

17.2 Medical Interview

Patient interview: The first step in the examination process. It allows the medical assistant to collect information and data pertinent to the patient's well-being.

Health history form: The medical office usually has a standard medical history form that it uses for all patients. The specific arrangement and wording of items vary from office to office.

Personal data: This information is obtained from the administrative sheet and includes basic data such as the patient's name, social security number, and birth date.

Chief complaint: Abbreviated as CC, it is the reason the patient came to visit the practitioner. It should be short and specific and cover subjective and objective data.

History of present illness: This includes detailed information about the chief complaint, including when the problem started and what the patient has done to treat the problem (including any medications taken). For example, a chief complaint might be "sore throat," and the history of the present illness would include when the sore throat began (e.g., three days ago), how severe the pain is on a scale of 1 to 10 (e.g., pain scale rating of 6 out of 10), and what treatments have been used (e.g., throat lozenges and four–six aspirin daily).

Past medical history: This section includes any and all health problems both present and past, including major illnesses and surgery. The past medical history also includes important information about medications and allergies. The abbreviation *NKDA* stands for *no known drug allergies.*

Family history: This section includes information about the health of the patient's family members. Many times the family history can help lead a practitioner to the cause of a current medical problem. Obtain specific information about family members' current ages and medical conditions or, if deceased, their age at death and the cause.

Social and occupational history: Information such as marital status, sexual behaviors and orientation, occupations, hobbies, and use of chemical substances help determine a patient's risk for disease. Patients should be asked about their use of alcohol, tobacco, recreational drugs, or other chemical substances. Marital status is an example of demographic data.

Six Cs of charting:

- Client's words—The patient's own phrasing must be recorded exactly.
- Clarity—Use precise medical terminology.
- Completeness—The chart must contain all pertinent information.
- Conciseness—Use abbreviations when possible, to save time and space.
- Chronological order—Date all entries.
- Confidentiality—Protect the patient's privacy.

Interviewing successfully:

- Do your research before the interview. Review the patient's medical history.
- Plan the interview. Plan what types of questions you want to ask.
- Approach the patient and request an interview. Make the patient feel part of the process.
- Make the patient feel at ease. Use icebreakers and casual conversation.
- Listen to the patient.
- Conduct the interview in private without interruption.
- Deal with sensitive topics with respect.
- Do not diagnose or give a diagnostic opinion. Never go beyond the scope of your practice.
- Formulate a general picture. Summarize key points, and let the patient ask questions.

Detect nonverbal clues and body language: During the pre-examination interview, you may note things that patients have not communicated to you verbally, such as anxiety, depression, signs of physical or psychological abuse, and signs of drug or alcohol abuse. If you suspect abuse, bring it to the physician's attention immediately.

17.3 Physical Examination

Purpose of the physical examination: The determination of the general state of health of the patient and the diagnosis of any medical problems and diseases the patient may have.

- The physician uses a variety of devices and laboratory tests to complete the physical findings. The majority of physicians begin at the patient's head and end at the feet.
- The physician may order some additional tests or procedures, such as blood sample testing, the collection of culture specimens, or X-rays.

Complete physical examination: Includes vital signs, examination of the patient's entire body, laboratory tests (complete blood count [CBC] and urinalysis); and diagnostic tests (X-rays).

Duty of a medical assistant: Preparing the room and equipment, getting the patient ready, and assisting the physician.

Emotional preparation: Begin by explaining what will happen during the examination. This step is especially important when dealing with children.

Physical preparation: The medical assistant is responsible for obtaining and recording weight, height, and vital signs; facilitating the examination; asking the patient to empty his or her bladder; asking the patient to disrobe completely; providing the patient with a full gown; and providing a drape sheet.

Examination methods: The six methods for examining a patient that are part of a complete physical examination are inspection, palpation, percussion, auscultation, manipulation, and mensuration.

Inspection: Observing the patient's body, overall appearance, and certain mental characteristics.

Palpation: Using pressure, commonly with the fingers, to assess tissues and organs not visualized during inspection.

Percussion: Tapping with the fingers and listening for sounds, particularly in the abdomen, back, and chest.

Auscultation: Listening to sounds with a stethoscope.

Manipulation: Skillful moving of the body parts, such as in range-of-motion, to assess functionality.

Mensuration: The act or process of measuring.

Symptoms: Subjective changes in the body felt or observed by the patient, such as headache, blurred vision, or dizziness.

Signs: Objective findings as perceived by another person, such as a physician or medical assistant. Examples of signs include fever, blood pressure, and heart murmurs.

Diagnose: To determine the cause and nature of an abnormal condition. It's important to remember that diagnosis is not within the scope or training of a medical assistant. You should never give a diagnosis to a patient. If patients ask you, refer them to the physician.

Clinical diagnosis: Using the signs and symptoms of a disease to determine its cause and nature.

Differential diagnosis: The process of ruling out certain possibilities, used to determine the correct diagnosis when two or more diagnoses are possible. A *differential* is also described as a diagnosis based on a comparison of signs and symptoms of similar diseases.

Plan of treatment: The treatment planned for a given diagnosis, which may include prescribed or discontinued medications, ancillaries, and any required follow-up examinations.

Prognosis: The outcome of a disorder, or a predication of the probable course of a disease in an individual and the chances of recovery.

Equipment

Examination tables: Usually adjustable to enable the patient to assume various positions. Tables are usually covered with disposable papers that must be changed after each patient.

Surfaces: Must be disinfected with products approved by the Environmental Protection Agency (EPA), such as 10% NaClO (sodium hypochlorite, the active ingredient in household bleach).

Accessibility: The ease with which people can move in and out of a space. The Americans with Disabilities Act of 1990 (ADA) requires:

- A doorway at least 36 inches wide to allow for the use of wheelchairs

- A clear space in rooms and hallways 60 inches in diameter to allow persons using a wheelchair to make a 180-degree turn

- Stable, firm, slip-resistant flooring

- Door-opening hardware that can be grasped with one hand and does not require the twisting of the wrist to use

- Door closers adjusted to allow time for a person in a wheelchair to enter and exit

- Grab bars in the lavatory

Instrument: A surgical device or tool to assist the physician in performing a specific function, such as measuring, examining, grasping, holding, cutting, or suturing. Some commonly used instruments are shown in Figure 17-1.

Gloves: Should always be worn if the hands will come in contact with a patient's nonintact skin, blood, body fluids, or moist surfaces and if the patient is suspected of having an infectious disease.

Tongue depressors: Used in the examination of the mouth and tongue.

Gooseneck lamp: A movable light used to focus on a body area for increased visibility during physical examination.

Penlight: A small flashlight used to provide additional light during an examination, for example, to check pupil response.

Reflex hammer: A percussion mallet with a rubber head, used to tap tendons, nerves, or muscles to elicit reflex reactions. It is used during a neurologic examination.

Lubricants: Used in examination of the rectum and female genitalia.

Anoscope: An instrument used to open the anus for examination.

Speculum: An instrument that expands and separates the walls of a cavity (such as the ear, nose, and vagina) to make examination possible.

Nasal speculum: Used to enlarge the opening of the nose to permit viewing. This type of speculum may consist of a reusable handle with a disposable speculum tip, or it may be a disposable one-piece unit.

Vaginal speculum: Used to enlarge the vagina to make the vagina and the cervix accessible to visual examination and specimen collection.

Thermometer: Used to measure body temperature.

Otoscope: An instrument used to examine the external ear canal and tympanic membrane.

Ophthalmoscope: A handheld instrument, equipped with a light, used to view inner eye structures.

Tuning fork: A small, metal instrument consisting of a stem and two prongs that produces a constant pitch when either prong is struck. It is used by physicians as a screening test of air and bone conduction.

Inspecting and maintaining instruments: Before examination, check all instruments and sanitize, disinfect, and sterilize as appropriate. Also, make sure that all of them are in good working order, and replace or repair instruments as necessary.

Arranging instruments: Arrange instruments so the physician may find them easily.

Disposable supplies used in physical examinations: Supplies that are used once and then discarded. They include:

- Cervical scraper

- Cotton balls

- Cotton-tipped applicators

- Curettes

- Disposable needles

- Disposable syringes

- Gauze, dressings, and bandages

- Glass slides

- Gloves, both sterile and exam (nonsterile)

- Paper tissues

- Specimen containers

- Tongue depressors

Consumable supplies: Supplies that can be emptied or used up in an examination. They include:

- Sprays (chemical spray used to preserve specimens)

- Isopropyl alcohol (used to cleanse the skin)

- Lubricants

Supply inventory: A list of all supplies used regularly in the medical office, usually kept in a notebook, on cards, or in an electronic spreadsheet file. It may be organized by type of supply, or by supplier. Lists are printed when supplies are counted,

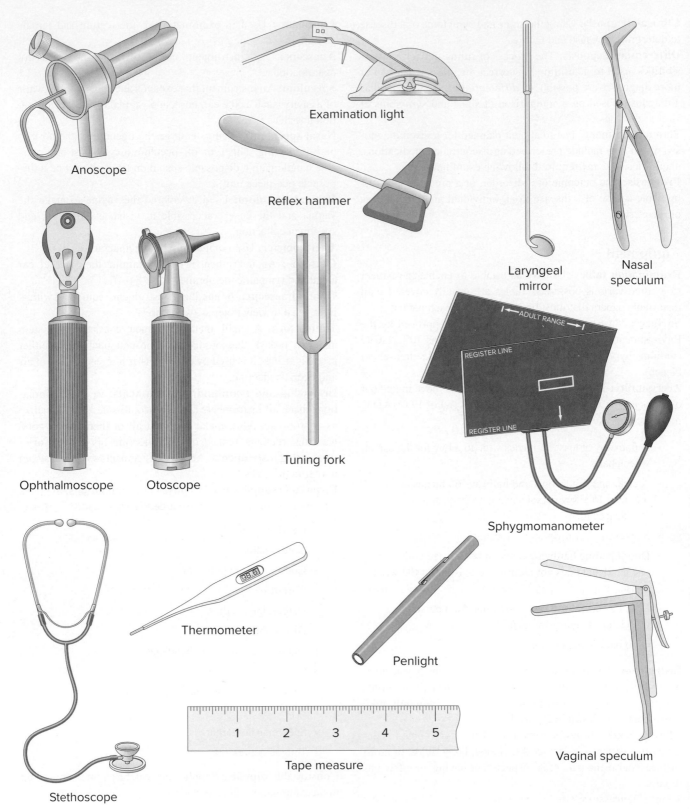

Anoscope

Examination light

Reflex hammer

Laryngeal
mirror

Nasal
speculum

Ophthalmoscope

Otoscope

Tuning fork

ADULT RANGE

REGISTER LINE

REGISTER LINE

Sphygmomanometer

Thermometer

Penlight

Stethoscope

Tape measure

Vaginal speculum

Figure 17-1 *These instruments may be used in a general physical examination.*

which the medical assistant usually does, once per month. Supply inventories should include item names, specific sizes, usual suppliers, cost per specific quantity, *reorder point* (the number that, when reached, means it is time to reorder the item), quantity ordered, order dates, dates of receipts, and initials of individuals placing or receiving orders.

Positioning and Draping

Draping: The placing of a sheet of fabric or paper during an examination to protect and cover all or a part of a patient's body, for the comfort and privacy of the patient.

Positioning: For physical examinations, the patient may need to be placed in a variety of positions to facilitate the examination of various parts of the body. The physician indicates which positions are needed for specific examinations, and the medical assistant helps the patient assume the positions. Cover the patient with a drape that will help keep the patient warm and maintain privacy.

Positions: Many positions are used for medical examinations, including sitting, supine, dorsal recumbent, lithotomy, Trendelenburg's, Fowler's, prone, Sims', knee-chest, proctological (jackknife), and standing. See Figure 17-2.

Sitting position: The patient sits at the edge of the examination table without back support. This position is used for examination of the head, neck, chest, heart, back, and arms. In this position, the physician can evaluate the patient's ability to fully expand the lungs and can check the upper body parts for symmetry.

Supine position: Also called the horizontal recumbent position. The patient lies flat on the back (face up). This position is used for examination of the head, neck, chest, breast, heart, abdomen, and arms and legs.

Dorsal recumbent: The patient lies face up while flexing the knees, with the soles of the feet flat on the table. This position is the same as the supine position except that the patient's knees are drawn up. It is used for examination of the head, neck, chest, heart, and lower extremities (vaginal, rectal, and perineal areas).

Lithotomy position: The patient lies on the back with the knees sharply flexed and the feet placed in stirrups that are set wide apart and away from the table. This position is used for examination of the vaginal and perineal areas. It is an embarrassing and physically uncomfortable position for most women, so you should not ask the patient to stay in this position any longer than necessary.

Trendelenburg's position: The patient lies flat on the back with the head lower than the legs. This position is used for abdominal surgery and for treatment of patients who are in shock, and to increase blood pressure in patients with hypotension.

Fowler's position: The patient lies face up on the examination table with the head elevated. Although the head of the table can be raised to 90 degrees, the most common position is 45 degrees. This position is used for examination and treatment of the head, neck, and chest. This position is best for people with lower-back injury or for those experiencing shortness of breath.

Prone position: The patient lies face down on the table. This position is used for examination of the back and feet. It is not suitable for patients who are obese, pregnant (in the late stage), or elderly or who have difficulties of the respiratory system.

Sims' position: Also called the lateral position. The patient lies on the left side with the left arm placed behind the body and the left leg slightly flexed. The right arm is flexed toward the head, and the right leg is flexed. This position is used for examination of the rectum.

Knee-chest position: The patient rests on the knees and chest with the thighs slightly separated. Patients who have difficulty in maintaining this position can be placed in a knee-elbow position. The knee-chest position is used for examination of rectal, sigmoid, and vaginal areas.

Proctological position: The patient lies face down with both the torso and the legs lowered. The hips of the patient are flexed at a 90-degree angle. Adjustable tables can be raised in the middle with both ends sloping down. This position is used for rectal examination. It is also known as the jackknife position.

Standing position: Used for examination of the musculoskeletal system, the neurological system, hernias, and the peripheral vascular system.

Eye and Ear Examination
Eye

Optometrist: A specialist who measures the eye's refractive power and prescribes correction of visual defects when needed. Optometrists treat and prescribe, but do not perform surgery.

Ophthalmologist: A medical doctor who specializes in diagnosing and treating disorders of the eye, including performing surgery.

Ophthalmic assistant: Provides administrative and clinical support for an ophthalmologist; works with patients; assists with surgery; keeps instruments and equipment in proper working order; and may conduct distance acuity, near acuity, and color perception tests.

Visual acuity test: Used to measure the degree of clarity or sharpness of vision. There are many types of tests for visual acuity. The test most commonly used in the medical office and performed by the medical assistant is the Snellen eye test.

Snellen letter chart: A chart used to test the distance vision of adults. The distance between the patient and the chart should be 20 feet. Normal vision is recorded as 20/20. If the patient misses only one or two letters on a line, record the results with a minus sign. For example, if one letter is missed on the 30-foot line from 20 feet away with the right eye, the result would be recorded as O.D. 20/30 –1. For adult patients who do not speak English, a *Snellen object chart* should be used. For children and nonreading adults, the *Snellen E chart* is used, which uses the letter "E" turned in various directions. See Figure 17-3.

Color blindness: The congenital or acquired inability to distinguish certain colors. Congenital color blindness is more common. This condition is seen in males more frequently than in females.

Color vision acuity test: Measures the patient's ability to determine and differentiate between colors. There are two common color tests, Ishihara and Richmond pseudoisochromatic, in which the individual must distinguish a figure made up of

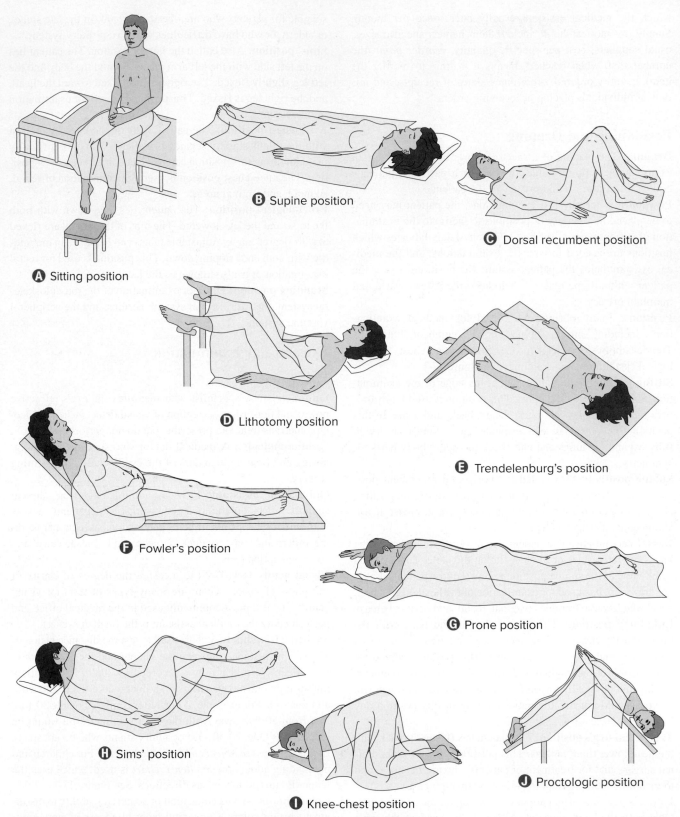

A Sitting position

B Supine position

C Dorsal recumbent position

D Lithotomy position

E Trendelenburg's position

F Fowler's position

G Prone position

H Sims' position

I Knee-chest position

J Proctologic position

Figure 17-2 *These positions may be used during the general physical examination.*

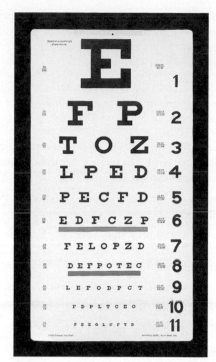

Figure 17-3 *The Snellen letter chart is used to test the ability to see objects that are relatively far away.*
© Good-Lite Company

colored dots from a background made up of dots of another color. A score of 10 or above indicates average color vision. A score of less than seven may represent a color vision deficiency.
Pelli-Robson contrast sensitivity test: A chart used to test ability to see large, faint objects. It has letters organized in groups of three, with two of these groups per line, with the dark-to-light contrast decreasing regularly. This test is used for cataracts, glaucoma, and even Parkinson's disease.
Tonometer: An instrument used in measuring tension or pressure of the intraocular region. It is used for the detection of glaucoma.
Eye irrigation: The flushing of foreign materials from the eye with a sterile solution formulated for this purpose.

Ear

Audiologist: A specialist who tests patients for hearing problems, under the direction of an ear specialist.
Hearing loss: An inability to perceive the entire range of sound heard by a person with normal hearing. There are two types: conductive and sensorineural. Most adults with hearing loss are unable to hear high-frequency sounds.
Conductive hearing loss: Caused by damage to, blockage of, or abnormalities of the middle ear.
Sensorineural hearing loss: Caused by damage to the inner ear (the cochlea or the auditory nerve).
Audiometer: An electronic device that measures hearing acuity by producing sounds in specific frequencies and intensities.

Audiology tests: Tests to determine the presence of conduction defects or nerve impairment. They are used to evaluate hearing loss.
Weber's test: A method of evaluating auditory acuity. The test is performed by placing the stem of a vibrating tuning fork against the center of a person's forehead, or the midline vertex. The loudness of the sound is equal in both ears if hearing is normal.
Rinne test: Compares bone conduction hearing with air conduction hearing. A vibrating tuning fork is held on the mastoid process of the ear until the patient no longer hears it. Then it is held close to the external auditory meatus.
Ear irrigation: Flushing of the ear canal to remove impacted cerumen, to relieve inflammation, or to remove a foreign body. The solution used should be warmed to room temperature before administration. To perform the irrigation for adults, the earlobe should be pulled upward and outward. For infants and children, the earlobe should be pulled down and back. See Figures 17-4 and 17-5.
Ear instillation: Applying eardrops to treat an ear disorder. The medication should be warmed to room temperature before application.

Cardiovascular Examination

Cardiologist: A physician trained in the treatment of heart diseases.
Medical assistant's role: To assist with and perform tests, to keep equipment properly maintained and calibrated, to educate patients about diet and exercise, and to provide emotional support to patients. However, the physician should always be present.
General cardiovascular examination: Taking a blood pressure reading, auscultation of heart sounds, palpating the chest wall and the vessels in the extremities, and recording an electrocardiogram (ECG).
Cardiac stress test: Recording an ECG while a patient is exercising on a treadmill, stationary bicycle, or stair-stepping ergonometer. The test determines the capacity of a patient to respond to an increased demand for energy.
Echocardiography: The process of obtaining echoes with the use of ultrasound and recording them on paper.
Phonocardiography: A process that graphically records the cardiac cycle sounds as heard through a stethoscope.
Cardiac catheterization: A diagnostic procedure in which a catheter is introduced through an incision into a large vein (in the arm or leg) and sent to the chambers of the heart. The procedure takes about one–three hours.
Angioplasty: The reconstruction of blood vessels damaged by disease or injury.
Pulse oximeter: A machine that measures the oxygen level of the blood. This device measures the pulse and oxygen saturation of the arterial blood. It is generally clipped onto a fingertip, and used to diagnose and evaluate cardiac and respiratory function. The sensor emits infrared light, passed from one side to the other. A photo detector measures amount of light absorbed by arterial hemoglobin. This measures oxygen saturation (i.e., percentage of hemoglobin bound with oxygen).

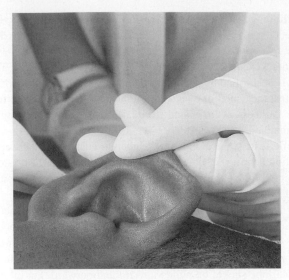

Figure 17-4 *Straighten an adult's ear canal by pulling the auricle upward and outward.*
© Terry Wild

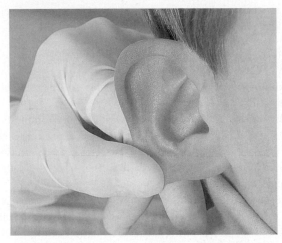

Figure 17-5 *Straighten an infant's or a child's ear canal by pulling the auricle downward and back.*
© Terry Wild

Respiratory System Examination

Eupnea: Normal breathing.

Throat culture: A commonly performed diagnostic test for determination of infection.

Sputum culture: Difficult to obtain. The patient must cough deeply and expectorate material from the lungs. Early morning is the best time to collect sputum.

Pulmonary function tests: Tests performed to measure the amount of air a patient can inhale and exhale.

Spirometer: An instrument that measures the air taken into and expelled from the lungs. Spirometers should be calibrated each day to ensure accurate readings. The medical assistant must use a standardized calibration syringe.

Spirometry: The measuring of breathing capacity (i.e., the air moving in and out of the lungs during specific respiratory maneuvers). It is used to determine air speed and volume, measured in liters, during inhalation and exhalation. The respiratory

cycle consists of lung *volumes* and *capacities*. A lung capacity is the total of two or more lung volumes. The medical assistant assists patients when spirometry is performed.

Patient preparation for spirometry:

- The medical assistant must inform the patient that any of the following may affect the accuracy of the spirometry test:

  - Viral infection or acute illness within the previous two–three weeks, or serious medical condition, such as a recent myocardial infarction

  - Recent myocardial infarction or other serious medical condition

  - Recent use of prescription medications if the test order requests spirometry before and after prescribed medications

  - Use of sedatives or opioids prior to the test

  - Smoking or eating a large meal within one hour of taking the test

- Weigh and measure the patient.

- Explain the procedure in simple terms.

- Loosen tight clothing so that breathing will not be restricted.

- Have the patient sit comfortably, with the legs uncrossed, and both feet flat on the floor.

- Offer a nose clip to the patient, or ask the patient to hold the nose tightly so that all breathing will be done through the mouth.

- If the test unit has a disposable mouthpiece, instruct the patient not to bite down on it, as this will obstruct airflow; make sure the patient forms a tight seal around the mouthpiece with the lips; if the patient wears dentures that make this difficult, ask him or her to remove them.

- Have the patient keep the chin slightly elevated and the neck slightly extended, and tell the patient that the initial force of exhalation must be strong enough to obtain a valid reading.

- Demonstrate the procedure so that the patient understands what to do.

- Have the patient take the deepest possible breath, insert the mouthpiece, form a tight seal, then blow into the mouthpiece as quickly and as hard as possible, to completely exhale for as long as possible to force air out of the lungs; "coach" the patient, encouraging to blow hard and continue blowing.

- Give the patient feedback and tell him or her how to improve during the next maneuver; three "acceptable" maneuvers are required.

- To be acceptable, the spirometry maneuver must not include any patient coughing, must have a quick and forceful start, must be for a minimum of six seconds, must have a consistent and quick flow with no variance, and must be consistent with other required maneuvers.

- If needed to avoid breathing difficulties, dizziness, or changes in blood pressure or pulse, allow the patient to rest briefly between maneuvers, and notify the physician immediately if there are any severe symptoms.

Forced vital capacity (FVC): The greatest volume of air that can be expelled when a person inhales as deeply as possible, and then performs rapid, forced expiration. *Forced expiratory volume in one second (FEV$_1$)* is the volume of air exhaled during the first second of the FVC maneuver, and is usually lower in obstructive airway diseases such as asthma or emphysema. The FEV$_1$/FVC ratio determines if the pulmonary function is normal, obstructive, or restrictive.

Diffusing capacity: Also called DLCO (diffusing lung capacity to transfer carbon monoxide), measures the lungs' ability to transfer gas. Diffusion is most efficient when alveolar-capillary surface area for gas transfer is high, and blood is able to accept the gas. Diffusing capacity is decreased in anemia, conditions that minimize blood's ability to accept and bind the gas, emphysema, pulmonary embolism, conditions that decrease alveolar-capillary surface area, pulmonary fibrosis, and conditions that alter membrane thickness or permeability. Carbon monoxide is used because it is more soluble in blood than in lung tissue. Normally, the volume of gas entering the blood *should* be limited by the lung's ability to transfer it.

Residual volume (RV): Air volume that remains in lungs after exhaling as long and hard as possible. It cannot be measured by spirometry but requires special tests. It is also called *static lung volume.*

Total lung capacity (TLC): The total volume when lungs are maximally inflated. It includes inspiratory capacity, functional residual capacity, tidal volume, expiratory reserve volume, and residual volume. TLC also cannot be measured by spirometry.

Laryngoscope: An endoscope for examining the larynx.

Bronchoscopy: Visual examination of the tracheobronchial tree by means of the standard rigid, tubular metal bronchoscope. The procedure also may be used for suctioning or biopsy.

Thoracentesis: The use of a needle or tube to remove excess fluid from the pleural space, which lies between the lungs and chest wall.

Cheyne-Stokes respiration: A breathing pattern marked by a period of apnea lasting 10–60 seconds, followed by gradually increasing depth and frequency of respirations. It is often related to congestive heart failure.

Nasal cannula: A device that delivers supplemental oxygen or increased airflow to a patient requiring respiratory assistance, as in oxygen therapy. Most cannulas provide low flow rates of up to five liters per minute, with an oxygen concentration of 28 to 44%.

Nebulizer: A device that delivers medication in the form of a mist inhaled into the lungs. It is used to treat asthma, cystic fibrosis, COPD, and other respiratory diseases. The medical assistant should educate patients about the proper use of these devices.

Gastrointestinal System Examination

Gastroenterologist: A physician who diagnoses and treats disorders of the entire gastrointestinal tract.

Proctology: The branch of medicine concerned with treating disorders of the colon, rectum, and anus.

Medical assistant's role: To tell patients how to prepare for examinations, to order informational brochures, and to answer patients' questions.

Endoscopy: Visual examination of the interior of cavities and organs of the body with an endoscope. The purpose of this procedure is the diagnosis of disorders. Endoscopy also can be used for biopsy. See Figure 17-6.

Gastroscopy: Examination of the stomach and abdominal cavity with a type of endoscope called a gastroscope.

Sigmoidoscopy: Inspection of the rectum and sigmoid colon with the aid of a sigmoidoscope. The medical assistant should assist the physician with the procedure and clean the equipment.

Colonoscopy: Visual examination of the large intestine by means of a colonoscope inserted through the anus.

Anoscope: A speculum used to examine the anus and lower rectum.

Proctoscopy: Examination of the lower rectum and anal canal by means of a proctoscope.

Cholecystogram: An X-ray of the gallbladder, made after injection of a radiopaque substance, usually a contrast medium containing iodine.

Barium swallow: Also called an upper GI series, used to diagnose abnormalities in the esophagus, stomach, and small intestine. The patient swallows a liquid containing barium, and X-rays are taken to record the diagnostic images.

Barium enema: Also called a lower GI series, used to detect abnormalities in the large intestine. Barium is given as an enema.

Gastric lavage: Obtaining a sample of stomach contents with an orogastric tube, which suctions the contents up for analysis.

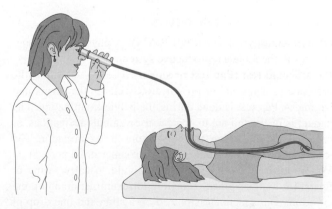

Figure 17-6 *To perform peroral endoscopy, the physician inserts a scope into the patient's mouth.*

Occult blood test: A chemical test or microscopic examination for blood, especially in the feces, that is not apparent on visual inspection.

Colonoscope: A long, flexible endoscope, usually fiber optic, that permits examination of the entire colon.

Laparotomy: Surgical incision into the peritoneal cavity.

Urinary System Examination

Urologist: A physician who specializes in the study of the urinary system.

Medical assistant's role: It is important to be thorough in taking a patient's history in order to obtain information about changes in frequency or urgency of urination, difficulty or pain with urination, and incontinence.

Urinalysis: Physical, chemical, and microscopic examination of urine to find bacteria, blood, or other substances and to monitor for dysfunctions of the prostate gland and for sexually transmitted diseases.

Urine culture: The placement of urine samples on special media that promote the growth of microorganisms and thus facilitate bacterial analysis.

Cystoscopy: Visual examination of the bladder and other urinary structures by means of a special instrument called a cystoscope.

Pyelogram: An X-ray image of the bladder made by using an opaque dye for visualization. The dye may be injected into the patient's vein, or the physician may insert a small catheter into the urethra through a cystoscope and inject the dye through the catheter.

Urinometer: A device for determining the specific gravity of urine. It is also called a urometer.

Vasectomy: A sterilization procedure for men in which a section of each vas deferens is removed.

Testicular self-exam: Because testicular cancer is common in men between the ages of 20 and 35, the medical assistant should teach males, once they enter puberty, about the importance of performing these self-exams because this type of cancer is often asymptomatic initially. They should be performed following a bath or shower, at least once a month, to check for painless nodules.

Gynecology and Obstetrics

Obstetrician/gynecologist (OB/GYN): A physician who specializes in the female reproductive system.

Papanicolau test (Pap test or smear): Used to determine the presence of abnormal or precancerous cells in the cervix and vagina. A Pap test is done during the pelvic examination. The patient is instructed not to douche, use vaginal medications, or have intercourse within 48 hours before the examination. The test should not be done during a patient's menstrual period.

Wet mount: A method of adding liquid, usually saline or formalin, to a specimen on a slide for examination and preservation. The specimen is placed on a slide and one drop of saline (for diagnosis of trichomonas vaginalis) or potassium hydroxide (for diagnosis of vaginal yeast infections, which is caused by *Candida albicans*) is applied and mixes with the specimen.

Pregnancy test: A test to determine whether the hormone human chorionic gonadotropin, which is produced during pregnancy, is present in a woman's blood or urine.

Ultrasonography: The process of imaging deep structures of the body by measuring and recording the reflection of pulsed or continuous high-frequency sound waves. It is a valuable tool to diagnose fetal abnormalities, gallstones, heart defects, and tumors. It is also called sonography.

Mammogram: A low-dose X-ray of breast tissue to detect early cancer. A mammogram is first taken on women between the ages of 35 and 40 years unless otherwise indicated.

Breast self-exam: Because breast cancer is the second most common type of cancer in women, the medical assistant should teach females, after age 20, about the importance of performing these self-exams. They should be performed in the shower, in front of a mirror, or lying down, at least once a month, to check for nodules or changes in breast texture and appearance.

Colposcopy: The examination of the vagina and cervix with a colposcope.

Schiller's test: Iodine staining of cervical and vaginal areas to diagnose cancer of the cervix or vagina.

Laparoscopy: Examination of the abdominal cavity with a laparoscope through one or more small incisions in the abdominal wall. The incisions are usually at the umbilicus. A general anesthetic is used. This procedure is also called an abdominoscopy.

Colpectomy: Partial or complete excision of the vagina, which is also known as *vaginectomy*.

Skin Examination

Dermatologist: A physician who diagnoses and treats skin diseases and disorders.

Whole-body skin examination: An examination of the entire surface of the skin, including the scalp and the areas between the toes, to look for lesions, especially suspicious moles or precancerous growths.

Wood's light examination: A type of dermatological examination in which a physician inspects the patient's skin under an ultraviolet lamp in a darkened room for certain fungal cultures.

Tuberculin skin test: Administered intradermally, a test performed to detect exposure to tuberculosis. Current TB testing involves intradermal injection to test for a skin reaction to tuberculosis. Two–three days after the injection, the result must be measured. The skin is observed for results after 48–72 hours. The tuberculin skin test is also known as the *Mantoux test*.

Scratch test: A test for specific allergies. The skin is scratched with a sterile lancet, and a drop of allergen (antigen) is added to the site. Results are recorded in 30 minutes. Another type of common allergy testing is the *radioallergosorbent test (RAST)*.

Patch test: A test for hypersensitivity allergy. Antigens are applied to the skin and covered with gauze patches and tape. The site is checked in 48 hours, and results are recorded. This type of test is used to discover the cause of contact dermatitis.

Tissue biopsy: There are three types, or methods: excision biopsy, punch biopsy, and shave biopsy.

Neurology Tests

Neurologist: A physician who diagnoses and treats diseases and disorders of the central nervous system and associated systems.

Myelogram: An X-ray taken after the injection of a radiopaque medium into the subarachnoid space to demonstrate any distortions of the spinal cord.

Electroencephalogram (EEG): A graphic chart on which the electrical potential produced by the brain is traced, detected by electrodes placed on the scalp. The resulting brain wave patterns are called alpha, beta, delta, and theta rhythms.

Carotid angiogram: A radiographic image of the carotid artery, into which a contrast medium has been injected.

Alpha-fetoprotein (AFP) testing: Measurements of AFP in amniotic fluid are used for early diagnosis of fetal neural tube defects, such as spina bifida and anencephaly.

Lumbar puncture: A diagnostic and therapeutic procedure done by a physician, involving the introduction of a hollow needle and stylet into the subarachnoid space of the lumbar part of the spinal canal. Also known as a *spinal tap*.

Infants and Children

Well-baby examination: Regular checkups when the infant is two weeks, one month, two months, four months, six months, nine months, 12 months, 15 months, and 18 months old. Starting at age two, children should have checkups every year.

Scoliosis examination: An assessment of a child 10 years of age or older for abnormal lateral curvature of the spine. See Figure 17-7.

Measurement: Examination and measurement of the circumference of the infant's head to determine normal growth and development.

- The size of the child's head reflects the growth of the brain.
- The circumference of the head should be measured during regular checkups, until the child reaches 36 months of age. The length and weight measurements in pediatrics are also important.
- The medical assistant may record and use a physical growth percentile chart to determine the growth value.

Immunizations: Usually given during routine office visits to protect children against hepatitis B, diphtheria, tetanus, pertussis, poliomyelitis, measles, mumps, rubella, chickenpox, and influenza. The child should not have an illness or fever at the time of immunization.

17.4 Minor Surgery

Outpatient surgery: A surgical procedure that requires less than one day and for which the patient does not need to stay in the facility overnight.

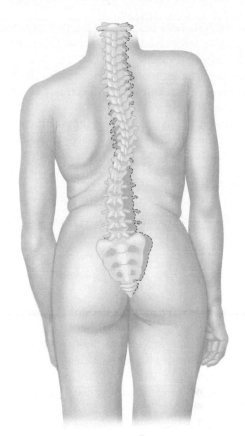

Figure 17-7 *Scoliosis causes the spine to curve into an S shape.*

Ambulatory surgery: A surgical procedure for which the patient is able to walk into and out of the surgical facility on the same day.

Invasive procedure: A diagnostic or therapeutic technique that requires entry into a body cavity or interruption of normal body functions. Examples include the Pap test, sigmoidoscopy, colonoscopy, and intravenous pyelography.

Anesthesia: Partial or complete loss of sensation. It is induced to permit the performance of surgery or other painful procedures. Local anesthesia provides loss of sensation in a particular location without loss of consciousness; it is used for diagnostic procedures or minor surgery. Techniques for administering local anesthetics include topical application, infiltration (injection into tissue), and block (injection into or around a nerve). Types of block anesthesia include regional, spinal, epidural, and saddle, which affect a group of nerves. General anesthesia is used for major surgery.

Anesthetic: A drug or agent used to prevent the sensation of pain and, depending on the situation, to achieve adequate muscle relaxation during surgery, to calm fear and anxiety, and to produce amnesia for the event.

Needle biopsy: The removal of a segment of living tissue for microscopic examination by inserting a hollow needle through the skin or the external surface of an organ or tumor.

Cautery: An agent or device used for scarring, burning, or cutting the skin or other tissues by means of heat, cold, electric current, or caustic chemicals.

Cauterization: The destruction of tissue with a cautery.

Electrocautery: An instrument for directing a high-frequency current through a local area of tissue.

Electrosurgery: The use of electrical current in surgical procedures such as electrocoagulation to cauterize blood vessels and electrocision to excise tissue.

Cryosurgery: The destruction of tissue (e.g., abnormal cells) by the use of freezing temperatures.

Laser: The acronym for *l*ight *a*mplification by *s*timulated *e*mission of *r*adiation. Thermal lasers are used to heat tissue at a microscopic level, causing vaporization and coagulation of the target area.

Surgical Asepsis

Disinfection: The destruction or inhibition of pathogenic organisms by physical means or by chemical germicides. Two common disinfectants are zephrin chloride and chlorophenyl. Contaminated instruments are completely immersed in a germicidal solution for 1–10 hours. The chemical disinfection process is referred to as a "cold" process because no heat is used.

Surgical asepsis: Used when sterility of supplies and the immediate environment is required. This technique is necessary during any invasive procedure. It requires sterile hand washing (surgical scrub), sterile gloves, special handling procedures, and sterilization of materials. Most dangerous bacteria are destroyed at a temperature of 50°–60°C (122°–140°F). Pasteurization of a fluid, which is the application of heat at about 60°C, destroys pathogenic bacteria. However, temperatures of 120°C are usually required to destroy spore cells. A sterile object that touches anything nonsterile is automatically considered contaminated and must not be used in surgery.

Surgical scrub: Hand washing to remove all dirt and microorganisms from the surface of the skin and the fingernails. Materials needed include a sterile surgical scrub brush, a dispenser with surgical soap, orange sticks, and sterile towels. The physician or surgical assistant must remove all jewelry, turn on warm water, keep the hands higher than the elbows, use surgical soap, scrub the hands with a brush for two minutes, rinse the hands, apply more surgical soap, and again scrub the hands for at least three minutes. Total hand-washing time should be approximately 10 minutes.

Sterilization: The process of destroying all microorganisms and their pathogenic products. Methods of sterilization include the application of steam under pressure, dry heat, bactericidal chemical compounds (in liquid or gas form), and radiation.

Moist heat sterilization: A method of sterilization that uses steam under pressure. This method kills all pathogens and spores and is the best and most accepted type of sterilization.

Autoclave: An appliance used to sterilize medical instruments.

- Autoclaving is one of the most effective methods for destruction of all types of microorganisms. The amount of time and the temperature necessary for sterilization depend on the articles to be sterilized.

- Wrapped items autoclaved with steam under pressure require 30 pounds of pressure at 132°C (270°F) for 20 minutes.

- Unwrapped items require only 10 minutes of autoclaving, which is known as flashing. The autoclave chamber must be cleaned after each load.

Dry heat sterilization: A method of sterilization that uses heated dry air at a temperature of 160°–180°C (320°–356°F) for 90 minutes–three hours.

Sterilization indicator: Any material that undergoes a change in appearance (usually a color shift) when it is exposed to a predetermined combination of temperature, pressure, and time. Indicators are used to confirm that the sterilization process has been completed. The most common forms of indicator include autoclave tape and sterilization indicator strips.

Autoclave indicator: A change of color or the appearance of dots on an indicator strip, tube, tape, or tag shows that steam has entered the chamber, not that the instruments are sterile. Autoclave indicator tape turns black after autoclaving.

Shelf life: The amount of time during which an item may be expected to retain its useful characteristics (such as sterility). Packages that have been autoclaved are stored with the date visible, and the oldest package is placed in front so that it is used first. Sterilized instruments are considered to have a shelf life of approximately one month. Autoclaved packages cannot be reautoclaved without washing, rinsing, drying, and rewrapping the items.

Clean gloves: Worn to protect health-care personnel from urine, stools, blood, saliva, and drainage from patients' wounds and lesions.

Sterile gloves: Used to prevent contamination of areas that need to be sterile on the patient.

Formalin: A dilute solution of formaldehyde used to preserve biological specimens.

Instruments

Surgical scissors: A sharp instrument composed of two opposing cutting blades, held together by a central pin on which the blades pivot, used to dissect and cut tissues. See Figure 17-8.

Operating scissors: Straight or curved, with a combination of blades such as sharp/sharp (s/s), blunt/blunt (b/b), or sharp/blunt (s/b).

Suture scissors: Used to remove sutures. The hook on the tip aids in getting under a suture, and the blunt end prevents puncturing of the tissues.

Bandage scissors: Inserted beneath a dressing or bandage to cut it for removal.

Scalpel: A small, straight surgical knife consisting of a handle and a sharp blade that has a convex edge used to make surgical incisions. There are both reusable and disposable scalpels. Blades are numbered according to size. A number 15 blade is often used in performing minor surgeries, such as draining abscesses.

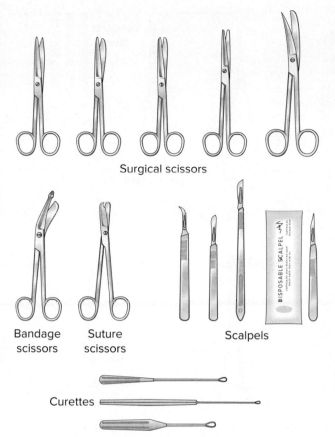

Surgical scissors

Bandage scissors   Suture scissors   Scalpels

Curettes

Figure 17-8 *These cutting and dissecting instruments are typically used in minor surgical procedures.*

Retractors: Used to hold tissue aside to improve the exposure of operative areas. See Figure 17-9.

Probes: Long, slender instruments used to explore wounds or body cavities.

Forceps: A surgical instrument with two handles, each attached to a dull blade, used to grasp, compress, pull, handle, or join tissue, equipment, or supplies. See Figure 17-10. Grasping types include thumb forceps and tissue forceps. (The word *forceps,* like *scissors,* is plural.)

Thumb forceps: Also called smooth forceps, used to pick up tissue or to grasp tissue between the adjacent surfaces of the blades.

Splinter forceps: Thumb forceps with sharp points that are useful in removing foreign objects.

Tissue forceps: Have teeth to prevent them from slipping. They are used to grasp tissue. The *teeth* are also called *serrations.*

Holding forceps: Have handles that can lock the blades closed.

Dressing forceps: Used in the application and removal of dressings.

Hemostatic forceps or hemostats: Used for clamping and grasping blood vessels.

Towel forceps: Used to keep towels in place during a surgical procedure.

Needle holders: Surgical forceps used to hold and pass a suturing needle through tissue. They are also called suture forceps and needle drivers.

Surgical suture needle: A sharp instrument used for puncturing and suturing. The needle carries suture material, also called

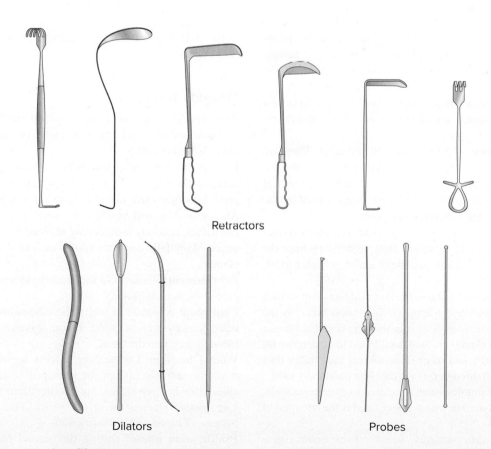

Retractors

Dilators   Probes

Figure 17-9 *These retracting, dilating, and probing instruments are typically used in minor surgical procedures.*

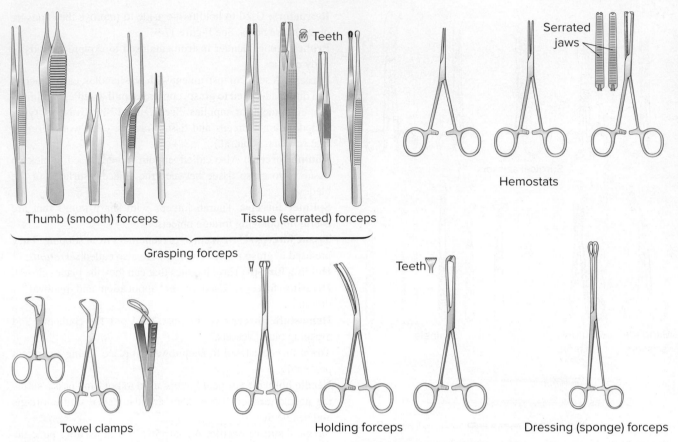

Figure 17-10 *These grasping and clamping instruments are typically used in minor surgical procedures.*

Thumb (smooth) forceps

Teeth

Tissue (serrated) forceps

Grasping forceps

Hemostats

Serrated jaws

Towel clamps

Holding forceps

Teeth

Dressing (sponge) forceps

ligature. Needles vary in their piercing ability (pointed or blunt-tipped), shape (straight or curved), and size, depending on their use. See Figure 17-11. A swaged needle has no eye; instead, the needle and suture material are combined in one length.

Suturing: Using sterile suture material and a needle to close a wound. Ligature (suture material) is of two types: absorbable and nonabsorbable.

Absorbable sutures: Used for internal suturing. They are digested by tissue enzymes and absorbed by body tissues. Absorption usually occurs 5–20 days after insertion. Surgical catgut made from the intestinal lining of sheep is used for the bladder, intestines, and subcutaneous tissue.

Nonabsorbable sutures: Generally used for outer tissues of the body. These types of suture must be removed after the wound begins healing. They may be made of polyester, steel, silk, nylon, or vicryl.

Suture size: In the United States, the size designation of sutures decreases as the thickness (diameter) decreases. Size 7 is the largest generally available. Size 3 is thinner; size 0 is thinner still. Sizes smaller than 0 are indicated by additional zeros: 00 (or 2-0), 000 (or 3-0), and so on. Few sutures are smaller than size 11-0. Sizes 2-0 through 6-0 are the most commonly used.

Staple: A piece of stainless steel wire used to close certain surgical wounds. It is used in major surgery and is the strongest of all suture material.

Suture removal: After surgery, nonabsorbable sutures generally remain in place from 5 to 6 days and then have to be removed. If they are not removed, they can cause infection and skin irritation.

Wounds and Bandaging

Puncture: A wound made by a sharp-pointed object, such as a needle, bullet, carpentry nail, knife, or animal tooth, that pierces the skin layers.

Laceration: A wound in which the tissues are torn apart rather than cut. The edges of the wound are irregular. Dull knife blades and other objects that tear into the skin produce lacerations.

Abrasion: A wound in which the outer layers of the skin are rubbed off, resulting in an oozing of blood from ruptured capillaries. Many falls cause abrasions, such as skinned knees and elbows.

Debridement: Removal of the dead tissue around a wound to expose the healthy tissue.

Contusion: A wound in which the tissues under the skin are injured, as by a blunt object. Blood vessels rupture, allowing blood to seep into the tissue.

Wound healing: The healing process serves to restore the structure and function of the damaged tissue. This process takes place in three phases: lag, proliferation, and maturation.

Lag phase: During the initial phase, bleeding is reduced because of blood vessel constriction.

Proliferation phase: During the second phase, new tissue forms.

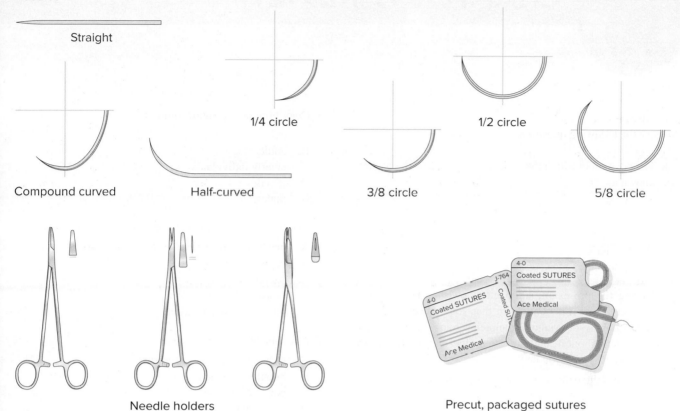

Needles

Straight

1/4 circle

1/2 circle

Compound curved

Half-curved

3/8 circle

5/8 circle

Needle holders

Precut, packaged sutures

Figure 17-11 *These instruments are typically used in suturing.*

Maturation phase: The last phase involves the formation of scar tissue.

Dressing: Sterile material used to cover a surgical or other wound.

Bandage: A strip of woven material used to wrap or cover a part of the body. A bandage causes pressure to control bleeding, protects a wound from contamination, holds a dressing in place, or supports or immobilizes an injured part of the body.

Types of bandage: Four types of bandage are often used in the medical office: roller, elastic, triangular, and tube gauze.

Roller bandages: Long strips of soft material that are coiled to form rolls. They are often used to apply pressure (i.e., as pressure bandages).

Elastic bandages: Made of woven cotton containing elastic fibers. They are typically used on swollen extremities or joints, on the chest to treat empyema, on fractured ribs, and on legs to support varicose veins. They are expensive, but they can be washed and reused.

Triangular bandages: Usually made of muslin and measuring approximately 55 inches across the base and 40 inches along the sides. They are frequently used in first aid.

Tube gauze bandage: Seamless tubular gauze bandage, with or without elastic, is superior material for covering round narrow surfaces such as fingers or toes. It can be used as either a dressing or a bandage. A tubular gauze bandage is applied with a cagelike applicator.

STRATEGIES FOR SUCCESS

▶ *Test-Taking Skills*

Answer the easy ones first!

Answering all the questions you know first will give you confidence and momentum to get through the rest of the exam. As you go through the exam, make a mark next to any questions that you want to come back to—questions you are uncertain about or difficult questions you don't want to answer right away. Go back to these questions once you've answered all the questions that you thought were easy. Often you will be surprised how your subconscious mind has continued to work on these questions, or perhaps how something later in the test has jogged your memory, and these hard questions won't seem that difficult anymore.

Instructions:

Answer the following questions.

1. The position in which the patient is lying flat on the back is known as

   A. prone.
   B. Sims'.
   C. supine.
   D. Fowler's.
   E. lithotomy.

2. During the pre-examination interview, you notice some cuts on an adult patient's arm that you suspect might be signs of abuse or even of attempted suicide. You try to ask the patient about it, but the patient doesn't want to talk to you. What should you do?

   A. Press the patient and explain how important it is that all your questions be answered.
   B. Call the police immediately and report that you have a victim of abuse to whom they need to talk.
   C. Tell the examining physician, and prepare a list of community resources that can provide advice and support to the patient even if the patient is not ready to talk to you.
   D. Ignore the problem because the patient obviously does not want to talk about it, and go on with assisting the physician as if you didn't see anything.
   E. Transfer the patient to a mental institution and notify immediate family members.

3. Which of the following positions is used for vaginal- and perineal-area examination?

   A. lithotomy
   B. Fowler's
   C. supine
   D. jackknife
   E. Trendelenburg's

4. Which of the following positions requires the examination table to be raised in the middle with both ends pointing down?

   A. Fowler's
   B. proctological
   C. knee-chest
   D. Sims'
   E. none of these

5. Color blindness is more common in

   A. children.
   B. adults.
   C. elderly individuals.
   D. females.
   E. males.

6. The best and most accepted method of sterilization is

   A. dry heat sterilization.
   B. zephrin chloride.
   C. bactericidal solution.
   D. moist heat sterilization.
   E. ultrasound sterilization.

7. A tonometer is used to detect

   A. nerve impairment of the ears.
   B. breathing capacity.
   C. contact dermatitis.
   D. glaucoma.
   E. heart rate.

8. A method of screening auditory acuity by placing the stem of a vibrating tuning fork against the center of the patient's forehead (to evaluate whether hearing is the same in both ears) is known as

   A. Weber's test.
   B. audiology test.
   C. audiometer.
   D. Schiller's test.
   E. none of these

9. In which of the following positions, used for the examination of the rectum, does the patient lie on the left side with the left leg slightly flexed?

   A. Sims'
   B. prone
   C. lithotomy
   D. dorsal recumbent
   E. Trendelenburg's

10. A drop of potassium hydroxide is added to a wet-mount preparation of vaginal secretions for which of the following reasons?

    A. to prevent overgrowth of microorganisms
    B. to determine *Neisseria gonorrhea*
    C. to sterilize the specimen
    D. to visualize *Candida albicans*
    E. to preserve *Trichomonas vaginalis*

CHAPTER 18

VITAL SIGNS AND MEASUREMENT

LEARNING OUTCOMES

18.1 Recall normal ranges, reason for, and process of obtaining a patient's temperature, pulse, respiratory rate, and blood pressure.

18.2 Describe the process of obtaining a patient's height and weight.

MEDICAL ASSISTING COMPETENCIES

COMPETENCY	CMA	RMA	CCMA	NCMA
Clinical				
Apply principles of aseptic techniques and infection control, including hand washing	X	X	X	X
Practice standard precautions	X	X	X	X
Obtain vital signs	X	X	X	X
General/Legal/Professional				
Determine the needs for documentation and reporting, and document accurately and appropriately	X	X	X	X
Conduct work within scope of education, training, and ability	X	X	X	X
Use appropriate medical terminology	X	X	X	X

18.1 Vital Signs

Vital signs: Also known as cardinal signs. They indicate that life is present. They are also indicators of the body's ability to maintain homeostasis. The vital signs include temperature (T), pulse (P), respiration (R), and blood pressure (BP). Pain assessment is also considered a vital sign. For normal ranges of vital signs, see Table 18-1.

Taking vital signs: OSHA has specific guidelines that must be followed in measuring vital signs. See Table 18-2.

Temperature

Celsius (°C): A scale for measurement of temperature in which 0°C is the freezing point of water and 100°C is the boiling point of water at sea level. Celsius is also known as centigrade.

Fahrenheit (°F): A scale for measurement of temperature in which the boiling point of water is 212°F. The freezing point of water is 32°F at sea level.

Converting Fahrenheit to Celsius: Subtract 32 from the Fahrenheit temperature, multiply the remainder by five, and divide by nine. See Table 18-3.

Converting Celsius to Fahrenheit: Multiply the Celsius temperature by nine, divide by five, and add 32. See Table 18-3. It is important that you know how to use these conversion formulas.

Body temperature: Controlled by the hypothalamus, located in the brain, and maintained through a balance of the heat produced in the body and the heat lost from the body. Most heat is produced in the body by muscle contractions and cell metabolism. Fever and strong emotional states increase heat production in the body. Radiation, evaporation, conduction, and convection all cause loss of heat from the body. Body temperature is measured with a thermometer.

AT A GLANCE   Normal Ranges for Vital Signs

	0–1 year	1–6 years	6–11 years	11–16 years	Adult
Temperature (°F)					
Oral	96–99.5	98.5–99.5	97.5–99.6	97.6–99.6	97.6–99.6
Rectal	99–100	99–100	98.5–99.6	98.6–100.6	98.6–100.6
Pulse (beats per minute)	80–160	75–130	70–115	55–110	60–100
Respirations (per minute)	26–40	20–30	18–24	16–24	12–20
Blood Pressure (mm Hg)					
Systolic	60–95	80–100	80–120	94–136	90–120
Diastolic	50–65	50–70	50–80	58–88	60–80

Table 18-1

AT A GLANCE   OSHA Guidelines for Taking Measurement of Vital Signs

Situation	OSHA Guideline
Before and after all patient contact	Clean the examination area according to OSHA standards.
Taking temperature orally or rectally, contact with a patient with lesions, contact with a patient suspected of having an infectious disease	Wear gloves. Use biohazard bags to dispose of thermometer sheaths, otoscope tips, alcohol swabs, dressings, and bandages.
In the presence of a patient suspected of having an airborne infectious disease	Wear a mask. The patient should be weighed, measured, and examined in a room away from staff and other patients. Wear protective clothing. Use biohazard bags for disposal of wastes.

Table 18-2

Converting From Celsius to Fahrenheit	Converting From Fahrenheit to Celsius
$°F = (°C \times 9/5) + 32$	$°C = (°F - 32) \times 5/9$
Note that, in this conversion, you may substitute the decimal 1.8 for the fraction 9/5 if desired.	Note that, in this conversion, you may substitute the decimal 0.55 for the fraction 5/9 if desired.

Table 18-3

Normal body temperature range: The range is from 97°F–99°F (36°C–37.2°C). The average temperature is 98.6°F (37°C).

Pyrexia: Fever, which is defined as any body temperature above 100.4°F (38°C). Causes of fever include infection, heat stroke, neoplasms, drug hypersensitivity, and central nervous system damage. Fevers are classified in five levels. See Table 18-4.

Hyperpyrexia: A temperature reading above 105.8°F (41°C). A body temperature above 106.0°F (41.1°C) is generally fatal.

Hypothermia: Occurs when the temperature falls below 97°F (36°C). In general, a body temperature below 93.2°F (34°C) is fatal.

Febrile: Having a body temperature above the normal range.

Afebrile: Having a body temperature within the normal range. The average normal value is 98.6°F (37°C).

Lysis: The gradual return of body temperature to normal after a period of fever; also, the gradual decline of a disease symptom.

Crisis: The sudden decrease of body temperature to normal levels. The patient may perspire profusely (diaphoresis). This term also refers to the turning point of a disease, when an important change has occurred.

Intermittent fever: A fluctuating fever that returns to or below baseline, then increases again.

Continuous fever: A fever that remains above the baseline; it does not fluctuate, but remains fairly constant.

Remittent fever: A fluctuating fever that does not return to the baseline temperature; it fluctuates, but remains increased.

Types of thermometers: Several types of thermometers are used in the ambulatory care setting, with digital thermometers being most common. Types of thermometers include reusable, disposable, and glass Galinstan (containing gallium or alcohol—these are not electronic or digital). Specific thermometers are available for a variety of locations on the body in order to measure temperature.

Electronic (digital) thermometer: The most prevalent type of thermometer used today, there are many varieties allowing quick, accurate temperatures to be taken in a number of body locations. See Figure 18-1.

Oral thermometer: Taking temperature orally is the most convenient method. An electronic (digital) thermometer should be placed in the mouth for at least 10 seconds.

Tympanic (aural) thermometer: Tympanic thermometers are used by inserting their shielded tip in the ear. Their benefits are speed and patient comfort. Accurate readings are obtained in approximately two seconds. Average temperature is 98.6°F. It is used with uncooperative patients of any age.

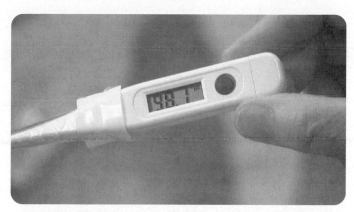

Figure 18-1 A: *An electronic (digital) thermometer.*
© McGraw-Hill Education

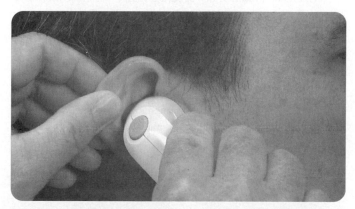

Figure 18-1 B: *The tympanic thermometer measures infrared energy emitted from the tympanic membrane. The result, converted to body temperature, is displayed within seconds of insertion of the shielded tip into the ear.*
© McGraw-Hill Education

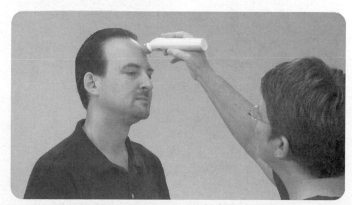

Figure 18-1 C: *A temporal artery thermometer, passed across the forehead, measures blood temperature in the temporal artery.*
© McGraw-Hill Education

Level	Fahrenheit (°F)	Celsius (°C)
Slight	99.6–101.0	37.5–38.3
Moderate	101.0–102.0	38.3–38.8
Severe	102.0–104.0	38.8–40.0
Dangerous	104.0–105.0	40.0–40.5
Fatal	Over 106.0	Over 41.1

Table 18-4

Axillary thermometer: The thermometer is placed in the middle of the axilla, with the shaft facing forward. The average normal value is 97.6°F. It is the least accurate measurement site for body temperature; 1° is added to the temperature.

Rectal thermometer: Rectal temperature is 1°F higher than oral (99.6°F). A rectal thermometer is used if a patient is unconscious, has had oral surgery, is very young, or is uncooperative. It is the most accurate method since it measures the body's core temperature.

Temporal artery (TA) thermometer: A new, noninvasive thermometer that is more accurate than most other thermometers. It is used on adults and children. The TA thermometer is fast and convenient to use. It is gently stroked across the patient's forehead, and uses infrared heat waves to measure the temperature from the temporal artery.

Mercury thermometer: An old type of thermometer that has been almost entirely replaced by digital thermometers of various types, because the risk for mercury poisoning is great if a mercury thermometer is broken and mercury escapes into the environment. The sale of mercury thermometers is now widely restricted. Additional information is available at http://www.epa.gov/mercury.

Antipyretic: Pertaining to a substance that reduces fever.

Pulse

Pulse: The throbbing of an artery caused by the flow of blood when the heart beats.

Pulse rate: The number of times the heart beats in a minute. The normal pulse rate in adults is 60–100 beats per minute.

- Several factors affect the pulse rate: age, sex, body size, physical exercise, health status, and medications. Infants and children have a faster pulse than adults. The pulse is usually faster in women than in men. Exercise increases the pulse rate. Anxiety, fever, anger, cancer, pregnancy, and hyperthyroidism can increase the pulse rate. Epinephrine increases and digitalis decreases the pulse rate.

- A stethoscope is used to auscultate the apical pulse.

Pulse oximetry: A noninvasive method of using photodetection technology to measure oxygen saturation of a patient. A sensory device is placed onto a fingertip or earlobe; or in infants, across a foot.

Tachycardia: A pulse rate above 100 beats per minute.

Bradycardia: A pulse rate below 60 beats per minute.

Pulse sites: A pulse can be taken at many locations on the body, including the temporal, carotid, brachial, radial, femoral, popliteal, posterior tibial, and dorsalis pedis arteries. See Figure 18-2.

Temporal artery: Located at the temple area of the skull. It is seldom used as a pulse site.

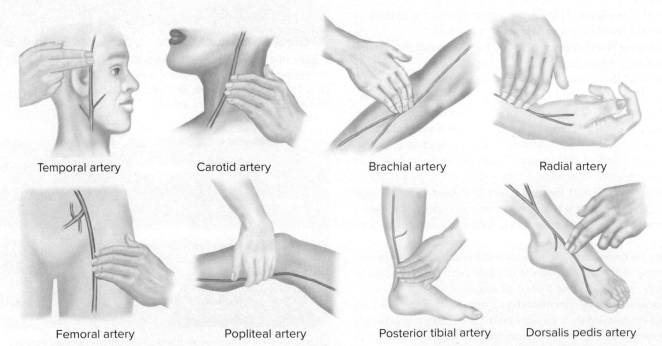

Temporal artery   Carotid artery   Brachial artery   Radial artery

Femoral artery   Popliteal artery   Posterior tibial artery   Dorsalis pedis artery

Figure 18-2 *There are many locations on the body where major arteries are close enough to the surface to allow a pulse to be felt and counted.*

Brachial artery: Located in the inner aspect of the elbow called the antecubital space. This site is the most commonly used site to obtain blood pressure measurements and pulse.

Carotid artery: Located between the larynx and the sternocleidomastoid muscle in the neck. This site is used in emergencies and during CPR.

Radial artery: Found in the groove on the thumb side of the inner wrist. It is the most commonly used site for measuring the pulse rate in adults.

Apical pulse: The pulse at the apex of the heart, located in the left fifth intercostal space on the midclavicular line. It must be heard with a stethoscope. This site is used commonly for newborns, infants, and children. The pulse is counted for 60 seconds. See Figure 18-3.

Popliteal artery: Located at the back of the knee. The patient must be in a supine position with the knee flexed for it to be felt because the artery is deep within the knee. This artery is the one used for leg blood pressure measurements and to monitor circulation.

Dorsalis pedis pulse: Felt on the top of the foot slightly to the side of midline. It is commonly used to monitor lower limb circulation.

Pulse deficit: The difference between the apical pulse rate and the radial pulse rate.

Blood stasis: Lack of circulation due to a stoppage of blood flow.

Respiration Rate

Respiration: The exchange of oxygen and carbon dioxide between living organisms or tissues and their surroundings; also, breathing (inhaling and exhaling, or inspiration and expiration). The control center for breathing is in the medulla oblongata (in the brain). There are two types of respiration: external and internal.

External respiration: The exchange of O_2 and CO_2 in the lungs.

Internal respiration: The exchange of O_2 and CO_2 at the tissue level.

Characteristics of respiration: The best way to check respiration is by watching the movement at the patient's chest, back, abdomen, or shoulders. Three important characteristics must be noted: rate, rhythm, and depth.

Respiratory rate: The number of respirations per minute. The normal adult range is 12–20 cycles per minute.

Increased respiratory rates: Occur because of asthma, heart attack, fever, hemorrhage, high altitudes, allergic reactions, nervousness, obstruction of air passages, shock, and pain.

Decreased respiratory rates: May occur as a result of the action of certain drugs (morphine), a decrease of CO_2 in the blood, stroke, and coma. The respiratory rate also can be affected by factors such as age.

Emphysema: An abnormal pulmonary condition with loss of lung elasticity, resulting in difficulty in exhaling.

Cyanosis: Bluish discoloration of the skin and mucous membranes due to oxygen deprivation.

Apnea: Temporary cessation of respirations that last more than 15 seconds.

Bradypnea: Slow respiration in an adult, fewer than 10 cycles per minute.

Hyperpnea: Rapid and deep breathing.

Dyspnea: Difficult or painful breathing.

Orthopnea: Difficulty in breathing when lying down.

Tachypnea: Fast breathing, more than 35 respirations per minute.

Depth of respiration: The amount of air being inhaled and exhaled.

Rales: Abnormal or crackling breath sounds that occur during the inspirational portion of breathing.

Stertorous: Characterized by a deep snoring sound that occurs with each inspiration.

Rhonchi: Whistling sounds made in the throat, also called gurgles. They are heard in patients with various respiratory disorders or conditions, such as asthma or chronic obstructive pulmonary disease.

Wheezing: High-pitched musical sound heard on expiration, often the result of an obstruction or narrowing of respiratory passage.

Stridor: Shrill, harsh respiratory sound heard during inhalation in the presence of a laryngeal obstruction or croup in children.

Spirogram: A visual record of respiratory movement made by a spirometer and used in the assessment of pulmonary function and capacity.

Spirometer: An instrument that measures and records the volume of inhaled and exhaled air.

Blood Pressure

Heart sounds: There are two basic heart sounds: The first, produced at systole, when the atrioventricular valves close is dull, firm, and prolonged (a "lubb" sound); the second, produced at diastole when the semilunar valves close, is shorter and sharper (a "dupp" sound). A "lubb dupp" is the sound of one heartbeat.

Blood pressure (BP): The pressure of the blood against the walls of the arteries. There are two BP readings: systolic pressure and diastolic pressure. Readings of BP give the systolic measure first, then the diastolic measure, in millimeters (mm)

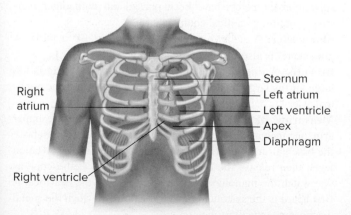

Figure 18-3 *A stethoscope is used over the apex of the heart to listen for the pulse in patients in whom pulse is difficult to detect.*

Right atrium
Right ventricle
Sternum
Left atrium
Left ventricle
Apex
Diaphragm

of mercury (Hg). BP readings should routinely be started at the age of five years.

Normal BP: Depends on age. The average normal BP in healthy persons of different ages is listed in Table 18-5.

Pulse pressure: The difference between the systolic and the diastolic pressure readings.

Systolic blood pressure: A measurement of the amount of pressure that blood exerts on arteries and vessels while the heart is beating.

Diastolic blood pressure: A measurement of the pressure exerted on the walls of various arteries in between heart beats, when the heart is relaxed.

Korotkoff's sounds: Heard during the taking of blood pressure by means of a sphygmomanometer and stethoscope. As air is released from the cuff, pressure on the brachial artery is reduced, and the blood is heard pulsing through the artery.

Factors affecting BP: Five physiological factors affect BP: blood volume, peripheral resistance of the vessels, condition of the heart muscle, vessel elasticity, and blood viscosity.

Blood volume and blood viscosity: BP elevates as the blood volume increases. Polycytopenia increases BP. Hemorrhage causes volume and BP to drop.

Peripheral resistance: The relationship of the lumen of the vessel and amount of blood flowing through it. Fatty cholesterol deposits narrow the lumen, resulting in high BP.

Heart muscle condition: The strength of the heart muscle affects the volume of blood flow.

Elasticity of vessels: The ability of blood vessels to expand and contract. It decreases with age.

Hypertension: High BP, defined as systolic pressure consistently above 140 mm Hg and diastolic pressure above 90 mm Hg. According to the American Heart Association, patients with systolic readings 130–139 mm Hg and diastolic readings 85–89 mm Hg are considered prehypertensive. Several factors contribute to hypertension, including hyperthyroidism, heart and liver disease, rigidity of blood vessels, smoking, anxiety, stress, and race. There are two types of hypertension: primary (essential) and secondary (nonessential). Hypertension should be found on at least two occasions before the patient is placed on medications, unless the diastolic reading is over 120 mm Hg.

Essential hypertension: The vast majority of patients with hypertension (90%) have essential hypertension. The actual cause of essential high BP is not known. It may be genetic.

Nonessential hypertension: Caused by disorders of other organs in the body, such as the kidney, as well as endocrine disorders.

Malignant hypertension: The most fatal form of hypertension. It is characterized by rapidly and severely elevated BP that commonly damages the intima of small vessels, the brain, the retina, the heart, and the kidneys. It is more common among African Americans and may be caused by genetic predisposition, stress, obesity, smoking, the use of contraceptives, and aging.

Hypotension: An abnormal condition in which the BP is not adequate for full oxygenation of the tissues. Several factors may cause hypotension. They include anemia, dehydration, shock, hemorrhage, cancer, starvation, infection, high fever, and certain medications. The common drugs that affect BP and cause hypotension are analgesics, narcotics, antihypertensives, and diuretics. Persistent readings of 90/60 mm Hg or below are usually considered hypotensive.

Orthostatic hypotension: Abnormally and temporarily low BP. It occurs when a patient rapidly moves from a lying to a standing position and is also called postural hypotension. Orthostatic hypotension can cause patients to experience vertigo or syncope. Some medications may cause orthostatic hypotension. Orthostatic blood pressure is ideally measured while the patient is lying down, then sitting, and then standing. For very frail patients, standing is avoided for measurement, and only lying-down and sitting BP is taken.

Stethoscope: A diagnostic instrument that amplifies sound, used to detect sounds produced by BP as well as heart sounds. This instrument consists of a chest piece consisting of a diaphragm and/or bell, flexible tubing, binaurals, a spring mechanism, and ear pieces.

Sphygmomanometer: An instrument used to measure BP. The components are the manometer, an inflation bulb with a control valve, and a pressure cuff. There are two types of sphygmomanometers: aneroid and digital (electronic). Mercury sphygmomanometers have been phased out with other mercury-containing medical equipment.

Manometer: A scale that registers the actual BP reading. A manometer is also called a pressure indicator.

BP cuffs: A thigh cuff is available when an adult arm is too large for the large arm cuff. When using a thigh cuff, the popliteal artery is palpated for a pulse.

Measuring BP: Wrap properly sized cuff around the upper arm, one inch above the elbow with center of the bladder above the brachial artery. Inflate the cuff to the maximum inflation level, then release the air, and listen with the stethoscope as you watch the manometer. The point at which the heartbeat is first heard is the systolic pressure; the point at which the sound disappears is the diastolic pressure.

Anthropometric: Relating to body size and proportion.

AT A GLANCE	Normal Blood Pressure at Different Ages
Age	**Average (mm Hg)**
Newborn	50/25
6–9 years	95/65
10–15 years	100/65
Young adult	118/76
Adult	120 to 129 / 80 to 84

Table 18-5

18.2 Body Measurements

Mensuration: A general term for the measurement of weight and height. Mensuration for infants also includes measuring the circumference of the head and chest.

First visit: Provides baseline or normal values for the patient's current condition. Weight and height measurements are taken at each office visit. Any sudden changes may be an indication of a medical problem.

Measuring weight (adult):

1. Identify the patient and introduce yourself.
2. Wash your hands and explain the procedure.
3. Check to see whether the scale is in balance by moving all the weights to the left side. The indicator should be level with the middle mark. If you are using a scale equipped to measure both kilograms and pounds, check to see that the scale is set to measure the desired units and that the upper and lower weights show the same units.
4. Place a disposable towel on the scale.
5. Ask the patient to remove shoes.
6. Ask the patient to step on the center of the scale, facing forward.
7. Place the lower weight at the highest number that does not cause the balance indicator to drop to the bottom.
8. Move the upper weight slowly to the right until the balance bar is centered at the middle mark, adjusting as necessary.
9. Add the two weight measurements together.
10. Record the patient's weight to the nearest quarter of a pound or tenth of a kilogram.

Measuring height (adult): See Figure 18-4.

1. Raise the height bar well above the patient's head and swing out the extension.

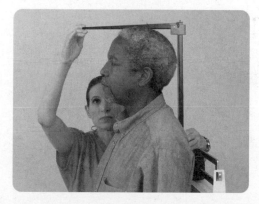

Figure 18-4 *The scale with attached height, bar at a 90-degree angle, is used for measuring the height and weight of children and adults.*
Courtesy of Shirley Zeiberg

2. Ask the patient to step on the center of the scale and stand up straight.
3. Gently lower the height bar until the extension rests on the patient's head.
4. Have the patient step off the scale before you read the measurement.
5. If the patient is fewer than 50 inches tall, read the height on the bottom part of the ruler. If the patient is more than 50 inches tall, read the height on the top, movable part of the ruler. Note that the numbers increase in opposite directions on the top and bottom, so make sure that you read the height in the right direction.
6. Record the patient's height.

Measuring height (infant):

1. The infant (this includes children under the age of two years) is measured while lying down, which is referred to as *recumbent length*. Two people should perform the measurement. The infant should be wearing only a clean diaper and an undershirt.
2. A flat, horizontal measuring table is covered with appropriate paper.
3. The measurer should stand at the infant's right side, while the assistant stands behind the infant's head.
4. Make sure that the infant is held sufficiently to remain as still as possible, and not roll off of the measuring table.
5. The assistant should cup the infant's ears and keep the head against the measuring table. The line from the infant's ear canals to the bottom of the eye sockets should be perpendicular to the table. The chin should not be lowered to meet the chest or raised too far back. The infant's body should be lying as flat against the table as possible.
6. The movable foot piece should be moved up, flat against the child's heels.
7. The infant's recumbent length should be read and called out, to the nearest 1/8 inch (0.1 centimeter), and recorded. It is common to take more than one measurement in order to account for movements and obtain the correct recumbent length.

Measuring weight (infant):

1. A calibrated infant scale is used to measure an infant's weight.
2. Ideally, the infant should be weighed nude, or only wearing a clean diaper.
3. Two people should perform the measurement. One weighs the infant and protects from falling, and so on, while the other records the measurement.
4. The infant should be placed in the center of the scale's tray. The weight should be recorded to the nearest ½ ounce (0.01 kilogram). The weight should be measured

at least twice to account for movements that can affect correct measurement. The measurements should agree within ¼ pound (0.1 kilogram) of each other.

5. The *tolerance of the measure,* which is multiple weight measurements that agree within ¼ pound (0.1 kilogram), should be recorded.

6. An alternative method is to zero out an adult scale, weigh the parent and record this weight, reset the scale to zero, then have the parent hold the child and weigh them together. The difference is the infant's weight. Note that adult scales are not as closely accurate, so this method should be used only if the suggested method is not possible for some reason.

Measuring head circumference of an infant:

1. Position the tape just above the eyebrows, above the ears, and around the largest part on the back of the infant's head.

2. Pull the tape tightly enough to compress the hair.

3. Read the measurement to the nearest 1/8 inch (0.1 centimeter).

4. Write the measurement on the chart or enter it appropriately if using an electronic charting method.

Instructions:

Answer the following questions.

1. The normal pulse rate (in beats per minute) for adults is
   A. 40–60.
   B. 60–100.
   C. 80–100.
   D. 100–120.
   E. 120–140.

2. The artery most commonly used for taking an adult patient's pulse is
   A. carotid.
   B. apical.
   C. temporal.
   D. celiac.
   E. radial.

3. A patient has an oral temperature of 100.5°F. The medical term for this condition is
   A. hyperpyrexia.
   B. pyuria.
   C. pyrexia.
   D. hypothermia.
   E. normal.

4. Which of the following respiratory terms means "difficulty breathing"?
   A. bradypnea
   B. orthopnea
   C. dyspnea
   D. apnea
   E. eupnea

5. The absence of respiration for periods lasting more than 15 seconds is called
   A. bradypnea.
   B. hyperpnea.
   C. shock.
   D. Cheyne-Stokes.
   E. apnea.

6. Which of the following refers to the process of determining the circumference of an infant's head?
   A. manipulation
   B. mensuration
   C. palpation
   D. inspection
   E. auscultation

7. Which of the following is an instrument used to amplify sounds?
   A. tympanoscope
   B. arthroscope
   C. stethoscope
   D. endoscope
   E. otoscope

8. How is orthostatic blood pressure ideally measured?
   A. when the patient is sitting, then lying down
   B. only when the patient is standing
   C. only when the patient is lying down
   D. with the patient lying, sitting, then standing
   E. when the patient is unconscious

9. Which of the following methods of obtaining body temperature utilizes infrared heat waves?
   A. temporal artery
   B. aural
   C. axillary
   D. oral
   E. gallium

10. Which of the following agents commonly causes hypotension?
    A. narcotics
    B. antihypertensives
    C. diuretics
    D. analgesics
    E. all of these

CHAPTER 19

PHARMACOLOGY

LEARNING OUTCOMES

19.1 Recognize the general terminology and concepts of pharmacology.

19.2 Identify drug forms, regulations for handling, and the effects of drugs in the human body.

19.3 Describe the different routes and methods of administering medication.

19.4 Identify types of antibiotics and their uses.

19.5 Identify the classifications, uses, and effects of drugs used to treat the integumentary system.

19.6 Identify the classifications, uses, and effects of drugs used to treat the musculoskeletal system.

19.7 Identify the classifications, uses, and effects of drugs used to treat the nervous system.

19.8 Identify the classifications, uses, and effects of drugs used to treat the cardiovascular system.

19.9 Identify the classifications, uses, and effects of drugs used to treat the respiratory system.

19.10 Identify the classifications, uses, and effects of drugs used to treat the digestive system.

19.11 Identify the classifications, uses, and effects of drugs used to treat the endocrine system.

19.12 Identify the classifications, uses, and effects of drugs used to treat the sensory system.

19.13 Identify the classifications, uses, and effects of drugs used to treat the urinary system.

19.14 Identify the classifications, uses, and effects of drugs used to treat the reproductive system.

MEDICAL ASSISTING COMPETENCIES

COMPETENCY	CMA	RMA	CCMA	NCMA
Clinical				
Apply principles of aseptic techniques and infection control, including hand washing	X	X	X	X
Practice standard precautions	X	X	X	X
Apply pharmacology principles to prepare and administer oral and parenteral (excluding IV) medications as directed by the physician	X	X	X	X
Maintain medication and immunization records	X	X	X	X
General/Legal/Professional				
Identify and respond to issues of confidentiality by maintaining confidentiality at all times and following appropriate guidelines when releasing records or information	X	X	X	X

MEDICAL ASSISTING COMPETENCIES (cont.)

General/Legal/Professional

Be aware of and perform within legal and ethical boundaries	X	X	X	X
Determine the needs for documentation and reporting, and document accurately and appropriately	X	X	X	X
Demonstrate knowledge of and monitor current federal and state health-care legislation and regulations, maintain licenses and accreditation	X	X	X	X
Dispose of controlled substances in compliance with government regulations	X	X	X	X
Perform risk management procedures	X	X	X	
Instruct individuals according to their needs	X	X	X	X
Provide patients with methods of health promotion and disease prevention	X	X	X	X
Conduct work within scope of education, training, and ability	X	X	X	X
Use appropriate medical terminology	X	X	X	X

STRATEGIES FOR SUCCESS

▶ *Study Skills*

Ask questions!

When you have trouble understanding a concept, don't be afraid to ask your instructor to explain it to you. If you are still unclear about something, go to your local library and try to find the answer in a reference book or check the Internet. The job of a medical assistant is complex, and it's easy to feel overwhelmed. Take control of your own education and success, and seek out the answers you need.

19.1 General Pharmacology Terms and Concepts

Pharmacology: The study of the origin, nature, chemistry, effects, and uses of drugs.

Drug: Any substance that may modify one or more of the functions of a living organism. Drugs have several uses, including therapeutic, palliative, preventive, replacement, and diagnostic. Table 19-1 provides information on drug uses. The 50 most commonly dispensed drugs in the United States are listed by category in Table 19-2.

Pharmacy: The art of compounding, preparing, dispensing, and correctly utilizing drugs for medicinal use; also, a drugstore.

AT A GLANCE Drugs and Their Uses

Type of Use	Purpose of Use
Therapeutic	To cure disease
Palliative	To relieve symptoms
Preventive	To prevent certain conditions
Replacement	To replace substances that the body is not producing sufficiently
Diagnostic	To diagnose disease

Table 19-1

Rank	Generic Name	Trade Name	Category
1	aripiprazole	Abilify®	Antipsychotic
2	esomeprazole	Nexium®	Proton pump inhibitor
3	adalimumab	Humira®	Biologic response modifier (tumor necrosis factor blocker)
4	rosuvastatin	Crestor®	Antihyperlipidemic, HMG-CoA reductase inhibitor
5	fluticasone, salmeterol	Advair Diskus®	Antiasthmatic combination drug
6	etanercept	Enbrel®	Biologic response modifier (tumor necrosis factor blocker)
7	infliximab	Remicade®	Biologic response modifier (tumor necrosis factor blocker)
8	duloxetine	Cymbalta®	Antidepressant, selective serotonin and norepinephrine reuptake inhibitor
9	glatiramer	Copaxone®	Amino acid combination drug used to treat multiple sclerosis
10	pegfilgrastim	Neulasta®	Colony stimulating factor used to prevent neutropenia caused by chemotherapy
11	insulin glargine	Lantus Solostar (Pen)®	Synthetic hormone used to treat type 1 or type 2 diabetes
12	rituximab	Rituxan®	Antineoplastic agent, used to treat non-Hodgkin's lymphoma or chronic lymphocytic leukemia
13	tiotropium	Spiriva Handihaler®	Anticholinergic
14	sitagliptin	Januvia®	Antidiabetic agent, dipeptidyl peptidase-4 inhibitor
15	efavirenz, emtricitabine, tenofovir	Atripla®	Combination drug used to treat HIV
16	insulin glargine	Lantus®	Antidiabetic, long-acting insulin
17	bevacizumab	Avastin®	Antineoplastic agent, usually combined with other agents, to treat brain, kidney, lung, colon, and rectal cancers
18	pregabalin	Lyrica®	Anticonvulsant, miscellaneous
19	oxycodone	OxyContin®	Narcotic analgesic
20	epoetin alfa	Epogen®	Synthetic protein used to treat anemia
21	celecoxib	Celebrex®	Nonsteroidal anti-inflammatory drug, COX-2 inhibitor
22	tenofovir, emtricitabine	Truvada®	Combination drug used to treat HIV
23	valsartan	Diovan®	Antihypertensive, angiotensin II receptor blocker
24	imatinib	Gleevec®	Antineoplastic agent, used to treat certain leukemias, stomach cancers, and other digestive system cancers
25	trastuzumab	Herceptin®	Antineoplastic agent, used to treat certain breast and stomach cancers
26	ranibizumab	Lucentis®	Human antibody used to treat macular degeneration and retinal swelling
27	memantine	Named®	Alzheimer's disease
28	lisdexamfetamine	Vyvanse®	CNS stimulant used to treat attention deficit hyperactivity disorder (ADHD)

Table 19-2

Rank	Generic Name	Trade Name	Category
29	ezetimibe	Zetia®	Antihyperlipidemic drug
30	insulin detemir	Levemir®	Synthetic insulin used to treat type 1 or type 2 diabetes mellitus
31	budesonide, formoterol	Symbicort®	Combination steroidal drug to treat asthma and COPD
32	sofosbuvir	Sovaldi®	Antiviral, used to prevent hepatitis C virus cells from multiplying
33	insulin aspart	NovoLog FlexPen®	Fast-acting rDNA-origin insulin used to treat type 1 diabetes mellitus (FlexPen is prefilled and disposable)
34	insulin aspart	NovoLog®	Fast-acting rDNA-origin insulin used to treat type 1 diabetes mellitus
35	dimethyl fumarate	Tecfidera®	Used to treat relapsing multiple sclerosis
36	buprenorphine, naloxone	Suboxone®	CNS stimulant
37	insulin lispro	HumaLOG®	Fast-acting insulin used to treat type 1 or type 2 diabetes mellitus
38	rivaroxaban	Xarelto®	Anticoagulant, used to treat deep vein thrombosis and atrial fibrillation to lower risk of stroke
39	quetiapine	Seroquel XR®	Antipsychotic (extended release) used to treat schizophrenia, bipolar disorder, and major depressive disorder
40	sildenafil	Viagra®	Used to treat erectile dysfunction
41	pemetrexed	Alimta®	Antineoplastic agent, used sometimes with other agents, to treat certain lung cancers
42	liraglutide	Victoza 3-Pak®	rDNA-origin medication used to treat type 2 diabetes mellitus when other medications have failed
43	interferon beta-1a	Avonex®	Natural protein used to treat multiple sclerosis
44	mometasone	Nasonex®	Steroid, used to treat and prevent nasal symptoms caused by allergies, and for nasal polyps
45	tadalafil	Cialis®	Used to treat erectile dysfunction and benign prostatic hypertrophy
46	fingolimod	Gilenya®	Immunosuppressant, used to treat relapsing multiple sclerosis
47	ustekinumab	Stelara®	Immunosuppressant, used to treat plaque psoriasis or psoriatic arthritis
48	fluticasone	Flovent HFA®	Steroid, used to prevent asthma attacks
49	darunavir	Prezista®	Protease inhibitor antiviral, used to treat HIV
50	epoetin alfa	Procrit®	Synthetic protein used to treat anemia

Table 19-2, concluded

Adapted from Top 100 Most Prescribed, Top Selling Drugs, Megan Brooks, *Medscape,* May 13, 2014. www.medscape.com/viewarticle/825053

Pharmacognosy: The branch of pharmacology dealing with natural drugs or natural products chemistry.

Pharmacodynamics: The study of the mechanisms of action of drugs on living organisms.

Pharmacokinetics: The study of the movement of drugs, metabolism, and action of drugs within the body, especially the processes of absorption, distribution, biotransformation, localization in tissue, and excretion.

Pharmacotherapeutics: The study of how drugs are used to treat disease. Also called *clinical pharmacology,* it includes drug categories, indications, labeling, safety, therapeutic value, and types of therapy.

Toxicology: The science that deals with poisons.

Prophylactic: An agent used to prevent disease.

19.2 Drugs and Their Effects

Drug process: A drug must pass through four basic stages: absorption, distribution, metabolism, and excretion.

Absorption: The process by which a drug is absorbed into circulation.

Distribution: The process by which the circulatory system transports drugs to the affected body parts.

Metabolism: The process by which drugs are broken down into useful by-products by enzymes in the liver. It is also known as biotransformation. The liver is the main body organ involved in the metabolism of drugs.

Excretion: The kidney is responsible for filtering out drugs from the blood. Drugs are also excreted through the lungs, sweat glands, and intestines.

Mechanism of action: The way in which a drug produces its effects.

Drug classification: Drugs are classified according to their effect on the body. See Table 19-3.

Synergism: The joint action of agents in which their combined effect is more intense than their individual effects.

Cumulation: The compound effect of an agent taken over time in individual small amounts.

Allergic reaction: An acquired, abnormal immune response to a substance that does not normally cause a reaction. It may develop within 30 minutes of administration of therapy. Symptoms of a mild allergic reaction include skin rashes, swelling, itchy eyes and skin, wheezing, and fever. Severe allergic reactions such as anaphylaxis include extreme weakness, nausea, vomiting, cyanosis, dyspnea, hypotension, shock, and cardiac arrest.

Adverse effect: A general term for an undesirable and potentially harmful drug effect.

Anaphylaxis: A severe allergic response to medication, involving respiratory distress.

Side effect: An adverse effect of a drug on another organ system that is not related to the main target of the drug.

Toxic effect: An adverse drug effect that can be harmful or life threatening.

Antagonism: The combined effect of two drugs that is less than the effect of either drug taken alone.

Tolerance: Increasing resistance to the usual effects of an established dosage of a drug as a result of continued use.

Dependence: A state of reliance on a drug, either psychological or physiological, that may result in withdrawal symptoms if drug use is discontinued.

Idiosyncrasy: An abnormal sensitivity to a drug. It usually refers to an individual patient's unique response to medication.

Factors that affect individual variation in a drug's effect: Age, weight, sex, and percentage of body fat; time of day, tolerance, genetic variation, emotional state, placebo effect, presence of a disease, and patient compliance.

Drug indications: Intended uses of any drug.

Contraindications: Situations or conditions under which a certain drug should not be administered.

Drug abuse: The use or overuse of any drug in a manner that deviates from the prescribed pattern.

Prophylaxis: A procedure or medication used to prevent a disease rather than to treat an existing disease.

Half-life: The amount of time required for 50% of the drug to be eliminated from the body.

Teratogen: A drug that causes birth defects. These drugs affect the X chromosome and therefore should not be given to pregnant women.

Placebo: A drug dosage form that has no pharmacological effect because it contains no active ingredients. Placebos are used in controlled clinical trials of new drugs.

Safety: A drug's potential for use in regard to acceptable adverse effects.

Efficacy: A drug's therapeutic value.

Potency: A measure of the strength or concentration of a drug required to produce the desired effect.

Posology: The study of the amount of drug that is required to produce therapeutic effects.

Drug therapy: The intended type of therapy to be achieved by a drug. Various drug therapies include *acute, empiric, maintenance, palliative, prophylactic, replacement, supportive,* and *supplemental* uses.

Polypharmacy: Multiple drug prescriptions. This situation is very common for elderly individuals, and it often increases confusion, forgetfulness, and noncompliance. Minimizing polypharmacy also should be an important consideration when trying to avoid harmful drug interactions.

Dosage: The amount of a drug prescribed for a given patient.

Dose: The measured portion of medication to be taken at one time.

Maintenance dose: The amount of medication needed to provide a consistent amount of drug in the blood or other tissues.

Dispense: To distribute a drug in properly labeled containers to a patient.

Labeling: Includes a drug's approved indications, its form, and other information as needed.

Administer: To give a drug directly to a patient by injection, by mouth, or by any route that introduces the drug directly into the patient's body.

Lethal dose 50 (LD_{50}): The dose that will kill 50% of the subjects tested.

Classification	Action	Examples
General		
Analgesic	Relieves pain	acetaminophen (Tylenol®); acetylsalicylic acid (aspirin); oxycodone HCl (Percocet®)
Anesthetic	Prevents sensation of pain	lidocaine HCl (Xylocaine®, Lidoderm®); tetracaine HCl (Pontocaine®)
Antibiotic (antibacterial)	Destroys or inhibits bacterial growth	amoxicillin (Amoxil®); ciprofloxacin (Cipro®); levofloxacin (Levaquin®)
Antihelmintic (or "antihelminthic")	Destroys or inhibits parasitic worms	mebendazole (Vermox®), pyrantel pamoate (Combantrin®, Antiminth®)
Antineoplastic	Poisons cancerous cells	bleomycin (Blenoxane®); dactinomycin (Cosmegen®); tamoxifen (Nolvadex®)
Antipyretic	Reduces fever	acetaminophen (Tylenol®); acetylsalicyclic acid (aspirin)
Antiseptic	Inhibits growth of microorganisms	isopropyl alcohol; povidone-iodine (Betadine®); chlorhexidine (PerioChip®)
Mydriatic	Constricts vessels, raises blood pressure, dilates pupils	atropine (Atropisol®); phenylephrine HCl (Alcon Efrin®, Neo-Synephrine®)
Integumentary System		
Antifungal	Treats fungal infections	amphotericin B (Fungizone®); fluconazole (Diflucan®); nystatin (Mycostatin®)
Antipruritic	Relieves itching	hydroxyzine HCl (Atarax®); diphenhydramine HCl (Benadryl®); hydrocortisone (Hydrocortisone Cream®)
Musculoskeletal System		
Muscle relaxant	Relaxes muscles on a short-term basis	carisoprodol (Rela®, Soma®); cyclobenzaprine HCl (Flexeril®)
Nonsteroidal anti-inflammatory drug (NSAID)	Reduces pain, inflammation, and fever	naproxen (Aleve®); ibuprofen (Motrin®, Advil®); celecoxib (Celebrex®)
Steroid	Reduces inflammation	dexamethasone (Decadron®); prednisone (Deltasone®); triamcinolone (Kenalog®)
Nervous System		
Antianxiety	Depresses the CNS	alprazolam (Alprazolam Intensol®); lorazepam (Ativan®); diazepam (Valium®)
Anticholinergic	Blocks parasympathetic nerve impulses	atropine sulfate (Isopto Atropine®); dicyclomine HCl (Bentyl®); ipratropium (Atrovent®)
Anticonvulsant	Prevents or relieves convulsions	clonazepam (Klonopin®); phenobarbital sodium (Luminol Sodium®); phenytoin (Dilantin®)
Antidepressant	Prevents or treats mental depression	amitriptyline HCl (Elavil®); phenelzine sulfate (Nardil®); fluoxetine HCl (Prozac®); venlafaxine HCl (Effexor XR®)
Antiepileptic	Treats epilepsy	carbamazepine (Tegretol®); ethosuximide (Zarontin®); felbamate (Felbatol®)
Antiparkinsonian	Treats Parkinson's disease	procyclidine (Kemadrin®); bromocriptine (Cycloset®); selegiline (Zelapar®)

Table 19-3

Common Drug Classifications and Actions

Classification	Action	Examples
Antipsychotic	Treats psychosis	chlorpromazine HCl (Thorazine®); clozapine (Clozaril®); haloperidol (Haldol®)
Sedative	Creates tranquilizing, soothing effects	chloral hydrate (Noctec®); secobarbital sodium (Seconal Sodium®); zolpidem (Ambien®)
Stimulant	Increases brain and other organ activity; decreases appetite	amphetamine sulfate (Benzedrine®); caffeine (No-Doz®); methylphenidate (Ritalin®)
Endocrine System		
Antidiabetic	Reduces glucose	metformin (Glucophage®); glipizide (Glucotrol®); pioglitazone HCl (Actos®)
Antisecretory	Inhibits secretion	omeprazole (Prilosec®), esomeprazole (Nexium®)
Insulin	Treats diabetes	insulin recombinant (Humulin®); insulin human (Exubera®); insulin glulisine (Apidra®)
Thyroid agent	Replaces thyroid function	levothyroxine sodium (Synthroid®, Levothroid®, Unthread®)
Cardiovascular System		
Antiarrhythmic	Regulates the heartbeat	disopyramide (Norpace®); propafenone HCl (Rythmol®); propranolol HCl (Inderal®)
Anticoagulant	Slows the coagulation process	enoxaparin (Lovenox®); heparin sodium (Hep-Lock®); warfarin sodium (Coumadin®)
Antihypercholesterolemic	Prevents or controls high cholesterol	gemfibrozil (Lopid®); atorvastatin (Lipitor®); rosuvastatin (Crestor®)
Antihypertensive	Prevents or controls high blood pressure	amlodipine (Norvasc®); metoprolol (Toprol XL®); valsartan (Diovan®)
Hemostatic	Promotes coagulation to control or stop bleeding	aminocaproic acid (Amicar®); phytonadione (Mephyton®); thrombin (Thrombogen®)
Vasoconstrictor	Constricts blood vessels, increasing blood pressure	dopamine HCl (Intropin®); norepinephrine (Levophed®); amphetamine (Adderall®)
Vasodilator	Dilates blood vessels, decreasing blood pressure	enalopril (Vasotec®); lisinopril (Prinivil®); nitroglycerin (Nitrostat®)
Respiratory System		
Antiasthmatic	Treats or prevents asthma attacks	montelukast (Singulair®); albuterol (ProAir HFA®); fluticasone, salmeterol (Advair Diskus®)
Antihistamine	Relieves allergies	cetirizine HCl (Zyrtec®); diphenhydramine HCl (Benadryl®); fexofenadine (Allegra®)
Antitussive	Relieves or prevents coughs	codeine; dextromethorphan hydrobromide (Robitussin DM®)
Bronchodilator	Dilates bronchi of the lungs	albuterol (Proventil®); epinephrine (Epinephrine Mist®); salmeterol (Serevent®)
Decongestant	Reduces mucus production	oxymetazoline HCl (Afrin®); phenylephrine HCl (Neo-Synephrine®); pseudoephedrine HCl (Sudafed®)
Expectorant (mucokinetic)	Liquefies mucus in bronchi	guaifenesin (Mucinex®); acetylcysteine (Mucomyst®); dornase alfa (Pulmozyme®)

Table 19-3, continued

Classification	Action	Examples
Digestive System		
Antacid/antiulcer	Neutralizes gastric acids	calcium carbonate (Tums®); esomeprazole (Nexium®); lanso-prazole (Prevacid®)
Antidiarrheal	Relieves diarrhea	bismuth subsalicylate (Pepto-Bismol®); kaolin, pectin (Kaopectate®); loperamide HCl (Imodium®)
Antiemetic	Controls nausea, vomiting, and motion sickness	prochlorperazine (Compazine®); promethazine (Phenergan®); trimethobenzamide HCl (Tigan®)
Laxative (cathartic)	Promotes evacuation of the intestines	bisacodyl (Dulcolax®); casanthranol (Peri-Colace®); magnesium hydroxide (Milk of Magnesia®)
Urinary System Diuretic	Increases urine excretion	bumetanide (Bumex®); furosemide (Lasix®); hydrochlorothiazide (HydroDIURIL®)
Reproductive System		
Androgen	Replaces male hormones	testosterone (AndroGel®, Testoderm®); testosterone undecanoate (Aveed®)
Antivenereal	Prevents or controls sexually transmitted (venereal) diseases	azithromycin (Azithromycin Dose Pack®); levofloxacin (Levaquin®); acyclovir (Zovirax®)
Contraceptive	Prevents conception	norgestrel (Ovrette®); ethinyl estradiol, norgestimate (Ortho Tri-Cyclen®); norethindrone, ethinyl estradiol (Ortho-Evra®)
Estrogen	Replaces female hormones	conjugated estrogens (Premarin®); conjugated estrogens, medroxyprogesterone (Prempro®); synthetic conjugated estrogens (Cenestin®)

Table 19-3, concluded

Effective dose 50 (ED_{50}): The dose that will produce an effect in 50% of the subjects tested.

Therapeutic index (TI): The ratio of the LD_{50} to the ED_{50}. TI = LD_{50}/ED_{50}. The ratio gives an estimate of the relative safety of a drug.

Drug names: There are three types of names for any drug: chemical, generic or official, and trade name or brand name.

Chemical name: The chemical structure of a drug that explains the composition of a drug.

Generic name: The official and nonproprietary name of a drug assigned by the U.S. Adopted Names (USAN) Council.

Trade name or brand name: A word, symbol, or device assigned to a drug (or other product) by its manufacturer, registered by the U.S. Patent Office, and approved by the U.S. Food and Drug Administration.

Prescription: An order written by a physician or licensed prescriber to be filled by a pharmacist. Physicians and licensed prescribers must sign their name and title to every prescription. Controlled-substance prescriptions also contain the DEA number of the prescriber.

Superscription: The part of a prescription that includes the patient's name, address, date, and the symbol *Rx,* which means "take thou" in Latin.

Inscription: The part of a prescription containing the names and quantities of the ingredients.

Subscription: The part of a drug prescription that gives directions to the pharmacist about how to prepare the drug.

Signature: The part of a prescription that gives instructions to patients. A signature tells the patient how to take the drug, when to take it, and how much to take.

Over the counter (OTC): Available without a prescription.

Drug Forms
Water-Based Solutions

Syrup (syr.): A solution of water and sugar to which a drug is added. Adding flavors also can eliminate the bitter taste of certain drugs. Examples include Robitussin®, a cough syrup.

Emulsion: Liquid medication that contains fats or oils suspended in water. They must be shaken before use. Cod liver oil used as a laxative is an emulsion.

Suspension: A solution containing finely divided solids that are dispersed (suspended) in a liquid (the dispersing medium). In various forms, they may be intended for oral, topical, or parenteral administration.

Magma: Heavy particles mixed with water to form a milky liquid. Magmas must be shaken before administration. Examples include Milk of Magnesia®.

Lotion: A suspension of drugs in a water base for external use. Lotions must be patted on the skin for protective, emollient, or antipruritic purposes. Examples include calamine lotion used as an antipruritic for poison ivy.

Liniment: A liquid suspension that is rubbed onto the skin. Liniments relieve pain and swelling. Examples include BENGAY®.

Aerosol: A liquid or semiliquid delivered as mist by pressurized gas, as with oral inhalers or nebulizers, which allows rapid absorption into the bloodstream. Examples include Proventil®, a bronchodilator used for asthma.

Alcoholic Solutions

Elixir (elix.): A fluid extract of drugs that are dissolved in various concentrations of alcohol, usually between 10% and 20%. Examples include phenobarbital elixir, an anticonvulsant, and Benadryl® elixir, an antihistamine.

Tincture: A potent solution made with alcohol. Examples include iodine, a strong antiseptic; belladonna tincture, an anticholinergic; and camphorated opium tincture, a laxative.

Injectable Forms

Ampule: A single dose of sterile solution contained in a glass bottle whose seal must be broken to draw up medication using a filter needle.

Vial: A bottle with a rubber stopper or other nonsterile seal. Vials provide multiple doses of medication.

Solids and Semisolids

Powder: Drugs dried and ground into fine particles. An example is potassium chloride (Kato® powder).

Tablet (tab.): Drug powders compressed into a convenient form for swallowing.

Troche or lozenge: A flattened tablet that is dissolved in the mouth. These medications are often used for colds and sore throats.

Capsule (cap.): A small gelatin enclosure containing powder or liquid drugs. The capsule dissolves in the stomach, releasing the drugs.

Delayed-release: Certain tablets and capsules are treated with special coatings so that various portions of the drug dissolve at different rates. In this way, drug effects can be extended over time.

Enteric coated: Certain tablets and capsules are coated with an acid-resistant substance so that the drug will be absorbed only in the less acidic portions of the intestine. Enteric-coated products need to be taken on an empty stomach with water, either one hour before or two hours after a meal.

Spheroidal Oral Drug Absorption System (SODAS): Pellets covered in a gelatin capsule that slowly release the drug, unaffected by food or the acid in the GI tract.

Gastrointestinal Therapeutic System (GITS): A two-compartment tablet. In the GI tract, water is drawn into the tablet forcing the drug out. This system delivers drugs at a constant rate over extended periods of time.

Suppository (supp.): Drugs mixed with a substance (cocoa butter) that will melt at body temperature. Suppositories are inserted into the rectum, urethra, or vagina.

Ointment or unguent (oint., ung.): A salve of soft, oily substances to which a drug has been added. It is applied to the skin.

Cream: A thick, smooth, water-based topical medication.

Transdermal: Administered through the skin with a bandage or a patch system. Patches are easy to apply and cause little or no discomfort, and they provide a continuous source of the drug over 24 hours or more.

Sources of Drug Information

Physicians' Desk Reference (**PDR**): The most widely used drug reference publication. It contains an index of manufacturers, a brand name and generic name index, a product category index, and a product identification guide. The brand name and generic name index makes up the pink section, the product classification or category index is the blue section, an alphabetical index by manufacturers is featured in the white section, a generic and chemical name index constitutes the yellow section, and diagnostic product information is found in the green section. The PDR is revised annually.

United States Pharmacopeia Dispensing Information (**USPDI**): Published in three volumes with monthly updates. Volume I provides in-depth information about prescription and OTC medications and nutritional supplements. Volume II contains advice for the patient. Volume III contains state and federal requirements for prescribing and dispensing drugs.

Drug Regulation

Controlled Substance Act of 1970: A law that controls the distribution and use of all drugs of abuse or potential abuse as designated by the DEA. It divides narcotics, stimulants, and some sedatives into five classes, called schedules. See Table 19-4 for examples.

Drug Regulation and Reform Act of 1978: Permits quicker investigation of new drugs, allowing consumers earlier access.

Orphan Drug Act of 1983: Speeds up the availability of drugs for patients with rare diseases.

Pregnancy categories: FDA-designated categories of the potential of a drug to cause birth defects if used during pregnancy. They include:

- Category A: Adequate, controlled studies have not demonstrated fetal risk in first trimester, and no evidence in later trimesters (examples: folic acid, levothyroxine, liothyronine, magnesium sulfate).
- Category B: Animal studies have not demonstrated fetal risk, and there are no adequate, controlled studies in pregnant women (examples: amoxicillin, cyclobenzaprine, hydrochlorothiazide, metformin).

Schedule	Abuse Potential	Prescription Requirement	Examples
I	High abuse potential; no accepted medical use	No prescription permitted	Heroin, hallucinogens, fenethylline, hashish, lysergic acid diethylamide (LSD), marijuana (except for in certain states), methaqualone (Quaalude®), peyote
II	High abuse potential; an accepted medical use	Prescription required; no refills permitted without a new written prescription	Narcotics, cocaine, morphine, opium, anabolic steroids, hydromorphone hydrochloride (Dilaudid®), amphetamines, short-acting barbiturates
III	Moderate abuse potential; an accepted medical use	Prescription required; five refills permitted in 6 months	Moderate-acting barbiturates, butabarbital (Butisol®), secobarbital (Seconal®), glutethimide, most preparations that include codeine combined with something else
IV	Low abuse potential; an accepted medical use	Prescription required; five refills permitted in six months	Chloral hydrate (Noctec®), diazepam (Valium®), alprazolam (Xanax®), pentazocine HCl (Talwin®)
V	Low abuse potential; an accepted medical use	No prescription required for individuals 18 or older with a few exceptions	Cough syrups with codeine (Cheracol® with codeine), guaifenesin (Naldecon Dx®), Lomotil®, Parepectolin®

Table 19-4

- Category C: Animal studies have not demonstrated adverse fetal effects, and there are no adequate, controlled human studies; potential benefit may warrant use of these drugs in pregnant women despite possible risks (examples: amlodipine, gabapentin, prednisone).
- Category D: Human studies, investigational studies, or marketing experiences have demonstrated evidence of fetal risk, yet potential benefits may warrant use (examples: alprazolam, clonazepam, lisinopril, lorazepam, losartan).
- Category X: Human or animal studies have demonstrated fetal abnormalities and/or there is positive evidence of fetal risk based on investigational or marketing experience; risks clearly outweigh potential benefits (examples: atorvastatin, finasteride, methotrexate, simvastatin, warfarin).
- Category NR: No rating is available.

Prescription drugs: One that can be used only by order of a licensed prescriber, such as a physician, and dispensed by a pharmacist, physician, podiatrist, midwife, or other licensed professional. Some prescription drugs are dispensed OTC, but in much weaker strengths.

Components of a prescription: These include seven basic categories:

- Prescriber information: name, address, telephone number, etc.
- Patient information: date, full name, date of birth, address, etc.
- Inscription (medication prescribed): generic or brand name, strength, quantity; placed after the "Rx" symbol
- Subscription: instructions to the pharmacist, including generic substitutions and refill authorizations
- Signa (transcription): instructions to the patient, usually following the abbreviation "Sig." which means *mark*
- Signature: the prescriber's signature on a handwritten prescription; a digital signature if the prescription is secure; if the prescription is printed, the signature is either hand-signed or otherwise authorized
- DEA number: used only on prescriptions that contain *controlled substances;* the DEA number is uniquely assigned to each prescriber

E-prescribing: The prescribing of medication that utilizes electronic entering and transmission between a prescriber and a pharmacy. Electronic prescriptions are never in the patient's possession. This is the most secure, efficient method of prescribing medications.

Record keeping: A doctor's office must maintain two types of records: dispensing and inventory. Dispensing records must indicate to whom, when, and how much of the drug was administered or dispensed. Inventory records involve counting the amount of each drug on hand. The controlled drug inventory must be completed at least every two years, with all the invoice copies from the drug suppliers included.

Registration: Doctor's offices that dispense or administer drugs must register with the DEA with a form called the "Application for Registration Under the Controlled Substances Act of 1970."

Storage: Some medications, such as antibiotics, may need to be refrigerated. All medications should be left in their original containers. Read drug labels and inserts for specific storage directions for each type of drug.

Security: Store controlled substances and prescription pads in a locked area. Be aware of and follow state guidelines and laws about keeping controlled substances secure.

Discarding drugs: Any medication that is out of date or without a label should be discarded. These drugs should be poured down a sink so that no one will be able to take them. However, the MA must follow the office policy and procedure manual prior to discarding drugs in any manner, to ascertain any rules and regulations for the disposal of specific drugs.

Patient Education

Patient education: Advise patients to provide your medical office with a complete list of drugs they use regularly or periodically—including alcohol and recreational drugs, as well as herbal medicines. Explain to patients how and when to take each drug to ensure safety and effectiveness. Explain how to identify possible adverse effects, and be prepared to answer any questions. Advise patients to report to the physician any adverse reactions or drug interactions.

Poisons

Poisons: All drugs will act as poisons if taken in excess. Only the dose separates the therapeutic effect from a toxic effect.

Antidote: An agent that counteracts a poison. There are four types: chemical, mechanical, physiological, and universal. Antidotes for some of the most common poisons are shown in Table 19-5.

Chemical antidotes: Neutralize the poison by changing its chemical nature.

AT A GLANCE	Poisons and Their Respective Antidotes
Poison	**Antidote**
Acetaminophen	N-acetylcysteine
Benzodiazepines	Flumazenil
Carbon monoxide	Oxygen
Cyanide	Amyl nitrite
Iron	Deferoxamine
Methanol	Ethanol
Opiates	Naloxone
Organophosphates	Atropine or pralidoxime

Table 19-5

Physiological antidotes: Counteract the effects of the poison by releasing opposing effects.

Mechanical antidotes: Prevent absorption of the poison.

Universal antidotes: Were supposedly effective against a wide range of toxins. These mixtures were formerly recommended as antidotes when the exact poison was not known. There is, in fact, no known universal antidote.

19.3 Drug Administration

Oral route: The drug is swallowed. This is the safest and most convenient route used for most medications. Oral medications may cause nausea and stomach irritation. They also have a slow absorption rate that can be affected by food. Examples include aspirin, sedatives, hypnotics, and antibiotics.

Buccal route (buc): The drug is placed between the gum and cheek and left there until it is dissolved. Examples include oxytocin (Pitocin®), which induces labor.

Sublingual route (subling, subl, SL): The drug is placed under the tongue and left there until it is dissolved. These drugs are used when rapid effects are needed. Examples include nitroglycerin for angina pectoris and ergotamine tartrate (Ergomar®) for migraines.

Topical route (T): The drug is rubbed into, patted on, sprayed on, swabbed on, or rinsed on skin. These drugs are used to soothe irritated areas or to cure local infections. Examples include most creams and ointments.

Transdermal route: A patch is applied to clean, dry, nonhairy skin. This is a convenient form that provides continuous absorption and effects that last over many hours. Estrogen and nitroglycerin can be administered in this way.

Inhalation route, inhalation therapy: The drug is inhaled to achieve local effects within the respiratory tract. Antiasthmatic medications such as epinephrine are administered in this way.

Ophthalmic route: Instillations of medications (usually drops) into the eye.

Otic route: Instillations of medications (usually drops) into the ear.

Nasal route: Nasal solutions act locally to treat minor congestion or infection.

Rectal route (R): A suppository is inserted into the rectum, or a solution is administered as an enema. This method is used when a patient cannot take oral medications or when local effects are desired. Analgesics and laxatives can be administered in this way.

Urethral route: A solution is instilled into the bladder by means of a catheter.

Vaginal route (p.v., vag): A solution is administered as a douche. Other forms are inserted into the vagina with an applicator. Examples include Mycostatin®.

Parenteral route: Drugs introduced into the body that bypass the gastrointestinal tract, usually by injection. Parenteral administration by way of injection is divided into four main categories according to the location of the injection: intradermal, subcutaneous, intramuscular, and intravenous.

Intradermal route: The drug is injected into the upper layers of the skin.

Subcutaneous route (SubQ, SC): The drug is injected into the subcutaneous layer of the skin.

Intramuscular route (IM): The drug is injected into a muscle. This method is used when a drug has poor oral absorption, when high blood levels are required, or when rapid effects are desired. Narcotic analgesics and antibiotics are administered in this way.

Intravenous route (IV): The drug is injected or infused into a vein. This method is used when an emergency situation exists, when immediate effects are required, and also when other medications are being administered by infusion. Examples include IV fluids (e.g., dextrose solution), nutrient supplementation, and antibiotics.

19.4 Antibiotics

Antibiotic: A chemical substance that destroys or interferes with the development of bacterial microorganisms. Antibiotics are divided into two groups: bactericidal and bacteriostatic. Examples of both are shown in Table 19-6.

AT A GLANCE	Examples of the Two Different Types of Antibiotics
Bactericidal	**Bacteriostatic**
Penicillins	Sulfonamides
Cephalosporins	Tetracyclines
Aminoglycosides	Chloramphenicol
Vancomycin	Clindamycin
Quinolones	Spectinomycin

Table 19-6

Bactericidal: Destructive to or killing bacteria.

Bacteriostatic: Inhibiting the growth of bacteria.

Antimicrobial: Killing or inhibiting the growth of microorganisms.

Broad spectrum: Effective against a wide variety of both gram-positive and gram-negative pathogenic bacteria.

Bacterial resistance: The ability of some bacteria to resist the actions of antibiotics.

Chemotherapy: The use of cytotoxic drugs to kill or to inhibit the growth of infectious organisms or cancerous cells.

Bactericidal Antibiotics

Penicillin: A large group of natural or synthetic antibacterial agents derived from fungi of the genus *Penicillium*. Penicillins were the first true antibiotics, and they are the most widely used class of antibiotics. They interfere with the synthesis of bacterial cell walls. Classifications of penicillin and examples (with generic names and brand names) are seen in Table 19-7. When used in high doses, penicillins may cause CNS disturbances, including convulsions. As a drug class, penicillins also cause the highest incidence of drug allergy. Patients must always be questioned about the possibility of a penicillin allergy and their medical history. It is possible to develop a penicillin allergy at a later time, even if a patient was not previously allergic to it.

Beta-lactamases: Bacterial enzymes that inactivate penicillin and cephalosporin antibiotics.

Penicillinase: An enzyme produced by some bacteria that inactivates penicillin, thus increasing resistance to the antibiotic. It is used in the treatment of reactions to penicillin.

Cephalosporin: One of a large group of broad-spectrum antibiotics from *Cephalosporium,* a genus of soil-inhabiting fungi.

AT A GLANCE	Classification of Penicillins	
Classification	**Example Generic Name (Brand Name)**	**Effectiveness**
First Generation Narrow spectrum	penicillin G (Pfizerpen®)	Gram-positive streptococci
Beta-lactamase sensitive	penicillin V (Penicillin VK®)	Gram-positive streptococci
Beta-lactamase resistant	oxacillin (Oxacillin®) nafcillin (Nafcillin Injection®) dicloxacillin (Dynapen®)	Gram-positive streptococci
Second Generation Broad spectrum	ampicillin (Principen®) amoxicillin (Amoxil®)	*Hemophilus Escherichia coli Neisseria*
Third Generation Extended spectrum	carbenicillin (Geocillin®)	*Pseudomonas*
Fourth Generation Widest spectrum, potent	piperacillin (Pipracil®)	Serious infections, *Pseudomonas aeruginosa, Proteus vulgaris, Klebsiella pneumoniae*

Table 19-7

Cephalosporins are similar in structure and action to penicillin. Like penicillins, they are classified into four generations. Common uses of cephalosporins include administration in patients allergic to the penicillins and treatment of certain urinary and respiratory tract infections. Side effects of cephalosporins include oral thrush, diarrhea, rashes, vaginitis, thrombophlebitis, and sometimes electrolyte imbalance. Intramuscular injections of cephalosporins are usually painful and may cause inflammation.

First-generation cephalosporins: Used to treat common gram-positive and gram-negative infections. Examples include cefazolin (Cefazolin Injection®).

Second-generation cephalosporins: Used for gram-negative infections. They are more resistant to the actions of penicillinase and cephalosporinase. Examples include cefamandole (Mandol®), cefotetan (Cefotan®), and cefoxitin (Mefoxin®).

Third-generation cephalosporins: Used for serious gram-negative infections. They have longer duration of action and are more potent than the first- or second-generation cephalosporins. Examples include cefotaxime (Claforan®) and ceftriaxone (Rocephin®).

Fourth-generation cephalosporins: Similar in spectrum to third-generation drugs. They have a greater resistance to beta-lactamase-inactivating enzymes. Examples include cefepime (Maxipime®).

Aminoglycoside: One of a group of bacterial antibiotics derived from the genus *Streptomyces* that irreversibly inhibit protein synthesis. All of the aminoglycosides are highly toxic. Types of aminoglycosides include amikacin (Amikin®), gentamicin (Garamycin®), kanamycin (Kantrex®), neomycin (Neo-Fradin®), streptomycin (Streptomycin®), and tobramycin (Tobi®). Aminoglycosides are used to treat infections caused by gram-negative organisms. They are often given in large doses before abdominal surgery to "sterilize" the bowel. They are also used for the treatment of resistant urinary tract infections. Streptomycin is used to treat tuberculosis, plague, and tularemia. Side effects include nausea, vomiting, diarrhea, ototoxicity (which can result in deafness), and nephrotoxicity. Aminoglycosides may interfere with normal renal function. They are contraindicated for use during pregnancy.

Quinolone: A general class of broad-spectrum antibiotics that interrupt the replication of DNA molecules in bacteria. They are well absorbed in the GI tract after oral administration. Examples include ciprofloxacin (Cipro®) and nalidixic acid (NegGram®). Common uses include treatment of urinary, GI, respiratory, bone and joint, and soft tissue infections. Quinolones are contraindicated for pediatric therapy because they cause permanent cartilage damage. Quinolones are also not recommended during pregnancy. Fluoroquinolones are synthetic quinolones.

Vancomycin (Vancomycin HCl Injection®): A miscellaneous antibacterial agent that does not fit into any of the preceding categories. It is effective only on gram-positive bacteria, particularly staphylococcal infections that are resistant to other antibiotics. It also is prescribed in the treatment of infectious diseases such as pneumonia, meningitis, endocarditis, septicemia, and osteomyelitis. Common side effects include ototoxicity, nephrotoxicity, and a flushing redness of the neck and trunk caused by histamines.

Bacteriostatic Antibiotics

Sulfonamides: Synthetic antibiotics that now have limited uses because of bacterial resistance. Examples include mafenide (Sulfamylon®) and sulfacetamide (Plexion®). Common uses include topical treatment of burns and treatment of urinary and GI tract infections. Common side effects include nausea, vomiting, diarrhea, crystalluria, anemia, leukopenia, and rashes.

Tetracyclines: Broad-spectrum antibiotics that are effective against both gram-negative and gram-positive microorganisms. They are bacteriostatic antibiotics. Foods containing calcium, mineral supplements, and antacids interfere with absorption of the tetracyclines. Tetracycline should not be administered in the last half of pregnancy and to children under eight years of age (because it discolors teeth). It is also secreted in breast milk. The use of outdated tetracycline may cause Fanconi's syndrome.

Chloramphenicol (Chloramphenicol Sodium Succinate®): A broad-spectrum antibiotic with specific therapeutic action against rickettsiae. Common uses include treatment of rickettsial infections, typhoid fever, and meningitis. It is reserved for serious or life-threatening infections. Side effects include aplastic anemia (bone marrow depression), oral thrush, and genital/anal pruritus (itching). Chloramphenicol is potentially a very toxic drug. In most cases, its effects are irreversible. It should not be administered to a newborn less than two weeks of age because it can result in a condition known as the gray baby syndrome, involving circulatory collapse, abdominal distention, and respiratory failure.

Clindamycin (Cleocin®): It is used for the treatment of a variety of gram-negative aerobic and gram-positive and gram-negative anaerobic organisms. Common uses include treatment against anaerobic organisms. Side effects include pseudomembranous colitis, severe gastrointestinal disturbances, and hypersensitivity.

Spectinomycin: An antibiotic that is often called by the trademark Trobicin®. It is used in the treatment of gonorrhea and certain other infections and in penicillin-allergic patients. Side effects include pain at the injection site and hypersensitivity.

Both Bactericidal and Bacteriostatic Antibiotics

Macrolide: An antibiotic that inhibits protein-synthesis in some bacteria. Macrolides are bactericidal and bacteriostatic. Examples include erythromycin (Benzamycin®), azithromycin (Zithromax®), and clarithromycin (Biaxin®). Common uses include treatment of diseases of the gastrointestinal tract, skin, and respiratory system and of sexually transmitted diseases. Side effects include thrombophlebitis, diarrhea, nausea, vomiting, and abnormal tastes in the mouth.

Antitubercular Agents

Antitubercular agents: A group of drugs used to treat tuberculosis. At least two drugs, and usually three, are required in various combinations in pulmonary tuberculosis therapy. Examples include isoniazid (Isoniazid Tablets®), rifampin (Rifadin®), ethambutol (Myambutol®), and streptomycin (Streptomycin®).

Isoniazid (Isoniazid Tablets®): A synthetic bactericidal drug used to treat tuberculosis. Common uses include prophylaxis and treatment of tuberculosis. Side effects include peripheral neuritis, hepatitis, numbness, nausea, vomiting, dizziness, ataxia, and hepatotoxicity.

Rifampin (Rifadin®): An antibiotic that prevents RNA synthesis. Common uses include treatment of tuberculosis and prevention of meningococci outbreaks. A common side effect is reddish-orange color in urine, saliva, feces, sputum, sweat, and tears that can permanently discolor soft contact lenses.

Ethambutol (Myambutol®): A bacteriostatic synthetic compound that inhibits the incorporation of mycolic acid into the bacterial cell wall. Side effects include confusion, fever, hallucinations, and blurred vision (red-green color changes).

Antifungal Agents

Antifungal: Destructive to fungi or inhibiting their growth. An antifungal drug is also called antimycotic. See Table 19-8 for a list of antifungal drugs.

Antiviral Agents

Amantadine (Symmetrel®): Prevents the virus that causes Asian influenza from penetrating human cells and releasing viral DNA into the cell. When administered after exposure to the flu, it also reduces the severity of the infection. It is recommended for high-risk patients only.

Acyclovir (Zovirax®): Inhibits viral DNA replication. It is used in the treatment of genital herpes, shingles, and chickenpox. Side effects include kidney damage, headache, confusion, irritability, nausea, and vomiting.

Valacyclovir (Valtrex®): Inhibits viral DNA synthesis by competing with deoxyguanosine triphosphate. It is used to treat herpes simplex keratitis.

Drugs used against HIV: Didanosine (Videx®), indinavir (Crixivan®), nelfinavir (Viracept®), saquinavir (Invirase®), zalcitabine (Hivid®), and zidovudine (Retrovir®). The frequency of HIV mutation and drug resistance results in poor clinical response.

19.5 Pharmacology of the Integumentary System

Anti-inflammatory drugs: Suppress inflammation and relieve itching (pruritus) and swelling (edema). Examples include betamethasone valerate (Luxiq®) and hydrocortisone. Anti-inflammatory drugs are classified as steroidal and nonsteroidal.

Astringents: Relieve itching, soothe mild sunburns, and dry the skin. They are used for poison ivy, insect bites, and mild sunburn. Examples include calamine and diphenhydramine hydrochloride.

Antipruritics: Relieve itching. They also have antihistamine, sedative, and drying effects. An example is trimeprazine tartrate.

Erythema: Redness caused by an expansion of the capillaries at the skin's surface.

Vasoconstrictors: Reduce swelling and edema (caused by buildup of fluid in the tissues) and increase venous flow. They are used to treat dermal ulcers. An example is DuoDERM® hydroactive gel.

Antiseptics: Kill germs and are used to treat surface infections, burns, minor wounds, and vaginitis. An example is povidone-iodine (Betadine®).

Keratolytics: Swell and soften excess keratin for easy removal and shedding. They are used for warts, corns, calluses, psoriasis, and seborrheic dermatitis. An example is salicylic acid, sold under many trade names.

AT A GLANCE | Antifungal Drugs

Generic Name	Trade Name	Uses
amphotericin B	Fungizone®	Systemic fungal infections, severe progressive fungal infections, cryptococcosis
fluconazole	Diflucan®	Systemic infection, oroesophageal candidiasis
ketoconazole	Nizoral®	Systemic infection
nystatin	Mycostatin®	Candidiasis, skin infections, GI infections
griseofulvin	Gris Peg®	Superficial fungal (dermatophytic) infections
butenafine	Mentax®	Athlete's foot
terconazole	Terazol-3®, Terazol-7®	Vulvovaginal candidiasis

Table 19-8

19.6 Pharmacology of the Musculoskeletal System

Centrally acting skeletal muscle relaxant: Inhibits skeletal muscle contraction by blocking conduction within the spinal cord. Examples include baclofen (Lioresal Intrathecal®), carisoprodol (Soma®), and tizanidine (Zanaflex®). Common uses include therapy for muscle strain and multiple sclerosis. Side effects include blurred vision, dizziness, lethargy, and decreased mental alertness.

Peripheral skeletal muscle relaxant: Inhibits muscle contraction at the neuromuscular junction or within the contractile process. An example is dantrolene (Dantrium®). It is commonly used during surgical procedures to relax the abdominal muscles, during shock therapy, and during tetanus. Side effects include toxicity-induced paralysis of the respiratory muscles.

19.7 Pharmacology of the Nervous System

Central Nervous System
Sedatives and Hypnotic Drugs

Hypnotic: A drug that causes insensitivity to pain by inhibiting the reception of sensory impressions in the brain, causing partial or complete unconsciousness. Sedative and hypnotic drugs produce their effects by increasing the inhibitory activity of gamma-aminobutyric acid (GABA), a neurotransmitter in the CNS.

Sedative: A hypnotic drug that exerts a quieting or tranquilizing effect. The most common sedatives and hypnotics are summarized in Table 19-9.

Barbiturate: A sedative drug that reduces brain activity and promotes sleep. The main sites of action of barbiturates are the reticular formation and the cerebral cortex. Barbiturates are used as sleep aids and as treatment for convulsions or seizures. Common side effects include drowsiness, dry mouth, lethargy, and lack of coordination. An overdose can result in extensive cardiovascular and CNS depression leading to coma, respiratory depression, and death. Prolonged and excessive use of barbiturates can result in tolerance and physical dependence. Patients who have acute intermittent porphyria should not take barbiturates because they may cause nerve damage, pain, and paralysis. Barbiturates should not be taken during pregnancy.

Nonbarbiturate: Unfortunately, prolonged abuse of these drugs will still result in physical dependence and tolerance. Chloral hydrate is a good example of a nonbarbiturate drug. Its mechanism of action is similar to alcohol, and it is used as a hypnotic, particularly in elderly individuals. Side effects involve excessive CNS depression and gastric irritation.

Benzodiazepines: A class of drugs used in the treatment of anxiety. They are commonly referred to as antianxiety drugs. They depress the reticular activating system to produce sedation and hypnosis. Benzodiazepines are well tolerated and produce few side effects. They do not interfere with REM sleep and produce less tolerance than barbiturates. Flurazepam, a type of benzodiazepine, may cause sedation or a "hangover effect" the following day after use. They are contraindicated during pregnancy.

AT A GLANCE Sedatives and Hypnotic Drugs

Classification • Drug	Uses	Side Effects	Contraindications
Sedative-Hypnotic Barbiturates			
• pentobarbital (Nembutal®) • secobarbital (Seconal Sodium®)	Sedation in smaller doses, promotion of sleep in larger doses; treatment of seizure disorders; control of epilepsy	Drowsiness, dry mouth, confusion, incoordination, respiratory depression, coma	Acute intermittent porphyria, pregnancy, suicidal tendencies
Sedative-Hypnotic Nonbarbiturates			
• chloral hydrate (Noctec®) • zolpidem (Ambien CR®)	Treatment of insomnia; sedation in elderly individuals	Nausea, vomiting, diarrhea, gastric irritation, dizziness	
Benzodiazepines			
• flurazepam (Dalmane®) • temazepam (Restoril®) • triazolam (Halcion®)	Treatment of anxiety	Flurazepam: hangover effect Triazolam: rebound insomnia and increased daytime anxiety	Pregnancy

Table 19-9

Antipsychotics

Antipsychotic drugs: Drugs that are used to treat schizophrenia and other psychotic mental disorders characterized by gross impairment in reality testing. Antipsychotic drugs are also referred to as neuroleptics. Most antipsychotics block dopamine D_2 receptors. The most important types of antipsychotic drugs are phenothiazines, butyrophenones, and thioxanthenes. See Table 19-10. Common side effects include sedation; dry mouth; constipation; visual disturbances; dystonic reactions with muscle spasms; akathisia with continuous body movement and restlessness. Antipsychotics are contraindicated during pregnancy.

Clozapine: Atypically blocks both dopamine (D_4) and serotonin receptors. It is the second-line drug used for the treatment of schizophrenia and psychosis. Common side effects include a reduction in the number of granulocytes.

Antidepressants, Psychomotor Stimulants, and Lithium

Antidepressant: A drug that prevents or relieves depression. Low levels of norepinephrine and serotonin are associated with mental depression, whereas high levels of norepinephrine and serotonin are involved in mania. Antidepressants increase the level of norepinephrine and serotonin in the brain. There are three major classes of antidepressants: monoamine oxidase (MAO) inhibitors, tricyclic antidepressants (TCAs), and selective serotonin reuptake inhibitors (SSRIs).

Monoamine oxidase (MAO) inhibitors: Increase the concentration of epinephrine, norepinephrine, and serotonin in storage sites in the nervous system. After 2 to 4 weeks of treatment, patients feel an increase in appetite and sleep and an elevation of mood. One of the disadvantages of MAO inhibitors is the dietary restriction of foods containing tyramine (wine, beer, herring, and certain cheeses). A combination of tyramine and MAO inhibitors may cause a hypertensive crisis or cerebral stroke. Other common side effects include postural hypotension, dry mouth, constipation, urinary retention, blurred vision, insomnia, tremors, convulsions, liver damage, and impotence in males. Examples include isocarboxazid (Marplan®), phenelzine (Nardil®), and tranylcypromine (Parnate®).

Tricyclic antidepressant (TCA) drugs: Block the reuptake of norepinephrine and serotonin into the neuronal nerve endings. These drugs get their name from their characteristic triple-ring structure. In addition to the antidepressant effect, they also produce varying degrees of sedation, anticholinergic effects, and alpha-adrenergic blockade. Common side effects include dry mouth, weight gain, constipation, urinary retention, rapid heartbeat, postural hypotension, blurred vision, drowsiness, restlessness, tremors, convulsion, mania, cardiac arrhythmias, and jaundice. Examples include imipramine (Tofranil®), doxepin (Sinequan®), desipramine (Norpramin®), and amoxapine (Amoxapine®).

Selective serotonin reuptake inhibitors (SSRIs): Newer antidepressant drugs that block the reuptake and inactivation of serotonin in the brain. They are the most widely used antidepressants. Fluoxetine (Prozac®) was the first drug of this class to be introduced. Fluoxetine is effective against depression and also obsessive-compulsive disorders. Other examples include fluvoxamine (Luvox®) and sertraline (Zoloft®). Common side effects include headache, nervousness, insomnia, tremors, nausea, diarrhea, dry mouth, weight loss, and anorexia.

Psychomotor stimulants: Include amphetamines and other closely related drugs. They are often used during the first few weeks of depression treatment until other antidepressants, such as the MAO inhibitors or tricyclics, begin their therapeutic effect. They are also used to treat narcolepsy and hyperkinesis. Amphetamines increase the activity of norepinephrine and dopamine in the brain. Common side effects include dry mouth, rapid heartbeat, increased blood pressure, restlessness, and insomnia. Examples include dextroamphetamine (Dexedrine®) and methylphenidate (Ritalin®).

Lithium: An antimanic drug prescribed in the treatment of manic episodes. Lithium decreases the excitability of nerve tissue, increases the reuptake of norepinephrine and dopamine, and decreases the release of neurotransmitters. Clinical use includes the treatment of bipolar affective disorder and acute manic conditions. Lithium also blocks relapse. Common side effects include hypothyroidism, polyuria, polydipsia, tremor, and teratogenesis. Other side effects are nausea, tremors, cardiac arrhythmias, and nephritis. Lithium is contraindicated during pregnancy.

AT A GLANCE — Common Antipsychotic Drugs

Classification	Uses	Side Effects	Contraindications
codeine meperidine (Demerol®) morphine pentazocine (Talwin®) propoxyphene (Darvon®)	Relief of severe acute and chronic pain; relief of pain associated with myocardial infarction, posttrauma, cancer, and chronic inflammatory conditions; suppression of coughing (codeine)	Sedation, confusion, euphoria, agitation, headache and dizziness, hypotension, bradycardia, nausea, vomiting, urinary retention, respiratory depression, physical and emotional dependence, convulsions with large doses	Bronchial asthma, heavy pulmonary secretions, convulsive disorders, biliary obstruction, head injuries, pregnancy

Table 19-10

Antiepileptic Drugs

Antiepileptic drugs: Reduce or prevent the severity of epileptic or other convulsive seizures. Antiepileptic drugs decrease the excitability of brain cells. The drug of choice for each type of seizure is shown in Table 19-11. Side effects of antiepileptic drugs are summarized in Table 19-12.

Valproic acid (Depakene®): One of the few drugs that can be used in all types of epilepsy. Its mechanism of action is related to its ability to increase levels of GABA, the inhibitory neurotransmitter in the CNS. Common side effects include nausea, vomiting, diarrhea, tremors, and liver toxicity.

Antiparkinsonian Drugs

Levodopa (Dopar®): The most effective drug available for Parkinson's disease. In the basal ganglia, levodopa is converted to dopamine, and increased levels of dopamine lessen Parkinsonian symptoms. Common side effects include nausea, vomiting, anorexia, orthostatic hypotension or fainting, irregular heartbeat, dystonias, and dyskinesias.

Selegiline (Eldepryl®): Inhibits the metabolism of dopamine in the brain. It slows the progression of Parkinson's disease.

Amantadine (Symmetrel®): An antiviral agent that is often effective in the treatment of Parkinson's disease. Common side effects include dry mouth, GI disturbances, visual disturbances, dizziness, skin discoloration, and confusion.

Atropine and scopolamine: Anticholinergic drugs that relieve some of the symptoms of Parkinson's disease because they decrease the level of cholinergic activity and thus reduce tremors, muscle rigidity, and postural disturbances. Side effects include dry mouth, constipation, urinary retention, rapid heartbeat, and pupillary dilation.

Anesthetics and Analgesics

Anesthetic: A substance that depresses all nervous tissue, inhibits voluntary and involuntary systems, and depresses respiratory function.

General anesthetics: Administered by inhalation or IV injection. Inhalation anesthetics include chloroform, ether, and nitrous oxide. Injectable anesthetics include barbiturates, etomidate, ketamine, midazolam, and propofol; they are usually administered intravenously. In addition to anesthetic agents, a variety of preanesthetic and postanesthetic medications are used to aid induction of general anesthesia, to counteract side effects, or to make recovery more comfortable. Side effects include dizziness, nausea, mental disorientation, and lack of coordination.

Narcotic (opioid) analgesics: Derivatives of opium or synthetic chemicals that relieve severe pain. Certain narcotic analgesics (codeine and dextromethorphan) are also antitussive. All narcotic analgesics produce tolerance and physical dependency with chronic use. Morphine and other narcotic analgesics mimic the effects of endorphins by blocking pain transmission to the brain. For a list of narcotic (opioid) analgesics, see Table 19-13.

Nonopioid analgesics: The most common drugs used for relieving pain. See Table 19-14.

AT A GLANCE	Antiepileptic Drugs
Type of Seizure	**Drugs of Choice**
Grand mal (tonic-clonic)	phenytoin (Dilantin®), carbamazepine (Tegretol®), phenobarbital (Phenobarbital®)
Status epilepticus	diazepam (Valium®), phenytoin (Dilantin®), phenobarbital (Phenobarbital®)
Complex partial (temporal lobe)	carbamazepine (Tegretol®), phenytoin (Dilantin®), primidone (Mysoline®)
Petit mal	ethosuximide (Zarontin®), valproic acid (Depakene®), clonazepam (Klonopin®)

Table 19-11

AT A GLANCE	Antiepileptic Drug Toxicities
Drug	**Side Effects**
Phenobarbital	Sedation, tolerance, dependence
Valproic acid	Nausea, vomiting, diarrhea, tremors, liver toxicity in young patients
Benzodiazepines	Sedation, dependence, tolerance
Phenytoin	Birth defects, gingival hyperplasia, nystagmus, anemias, hirsutism
Carbamazepine	Blood dyscrasias, diplopia, ataxia

Table 19-12

AT A GLANCE · Opioid Analgesics

Drug	Uses	Side Effects	Contraindications
codeine meperidine (Demerol®) morphine pentazocine (Talwin®) propoxyphene (Darvon®)	Relief of severe acute and chronic pain; relief of pain associated with myocardial infarction, posttrauma, cancer, and chronic inflammatory conditions; suppression of coughing (codeine)	Sedation, confusion, euphoria, agitation, headache and dizziness, hypotension, bradycardia, nausea, vomiting, urinary retention, respiratory depression, physical and emotional dependence, convulsions with large doses	Bronchial asthma, heavy pulmonary secretions, convulsive disorders, biliary obstruction, head injuries, pregnancy

Table 19-13

AT A GLANCE · Nonopioid Analgesics

Classification • Drug	Uses	Side Effects	Contraindications
Salicylates			
• aspirin (Bayer®, aspirin, Bufferin®, Anacin®)	Relief of mild-to-moderate pain and fever; treatment of inflammation; possible reduction in the risk of reinfarction and death following a myocardial infarction	Prolonged bleeding time, bleeding, gastric ulcer and bleeding, tinnitus, renal insufficiency, rash, hepatic dysfunction, stomach irritation, and nausea	GI ulcer and bleeding, asthma, bleeding disorders, influenza-like syndrome in children, pregnancy, vitamin K deficiency
N-Acetyl-P-Aminophenol			
• acetaminophen (Tylenol®)	Relief of fever, pain, and discomfort associated with the common cold and flu	Coma, respiratory failure, severe liver toxicity, renal insufficiency, rash	Renal or hepatic disease, anemia, cardiac or pulmonary disease
Synthetic Nonsteroidal Anti-Inflammatory Drugs (NSAIDs)			
• ibuprofen (Advil®, Motrin®, Nuprin®)	Relief of mild-to-moderate pain (headache, dental extraction, soft tissue injury, sunburn); treatment of chronic osteoarthritis and rheumatoid arthritis	Nausea, GI distress, ulceration, vertigo, confusion	

Table 19-14

Autonomic Nervous System

Autonomic nervous system drugs: Drugs that treat the body systems regulated by the autonomic nervous system. They are classified into four groups: adrenergics, adrenergic blockers, cholinergics, and cholinergic blockers. See Table 19-15.

Sympathetic Nervous System

Adrenergic drugs: Also called sympathomimetic agents, these drugs mimic or stimulate the sympathetic nervous system. They include epinephrine and dopamine. Adrenergic drugs have two effects: alpha and beta.

Alpha-adrenergic drugs: Cause the contraction of smooth muscle, thereby increasing blood pressure. The prototype alpha-adrenergic drug is norepinephrine. They are commonly used to increase blood pressure in hypotensive states (such as after surgery) and to reduce congestion of nasal and ocular mucosa. Side effects include excessive vasoconstriction of blood vessels, heart palpitations, hypertension, and tissue necrosis. Contraindications include hypertension and cardiac arrhythmias.

Adrenergics	Adrenergic Blockers	Cholinergic	Cholinergic Blockers
epinephrine (Adrenalin®)	methyldopa (Aldomet®)	neostigmine (Prostigmin®)	atropine (Atropine®)
dopamine (Dopamine®)	carvedilol (Coreg®)	pilocarpine (Salagen®)	scopolamine (Isopto Hyoscine®)
norepinephrine (Levophed®)	doxazosin (Cardura®)	bethanechol (Urecholine®)	hyoscyamine (Levsin®)
isoproterenol (Isuprel®)	propranolol (Inderal®)	cevimeline (Evoxac®)	oxybutynin (Anturol®)

Table 19-15

Beta-adrenergic drugs: Stimulate the heartbeat and act as bronchodilators. Isoproterenol is the most potent of these drugs; it acts as both a cardiac stimulant and a bronchodilator. A common use is treatment of acute allergic reactions, such as anaphylaxis. Common side effects include restlessness, tremors, anxiety, overstimulation of the heart, palpitation, and arrhythmias. These drugs should be used with caution in patients with existing heart disease.

Alpha-adrenergic blocking agents: Prevent norepinephrine from producing sympathetic responses resulting in vasodilation and lowered blood pressure. Doxazosin and methyldopa are common alpha-adrenergic blocking drugs. Common uses of these types of agents include treatment of hypertension, treatment of vascular disease, and diagnosis of pheochromocytoma. Common side effects include nasal congestion, increased GI activity, low blood pressure, and fainting.

Beta-adrenergic blocking agents (beta-blockers): Decrease the activity of the heart. An example is carvedilol, used for chronic heart failure. Another example, propranolol, is a common beta-adrenergic drug administered for cardiac arrhythmias, angina pectoris, and hypertension. Side effects include nausea, vomiting, diarrhea, bradycardia, and cardiac arrest. Antiadrenergic drugs are contraindicated in patients with asthma or other respiratory conditions.

Parasympathetic Nervous System

Cholinergic: An agent that allows the parasympathetic nerve fibers to liberate acetylcholine. Cholinergics are also called parasympathomimetic drugs. Examples include neostigmine, pilocarpine, and bethanechol. Common uses include treatment of myasthenia gravis (neostigmine), glaucoma (pilocarpine), and nonobstructive urinary retention (bethanechol). Side effects include nausea, vomiting, diarrhea, blurred vision, excessive sweating, weakness, hypotension, bronchospasm, and respiratory depression. Contraindications include asthma, cardiac disorders, peptic ulcer, and benign prostatic hypertrophy.

Cholinergic blocking agents: Drugs that block the action of acetylcholine. These agents, also called anticholinergics

or parasympatholytics, may be used by patients who have bradycardia. Examples include atropine, scopolamine, and hyoscyamine. These agents are commonly used as antispasmodics, as preanesthetics, and as antidotes for insecticide poisoning. Common side effects include fever or flushing, blurred vision, dry mouth, urinary retention, and tachycardia. Contraindications include asthma, chronic obstructive pulmonary disease, angle-closure glaucoma, gastrointestinal or genitourinary obstruction, hypertension, hypothyroidism, and hepatic or renal disease.

19.8 Pharmacology of the Cardiovascular System

Cardiac Glycosides

Cardiac glycosides: Used in the treatment of congestive heart failure (CHF), atrial fibrillation, and atrial tachycardia to increase the force of myocardial contractions. Glycosides slow and strengthen the heartbeat and increase cardiac output. Major side effects of overdose include arrhythmia, headache, visual disturbances, nausea, vomiting, and diarrhea. Examples include digitoxin and digoxin (Digibind®).

Antianginal Drugs

Nitroglycerin: The most common and widely used drug for angina pectoris. Nitroglycerin produces general vasodilation of systemic veins and arteries and decreases the preload and afterload of the heart, thereby reducing cardiac work and oxygen consumption. See Table 19-16.

Antihypertensive Drugs

Antihypertensive agents: Agents that are effective against hypertension. Some antihypertensives, such as calcium antagonists and sympathetic beta-blockers, are also antianginal agents. Some antihypertensive drugs and their side effects are listed in Table 19-17. Other antihypertensive drugs, indications, and contraindications are summarized in Table 19-18.

Antianginal Drugs (Vasodilators)

Drug	Effects
nitroglycerin (Nitrostat®, Nitro-Dur®)	Dilates veins in low doses. In high doses, it also dilates arterioles, so angina may get worse. It increases blood flow in the coronary arteries and thereby decreases angina and hypertension.
isosorbide dinitrate (Isordil®)	Dilates vessels; it is orally active but less potent than nitroglycerin.
nifedipine (Procardia®)	Relaxes arterioles; it is best for coronary artery spasm.
verapamil (Calan®, Isoptin SR®)	Slows the heart rate; its effect is partially overcome by reflex tachycardia. This drug is also widely used to treat supraventricular arrhythmias.

Table 19-16

Antihypertensive Drugs and Their Side Effects

Drug	Side Effects
Thiazide and Thiazide-Like Diuretics	
hydrochlorothiazide (Microzide®)	Hypokalemia, hyperuricemia, depression, slight hyperlipidemia
Sympathetic Blocking Drugs	
methyldopa (Aldomet®)	Positive Coombs' test, sedation
clonidine (Catapres®)	Dry mouth, sedation
propranolol (Inderal®)	Hypotension, palpitations, bradycardia
Angiotensin-Converting Enzyme (ACE) Inhibitors	
benazepril (Lotensin®)	Headache, dizziness, GI disturbances
captopril (Capoten®)	Leukocytopenia, tachycardia, hypotension
Calcium Antagonists	
diltiazem (Cardizem®)	Lethargy, arrhythmias, bradycardia, hypotension, photosensitivity
verapamil (Calan®)	Dizziness, hypotension, bradycardia
Vasodilator Drugs	
hydralazine (Apresoline®)	Nausea, vomiting, reflex tachycardia, rheumatoid arthritis, systemic lupus erythematosus
minoxidil (Loniten®)	Myocardial ischemia, pericardial effusion, hirsutism (growth of hair)

Table 19-17

Antihypertensive Drugs and Their Indications and Contraindications

Drug	Indications	Contraindications
Beta-blockers	Angina pectoris, postmyocardial infarction	Diabetes, asthma, peripheral vascular disease
Diuretics	Congestive heart failure, chronic renal failure	Diabetes, hyperlipidemia
Calcium channel blockers	Angina, hypertension, supraventricular tachycardia	Congestive heart failure

Table 19-18

Antiarrhythmic Drugs

Antiarrhythmic drug: An agent that prevents or alleviates cardiac arrhythmias. Some of these agents are useful in several types of cardiac diseases. There are four classes, listed in Table 19-19.

Anticoagulant Drugs

Anticoagulants: The two classes of anticoagulants used most frequently today are warfarin (Coumadin®) derivatives and heparin. They are employed to prevent venous thrombosis, especially pulmonary embolism. Anticoagulants such as

AT A GLANCE Antiarrhythmic Drugs

Drug	Mechanism of Action	Uses	Side Effects
Class 1			
quinidine (Quinidex®)	Depresses the myocardium and conduction system. Slows heart rate.	Ventricular arrhythmias, supraventricular tachycardia	Nausea, vomiting, diarrhea, cinchonism due to drug sensitivity or an overdose, hypotension, fatigue
procainamide (Pronestyl®)	Depresses the myocardium and conduction system. Slows heart rate.	Supraventricular arrhythmias, supraventricular tachycardia	Nausea, vomiting, anorexia, skin rashes
lidocaine (Xylocaine®)	Suppresses ectopic foci but does not depress normal impulse conduction. Depresses automaticity.	Ventricular arrhythmias (especially from a myocardial infarction or surgery); as a local anesthetic	Impaired liver function, convulsions due to stimulation of CNS
phenytoin (Dilantin®)	Appears to increase AV conduction and may eliminate AV blockage.	Ventricular arrhythmias induced by digitalis, epileptic seizure	Blurred vision, vertigo, nystagmus, hyperglycemia, gingival hyperplasia
Class 2			
propranolol (Inderal®)	Beta-blocker. Depresses cardiac membranes. Slows heart rate, decreases AV conduction, prolongs refractory period.	Supraventricular and ventricular tachycardia	Hypotension, bradycardia, possible cardiac arrest, skin rashes, mental confusion, visual disturbances
esmolol (Brevibloc®)	Selective beta-blocker.	Supraventricular and ventricular tachycardia	(With overdose): excessive bradycardia, delayed AV conduction, hypotension
Class 3			
amiodarone (Cordarone®)	Very potent local anesthetic. Blocks alpha-adrenergic, beta-adrenergic, and calcium receptors, prolongs refractory period.	Ventricular tachycardia	Corneal deposits, visual disturbances, dermatitis, skin discoloration, pulmonary fibrosis, liver dysfunction. Contraindications: pregnancy, nursing
bretylium (Bretylium®)	Adrenergic neuronal blocker. Prolongs refractory period of ventricles.	Ventricular tachycardia and ventricular fibrillation	GI disturbances, nausea, diarrhea, hypotension
Class 4			
verapamil (Calan®)	Affects pacemaker cells of the heart. Decreases sinoatrial node activity and AV node conduction.	Supraventricular tachycardia	Headache, dizziness, minor GI disturbances, constipation, hypotension

Table 19-19

heparin inhibit the function of clotting factors, and anticoagulants such as *coumarin* derivatives prevent the synthesis of normal clotting factors. They are used in the treatment of myocardial infarction, thrombophlebitis, and stroke. Heparin is the preferred drug to be given to pregnant women because it does not cross the placenta and affect the fetus. Examples include dalteparin (Fragmin®) and heparin.

Hypolipidemic Drugs

Hypolipidemic drug: Used as a dietary control and as a means to reduce cholesterol in the body. There are three main types of hypolipidemic drugs: bile acid sequestrants, HMG-CoA enzyme inhibitors, and drugs that alter lipid and lipoprotein metabolism. Examples include cholestyramine (Questran®) and simvastatin (Zocor®).

19.9 Pharmacology of the Respiratory System

Antihistamines

Histamine: A substance that creates a pharmacological reaction when it is released from an injured cell.
Antihistamine: A drug that counteracts the effects of histamine. Antihistamines are used to relieve the symptoms of allergic reactions, such as hay fever and other allergic disorders of the nasal passages. Sometimes antihistamines are also useful in the relief of motion sickness. Others have a sedative and hypnotic action and may be used as tranquilizers. Examples include cetirizine (Zyrtec®), clemastine (Tavist®), dimenhydrinate (Dramamine®), fexofenadine (Allegra®), and loratadine (Claritin®).

Antiallergic Drugs

Antiallergic drug: Prevents mast cells from releasing histamine and other vasoactive substances.
Prophylactic drug: Prevents the onset of exposure-induced symptoms before the reactive process can take place. Cromolyn sodium is such an antiallergic agent.

Asthma Drugs

Asthma drugs: The drug of choice for asthma depends on the severity of the condition. See Table 19-20.

19.10 Pharmacology of the Digestive System

Healing ulcers: Two primary mechanisms are involved in medication therapy for ulcers: reduction of gastric acidity and enhancement of mucosal barrier defenses. Antihistaminics, prostaglandins, proton pump inhibitors, and anticholinergic drugs reduce the volume and concentration of gastric acid. These drugs are known as antisecretory drugs.
Antisecretory drugs: Inhibit the secretion of digestive enzymes, hormones, or acid. Examples include famotidine (Pepcid®) and cimetidine (Tagamet®).
Antacids: Neutralize the acid present in the digestive system. Antacids react with hydrochloric acid (HCl) to form water and salts. Examples include Alka-Seltzer®, Maalox®, and Rolaids®.
H2-receptor antagonists: There are three types of histamine receptors. These drugs may be preferred to other antiulcer agents because of their convenience of use and lack of effect on GI motility. Examples include cimetidine (Tagamet®), famotidine (Pepcid®), and ranitidine (Zantac®).
Proton pump inhibitors: The final common pathway in gastric acid secretion is the proton pump—an H+/K+ adenosine triphosphatase. The proton pump inhibitors are more potent when they are taken orally and before meals. They are also absorbed more effectively in the morning. Examples include omeprazole (Prilosec®), lansoprazole (Prevacid®), and rabeprazole (Aciphex®).
Laxatives and cathartics: Agents that stimulate defecation. Laxatives produce a mild, gentle stimulus for defecation, and cathartics produce a more intense action on the bowel. They act directly on the intestine to alter stool formation. These drugs are used to relieve constipation and to evacuate the intestine prior to surgery or diagnostic examination.

19.11 Pharmacology of the Endocrine System

Adrenal steroids: Corticosteroids produced by the adrenal cortex. They are prescribed as treatment for Addison's disease when there is a hormone deficiency. This type of treatment is called replacement therapy. Examples include cortisone (Cortone®), prednisone (Deltasone®), and dexamethasone (Decadron®).

AT A GLANCE	Asthma
Indication	**Drug of Choice**
Acute, mild, intermittent symptoms	metaproterenol (Alupent®), albuterol (Proventil®, Ventolin®), terbutaline (Terbutaline Sulfate®)
More severe symptoms	theophylline (Theolair®), salmeterol (Serevent Diskus®), zafirlukast (Accolate®)
Prophylaxis	cromolyn sodium (Nasalcrom®)
Chronic; *status asthmaticus*	corticosteroids

Table 19-20

Anti-inflammatory effects of adrenal steroids: Steroids also are used in acute and chronic inflammatory conditions such as rheumatoid arthritis. Synthetic versions of glucocorticoids, which are adrenal steroids, are commonly used to treat inflammatory and allergic reactions. Side effects with long-term use include steroid addiction, mood changes, insomnia, personality changes, and psychological dependency.

Thyroid agents: Used in the treatment of two conditions: hyposecretion of the thyroid hormone (hypothyroidism) and hypersecretion of the thyroid hormone (hyperthyroidism). Thyroid hormone replacement therapy is used to treat hypothyroidism, and antithyroid drugs (iodide and iodine) are used for hyperthyroidism, which is often caused by a tumor. Examples include liothyronine sodium (Cytomel®), thyroglobulin (Proloid®), and liotrix (Thyrolar®).

Insulin: There are various types of insulin available for subcutaneous or intravenous injection. Insulin is used to treat type I diabetes mellitus and type II diabetes mellitus that cannot be controlled by diet and exercise or oral antidiabetics. Insulins also can reduce hyperkalemia. Side effects include blurred vision, hypoglycemia, headaches, fatigue, anxiety, nervousness, fainting, and convulsions.

Oral antidiabetic agents: Type II diabetic patients are treated with oral antidiabetic agents, diet, exercise, and, when necessary, insulin. Today, there are three types of oral antidiabetic agents: first- and second-generation sulfonylureas and a miscellaneous group that includes agents that differ from insulin in mode of action. Examples include chlorpropamide (Diabinese®), glipizide (Glucotrol®), and metformin (Glucophage®).

19.12 Pharmacology of the Sensory System

Eye Medications

Pilocarpine HCl (Isopto Carpine®): A topical medication that causes pupil constriction and reduces intraocular pressure. It is used in the treatment of glaucoma. Side effects include blurred vision, brow pain, eye irritation, and myopia.

Acetazolamide (Diamox Sequels®): Decreases the production of aqueous humor and is used to treat glaucoma. It is a carbonic anhydrase inhibitor (a diuretic). Side effects include myopia, paresthesia, drowsiness, nausea, and vomiting.

Betaxolol (Betoptic S®): A beta-adrenergic blocking agent that reduces the production of aqueous humor. It is used to treat glaucoma. Side effects include photophobia and overproduction of tears.

Atropine sulfate (Isopto Atropine®): Used for refraction during an eye exam. It dilates the pupil and causes the paralysis of muscles. Side effects include blurred vision and photophobia.

Ear Medications

Triethanolamine polypeptide (Cerumenex®): Used to soften ear wax (cerumen). Side effects include ear redness and itching.

19.13 Pharmacology of the Urinary System

Diuretics: Help the body eliminate excess fluids through urinary excretion. They decrease the reabsorption of salts and water from the kidney tubules, which results in more urine production. Some also help to dilate blood vessels and sometimes are given along with antihypertensive drugs to reduce high blood pressure.

Organic Acid or Loop Diuretics

Furosemide (Lasix®): A sulfonamide loop diuretic that prevents sodium and chloride ion transport in the loop of Henle, resulting in a greater loss of sodium, chloride, and water. Common uses include treatment of CHF, cirrhosis, nephrotic syndrome, and hypercalcemia. Side effects include ototoxicity, nephritis, gout, hypokalemia, and dehydration.

Thiazide and Thiazide-Like Diuretics

Hydrochlorothiazide (Microzide®): The most frequently prescribed diuretic because it is moderately potent and has relatively few side effects. It inhibits sodium transport in the distal portion of the nephron and increases chloride and potassium excretion. Common uses include treatment of hypertension, CHF, calcium stone formation, and diabetes insipidus. Side effects include hyponatremia, hypokalemic metabolic alkalosis, hyperglycemia, hyperlipidemia, hyperuricemia, and hypercalcemia.

Potassium-Sparing Diuretics

Potassium-sparing diuretics: Produce diuresis by blocking aldosterone receptors, thus inhibiting potassium secretion in the distal convoluted tubules. They do present a potential problem of hyperkalemia. Examples include spironolactone, triamterene, and amiloride. Common uses include treatment of hyperaldosteronism and potassium depletion. Side effects include hyperkalemia and gynecomastia.

19.14 Pharmacology of the Reproductive System

Use of Gonadal Hormones

Gonadal hormones: Sex hormones, produced by the ovaries in females and by the testes in males, which are under control of the anterior pituitary gland.

Androgen: Male sex hormone.

Estrogen and progesterone: Female sex hormones.

Common uses of female gonadal hormones: Hormone replacement therapy (HRT), oral contraception, fertility enhancement, treatment of breast cancers, and treatment after ovarectomy between ages 20–45 or at menopause. HRT in females may cause some side effects. For side effects of gonadal hormone therapies, see Table 19-21.

Hormone replacement therapy: Required in children with hypogonadism, primary ovarian failure, or incomplete puberty with resulting inadequate bone growth. In adults, the need for HRT arises from the removal of the ovaries or the cessation of ovarian activity at menopause. Estrogens are now also clinically indicated for the prevention and treatment of osteoporosis.

Oral contraceptives: Pills containing chemicals that are similar to natural estrogen and progesterone that prevent ovulation and thus prevent pregnancy. There are three main types: combined pill, phased pill, and mini pill.

Combined pill: Contains estrogen and progesterone in fixed doses.

Phased pill: Alternates pure estrogen and a combination of estrogen and progesterone.

Mini pill: Contains a fixed dose of progesterone only.

Morning-after pill: A contraceptive used after sexual intercourse. It contains only progesterone and is used as emergency contraception.

Spermicide: A foam, cream, jelly, or sponge that protects against pregnancy by killing the sperm.

Fertility drugs: Drugs that bring about ovulation. There are currently two types: one is synthetic and the other is a combination of three protein hormones extracted from human fluids. These drugs are prescribed for patients who desire to become pregnant but for some reason cannot ovulate or release an egg.

Cancer therapy: Certain cancers involving the breast, uterus, and prostate gland appear to be dependent on the presence of sex hormones. In some cases, the use of sex hormones seems to decrease tumor growth, whereas in others the removal of the ovaries or testes can produce beneficial results. Megestrol is specifically used in the treatment of breast cancer.

Androgens: Administered as replacement therapy to maintain male sex characteristics and organ function. Androgen replacement therapy is used for primary hypogonadism, hypogonadotropic hypogonadism, delayed puberty, and impotence that is the result of androgen deficiency. In women, androgens are used to treat metastatic inoperable breast cancer and postpartum breast engorgement.

Impotence

Sildenafil (Viagra®): An oral phosphodiesterase inhibitor indicated for erectile dysfunction in men. Common side effects include headache, flushing of the skin, upset stomach, nasal congestion, diarrhea, visual disturbances, and rash.

AT A GLANCE	Sex Hormones and Their Side Effects

Estrogens	Progesterones
Nausea	Weight gain
Vomiting	Depression
Breast tenderness	Hirsutism
Skin pigmentation	
Hypertension	
Breakthrough bleeding	

Table 19-21

STRATEGIES FOR SUCCESS

▶ *Test-Taking Skills*

Know where you're going!
After you register for the exam, find out where it's located and make sure that you can easily find your way there. On the day of the exam, leave early to account for any unforeseen problems and, if possible, try to arrive early. This approach will allow you to catch your breath and relax before the exam.

Instructions:

Answer the following questions.

1. The study of natural drugs is called
   A. pharmacology.
   B. toxicology.
   C. posology.
   D. pharmacognosy.
   E. pharmacokinetics.

2. Drugs with high abuse potential and no accepted medical use are classified in Schedule
   A. I.
   B. II.
   C. III.
   D. IV.
   E. V.

3. The combined effect of two drugs that is less than the effect of either drug taken alone is called
   A. synergism.
   B. dependence.
   C. antagonism.
   D. adverse effect.
   E. idiosyncrasy.

4. Which of the following is *not* a bacteriostatic antibiotic?
   A. sulfonamide
   B. tetracycline
   C. penicillin
   D. chloramphenicol
   E. clindamycin

5. Estrogen is often prescribed to treat
   A. osteoporosis.
   B. menarche.
   C. ovarian failure.
   D. myasthenia gravis.
   E. gynecomastia.

6. Cytomel® is a type of
   A. insulin.
   B. antidepressant.
   C. thyroid agent.
   D. cardiac glycoside.
   E. narcotic analgesic.

7. Cefazolin is a type of
   A. penicillin.
   B. cephalosporin.
   C. quinolone.
   D. aminoglycoside.
   E. vasodilator.

8. A controlled drug inventory must be completed at least every
   A. year.
   B. four years.
   C. three years.
   D. two years.
   E. six months.

9. In the *Physicians' Desk Reference,* the index of brand names and generic names for drugs is found in which section?
   A. white
   B. blue
   C. pink
   D. green
   E. red

10. Heroin is an example of a drug from which schedule?
    A. Schedule II
    B. Schedule I
    C. Schedule IV
    D. Schedule V
    E. Schedule III

CHAPTER 20

ADMINISTRATION OF MEDICATION

LEARNING OUTCOMES

20.1 Describe how drugs are classified.

20.2 Describe the process of measuring medication amounts and calculating proper dosages.

20.3 Recall the different methods of medication administration, including the "seven rights."

20.4 Describe the process of setting up medications prior to use.

20.5 Identify standard vaccines and the schedule for administration recommended by the CDC.

MEDICAL ASSISTING COMPETENCIES

COMPETENCY	CMA	RMA	CCMA	NCMA
CLINICAL				
Apply principles of aseptic techniques and infection control, including hand washing	X	X	X	X
Dispose of biohazardous materials	X	X	X	X
Practice standard precautions	X	X	X	X
Apply pharmacology principles to prepare and administer oral and parenteral (excluding IV) medications as directed by the physician	X	X	X	X
Maintain medication and immunization records	X	X	X	X
Screen and follow up on patient test results	X	X	X	X

MEDICAL ASSISTING COMPETENCIES (cont.)

GENERAL/LEGAL/PROFESSIONAL

Recognize and respond to verbal and nonverbal communications by being attentive and adapting communication to the recipient's level of understanding	X	X	X	X
Identify and respond to issues of confidentiality by maintaining confidentiality at all times and following appropriate guidelines when releasing records or information	X	X	X	X
Be aware of and perform within legal and ethical boundaries	X	X	X	X
Determine the needs for documentation and reporting, and document accurately and appropriately	X	X	X	X
Demonstrate knowledge of and monitor current federal and state health-care legislation and regulations; maintain licenses and accreditation	X	X	X	X
Dispose of controlled substances in compliance with government regulations	X	X	X	X
Perform risk management procedures	X	X	X	
Explain general office policies and procedures	X	X	X	X
Instruct individuals according to their needs	X	X	X	X
Provide patients with methods of health promotion and disease prevention	X	X	X	X
Be a "team player"	X	X	X	X
Have a responsible attitude	X	X	X	
Conduct work within scope of education, training, and ability	X	X	X	X
Be impartial and show empathy when dealing with patients	X	X		

STRATEGIES FOR SUCCESS

▶ *Test-Taking Skills*

Form study groups!
Find one or two well-prepared students in your class and arrange to meet for a study or homework session if possible. Working your way through questions and problems with other students will make you feel better about your own difficulties, and it will give you a chance to pose questions to your fellow students and combine your collective knowledge to help you understand material covered in class. You may find that another student can explain something better to you than the instructor could, or you may gain confidence in finding yourself explaining concepts to others that you didn't even realize you knew. During these study sessions, it's important that you know exactly why you are meeting. For example, you may want to work through some difficult practice questions, or you may want to review material covered in a chapter. Don't get bogged down on minor points or stray from the original goal of your meeting.

20.1 Drug Classifications

Drug classification: One method of classifying drugs is based on the form in which they are prepared (liquid or solid). See Table 20-1. Please also review this section in the "Pharmacology" chapter.

20.2 Measuring Medication and Dosage Calculations

Systems of measurement: Medical assistants must be familiar with the measurement of drug dosage. Three systems of measure are used in the United States for prescribing and administering medication: the metric system, the apothecaries' system, and the household system. Each has units of weight, volume, and length.

Metric system: The most commonly used, most accurate, and easiest to use of all the measuring systems.

- Used for most scientific and medical measurements; all pharmaceutical companies now use this system for labeling medications.
- It employs a uniform decimal scale (based on powers of 10). The basic metric units of measurement are the gram, liter, and meter.
- Prefixes added to the words *gram, liter,* and *meter* indicate smaller or larger units in the system. Example: the centimeter is 1/100 of a meter.
- For a list of metric system prefixes, see Table 20-2. The unit abbreviations of the metric system are summarized in Table 20-3.

AT A GLANCE Classification of Drugs Based on Preparation Form

Class	Definition	Example
Liquid		
Aerosol	A pressurized dosage form in which solid or liquid drug particles are suspended in a gas to be dispensed in a cloud or mist	Proventil HFA® inhaler
Elixir	A drug that is dissolved in a solution of alcohol and water	Tylenol® elixir
Emulsion	A mixture of oils in water	Cod liver oil
Liniment	A drug combined with oil, soap, alcohol, or water and applied externally	Camphor liniment
Lotion	An aqueous preparation that contains suspended ingredients	Nutraderm® lotion
Spirit	A drug combined with an alcoholic solution that is volatile	Aromatic spirit of ammonia
Spray	A fine stream of medicated vapor (to treat the nose and throat)	Dristan® nasal spray
Syrup	A drug dissolved in a solution of sugar and water	Robitussin® cough syrup
Tincture	An extract of a therapeutic material in alcohol	Tincture of benzoin
Solid		
Capsule	A drug contained in a gelatin capsule that is water soluble	Benadryl® capsule
Cream	A drug combined in a base that is generally nongreasy, resulting in a semisolid preparation	Aristocort® topical cream
Ointment	A drug combined with an oil base, resulting in a semi-solid preparation	Polysporin® ointment
Suppository	A drug mixed with a firm base, such as cocoa butter, that is designed to melt at body temperature	Nupercainal® suppository
Tablet	Powdered drugs that have been pressed into a disc shape	Aspirin tablet

Table 20-1

Prefix	Meaning
deca-	× 10
deci-	÷ 10
hect- / o	× 100
centi-	÷ 100
kilo-	× 1000
milli-	÷ 1000
mega-	× 1,000,000
micro-	÷ 1,000,000

Table 20-2

AT A GLANCE   Metric System Unit Abbreviations

Unit	Abbreviation
WEIGHT	
Microgram	μg
Milligram	mg
Gram	g
Kilogram	kg
VOLUME	
Milliliter	ml or mL
Cubic centimeter	cc
Liter	l or L
LENGTH	
Millimeter	mm
Centimeter	cm
Meter	m

Table 20-3

Gram: The basic metric unit of weight (for solids).
Liter: The basic metric unit of volume (for liquids).
Meter: The basic metric unit of length.
Cubic centimeter (cc): The amount of space occupied by one milliliter: one mL = one cc.
Apothecaries' system: An older and less accurate measuring system than the metric system.

- The basic unit of weight in the apothecaries' system is the grain (gr), derived from the weight of a large grain of wheat.

AT A GLANCE   Household System Liquid Equivalents

Measurement	Equivalent
1 teaspoon	60 drops or 5 milliliters
1 tablespoon	3 teaspoons
1 ounce	6 teaspoons = 2 tablespoons
1 teacup	6 ounces
1 glass or cup	8 ounces

Table 20-4

AT A GLANCE   Household System Abbreviations

Measurement	Abbreviation
Drop	gt, gtt
Teaspoon	tsp, t
Tablespoon	tbsp, T
Ounce	oz
Cup	c

Table 20-5

- The smallest unit of measurement of liquid volume is the minim (min), meaning "the least."
- A minim is approximately equivalent to a volume of water weighing one grain; 60 grains equal one dram, and eight drams equal one ounce.

Household system: More complicated and less accurate for administering liquid medication than the other systems.

- The only household units of measurement used in the administration of medication are based on volume.
- The basic unit of liquid volume is the drop (gt, plural gtt).
- One drop is approximately equal to 0.06 mL in the metric system and one minim in the apothecaries' system.
- See Tables 20-4 and 20-5. (There are also units called the ounce and cup for measuring dry weight; do not confuse them with the units of liquid volume.)

Conversions Between Systems of Measurement

Conversion chart: Lists approximate, not exact, equivalents between systems. For a list of approximate conversions between the metric and apothecaries' systems, see Table 20-6.

AT A GLANCE — Approximate Conversions Between the Metric and Apothecaries' Systems

Metric System	Apothecaries' System
2 g (2000 mg)	30 gr
1 g (1000 mg)	15 gr
600 mg (0.6 g)	10 gr
100 mg (0.1 g)	1½ gr
60 mg (0.06 g)	1 gr
30 mg (0.03 g)	½ gr
1 mg (0.001 g)	1/60 gr
0.1 mg (0.0001 g)	1/600 gr

Approximation formulas:

grams × 60 = milligrams

milligrams ÷ 60 = grains

grams × 15 = grains

grains ÷ 15 = grams

Table 20-6

Ratio method: To convert aspirin gr $\bar{x}$ to metric measurement (e.g., mg), follow these steps:

1. Set up the first ratio:

   unknown quantity : known quantity

   $x : 10$ gr

2. Set up the second ratio to show the standard equivalence between the desired unit of measurement (mg) and the given unit of measurement (gr). There are 60 mg in 1 grain, so the second ratio is:

   60 mg : 1 gr

3. Create a proportion using the ratios:

   x mg : 10 gr :: 60 mg : 1 gr ("x milligrams are to 10 grains as 60 milligrams are to 1 grain")

   Note that the x, which stands for our unknown measurement in milligrams, is in the same place in relationship to the 10 gr as the 60 mg is to the 1 gr. Your job now is to solve for x.

4. Multiply the outer and then the inner parts of the proportion and set them equal to each other:

   $x \times 1$ gr $= 10$ gr $\times 60$ mg

5. Divide both sides of the equation by 1 gr, and then do the arithmetic.

   $x = 600$ mg

   So 10 grains of aspirin is the same as 600 milligrams of aspirin.

   10 gr = 600 mg

Fraction method: To convert 300 mg of aspirin to an apothecaries' measure, follow these steps:

1. Set up a fraction with the known dose as the numerator (on the top) and the unknown amount, representing grains, as the denominator (on the bottom):

   300 mg$/x$

2. Set up a fraction with the standard equivalent, making sure that the units of measurement are in the same positions as in the first fraction:

   60 mg/1 gr

3. Set up a proportion with both fractions; in other words, set the two fractions equal to each other:

   300 mg$/x = 60$ mg$/1$ gr

4. Cross multiply:

   $x \times 60$ mg $= 300$ mg $\times 1$ gr

5. Divide both sides of the equation by 60 mg, and then do the arithmetic:

   $x = 5$ gr

(Notice that the two methods are interchangeable. The ratio method uses : and :: whereas the fraction method uses / and =, and the initial placement of the unknown quantity differs. But the results are the same.)

Calculating Drug Doses

Calculating drug doses: On occasion, it is necessary to calculate drug doses when the drug is not available in the exact amount the physician has prescribed. Drug doses can be calculated with either the ratio method or the fraction method.

Ratio method: If a physician orders 500 mg of a drug that comes in tablets of 250 mg, follow these steps to find the number of tablets you will need for the correct dose:

1. Set up a ratio of the unknown quantity (in this case, representing tablets) to the known quantity:

   $x : 500$ mg

2. Set up a ratio of the known conversion equivalence:

   1 tab : 250 mg

3. Put the ratios into a proportion:

   $x : 500$ mg :: 1 tab : 250 mg

4. Multiply the outer and then the inner parts of the proportion:

   $x \times 250$ mg $= 500$ mg $\times 1$ tab

5. To solve for x, divide both sides of the equation by 250 mg, and then do the arithmetic:

   $x = 2$ tabs

Fraction method: If a physician orders 30 mg of a drug that comes in capsules containing only 10 mg, follow these steps:

1. Set up a fraction with the dose ordered and the unknown number of capsules:

   30 mg/*x*

2. Set up a fraction with the known conversion equivalence. Make sure that the units of measurement are in the same position as in the first fraction:

   10 mg/1 cap

3. Set the two fractions equal to each other:

   30 mg/*x* = 10 mg/1 cap

4. Cross multiply:

   x × 10 mg = 30 mg × 1 cap

5. To solve for *x*, divide both sides of the equation by 10 mg, and then do the arithmetic:

   x = 3 caps

Pediatric Dose Calculations

Most pediatric dose calculations are based on the child's age or body weight. The common formulas used for pediatric dose calculations are Clark's rule and Young's rule.

Clark's Rule
weight of child/150 lb × average adult dose = child's dose

Young's Rule
age of child in years / (age of child in year + 12) × average adult dose = child's dose

Example: Katie has just turned three years old and weighs 30 pounds. Her mother wants to know how much cough syrup to give Katie. The directions have worn off the bottle, and she can only make out the dosage for adults: two teaspoons every four hours. How much cough syrup should Katie receive? The calculation based on Clark's rule would be like this:

   30/150 × 10 ml = Katie's dose

   1/5 × 10 mL = 2 mL

The calculation based on Young's rule would look like this:

   3/15 × 10 mL = Katie's dose

   0.24 ' 10mL = 2.4 mL

20.3 Methods of Administering Medications

"Seven rights" of drug administration: Never deviate from these seven principles: right patient, right drug, right dose, right time, right route, right technique, right documentation.

Right patient: Always check the name on the order, then ask the patient to tell you his or her name.

Right drug: Read the drug label before you take the container off the shelf, before you administer the drug, and before you put the container back on the shelf. Make sure to check the expiration date, and never use a drug that has passed this date.

Right dose: Compare the dose on the order with the dose you prepare.

Right time: If a drug must be taken after a meal, make sure that the patient has eaten recently.

Right route: Make sure that the route you are preparing to use matches the route the doctor ordered.

Right technique: Always use the proper administrative technique.

Right documentation: Document the procedure immediately after administering the drug. Include the date, time, drug name, dose, administration route, patient reaction, education of the patient about the drug, and your initials.

Route of administration: Medication may be administered by numerous routes, including oral, sublingual, buccal, inhalation, topical, rectal, urethral, vaginal, parenteral (intramuscular, subcutaneous, intradermal, or intravenous), ophthalmic, and otic.

Oral administration: The drug is given by mouth in either a solid form (tablet, capsule, or powder) or a liquid form (water-based solution, suspension, or alcohol solution). The drug is absorbed into the bloodstream through the lining of the stomach and intestine. This method is easy, safe, and economical, but drug absorption is slow and may be affected by the presence of food. Some medications may also cause nausea or stomach discomfort.

Sublingual administration: The medication must be placed under the tongue until it dissolves. See Figure 20-1. This method is faster than the oral method.

Buccal administration: The medication is placed in the mouth and absorbed in the buccal area. The patient should not chew or swallow the medication. See Figure 20-2.

Inhalation administration: The medication is given in the form of gases, sprays, or aerosol mists (fluid droplets). The respiratory tract absorbs medication more rapidly than any other mucous membrane. One inhalation medication that should be kept in every medical practice is oxygen.

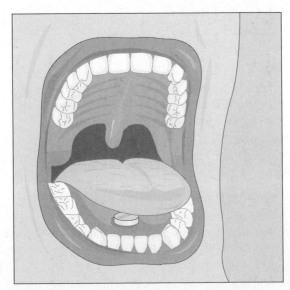

Figure 20-1 *Place a sublingual drug under the tongue.*

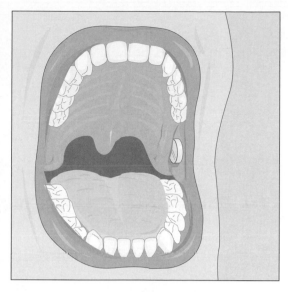

Figure 20-2 *Place a buccal drug between the cheek and gum.*

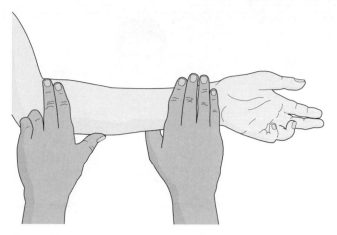

Figure 20-3 *This space is available for intradermal injection sites.*

Topical administration: Used in treating skin disorders. The medication is applied directly to affected areas of the skin. Topical medications come in the form of sprays, creams, lotions, ointments, transdermal patches, and compresses.

Transdermal drug delivery (TDD): A method of applying a drug to unbroken skin. The drug is absorbed continuously through the skin and enters the bloodstream. It is used particularly for the administration of nicotine, nitroglycerin, and scopolamine. To promote adhesion to the skin, the patch should be applied to a clean, dry area without hair.

Rectal administration: Useful if the patient is nauseated, vomiting, or unconscious. The best time to administer a rectal drug is after a bowel movement or the elimination of an enema. A suppository must be inserted one–two inches above the internal anal sphincter.

Vaginal administration: A liter or more of a solution of medication in warm water is introduced as a douche into the vagina under low pressure. Other forms of medication are inserted into the vagina with an applicator.

Parenteral administration: Medication is given outside the gastrointestinal tract. A common parenteral route is by injection. Drugs that are injected are absorbed more rapidly and completely than most other routes. In some cases, injection is the only way a drug can be given (e.g., to an unconscious patient). The disadvantages of the parenteral route are that all equipment must be sterile; that the method is often expensive, painful, and awkward for patients to administer themselves; and that there is a danger of injecting a drug incorrectly into a vein, which could cause serious harm or even death.

Intradermal (ID) injection: Given into the dermal layer of the skin. A very short needle of small gauge is used. The angle of insertion is 1015 degrees, nearly parallel to the skin. Absorption is slow. Only a small amount of medication may be injected (0.01–0.2 cc). The anterior forearm is the most common area for injection. See Figure 20-3. The gauge is usually 25–27. When an intradermal injection is correctly administered, a small wheal is raised on the skin. See Figure 20-4. The most common uses of intradermal injections are to administer allergy tests and tuberculin skin tests.

Subcutaneous (SC) injection: Given into the layer of fatty tissue that lies just below the skin. The most common sites for SC injections are the upper lateral part of the arm, anterior thigh, upper back, and abdomen. See Figure 20-5. The needle length varies ½–⅝ inch, and the gauge ranges 23–25. The needle should be inserted at a 45-degree angle to the skin. Drugs given subcutaneously must be isotonic, nonviscous, water soluble, and nonirritating. The amount of drug injected through the SC route should not exceed one mL. Medications commonly administered through this route include insulin, local anesthetics, epinephrine, and allergy treatments.

Intramuscular (IM) injection: Given deep into a muscle. Muscles can absorb a greater amount of fluid without discomfort to the patient, and IM injections are preferred for substances that can irritate the skin. The most common muscles used for this method of injection are the deltoid, gluteus medius, and vastus lateralis. See Figure 20-6. For injection of the gluteus muscle site, the patient must be in the prone position.

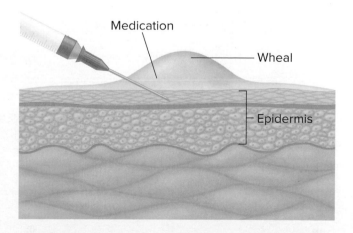

Figure 20-4 *Medication collects under the skin, forming a wheal, during an intradermal injection.*

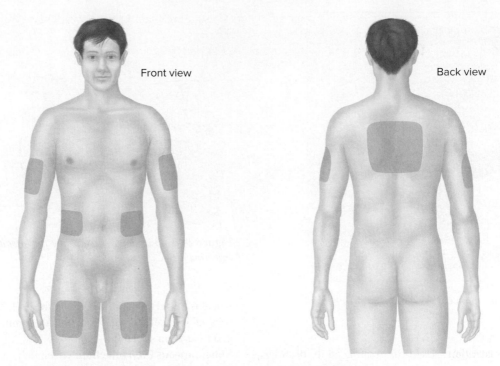

Front view

Back view

Figure 20-5 *Many sites are available for subcutaneous injections.*

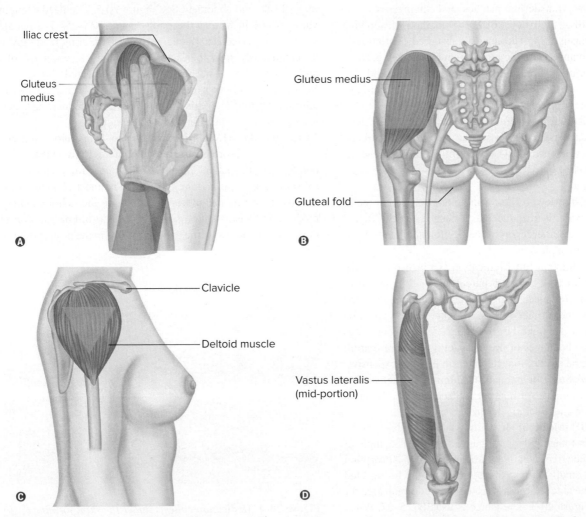

Iliac crest

Gluteus medius

Ⓐ

Gluteus medius

Gluteal fold

Ⓑ

Clavicle

Deltoid muscle

Ⓒ

Vastus lateralis (mid-portion)

Ⓓ

Figure 20-6 *For intramuscular injection in an adult, use (A) the ventrogluteal site, (B) the dorsogluteal site, (C) the deltoid site, or (D) the vastus lateralis site.*

For injection of the vastus lateralis site, the patient may be sitting or in the recumbent position. Most commonly, the needle used is 1–3 inches in length. The gauge of the needle ranges 18–23. The angle of insertion is 90 degrees. Dosage may vary from 0.5 to 5 mL. Dosages that exceed 3 mL should be split between two syringes, and two injections should be administered. The vastus lateralis muscle in the thigh is the preferred injection site for children under three years of age. Penicillin is often injected intramuscularly. A deep intramuscular injection into the dorsogluteal region may result in injury to the sciatic nerve. The deltoid muscle is used for intramuscular injections of 1 mL or less.

Z-track method: A type of IM injection in which a "zigzag" path is utilized to administer a medication into the gluteus maximus. It is used for medications that are irritating to SC or other skin tissue, or when they may cause discoloration of the skin. See Figure 20-7.

Intravenous (IV) injection: Given directly into a vein. IV injection is often used in an emergency situation for an immediate effect. In most cases, a physician or nurse must administer an IV drug. You may assist by gathering equipment and supplies. Examples of IV drugs include electrolytes, powerful antibiotics, emergency drugs, and chemotherapeutic drugs. Remember that the tourniquet must be removed immediately after the vein is punctured. The disadvantage is that painful infection may result. Rotation of the sites is necessary if injections are given repeatedly. Needles are 1–1½ inch in length. The gauges are usually 20–21.

IV drip: The insertion into a vein of a tube or a needle through which fluids are slowly added to the bloodstream over a period of time. It is also called infusion. The IV drip should not be confused with IV injection. To calculate an IV drip rate based on the volume of fluid to be infused over time, the *drops per minute* equal *the volume to be infused,* in cubic centimeters, multiplied by the *drop factor of the IV set.* This amount is then divided by the *time in minutes.*

Ophthalmic administration: Drugs are placed into the patient's eye.

Otic administration: Drugs are placed into the patient's ear.

Needles and Syringes

Needle: Consists of several parts: hub, hilt, shaft, lumen, point, and bevel. See Figure 20-8.

Needle gauge: The inside diameter of the needle. A larger gauge indicates a smaller diameter. The common range for administering medication is 18–27 gauge.

Needle length: Ranges between ⅛ of an inch and 3 inches. See Table 20-7.

Syringe: Used for inserting fluids into the body. It is usually made of plastic. A syringe consists of three parts: barrel, flange (rim), and plunger. See Figure 20-9.

Hypodermic syringes: Available in 2-, 2.5-, 3-, and 5-cc sizes. They are commonly used to administer IM injections.

Insulin syringe: Designed for an insulin injection. It is calibrated in units; 100 units = 1 mL. The most commonly used size is the 100-unit syringe (with a capacity of 100 units), divided into increments of 2 units.

Tuberculin syringe: Has a capacity of 1 cc. The calibrations are divided into tenths (0.1) and hundredths (0.01) of a cubic centimeter.

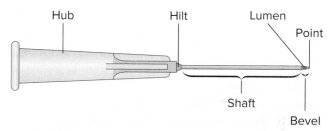

Figure 20-8 *Understanding the parts of a needle will help you use it correctly.*

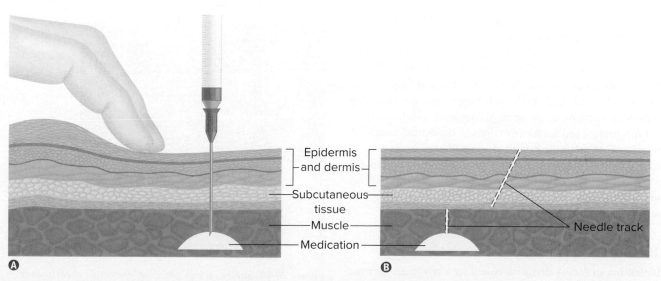

Figure 20-7 *Use the Z-track method for intramuscular injection of irritating solutions. (A) Pull the skin to one side before inserting the needle. (B) After injecting the drug, release the skin to seal off the needle track.*

Type of Injection	Gauge of Needle	Length of Needle
Intradermal	25–27 gauge	⅙–½ inch
Subcutaneous	23–27 gauge	½–⅝ inch
Intramuscular	18–25 gauge	1–3 inches

Table 20-7

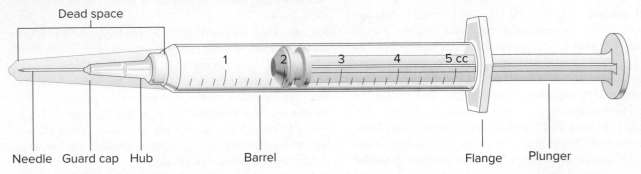

Figure 20-9 *Know the parts of a standard syringe.*

Prefilled syringe: Known as a cartridge. It is a sterile, disposable syringe. Needle units are packaged by the manufacturer with a single dose of medication inside, ready to administer.

Safety syringe: The commonly used type of syringe, which is equipped with a plastic guard or shield that may or may not move automatically into position over the needle as it is taken out of the skin. See Figure 20-10.

Needleless systems: Newer types of needle/syringe systems designed to decrease needlesticks. They include safety syringes and needleless IV line connection systems known as *lever locks* (see Figure 20-11).

Ampule: A small, sealed glass or plastic container that holds a single dose of medication.

Vial: A closed glass container with a rubber stopper protected by a soft metal cap. There are two types: single and multiple dose.

Deltoid muscle: Located at the top of the arm on the upper, outer surface. It is a good site for up to 1 mL of medication. The deltoid is commonly used for injections of tetanus boosters in adults, rabies vaccine after exposure, and vitamin B_{12}. Major blood vessels and nerves in the upper arm are located in the posterior portion of the arm. A 23-gauge, 1-inch needle is most frequently used for the injections in the deltoid muscle. A 25-gauge, ⅝-inch needle is used for a small arm.

Gluteus medius muscle: Most commonly used for deep IM injections, for injections of viscous medications (antibiotics), and for injections of irritating drugs. This site should not be used in infants.

Medication Orders

Medication order: A directive issued by a physician/licensed prescriber telling a nurse or another health-care worker which drug to administer. These orders should be written down so that

there is little chance of error. In an emergency situation, when there is no time to give written instructions, the order should be written down and signed by the prescriber within 24 hours. Orders are written on the physician's order sheet in a patient's chart. No medication should ever be given out without an order.

Prescription pads: Used to write medication orders for outpatients.

Medication order components: The patient's full name, date of the order, name of the drug preceded by the abbreviation *Rx*, dosage, route of administration, time and frequency, prescriber's signature (without which the medication order is not legal), number of refills and quantity (preceded by the word *repetatur*), and the prescriber's DEA number on all prescriptions for controlled substances.

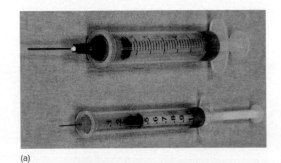

(a)

(b)

Figure 20-10 *Safety syringe showing protective sheaths that are pushed over the needle after each use.*
(a) © McGraw-Hill Education; *(b)* © Total Care Programming, Inc.

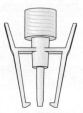

Figure 20-11 *Needleless lever-lock system.*
From Donna Gauwitz, Administering Medications, 7/e. Copyright ©
McGraw-Hill Education. Reprinted by permission of McGraw-Hill
Education.

Types of Drug Orders

Routine order: Specifies that a drug be administered until a discontinuation order is written or until a specified termination date is reached.

Standing order: Outlines a specific condition for which the drug is to be administered. These orders are frequently used in critical care units, where the patient's condition changes rapidly, and in long-term care facilities.

PRN order: Specifies that a drug be given only when the patient needs it, such as for pain or before an operation or diagnostic procedure. (PRN stands for *pro re nata*, roughly "for a circumstance that has come to be" or "as the situation requires.")

Stat order: A single order that is administered immediately, written usually for emergencies.

20.4 Setting Up Medications

Diligence: In setting up medication to be administered, be sure to observe the "seven rights" of drug administration. Get information from the Kardex®, medication record, or medicine cart, and concentrate on nothing but the task at hand. Do not engage in a conversation with someone else while you are trying to prepare and administer the medication.

Cleanliness: Clean up by washing your hands, and try never to touch the drugs. Never give a pill that has fallen on the floor. Keep unit doses sealed until you are ready to give them.

Tablets: After you have calculated the correct dose, you may find that you need only half or a quarter of a tablet. If you need to divide a tablet, use a pill cutter or a knife to make a quick, clean break. However, you should not divide a nonscored tablet due to potential medication errors. If you have to touch the pill to break it, use a tissue. Never open the tablet package until you administer the medication to the patient. If you need tablets from a bottle, pour them into the medicine cup without touching them. Sometimes tablets must be crushed or capsules opened. Check the reference book to make sure that such a procedure is permissible. Never crush enteric-coated or sustained-action medications.

Liquid medications: Remove the cap and place it upside down to prevent contamination. Hold the bottle so that the label is against the palm of your hand in order to prevent medication from running down the side of the bottle and damaging the label. Place the medication cup on a stable, flat surface at eye level to ensure accuracy. Do not hold the cup at eye level because you might tip the cup as you pour.

Recording Medication Administration

Kardex® file: A card-filing system that serves as a quick reference to the needs of a patient. Each card is folded once and lists up-to-date information about medications, treatments, and care. All information is written in pencil, so it can be erased and updated.

Medicine card: Used to record the patient's name, room and bed number, name of the drug, dose, route, and time at which the drug is to be given. One medicine card is written for each type of drug the patient is to receive; the information is copied over from the Kardex® file.

Medication administration record (MAR): A convenient way to document all the drugs administered to a patient every day, especially if there are several drugs given at different times. If the drug is to be given regularly, a complete schedule is written for all administration times. Each time a dose is administered, the health-care worker checks off the time at which it was given and initials the entry.

Patient chart or medical record: All events related to the treatment of a patient, including the administration of medications, need to be recorded in the patient's chart as a permanent record of care received. When medication is administered, you must record the drug's name, the strength and amount, the route, the times at which it is given, and the initials and signature of the health-care worker who administered it.

20.5 Vaccinations

Immunization: The process of rendering a person immune to a disease.

Artificial immunity: Produced by the administration of vaccines or other forms of immunization.

Vaccines: Made from dead or harmless infectious agents. They trigger the body's immune response to manufacture antibodies against the particular disease-causing agent. For a recommended schedule of vaccinations for children of all ages, see Figure 20-12.

Hepatitis (A and B)

Hepatitis A vaccine: Should be stored and shipped at temperatures ranging 35.6°F (2°C)–46.4°F (8°C) and should not be frozen. The vaccine should be administered intramuscularly into the deltoid muscle. A needle length appropriate for the patient's age and size should be used.

Hepatitis B vaccine: The vaccination schedule used most often for adults and children is three muscular injections, the second and third administered one and six months after the first, respectively.

Rotavirus (RV)

Rotavirus causes inflammation of the stomach and intestines (gastroenteritis), signified by severe watery diarrhea. In infants and young children, rotavirus can lead to dehydration and death. Two rotavirus vaccines were introduced in the United States in 2006. Though parts of the *porcine circovirus (PCV)* are present in both vaccines, no evidence shows that this virus causes

Figure 1. Recommended immunization schedule for persons aged 0 through 18 years – **United States, 2016.**
(FOR THOSE WHO FALL BEHIND OR START LATE, SEE THE CATCH-UP SCHEDULE [FIGURE 2]).

These recommendations must be read with the footnotes that follow. For those who fall behind or start late, provide catch-up vaccination at the earliest opportunity as indicated by the green bars in Figure 1. To determine minimum intervals between doses, see the catch-up schedule (Figure 2). School entry and adolescent vaccine age groups are shaded.

Vaccine	Birth	1 mo	2 mos	4 mos	6 mos	9 mos	12 mos	15 mos	18 mos	19–23 mos	2-3 yrs	4-6 yrs	7-10 yrs	11-12 yrs	13–15 yrs	16–18 yrs
Hepatitis B[1] (HepB)	1st dose	◄----- 2nd dose -----►			◄---------------- 3rd dose ---------------►											
Rotavirus[2] (RV) RV1 (2-dose series); RV5 (3-dose series)			1st dose	2nd dose	See footnote 2											
Diphtheria, tetanus, & acellular pertussis[3] (DTaP: <7 yrs)			1st dose	2nd dose	3rd dose		◄------ 4th dose ------►					5th dose				
Haemophilus influenzae type b[4] (Hib)			1st dose	2nd dose	See footnote 4		3rd or 4th dose, See footnote 4									
Pneumococcal conjugate[5] (PCV13)			1st dose	2nd dose	3rd dose		◄----- 4th dose -----►									
Inactivated poliovirus[6] (IPV: <18 yrs)			1st dose	2nd dose	◄-------------- 3rd dose --------------►							4th dose				
Influenza[7] (IIV; LAIV)					Annual vaccination (IIV only) 1 or 2 doses						Annual vaccination (LAIV or IIV) 1 or 2 doses		Annual vaccination (LAIV or IIV) 1 dose only			
Measles, mumps, rubella[8] (MMR)					See footnote 8		◄----- 1st dose -----►					2nd dose				
Varicella[9] (VAR)							◄----- 1st dose -----►					2nd dose				
Hepatitis A[10] (HepA)							◄----- 2-dose series, See footnote 10 -----►									
Meningococcal[11] (Hib-MenCY ≥ 6 weeks; MenACWY-D ≥9 mos; MenACWY-CRM ≥ 2 mos)			See footnote 11											1st dose		Booster
Tetanus, diphtheria, & acellular pertussis[12] (Tdap: ≥7 yrs)														(Tdap)		
Human papillomavirus[13] (2vHPV: females only; 4vHPV, 9vHPV: males and females)														(3-dose series)		
Meningococcal B[11]														See footnote 11		
Pneumococcal polysaccharide[5] (PPSV23)											See footnote 5					

Range of recommended ages for all children · Range of recommended ages for catch-up immunization · Range of recommended ages for certain high-risk groups · Range of recommended ages for non-high-risk groups that may receive vaccine, subject to individual clinical decision making · No recommendation

This schedule includes recommendations in effect as of January 1, 2016. Any dose not administered at the recommended age should be administered at a subsequent visit, when indicated and feasible. The use of a combination vaccine generally is preferred over separate injections of its equivalent component vaccines. Vaccination providers should consult the relevant Advisory Committee on Immunization Practices (ACIP) statement for detailed recommendations, available online at http://www.cdc.gov/vaccines/hcp/acip-recs/index.html. Clinically significant adverse events that follow vaccination should be reported to the Vaccine Adverse Event Reporting System (VAERS) online (http://www.vaers.hhs.gov) or by telephone (800-822-7967). Suspected cases of vaccine-preventable diseases should be reported to the state or local health department. Additional information, including precautions and contraindications for vaccination, is available from CDC online (http://www.cdc.gov/vaccines/recs/vac-admin/contraindications.htm) or by telephone (800-CDC-INFO [800-232-4636]).

This schedule is approved by the Advisory Committee on Immunization Practices (http://www.cdc.gov/vaccines/acip), the American Academy of Pediatrics (http://www.aap.org), the American Academy of Family Physicians (http://www.aafp.org), and the American College of Obstetricians and Gynecologists (http://www.acog.org).

NOTE: The above recommendations must be read along with the footnotes of this schedule.

Figure 20-12 *Recommended immunization schedule for persons ages 0–18 years—United States, 2016.*
Source: Centers for Disease Control and Prevention.

illness in humans. The RV-1 vaccine is a two-dose series, and the RV-5 vaccine is a three-dose series.

Diphtheria, Tetanus, and Acellular Pertussis (DTap and Tdap)

Diphtheria causes sore throat, fever, chills, the development of a thick coating that causes difficulty swallowing or breathing, and can lead to heart problems, paralysis, and death. Tetanus ("lockjaw") develops from a toxin in bacteria commonly found in soil. It causes headache, anxiety, muscle spasms, difficulty breathing, and paralysis. Pertussis ("whooping cough") causes prolonged, extreme coughing and severe coldlike symptoms that often require hospitalization. The DTap vaccine is given to children younger than seven years, and the Tdap vaccine is given to children age seven or older.

Haemophilus Influenzae Type B (Hib)

Haemophilus influenzae often causes severe bacterial infections in infants. The Hib vaccine prevents meningitis, pneumonia, epiglottitis, and other serious infections caused by the Hib virus. It is recommended for all children younger than five years of age, and is usually given to infants beginning at two months of age. It may be combined with other vaccines. Some brands contain Hib along with other vaccines in a single administration.

Pneumococcal Conjugate (PCV13)

This form of pneumococcal vaccine is recommended for all children under the age of 59 months, and for certain adults who have specific risk factors. Children who are 24 months or older, with high risk of pneumococcal disease, should also receive the PPSV23 vaccine. All adults who are age 65 or older, and those who are 19 or older with risk factors, should receive the PPSV23 vaccine as well.

Pneumococcal Polysaccharide (PPSV23)

Pneumococcal polysaccharide vaccine: Administer pneumococcal vaccine to children who are at risk and to adolescents who have chronic illnesses associated with increased risk for pneumococcal disease or its complications. Use adolescents' visits to providers to ensure that the vaccine has been administered to persons for whom it is indicated: one dose of 0.5 mL, IM or SC.

Inactivated Poliovirus (IPV)

Though polio has largely been eradicated in the United States, when the disease does occur, it has the potential to result in permanent disability and death. The inactivated polio vaccine is administered as an injection in the leg or arm, based on the patient's age. It may be given along with other vaccines. It is recommended for children under the age of 18, who receive four total doses, at the ages of two months, four months, six–18 months, and a final booster dose at four–six years. The formerly popular oral polio vaccine (OPV) has not been used in the United States since 2000, but is still used in other parts of the world.

Influenza (IIV; LAIV)

The inactivated influenza vaccine (IIV) is given to infants at a minimum age of six months, while the live attenuated influenza vaccine (LAIV) is given to children at a minimum age of two years. Beginning at age six months, the IIV is given to infants and children annually. For most healthy children (two–18 years) and nonpregnant individuals (up to age 49), either LAIV or IIV may be used. However, LAIV should not be administered to those with asthma, children age 2–4 years who have had wheezing in the past 12 months, or those with any other underlying medical conditions predisposing them to influenza complications. Most people require only one annual dose; however, certain annual influenza strains may require children to receive two doses, separated by at least four weeks, if they are receiving an influenza vaccine for the first time.

Measles, Mumps, Rubella (MMR)

Measles is a highly contagious respiratory viral disease that is also called *rubeola*. Mumps is a contagious viral disease that causes flulike symptoms, and can lead to meningitis, reproductive problems, and deafness. Rubella (German measles) is an acute viral disease that causes fever and rash for several days, which, in pregnant women, can cause fetal birth defects. The MMR vaccine was developed in 1971. The minimum age for the MMR vaccine is 12 months. It is usually first given 12–15 months of age, with a second dose given at age four–six years. However, the second dose may be given before age four, as long as at least four weeks have elapsed since the first dose. Infants and children being taken on international trips may require a different dosing schedule (see www.cdc.gov).

Varicella (VAR)

Shingles vaccine: In May 2006, the FDA licensed a new vaccine to reduce older patients' risk of shingles, which is a painful skin rash, often with blisters, that is also called "herpes zoster." It is caused by the varicella zoster virus, the same virus that causes chickenpox. This vaccine (trade name Zostavax) has

been shown to prevent shingles in about 50% of patients who are age 60 or older, and can also reduce the pain associated with shingles.

A single dose of this vaccine is indicated for adults ages 60 or older, and it is administered subcutaneously. No serious problems have been identified with the shingles vaccine. Its duration of protection is unknown, but protection from herpes zoster has been demonstrated through four years of follow-up. The shingles vaccine should not be administered to any immunocompromised patient, such as those with AIDS, cancer, or other conditions.

Chickenpox vaccine: This vaccine is primarily used for infants and children, and utilizes the trade name Varivax. A booster vaccine may be required within 10 years for certain age groups.

Human Papillomavirus (HPV)

HPV vaccine: In June 2006, the FDA licensed the first vaccine developed to prevent cancer and other diseases in women that are caused by certain types of the genital human papillomavirus (HPV). This vaccine (trade name Gardasil) protects against four HPV types (6, 11, 16, and 18) that are responsible for cervical cancer and 90% of genital warts. It is recommended for females 9–26 years.

The best time for females to receive this vaccine is ages 10–11 because, ideally, this vaccine should be administered before the onset of sexual activity. The recommendations for HPV vaccine are as follows: three IM injections over a six-month period, with the second dose given two months after the first dose, and the third dose given six months after the first dose.

Meningococcal (HibMenCY; MCV4-D; MCV4-CRM)

Neisseria meningitidis: Causes both endemic and epidemic disease, principally meningitis and meningococcemia. As a result of the control of *Haemophilus influenzae* type B infections (which can result in meningitis), *Neisseria meningitidis* has become the leading cause of bacterial meningitis in children and young adults in the United States. Persons who have other diseases associated with immunosuppression (e.g., HIV or *Streptococcus pneumoniae* infection) may be at higher risk for acquiring meningococcal disease and disease caused by some other encapsulated bacteria.

Meningococcal vaccine: Routine vaccination with the quadrivalent meningococcal polysaccharide vaccine is not recommended because of its relative ineffectiveness in children younger than two years of age (among whom risk for endemic disease is highest) and its relatively short duration of protection. However, the polysaccharide meningococcal vaccine is useful for controlling serogroup C meningococcal outbreaks.

Indications for use: In general, the use of polysaccharide meningococcal vaccine should be restricted to persons two years of age or older; however, children as young as three months of age may be vaccinated to elicit short-term protection against serogroup A meningococcal disease (two doses administered three months apart should be considered for children 3–18 months of age). Routine vaccination with the quadrivalent vaccine is recommended for certain high-risk groups, including persons who have terminal complement component deficiencies.

Administration: Primary vaccination, for both adults and children, is administered subcutaneously as a single 0.5-mL dose. The vaccine can be administered at the same time as other vaccines but at a different anatomical site (i.e., deltoid muscle or buttocks).

Rabies

Rabies: There are two types of rabies immunizing products. Rabies vaccines induce an active immune response that includes the production of neutralizing antibodies. Rabies immune globulins (RIGs) provide rapid, passive immune protection that persists for only a short time (a half-life of approximately 21 days).

Exposure to rabies: Rabies can be transmitted only when the virus is introduced into open cuts or wounds in skin or mucous membranes. Two categories of exposure (bite and nonbite) should be considered.

Bite: Any penetration of the skin by teeth constitutes a bite exposure. Bites to the face and hands carry the highest risk, but the site of the bite should not influence the decision to begin treatment.

Nonbite: Scratches, abrasions, open wounds, or mucous membranes contaminated with saliva or other potentially infectious material (such as brain tissue) from a rabid animal constitute nonbite exposure. If the material containing the virus is dry, the virus can be considered noninfectious.

Rabies vaccine: Studies conducted in the United States by the CDC have shown that a regimen of one dose of HRIG and five doses of HDCV over a 28-day period are safe and induce an excellent antibody response in all recipients. The schedule of the HDCV vaccinations is:

- First dose as soon as possible after exposure
- Second dose three days after the first
- Third dose seven days after the first
- Fourth dose 14 days after the first
- Fifth dose 28 days after the first

IM injection of rabies vaccine should be administered only in the deltoid muscle for postexposure. SC injection should be administered for preexposure.

Tuberculosis (TB)

Tuberculin skin test: Several methods are used. The most common is the Mantoux test.

Mantoux test: Administered by means of an intradermal needle and syringe. It must be read within 48–78 hours. The amount of solution that is injected is 0.1 mL. A short needle with a gauge of 26–27 is used.

Mantoux tuberculin skin test results: Induration of less than 10 mm is considered a negative reaction. According to the American Lung Association, induration of 5 mm or more is considered a positive reaction for infants, children, adults who have had close contact with active tuberculosis, persons with known or suspected HIV infection, and persons whose immune systems are suppressed. Induration of 10 mm or more is considered a positive reaction in persons who are foreign born from high-prevalence countries; persons with other medical risk factors; health-care workers; migrant workers; and residents of long-term care facilities, nursing homes, and correctional institutions. Induration of 15 mm or more is considered a positive reaction in all other persons.

Induration: An area of hardened tissue after a tuberculin test. Table 20-8 lists the routes of administration for the vaccinations discussed in this chapter.

Immunization records: The National Childhood Vaccine Injury Act of 1988 indicates that specific information belongs in each child's permanent medical record, concerning immunizations, as follows:

- Vaccine type, manufacturer, lot number
- Date of vaccine administration
- Name, address, and title of health-care provider who administered the vaccine
- Administration site and route
- Vaccine expiration date

Vaccine storage: The medical assistant is responsible for the proper storage of vaccines in order to ensure their safety and effectiveness, as follows:

- Once a vaccine arrives at your facility:
  - Store refrigerated vaccines 35°F –46°F (2°C–8°C).
  - Store frozen vaccines between −58°F and +5°F (−50°C and −15°C).
- Check and record refrigerator and freezer temperatures daily.
- Rotate vaccine supply so that those with shortest expiration dates are used first; place those with longest expiration dates behind those that will expire soonest.
- Any vaccine that has reached its expiration date must be removed from stock immediately.
- Prepare each vaccine just prior to administration to a patient.
- When preparing and administering vaccines, follow all infection control guidelines.

ROUTES OF ADMINISTRATION FOR VARIOUS VACCINATIONS

Vaccination	Route of Administration
Diphtheria, Tetanus, Acellular Pertussis (DTap; Tdap)	IM
Haemophilus Influenzae Type B (Hib)	IM
Hepatitis A (HepA)	IM
Hepatitis B (HepB)	IM
Human Papillomavirus (HPV)	IM
Inactivated Poliovirus (IPV)	IM, SC
Influenza (IIV; LAIV)	IM, intranasal spray
Measles, Mumps, Rubella (MMR)	SC
Meningococcal (HibMenCY; MCV4-D; MCV4-CRM)	IM, SC
Pneumococcal Conjugate (PCV13)	IM
Pneumococcal Polysaccharide (PPSV23)	IM, SC
Rabies	IM
Rotavirus (RV)	PO
Varicella (VAR)	SC

Table 20-8

STRATEGIES FOR SUCCESS

▶ *Test-Taking Skills*

Use all of the time allotted!
It may be tempting to submit your exam after you have answered the last question, but your score can be improved if you use all the time you are given. Look over your exam and make sure that you answered every question, and if a paper exam that the choices are clearly marked, and that the answer sheet numbers match the exam question numbers. If you have time, cover up your answers and rework some of the problems. Especially rework problems involving math or questions you originally thought were difficult. If a question still seems too complicated to decipher, try rephrasing and expressing it in your own terms. When a question involves math, make sure that you understand what the question is asking for. What do you need to calculate? Break down the question into its elements, list all the known variables, and name the unknown variable. Check your math to make sure that you didn't make any mistakes.

Instructions:

Answer the following questions.

1. Which of the following muscles is commonly used for intramuscular injections in the infant?

   A. deltoid
   B. internal oblique
   C. external oblique
   D. vastus lateralis
   E. gastrocnemius

2. Which of the following injection methods should be chosen for medications that are irritating or may cause discoloration of the skin?

   A. subcutaneous
   B. intravenous
   C. Z-track
   D. intradermal
   E. intramuscular

3. The needle gauges often used for intravenous injections are

   A. 18–19.
   B. 20–21.
   C. 23–24.
   D. 26–27.
   E. 28–32.

4. The doctor has ordered a dose of medicine to be 300 mg, but the medicine is available only in 50-mg tablets. What is the correct dose?

   A. five tablets
   B. six tablets
   C. 320 mg
   D. 75 mg
   E. none of these

5. The metric system employs a uniform scale based on powers of

   A. 1.
   B. 10.
   C. 50.
   D. 100.
   E. none of these

6. A physician orders ranitidine (Zantac®) 300 mg. If the drug is available in 150-mg tablets, how many tablets should be given to the patient?

   A. 1
   B. 1.5
   C. 2
   D. 2.5
   E. 3

7. The angle of insertion for intradermal injections is

   A. 5 degrees.
   B. 15 degrees.
   C. 45 degrees.
   D. 90 degrees.
   E. 30 degrees.

8. A major complication of a deep intramuscular injection into the dorsogluteal region is injury to which of the following structures?

   A. iliac artery
   B. gluteal nerve
   C. femoral artery
   D. sacroiliac joint
   E. sciatic nerve

9. Which of the following vaccines is recommended to be administered yearly?

   A. MMR
   B. PCV
   C. influenza
   D. varicella
   E. hepatitis B

10. A single order that is administered immediately and usually written for emergencies is known as a

    A. STAT order.
    B. standing order.
    C. routine order.
    D. PRN order.

ELECTROCARDIOGRAPHY

LEARNING OUTCOMES

21.1 Recall the structures and functions of the heart's conduction system.

21.2 Describe how to administer an ECG, troubleshoot inconsistencies, and perform basic interpretation.

21.3 Identify other tests used to record the activities of the heart.

21.4 Recall conditions of the heart and related procedures.

MEDICAL ASSISTING COMPETENCIES

COMPETENCY	CMA	RMA	CCMA	NCMA
Clinical				
Apply principles of aseptic techniques and infection control, including hand washing	X	X	X	X
Practice standard precautions	X	X	X	X
Perform electrocardiography	X	X	X	X
Prepare and maintain examination and treatment areas	X	X	X	X
Prepare the patient for and assist the physician with routine and specialty examinations, treatments, and minor office surgeries	X	X	X	X

MEDICAL ASSISTING COMPETENCIES (cont.)

General/Legal/Professional

Identify and respond to issues of confidentiality by maintaining confidentiality at all times and following appropriate guidelines when releasing records or information	X	X	X	X
Be aware of and perform within legal and ethical boundaries	X	X	X	X
Determine the needs for documentation and reporting, and document accurately and appropriately	X	X	X	X
Perform risk management procedures		X	X	
Explain general office policies and procedures	X	X	X	X
Instruct individuals according to their needs	X	X	X	X
Provide patients with methods of health promotion and disease prevention	X	X	X	X
Be a "team player"	X	X	X	X
Have a responsible attitude	X	X	X	
Be courteous and diplomatic	X	X	X	
Conduct work within scope of education, training, and ability	X	X	X	X
Be impartial and show empathy when dealing with patients	X	X		
Use appropriate medical terminology	X	X	X	X

STRATEGIES FOR SUCCESS

▶ *Study Skills*

Link to reality!

It might help you to remember concepts and terms better if you relate them to real life. Create a scenario in which you might need the information. What would your responsibilities be as a medical assistant? If the concept is a procedure, are there any situations in which there might be an exception to the established guidelines? Since reality is never as straightforward as textbook cases, can you think of situations in which it might be hard to decide what to do? Discuss these issues with your instructor, your coworkers, and your fellow students. The more you think about these concepts, practice them at work, and talk about them with the people around you, the better prepared you will be for the exam.

21.1 The Electrical System of the Heart

The heart and its structures: See Chapter 3.

Conduction system: Specialized electrical or pacemaker cells in the heart that are arranged in a system of pathways. Cardiac muscle differs from skeletal muscle in that it is able to contract rhythmically and conduct impulses. The pathways for the conduction system are shown in Figure 21-1.

Cardiac cells: There are two types: myocardial cells and pacemaker cells (specialized cells of the electrical conduction system). Cardiac cells have four primary characteristics: excitability (irritability), automaticity, conductivity, and contractility.

Pacemaker cells: Described as slow cells because their depolarization is dependent on calcium entry into the cells through slow channels. The primary properties of pacemaker cells of the heart are automaticity and conductivity.

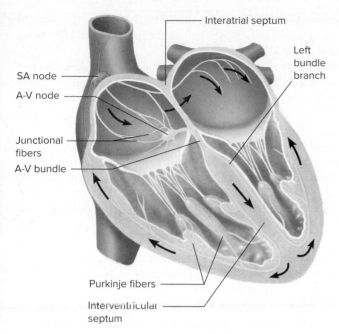

Figure 21-1 *The cardiac conduction system.*

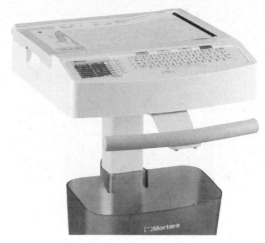

Figure 21-2 *Single-channel electrocardiograph.*
© Mortara Instrument

Myocardial cells: Described as fast cells because their depolarization is dependent on sodium entry into the cells through fast channels. The primary property of myocardial cells is contractility.

Excitability: The ability of cardiac muscle cells to respond to an outside stimulus. Excitability may be increased as a result of epinephrine and norepinephrine secretion by the adrenal medulla. All cardiac cells are characterized by excitability.

Automaticity: The ability of cardiac pacemaker cells to spontaneously initiate an electrical impulse without being stimulated from another source.

Contractility: The ability of cardiac cells to shorten, causing cardiac muscle contraction in response to an electrical stimulus. Contractility can be enhanced through the use of certain medications such as dopamine, epinephrine, and digitalis.

Conductivity: The ability of a cardiac cell to receive an electrical stimulus and conduct that impulse to an adjacent cell.

Action potential: Each muscle cell in the heart is stimulated to contract by going through an electrical process called the action potential. The action potential process is composed of five phases. These phases correlate with waveforms of the cardiac cycle recorded on the ECG. The recognition of abnormalities in the size of the waves or the various time intervals can aid in the diagnosis of certain types of heart problems.

21.2 The Electrocardiograph

Electrocardiograph: An instrument that measures the waves of electrical impulses that are responsible for the cardiac cycle. There are several types.

12-lead electrocardiograph: The standard machine, which simultaneously records the electrical activity of the heart from 12 different views. See Figure 21-2.

Single-channel electrocardiograph: Records information from one lead, giving one view of the heart's electrical activity.

Electrocardiogram (ECG or EKG): A record of the electrical impulses associated with cardiac contraction and relaxation. The two functions recorded are the amount of voltage generated by the heart and the time required for the voltage to travel through the heart.

Electrocardiography: The process by which a graphical pattern is created from the electrical impulses generated within the heart while it is pumping. It is commonly performed to evaluate heart disease or abnormal heart rhythms. It also evaluates the patient's status after a myocardial infarction (MI), or to verify effectiveness and adverse effects of medications. Occasionally, electrocardiography is done during a general examination.

Lead: An electrical connector (wire) between a specific combination of electrodes (sensors) attached to the body. Leads are used to record electrical activity. Each lead is given a specific designation and code. There are two types of leads: limb and precordial.

Limb lead: Six leads directly monitor electrodes on the arms and legs. Three are standard leads and three are augmented leads. They are also called bipolar leads because they monitor two electrodes.

Standard lead: Also called a bipolar lead because it directly monitors two electrodes. Leads I, II, and III are standard limb leads. If a patient has had a leg amputated, both leg electrodes should be placed on the thighs or abdomen.

Augmented lead: Also called a unipolar lead because it directly monitors only one electrode. The electrical activity recorded by an augmented lead is very slight. Leads aVR, aVL, and aVF are augmented limb leads.

Precordial lead: Also called a chest lead. The anodes, or positive (+) electrodes, of these six unipolar leads are placed across the chest in a specific pattern, along specific intercostal spaces. Each precordial lead is identified by the corresponding electrode, designated by the letter V with a numeral (V_1, V_2, V_3, V_4, V_5, and V_6). See Figure 21-3.

Unconventional leads: If P waves cannot be seen on the conventional 12-lead ECG, unconventional leads can be created. The intra-atrial lead is an example of an unconventional lead.

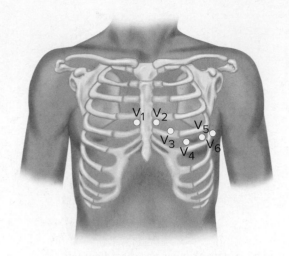

V_1 Fourth intercostal space (between the ribs), to the right of the sternum (breastbone)

V_2 Fourth intercostal space, to the left of the sternum

V_3 Fifth intercostal space, midway between V_2 and V_4

V_4 Fifth intercostal space, on the left midclavicular line

V_5 Fifth intercostal space, midway between V_4 and V_6

V_6 Fifth intercostal space, on the left midaxillary line

Figure 21-3 *Six precordial electrodes are arranged in specific positions on the chest. Note that electrode V_4 must be positioned before V_3 and V_6 before V_5.*

Intra-atrial lead: A specifically designed electrode wire (V lead) advanced intravenously (from the internal jugular, subclavian, or femoral vein) into the right atrial cavity.

Stylus: A penlike instrument that moves on the ECG paper and uses heat instead of ink to record the impulses that are received through electrodes as a result of the electrical activity of the heart.

Telemetry: The transmission of ECG signals via radio waves.

Oscilloscope: A monitor or TV-type device that shows the tracing of the electrical activity of the heart.

Administering an ECG

Electrocardiograph controls: Certain function controls are common on electrocardiographs: the standardization control, speed selector, sensitivity control, lead selector, centering control, stylus temperature control, marker control, and on/off switch. Some may need to be activated or adjusted before use.

Standardization control: This feature allows you to standardize the machine before use; a 1-mV impulse makes a standardization mark on the ECG paper. When this control is pressed, the stylus should move up 10 mm (10 small squares) and remain there for 0.08 second (2 mm).

Speed selector: ECG paper usually runs at 25 mm per second for adults, but this may be increased for children or others with a rapid heartbeat, because deflections would appear too close together at 25 mm. The speed selector allows you to adjust the speed to 50 mm per second. The peaks will then be separated

(easier to read). The paper should be written on to indicate if the speed was reset to 50 mm; otherwise, the speed of 25 mm is assumed.

Sensitivity control: This control adjusts the tracing height and the standardization mark. It is usually set on "1." If the height of the tracing is too great to fit completely, adjust this control to "1/2." This will reduce the tracing size and standardization mark by one-half.

Lead selector: This allows you to run each lead individually; normally, the ECG runs a 12-lead tracing automatically.

Centering control: This control allows adjustment of the stylus position so that it is centered on the paper.

Line control: This control allows adjustment of the stylus temperature; the higher the temperature, the heavier and thicker the line that is produced.

Preparing the patient's skin: Clean the skin with alcohol and rub it vigorously. If necessary, trim hair on the areas where the electrodes will be attached.

Electrode: A device that detects electrical charges. A reusable electrode may be cleaned with steel wool, warm water, or alcohol. Electrodes are also known as sensors.

Types of electrodes: There are three main types of electrodes: metal plate, suction bulb, and disposable electrodes. Disposable electrodes are the most commonly used type of electrode. This type of electrode has largely replaced the metal plate and suction bulb electrodes from previous models. Disposable electrodes come with the electrolyte product already applied; because the electrolyte gel is prepackaged and measured, artifacts occurring from the placement of unequal amounts of electrolyte have been minimized.

Anode: The positive electrode of an ECG lead.

Applying electrodes: Apply electrodes first to the fleshy portion of the limbs; then apply the precordial electrodes. You must position electrodes at 10 locations on the body. See Figure 21-4.

Electrolyte: Material applied to the skin to enhance contact between the skin and an electrode.

Attaching electrodes: Use electrolyte gel, lotion, or solution before placing reusable electrodes, and secure the electrodes with rubber straps or bulbs. For disposable electrodes, peel off the backings and press them into place.

Positioning electrodes: Precordial electrodes must be placed at specific locations, whereas the positions of limb electrodes need not be exact. Limb electrodes are most commonly placed on the inside of the fleshy part of the calf muscle and on the outside of the upper arm.

Einthoven's triangle: Electrodes placed on the right arm, left arm, and left leg form Einthoven's triangle. Leads I, II, and III record electrical activity between their two respective electrodes. One of these electrodes is always positive, and one is negative. The positive electrode is the recording electrode. The third electrode is a ground, which minimizes electrical activity from other sources. The right leg is never used for ECG tracings; it serves as an electrical ground. See Table 21-1.

Attaching the wires: Connect the limb wires first, then the precordial wires in sequence from V_1 to V_6. Make sure that the wires follow the patient's body contours and lie flat against the body. Drape the wires to avoid putting tension on the electrodes.

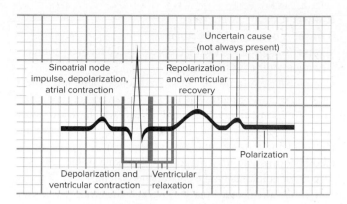

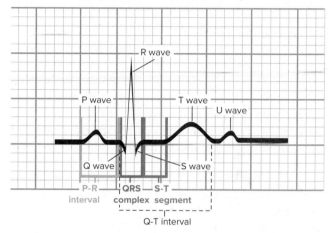

Figure 21-5 *This ECG tracing shows the pattern of one cardiac cycle in a normal heart. These specific electrical impulses (top) represent the cycle of cardiac contraction and relaxation. The waves and lines (bottom) represent specific parts of the pattern.*

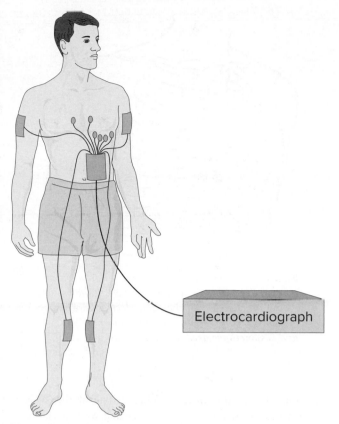

Figure 21-4 *There are 10 electrode positions for electrocardiography.*

Polarity: A positive or negative electrical state.

Polarization: The electrical state of the heart at rest, in which the electrical charge on the outside of muscle cells is negative in relation to the inside.

Depolarization: A change of polarity. It is the electrical discharge that precedes contraction. It flows from the SA node to the ventricles.

Baseline: An indication, as on an ECG tracing, of no electrical charge or activity between cardiac cycles. It is also known as an isoelectric line.

Repolarization: The restoration of a cell to its original pattern of charge. It is a return to polarization from the depolarized state (a return to rest).

Cardiac cycle: A complete phase of atrial contraction and ventricular contraction, followed by relaxation. It occurs about 60–100 times per minute. The contraction of the heart muscle is called systole. The ECG tracing of one heartbeat produces a pattern of waves designated as P, Q, R, S, T, and sometimes U, which correspond to certain electrical activities. See Figure 21-5.

P wave: A small upward curve that represents the contraction of the atria and is thus a measure of the atrial rate.

QRS complex: The Q, R, and S waves, which correlate with the contraction of the ventricles.

Q wave: A downward deflection.

AT A GLANCE Standard Limb Leads

Lead	Positive Electrode	Negative Electrode
I	Left arm	Right arm
II	Left leg	Right arm
III	Left leg	Left arm
MCL1	Right side of sternum, fourth intercostal space	Left arm

Table 21-1

R wave: A large upward spike.

S wave: A downward deflection.

T wave: An upward curve that represents the recovery (or repolarization) of the ventricles.

U wave: A small upward curve sometimes found after the T wave. The U wave represents the slow recovery (or repolarization) of Purkinje fibers, as seen in patients who have low potassium levels in their blood. It occurs between the T wave and the following P wave. A U wave taller than 2 mm is considered abnormal and may suggest hypokalemia or the effects of digoxin or quinidine on the conduction system.

P-R interval: Includes the P wave and the straight line connecting it to the QRS complex. It represents the time it takes for the electrical impulse to travel from the sinoatrial (SA) node, which initiates heart impulses, to the A-V node.

Q-T interval: Includes the QRS complex, S-T segment, and T wave. It represents the time it takes for the ventricles to contract and recover, or repolarize.

S-T segment: Connects the end of the QRS complex with the beginning of the T wave. It represents the time between contraction of the ventricles and recovery.

Asystole: Absence of cardiac electrical activity, represented as a straight (isoelectric) line on the ECG. It is also known as *flatline*.

Code Blue: The term used for an emergency in a hospital or other health-care facility when a person has a cardiac or respiratory arrest.

Cardiac rate: The pulse rate; the number of beats or contractions per minute.

Deflection: Deviation up or down from zero on the isoelectric line.

Refractory period: The period during repolarization when cells cannot respond normally to a second stimulus.

Cardiac output: The amount of blood ejected by the left ventricle into the aorta in one minute.

Amplitude: The height of a waveform on the ECG, showing the degree of voltage variation from zero (the baseline) up or down. It is measured in millimeters and is normally calibrated so that 10 mm represent 1.0 mV.

Pediatric ECG: An ECG for a child is performed with the same lead placement as for an adult. It may be necessary to move the V_3 lead to the right side of the chest. This is known as V_3 right (V_3R). See Figure 21-6.

Troubleshooting

Artifacts: Deflections caused by electrical activity from sources other than the heart. They are irregular and erratic markings caused by poor conduction, outside interference, improper handling of a tracing, a patient's movement (or talking), or dirty sensors. There are several types of artifacts: wandering baseline, flat line, and extraneous marks.

Wandering baseline: A shift in the baseline from the center position for that lead. It may be caused by electrodes that are too tight or loose, dried electrolyte gel, skin that is oily or excessively hairy, lotion on the skin, movement of the cables or patient, or dirty electrodes or cables.

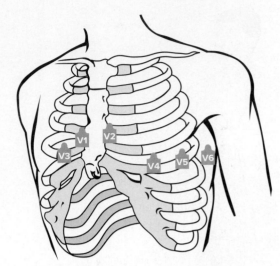

Figure 21-6 *For infants and small children, you may need to place V_3 on the right side of the chest to prevent crowding of the chest electrodes. This alternate method of placement is known as V_3R and is sometimes used on adults.*

Flat line: A flat line on the tracing of one of the leads is typically caused by a loose or disconnected wire. If flat lines occur on more than one lead, two of the wires may have been switched. If flat lines occur on all leads, there are two possible causes: The electrocardiograph unit or the connection to it is faulty, or the patient is in cardiac arrest.

Extraneous marks: Any marks on the paper that are not part of the tracing. The ECG graph paper is sensitive to heat and pressure. It can be easily damaged.

Line control: The ECG machine's stylus creates its line with heat. A higher temperature creates a darker, wider line while a lower temperature creates a lighter, thinner line. The medical assistant must monitor the line created by the stylus to determine if the line control needs to be adjusted.

Interference: The five types of interference that may occur during an ECG are (1) alternating current (AC) interference caused by other types of interference, (2) AC interference due to ground circuits or incorrect grounding, (3) AC interference due to differences in electrical potential, (4) shaking, and (5) zero-line fluctuations.

Interpreting the ECG

Heart rate: Can easily be determined by counting the number of QRS complexes in a six-second strip of the ECG tracing (30 large squares at 25 mm per second) and multiplying by 10.

Heart rhythm: The ECG is the best way to assess heart rhythm and the regularity of the heartbeat. A normal heart rhythm is indicated on the ECG by regularly spaced complexes (repeated intervals, such as between one P wave and the next P wave or between one R wave and the next R wave). The patient's rhythm is usually assessed by viewing the rhythm strip, the ECG tracing from lead II.

Arrhythmia: An irregularity, disturbance, or abnormality in heart rhythm. It is also called a dysrhythmia. Some arrhythmias do not cause problems.

Ectopy: Placement outside the usual location.

Ectopic beat: A beat having an ectopic focus.

Ectopic focus: A site of impulse formation located somewhere other than the SA node.

Bigeminy: A type of arrhythmia in which every other beat is ectopic or premature (or both).

Premature beat or premature contraction: A contraction that occurs early. Premature contractions are of three types: premature atrial contractions (PACs), premature junctional contractions (PJCs), and premature ventricular contractions (PVCs).

Premature ventricular contraction (PVC): Can occur normally in healthy persons with apparently normal hearts. Causes of abnormal PVCs include hypoxia; an increase in catecholamines; stimulants such as alcohol, tobacco, and caffeine; acid-base imbalance; electrolyte imbalance; digitalis toxicity; and drugs such as epinephrine, dopamine, phenothiazines, or isoproterenol. PVCs can cause ischemia, myocardial infarction, or congestive heart failure (CHF).

Acardia: The absence of the heart.

Acardiac rhythm: The absence of cardiac rhythm. It is also called asystole.

Bradyarrhythmia: An abnormally slow and irregular cardiac rhythm; irregular bradycardia.

Bradycardia: A heart rate slower than 60 beats per minute.

Tachyarrhythmia: An abnormally fast and irregular cardiac rhythm; irregular tachycardia.

Tachycardia: A heart rate faster than 100 beats per minute.

Atrial fibrillation: Incomplete, irregular, and rapid contraction of the atria 350–500 times per minute. The ventricular rate also may be rapid, or it may be relatively normal.

Atrial flutter: Contraction of the atria 250–350 beats per minute. The ventricular rate varies.

Ventricular fibrillation: Cessation of coordinated ventricular contraction. Untreated ventricular fibrillation leads to cardiac arrest. On an ECG, it appears as a "sawtooth" image.

Ventricular flutter: Contraction of the ventricles 150–300 times per minute. It is a dangerous rhythm and should be reported immediately.

Sinus rhythm: A heart rhythm established by impulses from the SA node. Irregularities include sinus bradycardia, sinus tachycardia, sinus arrest, and sinus arrhythmia.

Sinus arrest: The failure of the SA node to function. It is also called sinus pause. The complete cardiac complex is absent from the ECG tracing.

Sinus arrhythmia: A usually benign fluctuation of the heart rate occurring within the normal range of 60–100 beats per minute, distinguished by a vagally influenced slowing of the cardiac rate during respiratory expiration and an increase in the cardiac rate during inspiration.

Agonal rhythm: The rhythm of a dying heart, usually ventricular, extremely slow and irregular and becoming slower to the point of asystole. A rate of less than 10 beats per minute is common.

Automated external defibrillator: A machine that produces and sends an electrical shock to the heart, intended to correct the electrical pattern of the heart.

Pacemaker (electronic): A device that delivers a small measured amount of electrical energy to cause myocardial depolarization.

21.3 Other Tests

Holter monitor: A portable (ambulatory) electrocardiography device that includes a small cassette recorder worn around a patient's waist to record the heart's electrical activity during normal daily activities. This test is given over a 24-hour period. The tape is analyzed by a microcomputer in the physician's office or at a reference laboratory.

Exercise electrocardiography: Assessment of the heart's conduction system during physical exertion such as exercise. It is also known as stress testing. The patient is required to walk on a treadmill, pedal a stationary bicycle, or walk on a stair-stepping ergonometer while ECG readings are taken.

Echocardiography: Tests the structure and function of the heart through the use of reflected sound waves, or echoes. The echoes can indicate structural defects and fluid accumulation, among other conditions.

Heart catheterization: A diagnostic method in which a catheter is inserted into a vein or artery in an arm or leg and passed through blood vessels into the heart, so that blood samples may be taken, the pressure in the heart's chambers measured, and/or the heart's motions viewed.

Angiography: The X-ray examination of a blood vessel, after the injection of a contrast medium, to evaluate the function and structure.

Thallium stress test: An invasive type of exercise electrocardiography in which thallium, a radiopaque substance (one that is visible with an X-ray machine), is injected into the body to permit viewing the vessels around the heart.

Telemetry monitoring: The monitoring of the heart's electrical activity over 24–72 hours. Electrodes placed on the skin are connected to a small device that sends information to a remote monitoring station, where problems are assessed before or while they occur.

Cardiac stress test: It is most commonly known as a treadmill stress test because the exercise is usually performed on an exercise treadmill (see Figure 21-7). It is an effective test of diagnosing cardiac disorders. The procedure is performed with a cardiologist or other physician present.

21.4 Other Heart Conditions and Procedures

Cardiodynia: Pain in the heart. It is also called cardialgia.

Cardiomegaly: Enlargement of the heart. Cardiomegaly often occurs during the course of congestive heart failure (CHF).

Cardiorrhexis: Rupture of the heart wall.

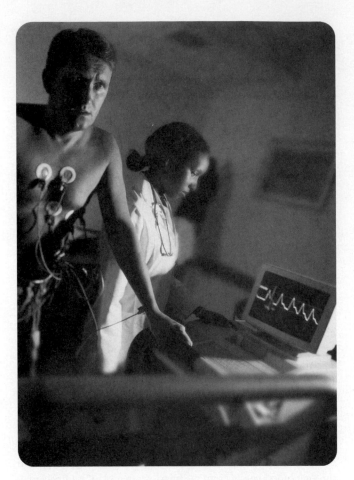

Figure 21-7 *A patient performing a treadmill stress test for a cardiologist.*
© Comstock Images/Picture Quest RF

Dextrocardia: Location of the heart in the right thorax as a result of a congenital defect or displacement by disease.

Cardioptosis: Drooping or falling of the heart at the normal location.

Hypertrophy of the heart: An increase in the size of the heart due to growth of the heart muscle tissue without an increase in the size of the heart chambers.

Heart blocks: Damage to the conduction system of the heart results in abnormal conduction patterns, causing dysrhythmias known as heart blocks. There are four types: first degree; two variants of second degree (Mobitz I and Mobitz II); and third degree, or complete.

Aortic aneurysm: Ballooning of the aorta.

Capture: The successful depolarization of an atrium or ventricle achieved, for example, by an artificial pacemaker.

Cardioversion: The administration of timed electrical shocks for the purpose of correcting certain arrhythmias or restoring normal rhythm, particularly in the ventricular beat.

Cardioplasty: Surgical repair of the heart.

Cardiorrhaphy: The suturing of the heart muscle.

Cardiomyopexy: A surgical procedure in which the blood supply from the nearby pectoral muscles of the chest is diverted directly to the coronary arteries.

STRATEGIES FOR SUCCESS

▶ *Test-Taking Skills*

Come prepared!

Always bring all the supplies you need to the exam. For a paper exam, bring a few number 2 pencils with you and a working eraser. Don't depend on someone else to give these supplies to you. Make sure that you have the CMA or RMA admission card you received after registering for the exam. You also need to bring at least two forms of identification, one of which should have a photo.

CHAPTER 21 REVIEW

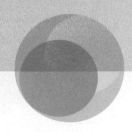

Instructions:

Answer the following questions.

1. The medical term meaning transmission of ECG signals via radio waves is

   A. telepathy.
   B. telemetry.
   C. telediagnosis.
   D. telocentric.
   E. telecardio.

2. On an ECG tracing, an indication of the absence of electrical charge or activity represents

   A. sinoatrial node.
   B. QRS complex.
   C. baseline.
   D. repolarization.
   E. none of these

3. A beat arising from a focus outside the SA node of the heart is known as

   A. ectopic beat.
   B. escape beat.
   C. uncontrolled beat.
   D. fusion beat.
   E. bigeminy.

4. The U wave represents

   A. repolarization of the Purkinje fibers.
   B. depolarization of an atrium.
   C. baseline.
   D. ectopic beat.
   E. contraction of the atria.

5. Which type of lead is lead III?

   A. bipolar lead
   B. unipolar (augmented) lead
   C. precordial lead
   D. intercostal lead
   E. none of these

6. Leads aVR, aVL, and aVF are

   A. standard leads.
   B. limb leads.
   C. intercostal leads.
   D. augmented leads.
   E. limb leads *and* augmented leads.

7. All of the following are causes of artifacts except

   A. a patient's talking.
   B. clean sensors.
   C. outside interference.
   D. poor conduction.
   E. improper handling of a tracing.

8. Augmented leads are also called

   A. standard leads.
   B. bipolar leads.
   C. unipolar leads.
   D. nonstandard leads.
   E. none of these

9. Which of the patient's limbs serves as an electrical ground?

   A. right leg
   B. left leg
   C. right arm
   D. left arm
   E. either arm

10. Which of the following waves on an ECG represent the slow recovery or repolarization of Purkinje fibers?

   A. Q wave
   B. QRS complex
   C. T wave
   D. U wave
   E. P wave

CHAPTER 22

DIAGNOSTIC IMAGING

LEARNING OUTCOMES

22.1 Recall terminology used in relation to diagnostic imaging.

22.2 Identify the different types of diagnostic imaging.

22.3 Identify types of radiation therapy.

22.4 Describe the role of the medical assistant in preparing the patient for diagnostic imaging.

22.5 Describe the proper techniques for safety and storage of radiographic materials.

MEDICAL ASSISTING COMPETENCIES

COMPETENCY	CMA	RMA	CCMA	NCMA
CLINICAL				
Apply principles of aseptic techniques and infection control, including hand washing	X	X	X	X
Practice standard precautions	X	X	X	X
Prepare and maintain examination and treatment areas	X	X	X	X
Prepare the patient for and assist the physician with routine and specialty examinations, treatments, and minor office surgeries	X	X	X	X
Screen and follow up on patient test results	X	X	X	X
GENERAL/LEGAL/PROFESSIONAL				
Be aware of and perform within legal and ethical boundaries	X	X	X	X
Instruct individuals according to their needs	X	X	X	X
Operate and maintain facilities, and perform routine maintenance of administrative and clinical equipment safely	X	X	X	X

22.1 Terminology

Radiology: The study of the uses of radioactive substances for visualizing the internal structures of the body in order to diagnose and treat disease. It is divided into three specialties: diagnostic radiology, radiation therapy, and nuclear medicine.

X-ray: An electromagnetic wave with a high energy level and short wavelength that can penetrate solid objects. X-rays can be used in diagnosis and therapy.

Digital X-ray: A form of X-ray imaging in which digital X-ray sensors are used instead of traditional photographic film. They reduce processing time and also require less radiation to produce images.

Magnetism: The ability of certain materials to attract iron and other metals.

Radioactive: Capable of emitting radiant energy; or giving off radiation as the result of the disintegration of the nucleus of an atom.

Nuclear energy: Energy produced by fission of an atomic nucleus.

Radiopaque: Refers to something that does not permit the passage of X-rays. Bones are relatively radiopaque.

Contrast media: Radiopaque substances used in radiography to permit visualization of internal structures.

- Contrast media include liquids, powders, and gases. They are administered orally, parenterally, and rectally.

- A positive contrast medium is more dense than the surrounding tissue. Barium sulfate and iodine are positive contrast media.

- A negative contrast medium is less dense than the surrounding area in the body. Air is a negative contrast medium.

Adverse effects of contrast media: Oral agents may cause skin rash, vomiting, diarrhea, abdominal pain, or constipation. IV agents can cause urticaria (rash), skin reddening, anaphylaxis, or death. Some individuals have allergies to iodine.

X-ray film: A special material with a sensitive emulsion layer that reacts when it is exposed to radiation and thereby produces an image. Single-emulsion film is used to create images of the extremities and the breasts.

Radiograph: An image recorded on film that has been exposed. An older term for radiograph is roentgenogram, named after the discoverer of X-rays, Wilhelm Conrad Roentgen.

Film fog: An unwanted increase in the density of the emulsion either before or after exposure to radiation. Heat, light, chemicals, and extraneous radiation can produce fogging, which appears as darkened areas on the finished radiograph.

Artifacts: Extraneous marks and areas of increased or decreased density on film. Artifacts interfere with the diagnostic value of the radiograph.

Cassette: A light-proof container that holds X-ray film and serves to intensify the image.

Contrast: The visible difference between any two areas of radiographic density.

Roentgen: A unit used to measure X-ray dosage in air.

Rem: A unit used to measure X-ray dosage in human beings. It is an abbreviation of *Roentgen equivalent (in) man.*

Rad: A unit used to measure the actual absorbed dose of radiation.

Ionization: The process by which an atom becomes ionized (gains or loses electrons).

Ionizing radiation: Radiation that causes ionization in the tissues that absorb it.

Scan: An image produced on film by a sweeping beam of radiation.

Isotopes: Variants of a single chemical element that have different atomic weights and different charges.

X-ray machine: Has four basic parts: table, control panel, X-ray tube, and high-voltage generator. The table is usually adjustable. The most important part of the machine is the tube.

Invasive procedure: Some radiological tests are invasive in that they require a radiologist to insert a catheter, wire, or other testing device into a patient's blood vessel or organ through the skin or body orifice. All invasive procedures require surgical aseptic technique.

Noninvasive procedure: A radiological test that does not require the insertion of devices or the breaking of skin. Examples include standard X-rays and ultrasonography.

Frequency: The repetition rate of electromagnetic radiation, measured in Hertz.

22.2 Types of Diagnostic Imaging

Diagnostic radiology: The use of X-ray technology for diagnostic purposes. It also includes the use of magnetic resonance imaging (MRI), ultrasound, computed tomography (CT), and nuclear medicine technologies, such as positron emission tomography (PET), among others. Table 22-1 provides a list of common radiological tests and the disorders these tests are used to diagnose or treat.

Magnetic resonance imaging (MRI): A noninvasive diagnostic modality allowing visualization of anatomic structures without using radioactive X-rays. It is contraindicated in patients with pacemakers or metallic prostheses.

Ultrasound: Directs high-frequency sound waves through the skin and produces an image based on the echoes. Ultrasound has many medical applications, including fetal monitoring, imaging of internal organs, and color imaging of blood vessels.

Tomography: Also called sectional imaging and body-section radiography. It allows the visualization of an organ or the body in cross section.

AT A GLANCE   Common Radiologic Tests and Disorders Diagnosed

Test	Disorders Diagnosed/Treated
Angiography Cardiovascular	Status of blood flow, collateral circulation, malformed vessels, aneurysm, narrowing or blockages of vessels, presence of hemorrhage
Cerebral	Aneurysm, hemorrhage, evidence of cerebrovascular accident, arteriosclerosis
Gastrointestinal (GI)	Upper GI bleeding
Pulmonary	Pulmonary emboli (especially when lung scan is inconclusive), evaluation of pulmonary circulation in some heart conditions before surgery
Renal	Abnormalities of blood vessels in urinary system
Arthrography	Joint conditions
Barium enema (lower GI series)	Obstructions, ulcers, polyps, diverticulosis, tumor, and motility problems of colon or rectum
Barium swallow (upper GI series)	Obstructions, ulcers, polyps, diverticulosis, tumor, and motility problems of esophagus, stomach, duodenum, and small intestine
Cholangiography, cholecystography	Gallstones, gallbladder, or common bile duct stones or obstructions, ability of gallbladder to concentrate and store dye
Computed tomography (CT) scan	Aortic and heart aneurysms, disorders of liver and biliary systems, renal and pulmonary tumors, brain abnormalities (tumors, blood clots, evidence of cerebrovascular accident, outlines of brain ventricles), GI tract lesions, GI disorders (acute pseudocyst of pancreas, abdominal abscesses, biliary obstruction), breast diseases and disorders, spinal disorders; to guide biopsy procedures
Fluoroscopy	Structure, process, and function of organs in motion to detect abnormalities
Intravenous pyelography (IVP) (excretory urography)	Urinary system abnormalities, including renal pelvis, ureters, and bladder (e.g., kidney stones); abnormal size, shape, or structure of kidneys, ureters, or bladder; space-occupying lesions; pyelonephrosis; hydronephrosis; trauma to the urinary system
KUB (*k*idneys, *u*reters, *b*ladder) radiography	Size, shape, and position of urinary organs; urinary system diseases or disorders; kidney stones
Magnetic resonance imaging (MRI)	Cancerous tissue, atherosclerotic tissue, blood clots, tumors, and deformities, particularly of the heart valves, brain, spine, and joints

Table 22-1

Test	Disorders Diagnosed/Treated
Mammography	Breast tumors and lesions
Myelography	Irregularities or compression of spinal cord
Nuclear medicine (radionuclide imaging)	Abnormal function (defects), lesions, or disorders of bone, brain, lungs, kidneys, liver, pancreas, thyroid, and spleen
Positron emission tomography (PET) scan	Brain-related conditions, such as epilepsy and Parkinson's disease
Radiation therapy	Treatment of cancer
Retrograde pyelogram	Obstruction of ureters, bladder, or urethra (including tumors, stones, strictures, or blood clots); perinephritic abscess
Stereoscopy	Fractures, dense areas that indicate a tumor or increased pressure within the skull
Thermography	Breast tumors, breast abscesses, fibrocystic breast disease
Ultrasound	Abnormalities of gallbladder, liver, spleen, heart, kidneys, gonads, blood vessels, and lymph system; fetal conditions (including number of fetuses, age and sex of fetus, fetal development, position, and deformities)
Xeroradiography	Breast cancer, abscesses, lesions, calcifications

Table 22-1, concluded

Computed tomography (CT) scan: A radiographic technique that shows a detailed, 360-degree cross section of tissue structure. It is a painless procedure.

Nuclear medicine: A branch of medicine that uses radionuclides in the diagnosis and treatment of disorders.

Radionuclide: A chemical substance (isotope) that exhibits radioactivity. A gamma camera is used to pick up its radioactive signals as it gathers in organs or tissues.

Positron emission tomography (PET): Involves the injection of isotopes combined with other substances, such as glucose. Positrons are emitted and are processed by a computer and displayed on a screen. It is useful for diagnosis of brain-related conditions, such as epilepsy and Parkinson's disease.

Angiography: X-ray visualization of blood vessels after the intravascular introduction of contrast media.

Arthrography: Used for joint conditions. It requires a contrast medium. Arthrography is performed by a radiologist and is usually done for knee, shoulder, or hip injuries. It also requires a local anesthetic.

Barium enema: The rectal infusion of barium sulfate (a radiopaque contrast medium), which is retained in the lower intestinal tract during X-ray studies. It is also called a contrast enema. The digestive tract must be totally empty for this procedure. Patients should thoroughly cleanse their digestive tract with a series of preparatory steps, including having nothing by mouth for eight hours before the test except for one cup of clear liquid on the morning of the test.

Barium meal, or barium swallow: The ingestion of barium sulfate. It is used for the radiographic examination of the esophagus, stomach, and intestinal tract. Before the test, the patient should have nothing to eat or drink for 12 hours.

Cholecystography: Radiological study of the gallbladder, not as frequently done as in the past. The preceding evening meal must be low fat, and an oral contrast medium is taken 12–15 hours before the procedure. The exam takes about 15 minutes.

Cholangiography: Similar to cholecystography and performed by a radiologist. The contrast medium is injected directly into the common bile duct (during gallbladder surgery).

Cystography: The radiographic examination of the urinary bladder after introduction of a radiopaque contrast medium.

Fluoroscopy: Radiological study, performed by a radiologist, that allows both structural and functional visualization of internal body structures directly on a screen. A contrast medium is needed. It is also called radioscopy.

Intravenous pyelography (IVP): Radiological study of the urinary system in which a series of X-rays is taken after a contrast medium has been injected into a vein. It is also known as excretory urography.

Mammography: Radiological study of the breast. It is used for the early diagnosis of breast cancer. The American Cancer Society recommends a baseline mammography at the age of 40 for all women. After age 40, women are urged to have a mammography every one–two years.

Hysterosalpingography: A special X-ray procedure that utilizes a contrast dye to examine the uterus and fallopian tubes.

Myelography: An X-ray study of the spinal cord, which produces a *myelogram*. The radiologist performs a lumbar puncture, removes some cerebrospinal fluid, and injects some radiopaque, water-soluble contrast medium. It is seldom used today, as tomography and MRI have largely replaced it.

Retrograde pyelography: Similar to IVP, except that the radiologist injects the contrast medium through a urethral catheter and takes a series of X-rays.

Sialography: Radiological study of the salivary gland duct. The patient sucks on a lemon wedge to open the duct. A catheter is inserted into the duct, and a contrast medium is introduced. The exam takes about one–two hours.

Stereoscopy: A rarely used X-ray procedure to study (primarily) the skull.

Thermography: A heat-sensing technique used for the detection of tumors. An infrared camera is used, which records variation in skin temperature. Warm areas appear light, and cool areas appear dark. Tomography is able to view a cross section of an organ.

Xeroradiography: A diagnostic X-ray technique in which an image is produced electrically rather than chemically. It permits shorter exposure times and lower radiation levels than ordinary X-rays. It is also called xerography. Xeroradiography is used primarily for mammography.

22.3 Therapeutic Uses of Radiation

Radiation therapy: The use of radiation to treat diseases such as cancer by preventing cellular reproduction.

Teletherapy: Radiation therapy administered by a machine that is positioned at some distance from the patient. Teletherapy permits deeper penetration and is used primarily for deep tumors. It is done on an outpatient basis.

Brachytherapy: The implanting of radioactive sources into localized tumor tissues that are to be treated for a specific period of time.

Radioiodine: A radioactive isotope of iodine used in nuclear medicine and radiotherapy. It is used especially in the treatment of some thyroid conditions.

22.4 Medical Assistant's Role

Extent of participation by the medical assistant: Varies by state. The responsibilities of the medical assistant may involve simply assisting the radiological technologist or radiologist, or they may involve operating certain X-ray equipment.

Timing of procedures: Procedures that require the patient to fast, such as barium enemas, are best scheduled in the morning, so that the patient sleeps through most of the period during which the digestive tract is empty.

Preprocedure care: Involves providing preparation instructions, such as diet restrictions or requirements; explaining the procedure to the patient; obtaining a medication history and other information from the patient; and instructing the patient to remove clothing, jewelry, and any other metals and to put on a gown.

Preparation for arthrography: Ask patients about possible allergies to contrast media, iodine, or shellfish. No other special preprocedure preparations are necessary.

Preparation for barium enema or IVP: Ask the patient about possible allergies to contrast media, iodine, or shellfish. The patient should follow an all-liquid diet starting the morning before the procedure and should take a prescribed amount of electrolyte solution or other laxative on a specified schedule. The patient may have one cup of coffee, tea, or water on the morning of the barium enema but should have no food or liquids after midnight before the IVP.

Preparation for cholecystography: Ask the patient about possible allergies to contrast media, iodine, or shellfish. The patient should eat a fat-free dinner the evening before the examination and should not smoke or have any foods or liquids after midnight. The oral contrast medium should be taken about two hours after dinner; tablets should be taken five minutes apart.

Preparation for tomography or CT scan: Ask the patient about possible allergies to contrast media, iodine, or shellfish. The patient must lie still while the scans are taken. For a CT scan, the patient may breathe normally, but it is necessary for the patient to hold his or her breath for a tomogram.

Preparation for MRI: If a contrast medium will be used, ask the patient about possible allergies to contrast media, iodine, or shellfish. Ask whether any internal metallic materials are present, such as a pacemaker, clips, shunts, heart valves, or slivers or chips from working with metal. Patients should avoid caffeine for four hours before the examination, and they should not wear eye makeup during the procedure.

Preparation for mammography: Avoiding caffeine 7–10 days prior to the procedure will reduce the possibility of swelling and soreness that will heighten discomfort. The patient should not use deodorant, powder, lotion, or perfume on the underarm area or breasts before the examination.

Positions: Patients need to be positioned in different ways, depending on the specific body part being X-rayed. The most common positions for taking X-rays are anteroposterior, posteroanterior, oblique, and lateral. See Figure 22-1.

Projections: A radiographic projection indicates relative body part positions to be X-rayed, along with location of the X-ray film and placement of the X-ray tube.

Frontal projection: The coronal plane of the body part or entire body is parallel to the film plane; the central ray is perpendicular to both. It is named either *anteroposterior* (supine, or facing the X-ray tube) or *posteroanterior* (prone, or facing the film).

Lateral projection: The sagittal plane is parallel to the film; named for the side of the patient closest to the film (left or right).

Oblique projection: The projection is neither frontal or lateral; this type is also named left or right.

Axial projection: The beam is projected at an angle, either cephalad (toward the head) or caudad (away from the head); also known as a *semiaxial projection*.

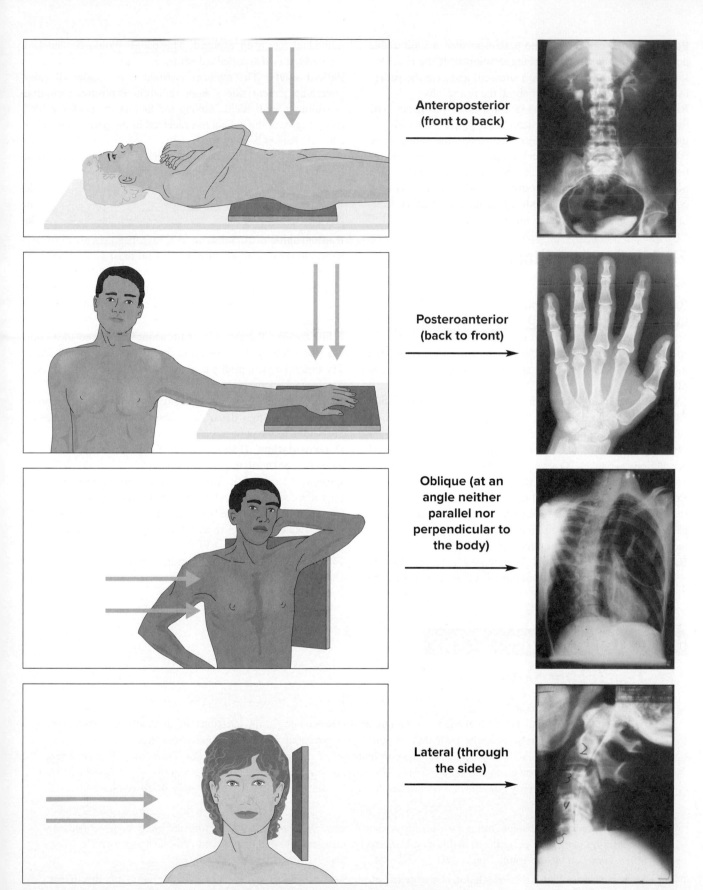

Figure 22-1 *Pathways and resulting projections for the most common types of X-rays.*
Photos: © Martin M. Rotker

Anteroposterior (front to back)

Posteroanterior (back to front)

Oblique (at an angle neither parallel nor perpendicular to the body)

Lateral (through the side)

Postprocedure care: Have the patient assume a comfortable position while the films are being developed. If the films are satisfactory, have the patient get dressed, and give the patient information on how to find out about the test results.

Radiographic equipment: This consists of the X-ray tube (where X-rays are formed), a lead-lined protective housing, a tube support (a ceiling mount or tube stand), the radiographic table (on which the patient lies), a *bucky* (moving grid device beneath the table surface), an upright cassette holder (that positions the X-ray film in an upright position), and a control console (inside the control booth, where the radiographer determines exposure factors to take the X-ray image).

22.5 Safety and Storage

Safety

Radiosensitivity: The susceptibility of cells, tissues, or any living substances to the effects of radiation; also, a biological organism's measure of response to radiation. Immature, non-specialized cells and cells that are growing rapidly are the most radiosensitive; mature, specialized cells are the most radioresistant.

Exposure: Exposure to radiation is cumulative, meaning that it adds up to a total dosage over the years. The amount of exposure is measured in units called roentgens.

Overexposure: Not likely from routine X-rays, especially if precautions are taken. Overexposure to radiation can produce a variety of symptoms, including nausea, fatigue, and bleeding.

Personnel safety: All medical personnel who work in facilities that perform radiological tests should wear radiation exposure badges, make sure that equipment is in good working order, and wear a lead shield when equipment is operating.

Radiation exposure badge: A sensitized piece of film, in a holder, that indicates the amount of radiation to which the individual has been exposed. The badge should be checked regularly. It is also called a dosimeter.

Patient safety: The medical assistant must follow all rules governing patient safety from radiation exposure, including providing a lead shield. Among the factors to check are how much exposure the patient has received in the past and whether a female patient is pregnant.

Absorbed dose: The amount of radiation energy absorbed in tissue.

Storage

Radiographic film: Sensitive to X-rays, heat, chemical fumes, light, moisture, and pressure. Fresh film must be kept on hand at all times. It must be properly stored and carefully handled.

Sensitometry: The measurement or study of how radiographic film responds chemically to radiation exposure and to processing conditions.

Film storage: Radiographic film should be stored in a cool, dry place. The best temperature for film storage is 60°–70°F. The best relative humidity is 40%–60%. Store packages on end; do not stack them on top of each other.

Ownership of radiographs: X-ray radiographs are the property of the radiology department where they are taken. They do not belong to the patient.

Documentation: Document the X-ray information on the patient record card or in the record book.

Labeling: Verify that film is labeled with the referring doctor's name, the date, and the patient's name. It is also critical to double-check that the film is labeled correctly with the right and left sides, in order to avoid improper diagnoses and other negative outcomes.

Filing: Place the processed film in a film-filing envelope, and file the envelope in the correct place in the filing cabinet.

STRATEGIES FOR SUCCESS

▶ *Test-Taking Skills*

If you must guess, guess!

You should know the material well enough to avoid having to guess on any of the questions. Realistically, however, there will be at least a few questions on the exam that you will be unsure about. When you come across these questions, try to make an educated guess at the correct answer and eliminate any of the answers that you know are wrong. Here are a few tips that will also help you eliminate some answers. However, before you apply them to every question you come across, remember that they are only guidelines, not hard and fast rules, so use them sparingly and only when you have no other option.

- Answers containing absolute terms such as *always, never, none, only, no one,* and *everyone* are often incorrect because most things cannot be generalized in this way. Conversely, answers that contain relative words such as *generally, most, often, some,* and *usually* are often correct.

- If the answer calls for the completion of a sentence, eliminate the answers that would not form grammatically correct sentences.

- The longest, most complete answer is often correct.

- If two answers are similar except for one or two words, one of these answers is usually the correct one.

Instructions:

Answer the following questions.

1. An image produced on film by a sweeping beam of radiation is known as
   A. MRI.
   B. cassette.
   C. radioactive.
   D. isotopes.
   E. scan.

2. The study of the gallbladder by X-ray with an oral contrast medium is called
   A. cholecystosonography.
   B. cholecystitis.
   C. cholecystokinin.
   D. cholecystography.
   E. cholangiography.

3. Radiation therapy for deeper tumors done on an outpatient basis is known as
   A. brachytherapy.
   B. cryotherapy.
   C. thermotherapy.
   D. teletherapy.
   E. xeroradiography.

4. Film artifacts are
   A. areas that interfere with the diagnostic value of the radiograph.
   B. desirable.
   C. films that are beyond their expiration dates.
   D. diagnostic areas of interest.
   E. none of these

5. A type of diagnostic radiology that uses high-frequency sound waves is
   A. magnetic resonance imaging.
   B. X-ray.
   C. tomography.
   D. arthrography.
   E. ultrasound.

6. The front-to-back position in radiology is known as
   A. posteroanterior.
   B. lateral.
   C. anteroposterior.
   D. oblique.
   E. supine.

7. In preparing patients for such tests as barium enemas and CT scans, the medical assistant should
   A. tell them that they will have to hold their breath.
   B. tell them to eat a fat-free dinner the night before.
   C. ask them whether internal metals are present.
   D. ask them whether they are allergic to contrast media, iodine, or shellfish.
   E. ask them whether they are wearing body lotion.

8. Which of the following is used in the patient's mouth for a sialography in order to open the salivary duct?
   A. an orange
   B. a grapefruit
   C. a lemon
   D. a grape
   E. none of these

9. Xeroradiography is useful to diagnose which of the following disorders?
   A. breast cancer
   B. compression of the spinal cord
   C. brain tumor
   D. skull fracture
   E. kidney stone

10. Which of the following types of radiology involves the injection of isotopes combined with glucose?
    A. ultrasound
    B. computed tomography
    C. positron emission tomography
    D. magnetic resonance imaging
    E. xeroradiography

PHYSICAL THERAPY

LEARNING OUTCOMES

23.1 Recall terminology used in relation to physical therapy.

23.2 Identify assessment techniques used in physical therapy.

23.3 Describe therapeutic treatments used in physical therapy.

23.4 Demonstrate the ability to educate the patient about the proper use of mobility-assisting devices.

MEDICAL ASSISTING COMPETENCIES

COMPETENCY	CMA	RMA	CCMA	NCMA
Clinical				
Apply principles of aseptic techniques and infection control, including hand washing	X	X	X	X
Practice standard precautions	X	X	X	X
Prepare and maintain examination and treatment areas	X	X	X	X
Prepare the patient for and assist the physician with routine and specialty examinations, treatments, and minor office surgeries	X	X	X	X
Screen and follow up on patient test results	X	X	X	X

MEDICAL ASSISTING COMPETENCIES (cont.)

General/Legal/Professional

Recognize and respond to verbal and nonverbal communications by being attentive and adapting communication to the recipient's level of understanding	X	X	X	X
Be aware of and perform within legal and ethical boundaries	X	X	X	X
Determine the needs for documentation and reporting, and document accurately and appropriately	X	X	X	X
Instruct individuals according to their needs	X	X	X	X
Provide patients with methods of health promotion and disease prevention	X	X	X	X
Be a "team player"	X	X	X	
Conduct work within scope of education, training, and ability	X	X	X	X

STRATEGIES FOR SUCCESS

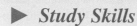

▶ Study Skills

Practice repetition! Practice repetition!
One of the most common ways to remember something is to repeat it often. If you have trouble remembering certain material, use any or all of these strategies: (1) Review your notes on the subject; try reading them aloud to yourself. (2) Create flash cards and test yourself often. (3) Write out summary sheets of the most important terms and concepts you want to remember. The very acts of reading silently, reciting aloud, and writing something over and over again will help you remember it when it's time for the exam.

23.1 Terminology

Physical medicine: The branch of medicine that uses physical devices or agents therapeutically for the diagnosis, treatment, management, and prevention of diseases. It is also called physiatry.

Rehabilitation: Restoration of those functions that have been affected by a patient's injuries or disease.

Sports medicine: The branch of medicine that specializes in the prevention and treatment of injuries caused by athletic participation. More than 2.6 million children alone are treated for sports injuries each year in the United States. Most sports injuries involve muscle strains, sprains, and tears. Sports medicine uses a number of different modalities that enable the patient to recover quickly and return to high levels of activity with minimal loss of fitness. [Source: http://www.niams.nih.gov (search for "child sports injuries").]

Body mechanics: The study of the action of muscles in producing motion or posture of the body.

Physiatrist: A physician specializing in physical medicine and rehabilitation.

Fitness: Overall good physical condition, including cardiovascular strength, muscular strength, and flexibility.

Range of motion (ROM): The degree to which a joint is able to move, measured in degrees with a protractor-like device called a goniometer.

Flexion: The bending movement allowed by certain joints of the skeleton, such as the elbow, that decreases the angle between the two adjoining bones.

Extension: The straightening movement allowed by certain joints of the skeleton, such as the knee, that increases the angle between the two adjoining bones.

Hyperextension: The position of maximum extension, or the extension of a body part beyond its normal limits.

Reduction: The correction of a fracture, dislocation, or hernia.

Lordosis (swayback): Exaggerated anterior curvature of the lumbar spine.

Kyphosis: Abnormally increased convex curvature of the thoracic spine. It is also colloquially called hunchback or humpback.

Scoliosis: Lateral deviation in the normal vertical curve of the spine.

Osteoporosis: A reduction in the mass of bone per unit of volume that interferes with the mechanical support function of bone, causing bone fractures in situations that would not normally damage the skeleton.

Luxation: Complete dislocation of the bone from the joint.

Subluxation: Incomplete dislocation of the bone from the joint.

Tendonitis: Inflammation of tendons. Tendonitis is one of the most common causes of acute pain in the shoulder.

Quadriplegia: Paralysis of all four extremities of the body and the trunk. This disorder is usually caused by spinal cord injury, especially in the area of the fifth to the seventh cervical vertebrae. Automobile accidents and sporting mishaps are common causes.

Paraplegia: Paralysis of the lower portion of the body, usually caused by spinal cord injury or disease. Paraplegia commonly results from automobile and motorcycle accidents, sporting accidents, falls, and gunshot wounds.

Hemiplegia: Paralysis of one side of the body. The three types of hemiplegia are cerebral, facial, and spastic.

Hemiparesis: Muscular weakness of one half of the body.

Cerebral palsy: Nonprogressive paralysis due to defects in or trauma to the brain, especially at birth. Spastic cerebral palsy is characterized by hyperactive reflexes, rapid muscle contraction, muscle weakness, and underdevelopment of the limbs. Mental retardation, seizure disorders, and impaired speech are also common with this condition. Treatment may include the use of braces, adaptive appliances, and ROM exercises.

23.2 Patient Assessment

Gait: A style of walking. A normal gait consists of two phases: stance and swing. Generally, a physician or physical therapist assesses a patient's gait. The patient is asked to walk away, turn around, and walk back. Assessment includes an appraisal of the patient's length of stride, balance, coordination, direction of knees (inward or outward), and direction of feet (inward or outward).

Goniometry: The measurement of joint mobility. Goniometric tests are noninvasive. The movements measured by goniometry are explained in Table 23-1.

Goniometer: A device used to measure the degree of joint movement. See Figure 23-1.

Using a goniometer: The medical assistant may be asked to assist with or perform goniometry. Have the patient move each body part in a specified manner, and position the goniometer to measure degrees of movement.

Muscle testing: Consists of ROM tests (with a goniometer), strength tests, and task skill tests.

Muscle strength testing: Determines the amount of muscle force. This test is usually done from head to foot, usually in combination with ROM testing. The patient is asked to resist pressure that the physician or medical assistant applies to each muscle or group of muscles. Strength is rated according to a five-point scale, as shown in Table 23-2.

Posture testing: The physician looks at the patient's spinal curve from the sides, back, and front; notes the symmetry of alignment of the shoulders, knees, and hips; assesses alignment and degree of straightness as the patient bends at the waist; and assesses knee position by having the patient stand with both feet together.

Electromyography (EMG): A process of electrically recording muscle action potentials. The patient may receive sedation before this test because the electric current can be painful. Abnormal EMG test results can indicate a congenital or an acquired disease condition of the muscles.

23.3 Treatment

Physical therapy: The treatment of disorders with physical agents and methods such as massage, manipulation, therapeutic exercise, cold, heat, hydrotherapy, and electrical stimulation. Physical therapy includes rehabilitative treatment to restore function after an illness or an injury. It is also called physiotherapy.

Thermotherapy

Thermotherapy: The treatment of disease by the application of heat. Thermotherapy is used to relieve pain, to relax spasms of muscles, to relieve localized swelling, to increase tissue metabolism and repair, and to increase drainage from an infected area. Heat therapy should not be used on pregnant or menstruating women, and it also should not be used longer than ordered by the physician. Thermotherapy should not be used longer than 30 minutes.

Types of heat therapy: The main types are dry heat, moist heat, and diathermy.

Dry heat therapy: Includes the use of heating pads, hot-water bottles, chemical hot packs, heat lamps, and fluidotherapy.

Heating pad: A therapeutic warming pad that contains a heating element powered by electricity, usually with several temperature settings. The patient lies on a towel or pillowcase, which is placed over the pad.

Hot-water bottle: A rubber or plastic bottle filled with hot water, and used for therapeutic warmth. Fill the bottle halfway, and expel the air. Cover the bottle with a cloth or pillowcase before applying.

Chemical hot pack: A disposable, flexible pack of chemicals that becomes hot when activated (kneaded or slapped). After activating the pack, cover it with a cloth and place it on the patient's skin in the area being treated.

Heat lamp: Uses an infrared or ultraviolet bulb. Place the lamp two–four feet from the area being treated. Treatment usually lasts 20–30 minutes.

Infrared therapy: Treatment by exposure to various wavelengths of infrared radiation. Infrared treatment is performed to relieve pain and to stimulate blood circulation.

Ultraviolet therapy: Used in the treatment of rickets and certain skin conditions such as psoriasis.

- This therapy is also useful in the control of infectious airborne bacteria and viruses. Ultraviolet ray lamp treatments must be carefully controlled because they can cause severe sunburn and even second- or third-degree burns.

- The time and the distance of the lamp from the patient must be controlled. Treatment is prescribed by the second, for example, 10–20 seconds of exposure.

- The patient should cover his or her eyes with dark goggles.

Fluidotherapy: A relatively new technique in which the patient places the hand or foot in a container of glass beads that are heated and agitated with hot air.

Term	Description	Example
Abduction	Movement away from the midline of the body or away from the axis of a limb	Raising an arm straight out to the side
Adduction	Movement toward the midline of the body or toward the axis of a limb	Lowering a raised arm to the side
Circumduction	Circular movement of a body part	Performing arm circles
Dorsiflexion	Upward or backward movement of a body part	Flexing a foot so that the toes point upward
Eversion	Outward movement of a body part	Moving an ankle so that the sole of the foot turns outward
Extension	Movement that spreads two body parts or that opens a joint	Straightening a leg by unbending the knee
Flexion	Movement that brings together two body parts or that closes a joint	Bending a leg at the knee
Inversion	Inward movement of a body part	Moving an ankle so that the sole of the foot turns inward
Plantar flexion	Downward movement of a body part	Flexing a foot so that the toes point downward
Pronation	Twisting movement that brings a palm facing downward	Turning a wrist so that the palm faces downward
Rotation	Movement of a body part around its axis	Turning the head from side to side
Supination	Twisting movement that brings a palm facing upward	Turning a wrist so that the palm faces upward

Table 23-1

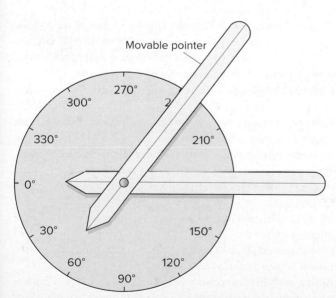

Figure 23-1 *A universal goniometer is a protractor with a movable pointer that measures degrees of joint movement.*

Moist heat therapy: There are several types of moist heat applications, including hot soaks, hot compresses, hot packs, and paraffin baths.

Hydroculator: The device used to keep moist/wet packs at a constant temperature.

Hot soak: Often used on arms or legs. The patient places the body part being treated in a container of plain or medicated water heated to not more than 110°F. A hot soak should last about 15 minutes.

Hot compress: Soak the gauze or cloth in hot water, wring it out, and apply it to the area being treated. Either place a hot-water bottle on top of it or frequently rewarm the compress in hot water.

Hot pack: A moist, hot pack is covered with a towel and placed over the area being treated.

Paraffin bath: Utilizes a receptacle of heated wax and mineral oil to reduce pain, muscle spasms, and stiffness in patients with arthritis. A thick coat of wax remains on the area for about 30 minutes and then is peeled off.

Diathermy: The production of heat in body tissues for therapeutic purposes by high-frequency currents that are

Muscle Response	Rating	Meaning
No response	0	Paralysis
Slight contraction felt	1	Severe weakness
Passive ROM when resistance is removed	2	Moderate weakness
Active ROM against gravity or light resistance	3 or 4	Mild weakness
Active ROM against heavy resistance	5	Normal strength

Table 23-2

insufficiently intense to destroy tissues. Diathermy is useful in treating muscular disorders, tendonitis, arthritis, and bursitis. Diathermy cannot be used in patients with metal implants, such as hip replacements, because of the electrical field it creates and the consequent danger of burns. Patients must remove all metal jewelry and buckles before treatment, which usually lasts 15–30 minutes. There are three basic methods of diathermy: ultrasound, microwave, and shortwave.

Ultrasound: Projects high-frequency sound waves that are converted to heat in muscle tissue. The most common type of diathermy, it is administered by rubbing a gel-covered transducer over the skin in circular patterns. It is used to treat sprains, strains, and other acute ailments. Ultrasound treatments should not be used in areas where bones are near the skin's surface.

Microwave: Electromagnetic radiation that is converted into heat in tissues. It should not be used on patients with pacemakers, in combination with wet dressings, or near metal implants.

Shortwave: Provides heat deep in the body by means of radio waves that travel between two condenser plates. It is used to treat chronic arthritis, bursitis, sinusitis, and other conditions.

Cryotherapy

Cryotherapy: Treatment using dry-cold or wet-cold applications to:

- Prevent swelling by limiting fluid accumulation in body tissue
- Control bleeding by constricting blood vessels
- Reduce inflammation by slowing blood and fluid movement
- Provide an anesthetic effect by reducing inflammation
- Reduce pus formation by inhibiting microorganisms
- Lower body temperature

For best results, cryotherapy should be used frequently, for example, about 20 minutes every hour for acute conditions or injuries (during the first 48 hours).

Dry-cold applications: Ice bags (or ice collars) and chemical ice packs.

Ice bag or ice collar: Place ice chips or small ice cubes in the device, filling it two-thirds full; compress the container to expel air; dry the container; and cover it with a towel to absorb moisture. Ice bags are used to prevent edema immediately after an injury.

Chemical ice pack: A flat plastic bag containing semifluid chemicals. Most chemical ice packs remain cold 30–60 minutes. Check the pack for leaks, and shake or squeeze it to activate the chemicals. Cover the pack with a towel.

Wet-cold applications: Cold compresses and ice massage.

Cold compress: Place large ice cubes and a small amount of water in a basin. Place a washcloth or gauze square in the basin to moisten it, wring it out, and apply it to the area being treated.

Ice massage: Wrap an ice cube in a plastic bag, or freeze water in a paper cup, then use the device to massage the area.

Other Therapy

Hydrotherapy: The use of water in the treatment of various disorders. Hydrotherapy may include continuous tub baths, wet sheet packs, or shower sprays.

Whirlpool: A tank in which water is agitated by jets of air under pressure, used to relax muscles and to increase circulation. Also used to cleanse and debride the skin of patients with wounds, ulcers, or burns.

Contrast bath: Two baths, one filled with hot water and the other with cold water. The patient quickly moves the affected body part from one to the other. It is used to induce relaxation, stimulate circulation, and improve mobility.

Underwater exercises: Generally performed in a warm swimming pool by patients with joint injuries, burns, and arthritis.

Exercise therapy: A technique for helping patients prevent deformities, regain body movement, improve muscle strength, stimulate circulation, retain neuromuscular coordination, and resume normal daily activities. Therapeutic exercises are ordered by the physician after complete evaluation of the physical problem.

Medical assistant's role in exercise therapy: To provide information for the patient and family, to provide support and encouragement, to assist with ROM exercises, and to teach the patient how to perform them at home.

Active mobility exercises: Self-directed exercises a patient performs without assistance to increase muscle strength and function. They may require such equipment as a stationary bicycle or treadmill.

Passive mobility exercises: Used for patients with neuromuscular disabilities or weaknesses. The physical therapist or a machine moves the body part.

Aided mobility exercises: Self-directed exercises performed with the help of such devices as exercise machines or therapy pools.

Active resistance exercises: The patient works against resistance, which is provided by a therapist or by an exercise machine, to increase muscle strength.

ROM exercises: Exercises that slowly move each joint through its full range of motion. They may be active (performed by the patient without assistance) or passive (performed with the help of another person or a machine). Typical ROM exercises are shoulder abduction, back rotation, hip flexion, and toe abduction.

Electrical stimulation: The delivery of controlled amounts of low-voltage electric current to motor and sensory nerves to stimulate muscles. It is used to help retrain a patient to use injured muscles.

Massage: The application of pressure with the hands on the soft tissue of the body through stroking, rubbing, kneading, or tapping, in order to increase circulation, improve muscle tone, and relax the patient. It is one of the oldest known methods for promoting healing. The most common sites for massage are the back, knees, elbows, and heels. Stroking is the most common massage modality used in the medical office.

Immobilization: The restriction of movement of a body part in order to promote healing. Devices such as splints and slings are prescribed by the physician and used by the physical therapist to immobilize damaged tissues and bones.

Manipulation: The application of rapid thrusting motions in order to stabilize, stretch, or reposition a joint.

Traction: The process of pulling or stretching a part of the body. It is applied by a physical therapist to create proper bone alignment, reduce joint stiffening and abnormal muscle shortening, correct deformities, relieve compression of vertebral joints, and reduce or relieve muscle spasms.

Chiropractic: An alternative therapy in which the hands or tools are used to manipulate the spinal vertebrae to relieve disruptions in nerve transmission and musculoskeletal pain.

Acupuncture: An alternative therapy in which needles are inserted in specific points on the body to manipulate the flow of energy and relieve pain.

Acupressure: An alternative therapy in which manual pressure, usually with the fingertips, is applied to specific points on the body to manipulate the flow of energy and relieve pain.

23.4 Mobility-Assisting Devices

Cane: A sturdy wooden or aluminum shaft or walking stick, used to give support and greater mobility to a person who is ambulatory but needs some assistance.

Standard cane: A cane with a single leg, used by someone who needs only a small amount of support in walking.

Tripod and quad-base canes: Canes with bases having three and four legs, respectively, that provide greater support and stability.

Cane height: When the patient is holding the cane and standing up straight, the cane should be level with the top of the patient's femur, and the elbow should be bent at a 20- to 25-degree angle.

Teaching a patient to use a cane: The medical assistant may be asked to teach a patient how to use a cane. Table 23-3 explains how to use a cane to stand up, walk, and climb stairs.

Crutch: A metal or wooden staff used to aid a person in walking. It is important that the person be taught how to use the crutch(es) safely and how to achieve a stable and acceptable gait.

Types of crutches: The two basic kinds of crutches are axillary crutches (which reach from the ground almost to the armpit) and forearm crutches (which reach from the ground to the forearm and are also called Lofstrand or Canadian crutches).

Measuring a patient for crutches: Crutches must be measured to fit the patient. Crutches that are too long or too short can cause muscle weakness, back strain, crutch palsy, or imbalance. When the patient is standing erect, with feet slightly apart, and the crutch tips are positioned two inches in front of the feet and four–six inches to the side of each foot, there should be two–three finger-widths between the axillary supports and the armpits (for axillary crutches), and the handgrips should be positioned to create a 30-degree flexion at the elbows.

Using crutches: In teaching patients how to use crutches, emphasize the following points:

- Support body weight with the hands.
- Stand erect.
- Look straight ahead.
- Move crutches no more than six inches at a time.
- Wear flat, well-fitting, nonskid shoes.
- Remove throw rugs and other unsecured articles from traffic areas.
- Check the tips regularly for wear and wetness.
- Check all wing nuts and bolts for tightness.

Crutch gaits: Begin with the standing or tripod position, in which the patient places the crutch tips four–six inches in front of the feet and four–six inches away from the side of each foot. Patients should use a slow gait in crowded areas or when feeling tired.

Four-point gait: A slow gait used by persons who can bear weight on both legs. The patient should begin in the tripod position, then move the right crutch forward, move the left foot forward to the level of the left crutch, move the left crutch forward, and move the right foot forward to the level of the right crutch.

Three-point gait: Used by persons who can bear full weight on one leg and no weight on the other. It requires good muscle coordination and arm strength. The patient begins in the tripod position, moves both crutches and the affected leg forward, then balances weight on both crutches and moves the unaffected leg forward.

Two-point gait: A faster gait used by persons who can bear some weight on both feet and have good muscle coordination and balance. The patient begins in the tripod position, then moves the left crutch and right foot forward at the same time, followed by the right crutch and left foot.

Swing-to gait: A modified three-point gait often used by persons with physical disabilities. The patient begins in the tripod

Standing from a chair

1. Instruct the patient to slide his buttocks to the edge of the chair.
2. Tell the patient to place his right foot against the right front leg of the chair and his left foot against the left front leg of the chair.
3. Instruct the patient to lean forward and use the armrests of the chair to push upward. Caution the patient not to lean on the cane.
4. Have the patient position the cane for support on the strong side of the body.

Walking

1. Teach the patient to hold the cane on the strong side of her body with the tip(s) of the cane four–six inches from the side of her strong foot. Remind the patient to make sure to keep the tip(s) flat on the ground.
2. Have the patient move the cane forward approximately 12 inches and then move her affected foot forward, parallel to the cane.
3. Next have the patient move her strong leg forward past both the cane and her weak leg.
4. Observe as the patient repeats this process.

Going up stairs

1. Instruct the patient always to start with his strong leg when going up stairs.
2. Advise the patient to keep the cane on the strong side of his body and to use the wall or rail for support on the weak side.
3. After the patient steps on the strong leg, instruct him to bring up his weak leg and then the cane.
4. Remind the patient not to rush.

Going down stairs

1. Instruct the patient always to start with her weak leg when going down stairs.
2. Advise the patient to keep the cane on the strong side of her body and to use the wall or rail for support on the weak side.
3. Have the patient use the strong leg and wall or rail to support her body, bending the strong leg as she lowers her weak leg and cane to the next step. She can move the cane and weak leg simultaneously, or she can move the cane first, followed by the weak leg.
4. Instruct the patient to step down with the strong leg.

Table 23-3

position and then moves both crutches forward at the same time. The patient then lifts the body and swings it to the crutches.

Swing-through gait: Also often used by persons with physical disabilities. It is like the swing-to gait, but the patient swings the body past the crutches.

Walker: An extremely light, movable apparatus, about waist high, made of metal tubing (usually aluminum), used to aid a patient in walking. There are two types: standard (with four widely placed legs ending in rubber tips) and rolling (with wheels).

Walker height: The top of the walker should be just below the patient's waist or at the same height as the top of the hip bone, so that when the patient holds the handgrip, the elbow is bent at a 30-degree angle.

Using a walker: Although a physical therapist usually trains patients in the use of walkers, medical assistants may be asked to do it or to reinforce the information. Table 23-4 provides information on how to teach a patient to use a walker.

Wheelchair: A mobile chair equipped with large wheels and brakes. If long-term use of the chair is expected, a physical therapist may prescribe particular features, such as seat size and height, left- or right-hand propulsion, brake type, armrest height, footrest style (e.g., fixed, swing-away, elevating), and special seat pads.

Using a wheelchair: To get into the wheelchair, the patient should lock the chair and fold back the footplates, then back into the chair, supporting the body on the armrests while lowering into the chair.

Transferring a patient from a wheelchair to a table: If the patient is weak, heavy, or unstable, ask for help. Make sure that the wheelchair is in the locked position and that the patient is sitting at the front of the wheelchair seat. Face the patient, spread your feet apart, and bend slightly at the knees. Have the patient hold on to your shoulders, and place your arms around the patient under the arms. At the count of "3," lift and pivot the patient to bring the back of his or her knees against the table. Gently lower the patient into a sitting or supine position on the table. The medical assistant must inform the patient's family if the patient is not using the wheelchair correctly.

1. Instruct the patient to step into the walker.
2. Tell the patient to place the hands on the handgrips on the sides of the walker.
3. Make sure that the patient's feet are far enough apart to feel balanced.
4. Instruct the patient to pick up the walker and to move it forward about six inches.
5. Have the patient move one foot forward and then the other foot.
6. Instruct the patient to pick up the walker again and to move it forward. If the patient is strong enough, explain that he or she may advance the walker after moving each foot rather than waiting until after having moved both feet.

Table 23-4

STRATEGIES FOR SUCCESS

▶ *Test-Taking Skills*

Do a mind dump!

As soon as the exam starts, you may find it helpful to do a mind dump. Briefly look over the questions and quickly write down all the information that is fresh in your head. Write out any lists that you have memorized. All the concepts and formulas that you always had trouble remembering and those that you were still going over and memorizing as the exam began should be written down as soon as possible so that you don't forget them. Then you can focus on the exam with more confidence. A mind dump doesn't work for everyone, and it should not take valuable time away from your exam. Note that on the CMA exam, no scratch paper or other extraneous items are allowed to be brought into the testing room.

CHAPTER 23 REVIEW

Instructions:

Answer the following questions.

1. The branch of medicine that uses physical devices or agents therapeutically for the diagnosis, treatment, management, and prevention of diseases is

   A. physical therapy.
   B. physiatry.
   C. sports medicine.
   D. manipulation.
   E. none of these

2. The degree to which a joint is able to move is known as

   A. goniometer.
   B. goniometry.
   C. range of motion.
   D. range of reach.
   E. universal goniometer.

3. Which of the following is paralysis of the lower portion of the body?

   A. hemiplegia
   B. paraplegia
   C. quadriplegia
   D. hemiparesis
   E. parapraxia

4. Cryotherapy is used for all of the following purposes *except*

   A. to lower body temperature.
   B. to reduce swelling.
   C. to reduce bleeding.
   D. to reduce pus formation.
   E. to reduce clotting.

5. Patients instructed on how to use crutches should be told to

   A. move crutches no more than six inches at a time.
   B. look down at the ground to check where they place the crutches.
   C. balance their body weight between their feet and hands.
   D. move crutches approximately a foot at a time.
   E. stand bent over the crutches at a 30-degree angle for increased support.

6. Diathermy is useful in treating patients with all of the following conditions *except*

   A. tendonitis.
   B. metal implants.
   C. muscular disorders.
   D. arthritis.
   E. bursitis.

7. Exaggerated anterior curvature of the lumbar spine is called

   A. lordosis.
   B. kyphosis.
   C. scoliosis.
   D. luxation.
   E. none of these

8. A modified three-point gait often used by persons with physical disabilities is called a

   A. four-point gait.
   B. two-point gait.
   C. swing-to gait.
   D. swing-through gait.
   E. none of these

9. Which of the following methods of measurement is used to assess the range of motion of a joint?

   A. mensuration
   B. goniometry
   C. palpation
   D. percussion
   E. inspection

10. A patient comes to the medical office for an annual physical examination. While walking into the office, the patient trips and falls on his right knee. Which of the following is the most likely effect of immediately applying ice to the patient's knee?

    A. faster tissue repair
    B. increased blood flow
    C. decreased deformity
    D. relaxation of muscles
    E. prevention of swelling

MEDICAL EMERGENCIES AND FIRST AID

LEARNING OUTCOMES

24.1 Recognize medical situations that require emergency treatment.

24.2 Describe the medical assistant's role in handling medical emergencies.

24.3 Recall information about injuries resulting from exposure to extreme temperatures.

24.4 Describe the different types of burns and the rule of nines.

24.5 Identify the different types of open and closed wounds.

24.6 Describe the proper treatment of bites and stings.

24.7 Identify the types and treatments of orthopedic injuries.

24.8 Identify the types and treatments of head and related injuries.

24.9 Describe the types and treatments of diabetic emergencies.

24.10 Describe the types and treatments of cardiovascular emergencies, including shock, bleeding, and heart attack, and when and how to initiate CPR.

24.11 Identify the types and treatments of respiratory emergencies.

24.12 Identify the types and treatments of digestive emergencies.

24.13 Recognize emergencies of the reproductive system, including emergency childbirth.

24.14 Describe the proper treatment of the different types of poisoning emergencies.

24.15 Identify biological agents that may be used as weapons of bioterrorism.

MEDICAL ASSISTING COMPETENCIES

COMPETENCY	CMA	RMA	CCMA	NCMA
Clinical				
Apply principles of aseptic techniques and infection control, including hand washing	X	X	X	X
Practice standard precautions	X	X	X	X
Obtain vital signs	X	X	X	X
Interview the patient to obtain and record the patient's history	X	X	X	X
Recognize emergencies; perform first aid and CPR	X	X	X	X

MEDICAL ASSISTING COMPETENCIES (cont.)

General/Legal/Professional

Recognize and respond to verbal and nonverbal communications by being attentive and adapting communication to the recipient's level of understanding	X	X	X	X
Be aware of and perform within legal and ethical boundaries	X	X	X	X
Determine the needs for documentation and reporting, and document accurately and appropriately	X	X	X	X
Instruct individuals according to their needs	X	X	X	X
Provide patients with methods of health promotion and disease prevention	X	X	X	X
Identify community resources and information for patients and employers	X	X	X	
Project a positive attitude	X	X	X	
Adapt to change	X	X	X	X
Have a responsible attitude	X	X	X	X
Be courteous and diplomatic	X	X	X	
Conduct work within scope of education, training, and ability	X	X	X	X
Be impartial and show empathy when dealing with patients	X	X	X	

STRATEGIES FOR SUCCESS

► *Study Skills*

Rephrase!
When a concept seems complicated, look up any words you don't understand in a medical dictionary or a reference book, and try rephrasing the definition in your own words. Be sure that you only make the definition clearer and that you are not actually changing what the definition says. Rephrasing will help you understand the subject matter, and the concept will be easier to recall on an exam.

24.1 Emergencies

Medical emergency: A situation in which an individual suddenly becomes ill or has an injury that requires immediate attention and help by a health-care professional.

First aid: Immediate care given to a person who has suddenly become injured or ill. First aid can save a life, reduce pain, prevent further injury, reduce the risk of permanent disability, and increase the chance of early recovery.

Emergency Medical Services (EMS): A network of qualified police, fire, and medical personnel who use community resources and equipment to provide emergency care to victims of injury or sudden illness. Post the EMS telephone number, which is 911 in many communities, at every telephone and on the crash cart or first-aid tray.

Involving the EMS: To involve the EMS in an emergency, it is necessary to

1. Recognize that an emergency exists.
2. Decide to act.
3. Call the local emergency telephone number.
4. Provide care until help arrives.

Universal emergency identification symbol: Represents a person who has a life-threatening health condition.

24.2 Handling Emergencies

Medical assistant's responsibilities: You may be responsible for providing first aid, but you are never responsible for diagnosing or providing other medical care. Note the presence of serious conditions and take the appropriate action. Perform only procedures that you have been trained to perform. See Table 24-1.

Emergency triage: The classification of injuries according to severity, urgency of treatment, and place for treatment. The MA must understand the severity and urgency of each patient's condition. For example, patients with arrhythmia, hemorrhaging, or respiratory distress would be treated before patients with fractures, sprains, or minor burns.

Personal protection: Universal precautions include wearing gloves and other personal protective equipment (PPE). If you have been exposed to blood or other body fluids, tell the physician so that you can obtain postexposure treatment.

Documentation: Document all office emergencies in the patient's chart, including information on assessment, treatment, and the patient's response.

Good Samaritan law: Permits emergency care on the condition that it is within the scope of competence of the person administering first aid. It holds individuals giving first aid responsible for any injury they cause as a result of negligence or failure to exercise reasonable care. If the victim is conscious or a family member is present, obtain verbal consent. If the victim is unconscious, consent is implied. State laws also apply.

Crash cart: A rolling cart that contains basic drugs, supplies, and equipment for medical emergencies. Most crash carts also contain a first-aid kit with supplies for managing minor injuries and ailments. See Table 24-2.

24.3 Injuries Caused by Extreme Temperatures

Hypothermia: The body temperature is dangerously reduced below the normal range, below 95°F (rectal, child/adult) or 97.7°F (rectal, newborn). Major symptoms include mild shivering, cool skin, and pallor. Risk factors include exposure to a cool or cold environment, trauma, malnutrition, consumption of alcohol, specific medications, decreased metabolic rate, aging, and inactivity.

Frostbite: The traumatic effect of extreme cold on skin and subcutaneous tissues, particularly the toes, fingers, ears, and nose. Vasoconstriction of blood vessels causes anoxia, edema, vesiculation, and necrosis. Symptoms include white, waxy, or grayish yellow skin that may feel crusty, with possible softness in the underlying tissue. The body part experiences sensations of cold, tingling, and pain. To treat frostbite, wrap warm clothing or blankets around the affected body part, or place the affected area in warm but not hot water (100°–105°F). Do not rub or massage the affected area. Obtain medical assistance.

Hyperthermia: Body temperature elevated above the normal range. Skin is warm to the touch and appears flushed. The patient may experience tachypnea, tachycardia, seizures, or convulsions. Major factors include exposure to a hot environment, vigorous activity, medications or anesthesia, increased metabolic rate, trauma or illness, and dehydration. Individuals who are in poor health, alcoholic, obese, very young, or elderly are less able to tolerate heat waves and constant high temperatures.

Heatstroke: A severe and sometimes fatal condition generally caused by prolonged exposure to high temperatures. Symptoms include hot, dry skin; high body temperature; altered mental

---

AT A GLANCE Performing Emergency Assessment

1. Wash your hands and put on examination gloves if possible.
2. Talk to the patient to determine level of consciousness.
3. If the patient can communicate clearly, ask what happened. If the patient can't talk, ask someone who observed the incident.
4. If you cannot determine the patient's medical history by talking to the patient, check for a medical identification card or a bracelet.
5. Assess the patient's ABCs (*a*irway, *b*reathing, and *c*irculation), and begin rescue breathing or CPR as needed. NOTE: The American Heart Association's new recommendations require that chest compressions begin first, before rescue breathing. Therefore, the actual order of this process is now considered to be "C-A-B" rather than "A-B-C". If a person is not trained in CPR, he or she should perform 100 chest compressions per minute until other help arrives, and avoid attempting rescue breathing
6. Assess for injury, observing the body from head to toe. Palpate gently.
7. Observe the skin for pallor (paleness) or cyanosis (a bluish tint). If the patient is dark-skinned, observe for pallor or cyanosis on the inside of the lips and mouth.
8. Check the pulse for regularity and strength.
9. Check the eyes for pupil size. Using a penlight, assess pupil response to light.
10. Document your findings and report them to the doctor or emergency medical technician (EMT).
11. Assist the doctor or EMT as requested.
12. Remove the gloves and wash your hands.

Table 24-1

1. Review the office protocol for a list of items that should be on the crash cart.
2. Check the *drugs* on the cart against the list. Restock as necessary, and replace any drugs that have passed their expiration date. The following drugs are often included on the cart:

- Activated charcoal
- Amobarbital sodium (Amytal Sodium®)
- Apomorphine hydrochloride
- Atropine
- Dextrose 50%
- Diazepam (Valium®)
- Digoxin (Lanoxin®)
- Diphenhydramine hydrochloride (Benadryl®)
- Epinephrine, injectable
- Furosemide (Lasix®)
- Glucagon
- Glucose paste or tablets
- Insulin (regular or a variety)
- Narcotics

- Intravenous dextrose in saline and intravenous dextrose in water
- Isoproterenol hydrochloride (Isuprel®), aerosol inhaler and injectable
- Lactated Ringer's IV solution
- Lidocaine (Xylocaine®), injectable
- Metaraminol (Aramine®)
- Methylprednisolone tablets
- Nitroglycerin tablets
- Phenobarbital, injectable
- Phenytoin (Dilantin®)
- Saline solution, isotonic (0.9%)
- Sodium bicarbonate, injectable
- Sterile water for injection

3. Check the *supplies* on the cart against the list. Restock used items, and make sure that all packaging of supplies on the cart is still intact. Crash cart supplies typically include:

- Adhesive tape
- Constricting band or tourniquet
- Dressing supplies (alcohol wipes, rolls of gauze, bandage strips, bandage scissors)
- IV tubing, venipuncture devices, and butterfly needles
- Padded tongue blades
- Personal protective equipment
- Syringes and needles in various sizes

4. Check the *equipment* on the crash cart against the list, and examine everything to make sure that it is in working order. Restock equipment that is missing or broken. The equipment usually consists of:

- Airways in assorted sizes
- Ambu-bag™, a trademark for a breathing bag used to assist respiratory ventilation
- Defibrillator (electrical device that shocks the heart to restore normal breathing)
- Endotracheal tubes in various sizes
- Oxygen tank with oxygen mask and cannula

5. Check *miscellaneous items* on the cart against the list, and restock as needed. These items usually include:

- Orange juice
- Sugar packets

Table 24-2

state; rapid pulse; rapid breathing; dizziness; and weakness. To treat heatstroke, call the EMS system. Move the patient to a cool place and remove the patient's outer clothing. Cool the patient, using any means available. Keep the patient's head and shoulders slightly elevated.

Heat cramps: Painful spasms of the voluntary muscles in the leg, abdomen, or arm, which may be caused by depletion in the body of both water and salt. It occurs in an extremely hot environment.

Heat exhaustion: Characterized by muscle cramps, weakness, nausea, dizziness, and loss of consciousness, caused by depletion of body fluids and electrolytes. It is the most frequent heat-related injury. Treatment includes moving the patient to a cool place and starting fluid and electrolyte replacement.

24.4 Burns

Burn: An injury to the tissues of the body caused by heat, electricity, chemicals, radiation, or gases. The severity of a burn depends on the depth of the burn and the percentage of the body involved. Burns are classified according to the depth of tissue injured. There are three types: first degree, second degree, and third degree. See Figure 24-1.

Superficial (first-degree) burns: The most common type of burn. They cause pain and make the surrounding skin turn red. A superficial burn damages only the epidermis and causes edema. Sunburn is a common example of a superficial burn.

Partial-thickness (second-degree) burns: These burns extend deeper into the skin than first-degree burns, damaging the epidermis and dermis. The injured area appears blistered, with redness and pain. The blisters should not be broken. They prevent infection of the burned area. They are usually very painful and heal within three–four weeks. To treat a partial-thickness burn, immerse the burned area in cold water until the pain subsides, pat the area dry, and apply a dry, sterile dressing.

Full-thickness (third-degree) burns: These burns involve all layers of skin and completely damage both the epidermis and the dermis, extending into the underlying connective tissues, such as fat, muscle, and even bone. A full-thickness burn is an emergency condition. Spontaneous healing is impossible. These burns require the removal of scars and the application of skin grafts. The most severe and major complication is infection.

Estimating the extent of the burn: To calculate the amount of skin surface burned on an adult, use the rule of nines. Each of the following parts of the body is considered to be 9% of the body's surface: the head and neck, each upper limb, the chest, the abdomen, the upper back, the lower back and buttocks, the front of each lower limb, and the back of each lower limb. The remaining 1% is the genital area. See Figure 24-2, which also shows the percentages to use when making calculations in children.

Chemical burns: To treat a chemical burn, flood the area with large amounts of cool water for at least 15 minutes, and cover it with a dry dressing. Call the EMS system.

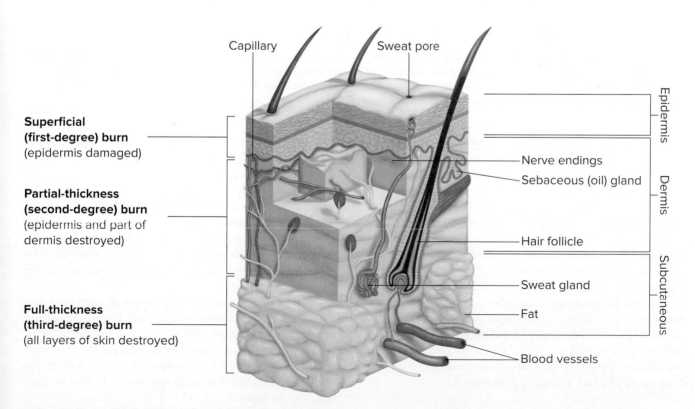

Capillary   Sweat pore

Superficial (first-degree) burn (epidermis damaged)

Partial-thickness (second-degree) burn (epidermis and part of dermis destroyed)

Full-thickness (third-degree) burn (all layers of skin destroyed)

Nerve endings
Sebaceous (oil) gland
Hair follicle
Sweat gland
Fat
Blood vessels

Epidermis
Dermis
Subcutaneous

Figure 24-1 *The depth of skin damage is one factor used to determine the severity of burns.*

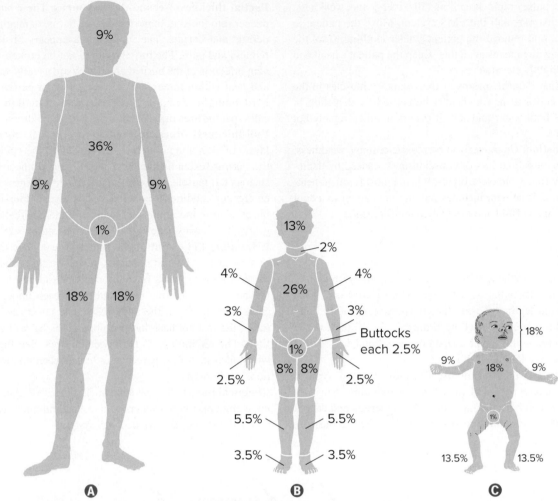

Figure 24-2 *(A) Use the rule of nines to calculate the percentage of body surface affected by burns in adults. Except for the genital region, percentage figures combine front and back surfaces. (B) In children, use the percentages based on the Lund and Browder chart. These numbers take into account that children's body proportions differ from those of adults. (C) In infants, the rule of nines is used. These numbers take into account an infant's properties.*

Thermal burns: Caused by contact with hot liquids, steam, flames, radiation, excessive heat from fire, or hot objects. Call the EMS system. Use water to cool a burning substance, or use a wet cloth or blanket to put out a flame.

Electrical burns: Injuries from exposure to electrical currents, including lightning. These burns occur at the site where the electricity enters the body and where the current exits the body and enters the ground. Along the current's pathway, extensive tissue damage can occur from heat, followed by chemical changes to nerve, muscle, and heart tissue. Call the EMS team immediately for these types of injuries.

Sunburn: Causes redness, tenderness, pain, swelling, blisters, and peeling skin and can lead to skin damage or cancer. To treat sunburn, soak skin in cool water and apply cold compresses and calamine lotion. Have the patient elevate the legs and arms, drink plenty of water, and take a pain reliever.

24.5 Wounds

Wound: A physical injury in which the skin or tissues under the skin are damaged. There are two types of wounds: open and closed.

Open wounds: Include punctures, lacerations, abrasions, and incisions (see Figure 24-3).

Incision: A clean and smooth cut.

Laceration: A cut with jagged edges.

Treating incisions and lacerations: See Table 24-3 for the way to treat minor incisions and lacerations. For deeper wounds that involve muscle, tendons, the face, the genitals, the mouth, or the tongue, control the bleeding with direct pressure to the wound, elevation, and the use of pressure points; contact the physician or EMS system.

Abrasion: A scraping of the skin. Wash with soap and water, making sure to remove all dirt and debris. Use a bandage on a large abrasion. See Figure 24-4.

Puncture: A small hole created by a piercing object. Allow the wound to bleed freely for 15 minutes, then clean it with soap and water and apply a dry, sterile dressing. A tetanus immunization may be required.

Closed wound: An injury that occurs inside the body without tearing the skin. Closed wounds are called contusions or bruises. They are caused by a sudden blow or force from a blunt object. Apply cold compresses to reduce swelling.

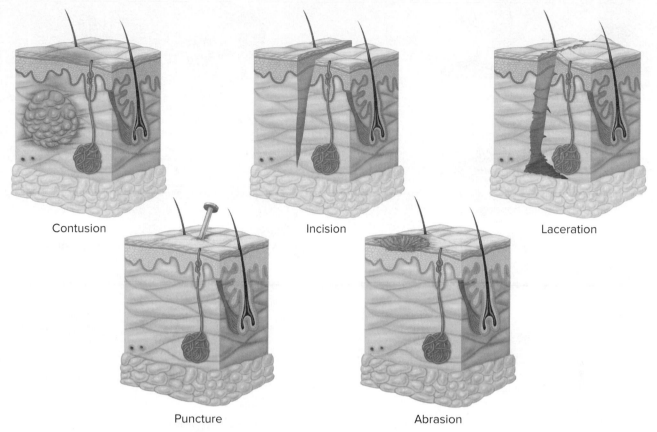

Contusion   Incision   Laceration

Puncture   Abrasion

Figure 24-3 *Different types of wounds produce different degrees of tissue damage.*

AT A GLANCE | Cleaning Minor Wounds

1. Wash your hands and put on examination gloves.
2. Dip several gauze squares in a basin of warm, soapy water.
3. Wash the wound from the center outward to avoid bringing contaminants from the surrounding skin into the wound. Use a new gauze square for each cleansing motion.
4. As you wash, remove debris that could cause infection.
5. Rinse the area thoroughly, preferably by placing the wound under warm, running water.
6. Pat the wound dry with sterile gauze squares.
7. Cover the wound with a dry, sterile dressing. Bandage the dressing in place.
8. Properly dispose of contaminated materials.
9. Remove the gloves and wash your hands.
10. Instruct the patient on wound care.
11. Record the procedure in the patient's chart.

Table 24-3

Avulsion: The forcible separation of a part of the body from the remainder, because of trauma or surgery.

Changing dressings: After washing hands and putting on gloves, remove the old dressing. Assess the wound by measuring it, and indicating its deepest point. Assess phase of wound healing, and qualities of any present drainage. Cleanse the wound if needed and apply a sterile dressing, using gauze, medical tape, and other appropriate materials.

Bandages: Strips of woven material used to cover or wrap body parts. Bandages may control bleeding, protect wounds from

contamination, keep dressings in place, or immobilize and support body parts. Basic types of bandages include:

- Elastic bandages: made of woven cotton containing elastic fibers; they can be washed and reused. Medical assistants must carefully apply these since they can be wrapped too tightly and impede circulation. There are also elastic adhesive bandages available.

- Roller bandages: long strips of soft material, usually sterilized gauze, that range 0.5–6 inches in width, and

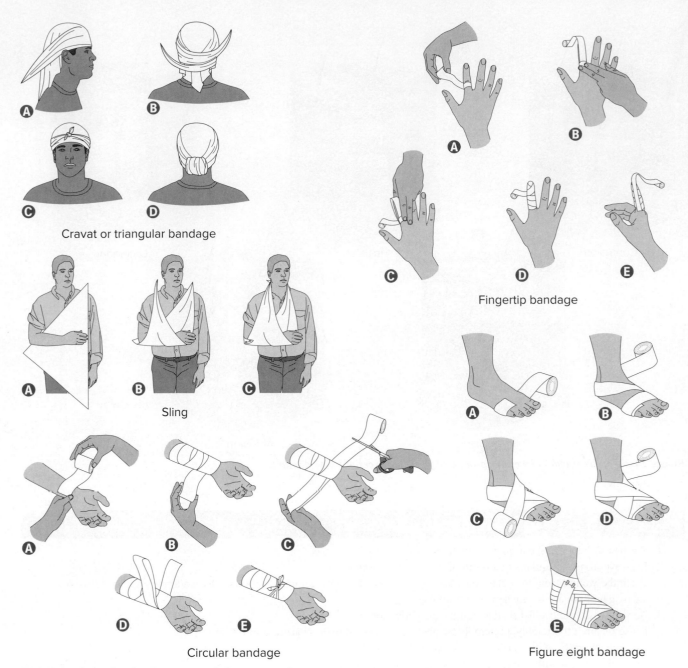

Cravat or triangular bandage

Sling

Circular bandage

Fingertip bandage

Figure eight bandage

Figure 24-4 *Apply a bandage, as needed, to a wound.*

two–five yards in length. The width chosen is based on the size of the body part being bandaged. These bandages are porous, lightweight, and disposable.

- Kling gauze: a special type of gauze that stretches, so that it clings to body parts better than ordinary gauze.

24.6 Bites and Stings

Animal bites: May range in severity from minor to serious. A wound that tears the skin should be seen by a physician and may need to be reported to the police, animal control office, and local health department. If the animal can be found, it should be checked for rabies.

Treating animal bites: If the bite is a puncture wound, try to make it bleed to flush out bacteria. Wash the area thoroughly with antiseptic soap and water. Apply an antibiotic ointment and a dry, sterile dressing. The physician will administer a tetanus shot if the patient has not had one for 7–10 years.

Rabies: A viral infection normally transmitted through the saliva of rabid animals. Dogs, cats, skunks, squirrels, raccoons, bats, and foxes are more likely to carry rabies than other animals. Prevention involves vaccinating house pets. Immunization of a person who has been exposed to rabies should be started as soon as possible because treatment is ineffective once clinical symptoms develop. If left untreated, rabies can cause paralysis and death.

Snakebite: A wound resulting from penetration of the skin by the fangs of a snake. Not all snakebites are poisonous. Symptoms of a poisonous snakebite include puncture marks, pain, swelling, rapid pulse, nausea, vomiting, and possibly unconsciousness and seizures. Bites from snakes known to be nonvenomous are treated as puncture wounds. Bites from poisonous or unidentified snakes require immediate attention. Call a doctor or the EMS system. The bitten area should be immobilized and positioned below heart level, and the patient should not walk. Wash the bite area with soap and water. Do not apply a tourniquet or ice, and do not cut or suction the wound.

Spider bite: A puncture wound produced by the bite of venomous spiders, which in the United States include the black widow and the brown recluse. Symptoms include swelling, pain, nausea, vomiting, rigid abdomen, fever, rash, and difficulty breathing or swallowing. Any patient bitten by a spider should be seen by a doctor. Wash the area thoroughly with soap and water, apply an ice pack, and keep the area below heart level.

Scorpion stings: Of the different scorpion types in the American Southwest, some are more poisonous to young children. Antivenin may be available in some areas. Scorpion stings are treated similarly to spider bites.

24.7 Orthopedic Injuries

Strain: Overstretching of muscles or tendons caused by trauma. The neck, back, thigh, and calf are the most common sites for muscle injuries caused by excessive physical force.

Sprain: An acute partial tear of a tendon, muscle, or ligament, characterized by pain and edema. The joints most commonly sprained are ankles, knees, wrists, and fingers.

Dislocation: The displacement of a bone from its normal articulation with a joint. It is caused by a violent pulling or pushing force that tears the ligaments.

Fracture: A break in a bone. Review this section in Chapter 4.

Treating fractures and dislocations: To reduce pain and continuing damage to soft tissue, immobilize the body area by the application of a splint or cast. In some cases, it is necessary to move the bone back into the proper position.

Splint: An orthopedic device for immobilization or support of any part of the body. It may be rigid (made of metal, plaster, or wood) or flexible (made of leather, rolled newspapers, or magazines). The body part should be splinted in the position in which it was found. The splint should immobilize the area above and below the injury.

Sling: A wide piece of cloth suspended from the neck for supporting an injured hand or arm across the front of the body.

Cast: A rigid external dressing, usually made of plaster or fiberglass, that is molded to the contours of the body part. The basic elements of cast care, which should be communicated to the patient, are:

- Tell the physician about any pain, swelling, discoloration, lack of pulsation and warmth, or inability to move exposed parts.
- Keep the extremity elevated for the first day.

- Avoid allowing the affected limb to hang unsupported for any length of time.
- Take care to avoid indenting the cast until it is dry.
- Restrict strenuous activity for the first few days.
- Do not put anything inside the cast.
- Keep the cast dry.

24.8 Head and Related Injuries

Head injury: Scalp hematoma, scalp laceration, concussion. Severe head injuries include contusion, fracture, and intracranial bleeding. Some head injuries can be life threatening.

Scalp hematoma: A bump on the head caused by a buildup of blood under the skin. The swelling can be reduced by applying ice.

Scalp laceration: A wound that usually bleeds profusely. Direct pressure should be applied to stop the bleeding.

Contusion: Bruising of the head, which may include *cerebral contusion,* in which the brain tissue itself is bruised. Contusion occurs in 20–30% of head injuries.

Concussion: A jarring injury to the brain, which is the most common type of head injury. Symptoms include loss of consciousness, temporary loss of vision, pallor, listlessness, memory loss, and vomiting. Symptoms may disappear rapidly or last up to 24 hours. The patient should refrain from strenuous activity, rest, and then return to regular activity gradually. The patient should eat lightly and a family member should check on the patient every few hours.

Fainting: A brief loss of consciousness, also called syncope, that can result from a variety of causes. The most common direct cause of syncope is decreased cerebral blood flow. Have the patient lower his or her head between the legs and breathe deeply. Lay a patient who has fainted on his or her back with feet slightly elevated; loosen tight clothing, and apply a cold cloth to the face. Notify the physician.

Convulsions: May be caused by injury, trauma, fever, infection, hypocalcemia, hypoglycemia, or idiopathic factors. Convulsions, also called seizures, usually last only a few minutes.

Cerebrovascular accident (CVA): Also known as a stroke. An abnormal condition of the brain characterized by occlusion by an embolus, thrombus, or cerebrovascular hemorrhage. Possible effects of stroke include paralysis, weakness, speech defects, aphasia, and death.

24.9 Diabetic Emergencies

Diabetes: A fairly common disorder of carbohydrate metabolism, diabetes can cause hyperglycemia and hypoglycemia, both of which may become medical emergencies.

Hypoglycemia: A lower-than-normal level of glucose in the blood, usually caused by the administration of too much insulin, excessive secretion of insulin by the pancreas, or dietary deficiency. Symptoms of hypoglycemia include weakness, headache, hunger, ataxia, anxiety, and visual disturbances. Untreated hypoglycemia can result in delirium, coma, and death.

Insulin shock: Very severe hypoglycemia. The symptoms include weakness, tachycardia, cold skin, tremors, convulsions, restlessness, confusion, and fainting. The treatment is the administration of some form of sugar.

Hyperglycemia: A higher-than-normal level of blood glucose. Symptoms include dry mouth, intense thirst, muscle weakness, and blurred vision.

24.10 Cardiovascular Emergencies

Shock

Shock: A life-threatening state associated with failure of the cardiovascular system.

Hypovolemic shock: Inadequate intravascular volume producing diminished ventricular filling and reduced stroke volume, which results in decreased cardiac output. It occurs after an injury that causes major fluid loss.

Cardiogenic shock: Results from reduction in cardiac output due to factors other than inadequate intravascular volume (e.g., cardiac tamponade, pulmonary embolism, myocardial infarction, myocarditis, drugs, tachycardia, and bradycardia).

Neurogenic shock: May occur following severe cerebral trauma or hemorrhage.

Septic shock: May be partly due to the effects of endotoxin or other chemical mediators on resistance vessels, resulting in vasodilation and decreased vascular resistance.

Anaphylactic shock: Occurs following allergic reactions. Also called anaphylaxis, it is severe and often fatal.

Symptoms of shock: Restlessness; irritability; fear; rapid pulse; pale, cool skin; and increased respiratory rate.

Treating shock: Elevate the patient's feet 8–12 inches, unless there is head injury. Monitor airways, breathing, and circulation, and control bleeding if necessary.

Bleeding

Bleeding: The release of blood from the vascular system as a result of damage to a blood vessel. It is also called hemorrhaging and can be minor or very severe. There are two types of bleeding: external and internal.

Internal bleeding: Hemorrhaging from an internal organ or tissue, such as intraperitoneal bleeding into the peritoneal cavity, or intestinal bleeding into the bowel.

Hematemesis: The vomiting of bright red blood, indicating rapid upper GI bleeding. The most common causes are esophageal varices and peptic ulcer.

Hemoptysis: The coughing up of blood from the respiratory tract.

Controlling internal bleeding: Cover the patient with a blanket, keep the patient quiet and calm, and get medical help immediately.

External bleeding: Bleeding that can be seen outside the body, such as bleeding from wounds, open fractures, and nosebleeds. The most common type of external bleeding is capillary bleeding. The most serious and least common type of external bleeding is arterial. Ask the victim to pinch the nostrils together just below the bridge of the nose for 10 minutes. Ask the victim to breathe through the mouth and not speak, swallow, cough, or sniff; then place a cold compress on the bridge of the nose.

Epistaxis (nosebleed): A common type of external bleeding usually caused by trauma, hypertension, exposure to high altitudes, or an upper respiratory infection.

Controlling external bleeding: If time permits, wash your hands and put on personal protective equipment. Apply direct pressure over the wound, using a clean or sterile dressing.

Heart Attack

Chest pain: A symptom that may be indicative of cardiac disease, such as myocardial infarction, angina pectoris, or pericarditis; of respiratory disorders, such as pleurisy, pneumonia, or pulmonary embolism; or of nonmyocardial infarction. Another source of chest pain can be cocaine use.

Myocardial infarction (MI): Ischemic myocardial necrosis of a portion of the cardiac muscle caused by obstruction in a coronary artery. It is also known as a heart attack. In more than 90% of patients with acute MI, an acute thrombus, often associated with plaque rupture, occludes the coronary artery. Chest pain is the major symptom of a heart attack. The pain may radiate down the left arm or into the jaw, throat, or both shoulders, and it may be accompanied by shortness of breath, sweating, nausea, and vomiting.

Cardiac arrest: The sudden cessation of cardiac output and effective circulation, usually followed by ventricular fibrillation or ventricular asystole. It is also called cardiac standstill. Immediate initiation of CPR is required to prevent heart, lung, kidney, and brain damage.

Chain of Survival: The American Heart Association's term *Chain of Survival* provides useful information for emergency cardiovascular care (ECC). The ECC systems concept summarizes the present understanding of the best approach to the treatment of persons with sudden cardiac arrest. The five links in the adult *Chain of Survival* are:

- Immediate recognition of cardiac arrest and activation of the emergency response system
- Early cardiopulmonary resuscitation with emphasis on chest compressions
- Rapid defibrillation
- Effective advanced life support
- Integrated postcardiac arrest care

Cardiopulmonary resuscitation (CPR): In collapsed or unconscious persons, the state of ventilation and circulation must be determined immediately. Speed, efficiency, and proper application of CPR directly affect success. Tissue anoxia for more than four–six minutes can result in irreversible brain damage or death. After establishing unresponsiveness of the victim, call for help, note the exact time of arrest, and position the victim horizontally on a hard surface. The American Heart Association has changed the order of the steps required in assessing a patient from "A-B-C" to "C-A-B." This means that a primary survey should assess the patient's *c*irculation, *a*irway, and *b*reathing. NOTE: This is not true for neonatal CPR technique (see www.heart.org/cpr for complete information).

The reason for changing the order from "A-B-C" to "C-A-B" is because chest compressions are initiated sooner rather than later in the process. Chest compressions are more critical *early* in the process, in *most cases,* than the establishment of an airway. Since most cardiac arrests occur in adults, and those who are successfully treated receive early chest compressions and defibrillation, it has been determined that chest compressions need to occur first in the process. It is important to allow the chest to fully recoil after each hard, fast compression.

CPR involves three basic components: chest compressions, opening the airway, and rescue breathing. See Figures 24-6 through 24-10. Table 24-4 gives a summary of steps of CPR for adults, children, and infants. CPR must be continued until the cardiopulmonary system is stabilized, the patient is pronounced dead, or resuscitation cannot be continued (because of rescuer exhaustion). Resuscitation efforts can be divided into basic life support (BLS), which is carried out with techniques and equipment that are immediately available, and advanced cardiac life support (ACLS), which involves drug therapy, cardiac monitoring, and other specialized techniques and equipment.

For adults, the following steps should be performed in order to maintain BLS:

1. Determine if the patient is responsive and call, or have someone else call, 9-1-1.

2. Start CPR immediately, with chest compressions of at least 100 per minute, allowing full chest recoil. Each compression should be at least two inches (five centimeters) deep for adult patients.

3. If possible, ask someone to get an AED while continuing CPR for two minutes.

4. If no response, open the airway and give two breaths. Check the patient's pulse. The best location to use is the carotid artery of the neck.

5. If there is a pulse, give 8–10 breaths per minute.

6. If there is no pulse, give 30 chest compressions to every two breaths, and repeat until the AED arrives.

NOTE: The American Red Cross currently advises that continual chest compressions should occur until either an AED or EMS arrives.

The reason for chest compressions is to provide adequate blood circulation to the brain. Faster chest compressions of adequate depth have been shown to result in a higher survival rate than slower, shallower compressions. Chest compressions create blood flow mostly by increasing intrathoracic pressure, which directly compresses the heart.

Automated external defibrillator: A device that delivers an electrical shock at a preset voltage to the myocardium through the chest wall (see Figure 24-11). It is used for restoring the normal cardiac rhythm and rate when the heart has stopped beating or is fibrillating. This defibrillator is portable and is powered by standard 110V current or batteries. NOTE: The American Heart Association now advises that for defibrillation of children one–eight years of age, the rescuer should utilize a *pediatric dose-attenuator system* if available instead of an automated external defibrillator (AED). For infants (under

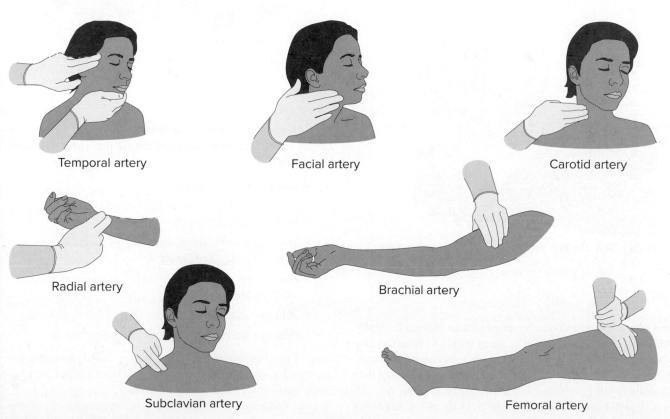

Temporal artery

Facial artery

Carotid artery

Radial artery

Brachial artery

Subclavian artery

Femoral artery

Figure 24-5 *Different pulse points.*

Source: From 2015 AHA Guidelines for CPR & ECC. © 2015, American Heart Association, Inc.

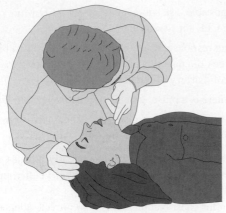

Figure 24-6 *Use the head tilt–chin lift maneuver to open an airway.*

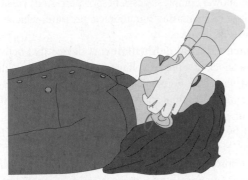

Figure 24-7 *Use the jaw thrust maneuver for a patient with a neck injury.*

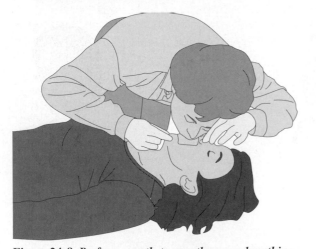

Figure 24-8 *Perform mouth-to-mouth rescue breathing.*

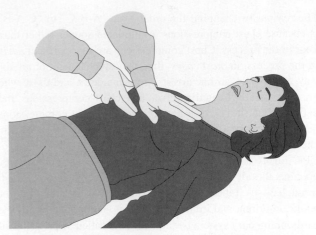

Figure 24-9 *Place your hands in the center of the chest (above the xiphoid process).*

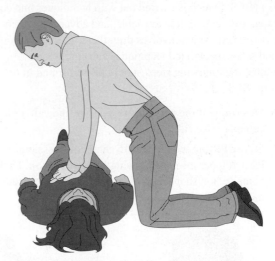

Figure 24-10 *Align your shoulders directly over the victim's sternum, with your elbows locked.*

Modifications to CPR for children: Although the steps for giving CPR to an adult and child are similar, there are a few differences:

- Amount of air for breaths
- Possible need to try more than twice to deliver two breaths that make the chest rise
- Depth of compressions; note that this should be one-third of the depth of the chest
- Possible use of one-handed chest compressions for very small children
- When to attach an AED
- When to activate the emergency response system

Note: The American Heart Association (in 2010) recommended that cycles of compressions and ventilations for adults, children, and infants include the 30:2 ratio.

If two people are assisting in CPR involving cardiac arrest, the use of *cricoid pressure* is no longer recommended. Cricoid pressure involves the application of pressure to the patient's cricoid cartilage to push the trachea posteriorly. This compresses the

one year of age), a manual defibrillator is preferred. Ideally, AEDs should be available in as many public locations as possible, including airports, sports facilities, hotels, cruise ships, etc. For children older than one year or who weigh more than 22 pounds (10 kilograms), adult automated external defibrillator paddles (eight centimeters in size) should be used. For infants and children up to one year, or who weigh less than 22 pounds, pediatric paddles (4.5 centimeters in size) should be used.

AHA Summary of Key Basic Life Support Components for Adults, Children, and Infants

Component	Adults	Children	Infants
Scene safety	Make sure the environment is safe for rescuers and victim		
Recognition	Unresponsive (for all ages)		
	No breathing or no normal breathing (i.e., only gasping)	No breathing or only gasping	
	No pulse palpated within 10 seconds for all ages (HCP only)		
	(Breathing and pulse check can be performed simultaneously in less than 10 seconds)		
Activate emergency response system	If you are alone with no mobile phone, leave victim to activate ERS and get the AED before beginning CPR. Otherwise, send someone and begin CPR immediately. Use AED as soon as it is available. **Witnessed collapse:** Follow steps for adults and adolescents on the left. **Unwitnessed collapse:** Give two minutes of CPR. Leave victim to activate ERS and get the AED. Return to child or infant, resume CPR. Use AED as soon as it is available.		
CPR sequence	C-A-B		
Compression rate	100–120/min		
Compression depth	At least two inches (five cm). Compression depth should be no more than 2.4 inches (six cm).	At least ⅓ AP diameter of chest About two inches (five cm)	At least ½ AP diameter of chest About 1 and ½ inches (four cm)
Hand placement	Adults: two hands on lower half of breastbone (sternum). Children: two hands or one hand (optional for very small child) on lower half of breastbone (sternum). Infants: **one rescuer:** two fingers in center of chest, just below nipple line; **two rescuers:** two thumb-encircling hands in center of chest, just below nipple line.		
Chest wall recoil	Allow full recoil of chest after each compression—do not lean on chest after each compression Minimize interruptions in chest compressions Attempt to limit interruptions to <10 seconds		
Airway	Head tilt–chin lift (HCP suspected trauma: jaw thrust maneuver, which is putting the fingers behind the jawbone just below the ear, and pushing the jaw forward)		
Compression to ventilation ratio (until advanced airway placed)	30:2 one or two rescuers	30:2 Single rescuer 15:2 two HCP rescuers	
Ventilations: When rescuer untrained or trained and not proficient	Compressions only		
Ventilations with advanced airway (HCP)	One breath every six seconds (10 breaths per minute) Asynchronous with chest compressions (continuous compressions at a rate of 100–120/min) About one second per breath Visible chest rise		
Defibrillation	Attach and use AED as soon as available. Minimize interruptions in chest compressions before and after shock; resume CPR beginning with compressions immediately after each shock.		

Table 24-4

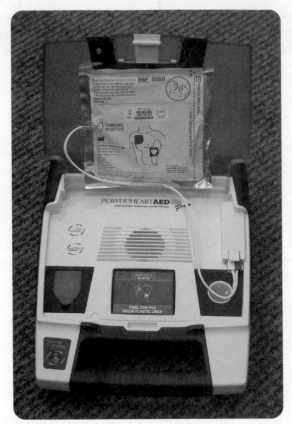

Figure 24-11 *An automated external defibrillator.*
© McGraw-Hill Education

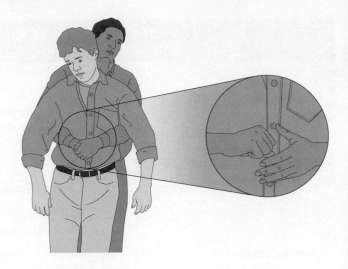

Figure 24-12 *Perform abdominal thrusts on a conscious choking victim.*

esophagus against the cervical vertebrae, which can prevent gastric inflation and reduce risk of regurgitation and aspiration if bag-mask ventilation is being used. However, it may also impede ventilation. Therefore, untrained individuals should completely avoid using cricoid pressure in cardiac arrest patients. Also, rescuers should suspect cardiac arrest if the patient is not breathing or only gasping.

24.11 Respiratory Emergencies

Choking: A condition in which the respiratory passage is blocked by an obstruction, usually food in the trachea. If the victim is coughing forcefully, do nothing but observe. If the victim is conscious but cannot speak, breathe, or cough, use the Heimlich maneuver. Give upward subdiaphragmatic abdominal thrusts until the foreign body is expelled. See Figure 24-12. If the victim loses consciousness, lay the person down slowly on his or her back. Check the mouth for a foreign body, and sweep it out with your fingers if possible. Continue to administer upward abdominal thrusts, with the heel of one hand between the xiphoid process and the navel and the second hand on top of the first, until the foreign body is expelled. If the person is still not breathing independently when the airway is clear, perform CPR. The objectives of emergency treatment are (1) removal of the obstruction and (2) resuscitation if necessary.

Respiratory arrest: Lack of breathing, usually preceded by symptoms of respiratory distress.

Asthma: A respiratory disorder characterized by (1) airway constriction that is reversible, either spontaneously or with treatment; (2) airway inflammation; and (3) increased airway sensitivity to a variety of stimuli.

Hyperventilation: Breathing too rapidly and too deeply, which can cause patients to feel light-headed and as if they cannot get enough air. Move the patient to a quiet area, and have the patient breathe into a paper bag that is held tightly around the nose and mouth. Encourage the patient to take slow, normal breaths.

24.12 Digestive Emergencies

Abdominal pain: Acute and severe pain nearly always is a symptom of intra-abdominal abnormality. It may be the most important indication that an emergency operation or treatment is needed, such as for appendicitis, perforated peptic ulcer, intestinal obstruction, general peritonitis, twisted ovarian cyst, or ectopic pregnancy.

Treating abdominal pain: Call for transport, and have the patient lie on the back with the knees flexed. Keep the patient warm and quiet. Do not apply heat. Monitor the patient's pulse and consciousness, and check for signs of shock.

Melena: Abnormal black, tarry stool that has a distinctive odor and contains digested blood. It usually results from bleeding in the upper GI tract. In adults, it is often a sign of peptic ulcer or small bowel disease.

24.13 Reproductive System Emergencies

Vaginal bleeding: If a patient experiences gushing vaginal bleeding, call the EMS system, and have her lie down with her feet elevated.

Emergency childbirth: If a physician is not present, the medical assistant should summon help and begin the procedure. Ask the woman how far apart her contractions are, whether her water has broken, and whether she feels straining or pressure as if the baby is coming. Always explain to the woman what you are doing and reassure her. Do a visual examination of the vagina to see whether there is crowning (a bulging caused by the baby's head). If the head is crowning, childbirth is imminent. Place clean cloths under the woman, and use sterile sheets or towels (if available) to cover her legs and stomach. Wash your hands thoroughly, and put on examination gloves if possible. If a physician is available, position yourself at the woman's head and provide emotional support and help if she vomits. If no physician is available, position yourself at the woman's side so that you can see the vaginal opening. Place one hand below the baby's head as it is delivered. Never pull on the baby. If the umbilical cord is wrapped around the baby's neck, gently loosen it and slide it over the head. If the amniotic sac has not broken, use your finger to puncture the membrane and pull the membranes as well as blood and mucus away from the baby's mouth and nose. After the feet are delivered, lay the baby on his or her side, with the head slightly lower than the body. Keep the baby at the same level as the mother until you cut the umbilical cord. The infant must be breathing independently before you clamp and cut the cord. Wait several minutes until the pulsation of the umbilical cord stops, then use clamps or pieces of string to close off the cord in two places: 6 and 12 inches from the baby. Cut the cord between the two clamps with sterilized scissors. Within 10 minutes of birth, expulsion of the placenta will begin. Keep it in a plastic bag for further examination. Keep the mother and baby warm by wrapping them in towels and blankets. Massage the mother's abdomen just below the navel every few minutes to control internal bleeding.

24.14 Poisoning

Poison: A substance that impedes biological functions when taken into the body. The majority of accidental poisonings occur at home in children under the age of 5 years. A poison may enter the body by ingestion, absorption, injection, or inhalation. Clinically, poisons are divided into those that respond to specific antidotes or treatment and those for which there is no specific treatment.
Symptoms of ingested poisons: Abdominal pain; cramping; nausea; vomiting; diarrhea; odor, stains, or burns around the mouth; drowsiness; and unconsciousness.
Treating ingested poisons: Call a poison control center, hospital emergency room, physician, or the EMS system for instructions.

Inducing vomiting: Induce vomiting only if directed to do so by a medical authority. When vomiting has stopped, administer 30–50 g of activated charcoal to absorb residual poison.
Treating absorbed poisons: Call a poison control center. Have the patient remove all contaminated clothing. Wash infected skin thoroughly with soap and water, drench it with alcohol, and rinse well. Apply wet compresses soaked in calamine lotion and suggest a bath in colloidal oatmeal or the application of a paste of baking soda and water to soothe the itching.
Symptoms of inhaled poisons: Headache, tinnitus, angina, shortness of breath, muscle weakness, nausea, vomiting, confusion, dizziness, blurred or double vision, unconsciousness, and cardiac arrest. Carbon monoxide is the most commonly inhaled poison.
Treating inhaled poisons: Get the patient into fresh air. Call the EMS system or a poison control center. Loosen tight-fitting clothing, and wrap the patient in a blanket to prevent shock.
Lavage: The process of washing out an organ by first instilling, then removing large amounts of fluid. The organs most commonly lavaged include the urinary bladder (sometimes called bladder irrigation), the bowels (enema), and the stomach. The most common reason for stomach lavage is the removal of poisons.

24.15 Bioterrorism

Bioterrorism: The intentional release of a biological agent with the intent to harm individuals. The CDC defines a biological agent as a weapon when it is easy to disseminate, has a high potential for mortality, can cause a public panic or social disruption, and requires public health preparedness. There are numerous biological agents identified as weapons, including anthrax, tularemia, smallpox, plague, and botulism. The CDC maintains an Internet site with current information about identified biological agents at http://www.emergency.cdc.gov/agent/agentlist.asp.

In recent years, terrorists have used many different substances aside from explosives. These include chemical and biologic agents. Examples of chemical agents have included vesicants (blistering agents), pulmonary (choking) agents, and nerve agents (such as sarin). Biologic agents include viruses, bacteria (most recently, anthrax), and neurotoxins (most recently, ricin).

CHAPTER 24 REVIEW

Instructions:
Answer the following questions.

1. What percentage of the body is involved in a burn that covers one arm and the head of an adult?

   A. 1%
   B. 9%
   C. 18%
   D. 36%
   E. 40%

2. The Good Samaritan law explicitly allows medical assistants

   A. to administer first aid within the scope of their competence.
   B. to call the EMS system and stay with the victim until EMS personnel arrive.
   C. to act freely in an emergency situation to save the victim's life.
   D. to diagnose the patient at the scene of an accident or emergency.
   E. only to call the EMS system and wait for authorized personnel but not to touch or communicate with an accident victim.

3. To treat frostbite, a medical assistant can

   A. massage the affected area gently.
   B. rub the affected area with a warmed towel.
   C. keep the patient's head and shoulders slightly elevated.
   D. wash the area with soap and water.
   E. place warm clothing and blankets around the affected area.

4. When Bill Williams scraped his skin, he most likely got a(n)

   A. incision.
   B. laceration.
   C. abrasion.
   D. puncture.
   E. bruise.

5. Irreversible brain damage can be caused by tissue anoxia lasting more than

   A. two minutes.
   B. three minutes.
   C. four–six minutes.
   D. 45 minutes.
   E. three hours.

6. One possible cause of stroke is

   A. occlusion in the brain by a thrombus.
   B. decreased cerebral blood flow.
   C. ingested poisons.
   D. hypocalcemia.
   E. hyperthermia.

7. The Heimlich maneuver is used for which of the following?

   A. convulsion
   B. epistaxis
   C. hematemesis
   D. shock
   E. choking

8. The most severe and major complication for burn victims is

   A. pain.
   B. anemia.
   C. infection.
   D. malignant fever.
   E. none of these

9. Which of the following should not be done when a patient complains of abdominal pain?

   A. Have the patient lie on the back.
   B. Apply heat to the patient's abdomen.
   C. Have the patient flex the knees.
   D. Monitor the patient's pulse.
   E. Check for signs of shock.

10. When you suspect neck injury, what action should you take to open the patient's airway before administering rescue breathing?

   A. Place your mouth over the patient's nose and blow air into it until the patient's chest rises.
   B. Put your fingers behind the jawbone just below the ear and push the jaw forward.
   C. Wait for EMS personnel, and do not administer rescue breathing.
   D. Hold the patient's neck rigidly while you lift the patient's chin up and push back on the forehead.
   E. Open an airway in the patient's neck with a sterile instrument.

CHAPTER 25

CLINICAL LABORATORY

LEARNING OUTCOMES

25.1 Describe the medical assistant's role in collecting and testing blood samples in the physician's office laboratory.

25.2 Describe the medical assistant's role in collecting, processing, and testing urine specimens.

25.3 Recall the process of collecting and preparing specimens for microbiological examination.

MEDICAL ASSISTING COMPETENCIES

COMPETENCY	CMA	RMA	CCMA	NCMA
Clinical				
Apply principles of aseptic techniques and infection control, including hand washing	X	X	X	X
Dispose of biohazardous materials	X	X	X	X
Practice standard precautions	X	X	X	X
Perform venipuncture	X	X	X	X
Perform capillary puncture	X	X	X	X
Obtain specimens for microbiological testing, including throat specimens and wound cultures	X	X	X	X
Instruct patients in the collection of a clean-catch midstream urine specimen	X	X	X	X
Instruct patients in the collection of fecal specimens	X	X	X	X

MEDICAL ASSISTING COMPETENCIES (cont.)

Clinical

Perform electrocardiography	X	X	X	X
Perform respiratory testing	X	X	X	X
Perform selected CLIA-waived tests (i.e., "kit tests")	X	X	X	X
Perform urinalysis	X	X	X	X
Perform hematological testing	X	X	X	X
Perform chemistry testing	X	X	X	
Perform immunology testing	X	X	X	
Perform microbiology testing	X	X	X	
Screen and follow up on patient test results	X	X	X	X

General/Legal/Professional

Identify and respond to issues of confidentiality by maintaining confidentiality at all times and following appropriate guidelines when releasing records or information	X	X	X	
Be aware of and perform within legal and ethical boundaries	X	X	X	X
Determine the needs for documentation and reporting, and document accurately and appropriately	X	X	X	X
Demonstrate knowledge of and monitor current federal and state health-care legislation and regulations; maintain licenses and accreditation	X	X	X	X
Perform risk management procedures	X	X	X	
Explain general office policies and procedures	X	X	X	X
Instruct individuals according to their needs	X	X	X	X
Perform quality control procedures	X	X	X	X
Conduct work within scope of education, training, and ability	X	X	X	X
Understand allied health professions and credentialing	X	X	X	X

STRATEGIES FOR SUCCESS

▶ *Study Skills*

Take study breaks!
Long periods of uninterrupted studying can dull your concentration, make your mind wander, and lead you to daydream. So, after a few hours of studying, treat yourself to a mental break. Giving yourself short, well-defined breaks will help prevent burnout and keep your energy focused. Take a walk outside, read an article in a magazine, or do something that relaxes and refreshes you. Then get back to studying.

25.1 Collecting and Testing Blood

Medical assistant's role: In the physician's office laboratory (POL), the medical assistant's roles include preparing patients for tests, collecting samples, completing testing, and reporting results to the physician. The degree of federal or state regulation depends on the complexity of tests performed.

Hematology

Hematology: The study of blood and blood-forming tissues.

Functions of blood: To distribute oxygen, nutrients, and hormones to body cells; to eliminate waste products from body cells; to attack infecting organisms or pathogens; to maintain the body's acid-base balance; and to regulate body temperature.

Hematopoiesis: The normal formation and development of blood cells in the bone marrow.

Whole blood: Consists of plasma and the formed elements. In adults, total blood volume normally makes up 7–8% of body weight, or 70 mL/kg of body weight in men and about 65 mL/kg in women. Blood is pumped through the body at a speed of about 30 cm per second, with complete circulation in 20 seconds.

Plasma: The liquid in which the other components of blood are suspended. Plasma accounts for 55% of the body's total blood volume. Water makes up about 90% of plasma. About 9% is protein and 1% is other substances, including carbohydrates, fats, gases, mineral salts, protective substances, and waste products. Free of its formed elements and particles, plasma is a clear, yellow fluid. When a tube of blood is centrifuged, the plasma rises to the top.

Formed elements, or blood cells: Red cells (erythrocytes), white cells (leukocytes), and platelets (thrombocytes). Blood cells constitute about 45% of the body's total volume of blood. An older term for a formed element is blood corpuscle. See Figure 25-1.

Blood gas: Dissolved gas in the liquid part of the blood. Blood gases include oxygen, carbon dioxide, and nitrogen.

Bone marrow: Found in the cavities of all bones. It may be present in two forms: red and yellow. Yellow marrow is inactive and is composed mostly of fat tissue. Red marrow is active in the production of most types of blood cells. By age 18, red marrow is found only in the vertebrae, ribs, sternum, skull bones, and pelvis.

Erythrocytes

Erythrocyte: Also known as a red blood cell (RBC). A mature RBC is made up of lipids and proteins to which hemoglobin molecules are attached. RBCs play a vital role in internal respiration, the exchange of gases between blood and body cells. They are disk shaped and have concave sides.

Red blood cell indices: Using blood from a CBC, these are used to classify anemias, select more tests to determine their causes, and to monitor anemia treatments. They include *mean corpuscular volume (MCV), mean corpuscular hemoglobin (MCH),* and *MCH concentration or content (MCHC).*

Mean corpuscular volume (MCV): The most important index for classifying anemias as macrocytic or microcytic, it measures the size of RBCs. Normal reference range is 82–108 femtoliters (fL). A femtoliter is equivalent to one cubic micrometer.

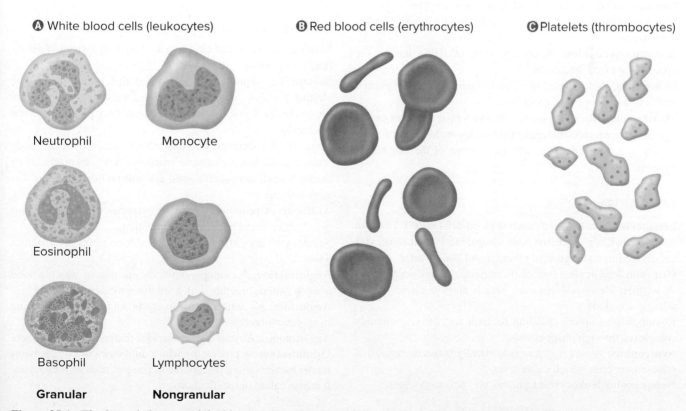

A White blood cells (leukocytes)

Neutrophil Monocyte

Eosinophil

Basophil Lymphocytes

Granular **Nongranular**

B Red blood cells (erythrocytes)

C Platelets (thrombocytes)

Figure 25-1 *The formed elements of the blood are (A) white blood cells, (B) red blood cells, and (C) platelets.*

Mean corpuscular hemoglobin (MCH): Calculates the average weight of hemoglobin in a single red blood cell.

MCH concentration or content (MCHC): Calculates the average weight of hemoglobin compared with the RBC size.

Erythropoiesis: The process of erythrocyte production. This process develops in the embryonic yolk sac, liver, and spleen. It is ultimately located in the red bone marrow during late fetal development, childhood, and adult life.

Erythropoietin: A glycoprotein hormone, produced primarily by the kidneys and also secreted by the liver, that stimulates erythropoiesis. It can cross the placental barrier.

Reticulocyte: The last stage of the immature erythrocyte. This cell has a nucleus and is found both in the bone marrow and, often, in peripheral blood.

Anisochromia: A difference in color in two structures or parts of the same color that are normally identical; also known as *heterochromia*.

Anisocytosis: Presence in the blood of erythrocytes showing excessive variations in size.

Poikilocytosis: Presence in the blood of erythrocytes showing abnormal variations in shape.

Polychromasia: Variation in the hemoglobin content of erythrocytes; also known as *polychromatophilia*.

Spherocytosis: The presence of spherocytes in the blood, which are small, spherical RBCs characteristic of certain hemolytic anemias.

Transferrin: A specific transport protein in the blood. It binds iron and transports it back to the bone marrow for hemoglobin synthesis.

Hemoglobin: The iron-containing pigment of RBCs that carries oxygen from the lungs to the tissues.

Hemagglutination: The coagulation of erythrocytes.

Hemagglutinin: A type of antibody that agglutinates erythrocytes.

Rouleaux formation: A configuration of RBCs having the appearance of stacked coins.

Hematocrit: Abbreviated *Hct,* this is a measurement of packed RBCs in a certain volume of blood.

Microhematocrit: The *spun microhematocrit test* utilizes centrifugation to separate cellular elements from plasma. Microhematocrits should be performed twice, with the average of the two results reported.

Leukocytes

Leukocyte: Also known as a white blood cell (WBC). Through phagocytosis, it protects the body against infection. Leukocytes are divided into two groups: granular and nongranular.

Granular leukocytes: Basophils, eosinophils, and neutrophils.

Basophils: Produce histamine, which plays a major role in allergic reactions.

Eosinophils: Capture invading bacteria and antigen-antibody complexes through phagocytosis.

Neutrophils: Attack invaders (specifically target bacteria) and release pyrogens, which cause fever.

Nongranular leukocytes: Lymphocytes and monocytes.

Lymphocytes: The smallest leukocytes, which contain the largest nuclei. They include B cells and T cells. B lymphocytes produce antibodies to combat specific pathogens. T lymphocytes regulate the immune response.

Monocytes: Large leukocytes in the bloodstream with oval or horseshoe-shaped nuclei. Their major functions are phagocytosis and synthesis of various biological compounds, including transferrin, complement, interferon, and certain growth factors.

Macrophages: Monocytes that mature outside the circulatory system, distributed in tissues throughout the body. They have a variety of names (often depending on their location in the body), such as histiocytes, Kupffer cells, osteoclasts, and microglial cells.

Phagocytes: Cells that have the capacity for phagocytosis. Macrophages, as well as most of the leukocytes, are phagocytes. Large phagocytes can destroy worn-out RBCs or bacteria. They are found in the spleen, thymus, and lymphoid tissues.

Phagocytosis: The process by which cells engulf and ingest microorganisms.

Thrombocytes

Platelets: Metabolically active anuclear cell fragments produced in the bone marrow that assist in blood coagulation and clotting. They are also called thrombocytes. Normally, 130,000,400,000 platelets are found in one cubic milliliter of blood.

Megakaryocytes: Precursors of platelets. They are the largest cells found in the bone marrow, and they have a nucleus with many lobes. They are normally not present in circulating blood.

Serology and Immunology

Serology: The study of blood serum based on antigen-antibody reactions in vitro.

Serum: The liquid portion of blood that remains after the clotting proteins and cells have been removed. It differs from plasma in that it does not contain fibrinogen, a protein involved in clotting.

Antigen: A substance on cells whose presence in the body stimulates the body's immune response. Antigens produced by the body itself are autoantigens; antigens on other cells are foreign antigens.

Antibody: A protein produced in response to a specific antigen. It defends the body against infection.

Serology abbreviations: Common abbreviations are listed in Table 25-1.

Agglutination: An antigen-antibody reaction in which a solid antigen clumps together with a soluble antibody.

Agglutinin: An antibody that interacts with antigens, resulting in agglutination.

Agglutinogen: Any antigenic substance that causes agglutination.

Opsonization: A process by which antibodies or complements render bacteria more susceptible to phagocytosis by leukocytes. It is also called opsonification.

Ab	antibody		CHE	cholinesterase
ABO	classification system for four blood groups		CK	creatine kinase
AcAc	acetoacetate		CMV	cytomegalovirus
ACE	angiotensin-converting enzyme		CN−	cyanide anion
ACT	activated coagulation time		CO	carbon monoxide
ACTH	adrenocorticotropic hormone		CO_2	carbon dioxide
ADH	antidiuretic hormone		COHb	carboxyhemoglobin
AFB	acid-fast bacillus		Cr	creatinine
AFP	alpha-fetoprotein		CrCl	creatinine clearance
Ag	antigen		CT	calcitonin
AG	anion gap		DAF	decay accelerating factor
A/G R	albumin-globulin ratio		DHEA	dehydroepiandrosterone, unconjugated
AHF	antihemolytic factor		Diff	differential (blood cell count)
Alb	albumin		EBNA	Epstein-Barr virus nuclear antigen
Alc	alcohol		EBV	Epstein-Barr virus
ALG	antilymphocyte globulin		EDTA	ethylenediaminetetraacetic acid
ALP; alk phos	alkaline phosphatase		Eos	eosinophil
ALT	alanine aminotransferase		EP	electrophoresis
ANA	antinuclear antibody		Eq	equivalent
APAP	acetaminophen		ERP	estrogen receptor protein
APTT	activated partial thromboplastin time		ESR	erythrocyte sedimentation rate
ASA	acetylsalicylic acid (aspirin)		FBS	fasting blood sugar
AST	aspartate aminotransferase		FFA	free fatty acids
AT-III	antithrombin III		FSH	follicle-stimulating hormone (follitropin)
B	blood (whole blood)		FT_4	free thyroxine
Baso	basophil		FT_4I	free thyroxine index
BCA	breast cancer antigen		GFR	glomerular filtration rate
BJP	Bence Jones protein		GH	growth hormone
BT	bleeding time		GHRH	growth hormone–releasing hormone
BUN	blood urea nitrogen		GnRH	gonadotropin-releasing hormone
Ca; Ca^{++}	calcium		GTT	glucose tolerance test
CA	cancer antigen		HA	hemagglutination
CBC	complete blood (cell) count		HAI	hemagglutination inhibition test
CEA	carcinoembryonic antigen		HAV	hepatitis A virus
Hb; Hgb	hemoglobin		P	plasma
HbCO	carboxyhemoglobin		PAP	prostatic acid phosphatase
HBV	hepatitis B virus		PB	protein binding

Table 25-1 continued

HCG; hCG	human chorionic gonadotropin		PBG	porphobilinogen
Hct	hematocrit		PCT	prothrombin consumption time
HCV	hepatitis C virus		PCV	packed cell volume (hematocrit)
HDL	high-density lipoprotein		P_i	inorganic phosphate
HDV	hepatitis delta virus		PKU	phenylketonuria
HGH; hGH	human growth hormone		PLT	platelet
HIV	human immunodeficiency virus		PMN	polymorphonuclear (leukocyte; neutrophil)
HLA	human leukocyte antigen		PRL	prolactin
HPV	human papilloma virus		PSA	prostate-specific antigen
HSV	herpes simplex virus		PT	prothrombin time
HTLV	human T-cell lymphotrophic virus		PTH	parathyroid hormone
Ig	immunoglobulin		PTT	partial thromboplastin time
IgE	immunoglobulin E		PV	plasma volume
INH	inhibitor		PZP	pregnancy zone protein
IV	intravenous		RAIU	thyroid uptake of radioactive iodine
L	liver		RBC	red blood cell; red blood (cell) count
LD; LDH	lactate dehydrogenase		RBP	retinol-binding protein
LDL	low-density lipoprotein		RCM	red cell mass
LH	luteinizing hormone		RCV	red cell volume
LMWH	low-molecular-weight heparin		RDW	red cell distribution of width
Lytes	electrolytes		Retic	reticulocyte
MCV	mean corpuscular volume		RF	rheumatoid factor; relative fluorescence unit
MetHb	methemoglobin		Rh	rhesus factor
MLC	mixed lymphocyte culture		RIA	radioimmunoassay
MONO	monocyte		rT_3	reverse triiodothyronine
MPV	mean platelet volume		S	serum
MSAFP	maternal serum alpha-fetoprotein		Segs	segmented polymorphonuclear leukocyte
NE	norepinephrine		SPE	serum protein electrophoresis
NPN	nonprotein nitrogen		T_3	triiodothyronine
OGTT	oral glucose tolerance test		T_4	thyroxine
TBG	thyroxine-binding globulin		VDRL	Venereal Disease Research Laboratory (test for syphilis)
TBV	total blood volume		VLDL	very-low-density lipoprotein
TG	triglyceride		WB	Western blot
TRH	thyrotropin-releasing hormone		WBC	white blood cell; white blood (cell) count
TSH	thyroid-stimulating hormone			

Table 25-1, concluded

Immunology: The study of the reaction of immune system tissues to antigenic stimulation.

Immune: Protected by antibodies against infective or allergic disease.

Immune response: A defense function of the body that produces antibodies to destroy invading antigens and cancer cells.

Antiserum: A serum of animal or human origin that contains antibodies against a specific disease. It is also called immune serum. Antiserums (or antisera) do not provoke the production of antibodies. There are two types: antitoxin and antimicrobial.

Complement: Protein molecules that are chief humoral mediators of antigen-antibody reactions in the immune system. Complement proteins stimulate phagocytosis and inflammation.

Classification of immunoglobulin: In response to specific antigens, immunoglobulins are formed in the bone marrow, the spleen, and all lymphoid tissue of the body except the thymus. All antibodies are immunoglobulins.

Collecting Blood

Collecting blood: The two common ways to collect blood are phlebotomy and capillary puncture. Some, but not all, states permit medical assistants to obtain blood samples. You should know the appropriate laws of your state.

Phlebotomy: The insertion of a needle or IV catheter into a vein to draw blood. It is also called venipuncture or venesection. Phlebotomy is the most common method of collecting blood for hematological testing. The most common site for venipuncture is the median cubital vein. The cephalic vein of the forearm, the basilic vein of the forearm, and the veins in the back of the hand are also sometimes used. See Figure 25-2.

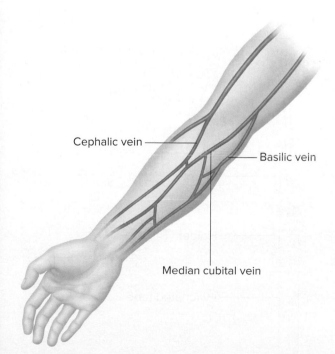

Cephalic vein

Basilic vein

Median cubital vein

Figure 25-2 *Veins commonly used for venipuncture include the cephalic vein, the basilic vein, and the median cubital vein.*

Capillary puncture: A superficial puncture of the skin with a sharp point that releases a smaller amount of blood than venipuncture. It is also called a finger stick. Capillary puncture in adults and children is usually performed on the great (middle) finger or the ring finger. Try to use the patient's nondominant hand, and do not reuse a previous puncture site. Capillary puncture in infants is usually performed on one of the outer edges of the underside of the heel. The rear curve of the heel should never be punctured. An alternate site for both children and adults is the lower side of a nonpierced earlobe. A puncture should not be deeper than 2.4 mm (0.1 in). Puncturing skin that is still wet from an alcohol swab will be painful, and can hemolyze the specimen. Capillary puncture is indicated for older patients, children (especially under age two years), when the patient has burns or scars in venipuncture sites, when the patient requires frequent glucose monitoring, for obese patients, for patients receiving IV therapy, for postmastectomy patients, for severely dehydrated patients, for those at risk for venous thrombosis, and when only a small amount of blood is needed for testing. Capillary blood is a mixture of arterial and venal blood, as well as small amounts of tissue fluid (especially in the first drop following puncture). In capillary blood, hemoglobin and glucose values are higher, while calcium, potassium, and total protein are lower.

Needlestick Safety and Prevention Act: In response to the Needlestick Safety and Prevention Act, which was signed into law in November 2000, OSHA revised the Blood-Borne Pathogens Standard. The additional provisions to the standard are:

- Health-care employers must evaluate new safety-engineered control devices on an annual basis and implement the use of devices that reasonably reduce the risk of needlestick injuries.

- Health-care facilities must maintain a detailed log of sharps injuries that are incurred from contaminated sharps.

- Health-care employers must solicit input from employees involved in direct patient care to identify, evaluate, and implement engineering and work practice controls.

Quality Control Procedures

Quality control: When taking a blood specimen, follow quality-control procedures.

1. Review the request form, verify the procedure, and prepare the equipment, paperwork, and work area.

2. Identify the patient, confirm the patient's identification, and explain the procedure.

3. Confirm that the patient has followed pretest preparation requirements.

4. Collect the specimen properly, using sterile equipment and proper technique.

5. Use the correct specimen collection containers and preservatives.

6. Immediately label the specimens with the patient's name, date and time of collection, test name, and name of the person collecting the specimen.

7. Follow correct procedures for disposing of hazardous waste and decontaminating the work area.

8. Prepare the specimen for transport in the proper container, following OSHA regulations.

Documentation: Maintain the quality control log, reagent control log, equipment maintenance log, reference laboratory log, and daily workload log, as applicable.

Quality control log: Shows the completion of every quality control check conducted on a piece of equipment. The testing equipment must be calibrated regularly in accordance with manufacturer's guidelines. Calibration routines are performed on a set of standards, the values of which are already known.

Control sample: A specimen with a known value that is used every time a patient sample is processed. Using a control sample serves as a check on the accuracy of the test.

Reagent: A chemical or chemically treated substance that reacts in specific ways when exposed under specific conditions.

Reagent control log: Shows the quality testing performed on every batch or lot of reagent products. Control samples or standards are run every time you open a new supply of testing products, such as staining materials, culture media, and reagents.

Equipment maintenance record: Documents any maintenance done on laboratory equipment.

Reference laboratory log: Lists specimens sent to another laboratory for testing.

Daily workload log: Shows all procedures completed during the workday.

Laboratory requisition form: The completed form should be included with the specimen collected or sent with the patient to the laboratory. Be sure to include the following information on all requisitions:

- Patient's full name, sex, date of birth, and address
- Patient's insurance information
- Physician's name, address, and phone number
- Source of the specimen
- Date and time of the specimen collection
- Test(s) requested
- Preliminary diagnosis
- Any current treatment that might affect the results

Patient record: Record test results in the patient's record, and properly identify any unusual findings. Remember that only a physician is qualified to interpret test results, so these results should not be communicated to the patient until the physician has had an opportunity to review the information.

Blood Collecting Equipment

Equipment needed: Typically includes a needle, syringe, tube, or lancet to draw blood; alcohol and cotton balls or alcohol wipes; sterile gauze; adhesive bandages; and a tourniquet.

Venipuncture collection needle: Specially designed needle used with an evacuated tube blood collection system ranging from 19–23 gauge and 1–1.5 inches in length. A 21-gauge needle is used most commonly for a routine venipuncture. Using a small-gauge needle such as 25 gauge can cause hemolysis.

Blood lancet: A small, sterile, disposable instrument used for skin or capillary puncture.

Automatic puncturing device: A spring-loaded mechanism equipped with a disposable lancet for capillary puncture.

Micropipette: A calibrated glass tube for measuring small, precise volumes of fluids used in capillary puncture.

Unopette®: A disposable micropipette blood-diluting system used to perform manual blood counts. (It is manufactured by Becton Dickinson Vacutainer® Systems.)

Reagent strip: Used with freshly collected blood droplets in capillary puncture. It is also referred to as a dipstick. Blood is dropped or smeared on the strip. Some of the blood tests performed in this way are those for determining blood glucose levels, sickle cell anemia, infectious mononucleosis, and rheumatoid arthritis.

Smear slide: A prepared microscope slide to which freshly collected blood is applied.

Butterfly needle set: A device used to collect blood samples from individuals with small or fragile veins. It consists of a needle with plastic wings, flexible tubing, an adapter, and a collection device. A butterfly system generally uses a smaller needle (23–25 gauge) than other venipuncture techniques do. Once inserted, the needle is held in place by holding the wing of the needle while the collection device is manipulated.

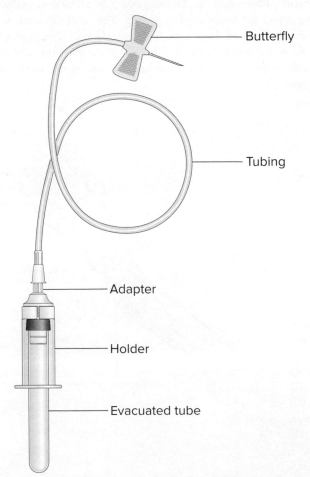

Figure 25-3 *A butterfly system is used to collect blood from individuals with fragile or small veins.*

The needle causes less trauma to the vein and surrounding tissue if the patient moves during the collection of the specimen. See Figure 25-3.

Engineered safety devices: In response to the Needlestick Safety and Prevention Act, a number of engineered safety devices have been developed. These devices are intended to reduce the possibility of needlestick injuries. According to the National Institute for Occupational Safety and Health (NIOSH), the desired characteristics of engineered safety devices include the following:

- The performance of the device is reliable.
- The device is easy to use, safe, and effective.
- The device should be needleless when possible.
- The device either should not have to be activated by the user or may be activated with only one hand.
- Once the safety feature is activated, it cannot be deactivated.

In certain circumstances, some of these characteristics are not feasible. Drawing blood from an artery or a vein is not possible without the use of a needle. Several types of safety devices for collecting blood specimens have been developed. These include:

- Retracting needles
- Shields that are hinged or sliding that cover phlebotomy needles and winged-steel (butterfly) needles
- Self-blunting phlebotomy and winged-steel needles
- Retractable lancets

In addition to the use of appropriate safety-engineered devices, NIOSH also recommends that health-care workers follow these precautions:

- One-handed recap of needles should only be done when absolutely necessary.
- Ensure the safe handling and disposal of sharps before beginning a procedure.
- Dispose of used sharps promptly, using approved sharps containers.
- Report all needlestick injuries.
- Inform their employer of workplace hazards.
- Attend yearly blood-borne pathogen training.
- Follow recommended infection control practices.

Evacuation tube: The most common evacuation system is the Vacutainer® system (manufactured by Becton Dickinson Vacutainer® Systems). It uses a special needle, a needle holder/adapter, and collection tubes that have been sealed to maintain a slight vacuum. See Figure 25-4. Some tubes are prepared with additives needed to process the blood sample for testing, such as anticoagulants. The tube stoppers are color-coded according to the type of additive used. See Table 25-2. Expired tubes may no longer have a vacuum.

Collection tubes: No matter which method is used to collect blood, the samples must immediately be mixed with the appropriate additives in the correct collection tubes before they are transported to the laboratory for testing. Each laboratory may choose which tubes to use for a particular test.

Anticoagulants: Substances that prevent blood clotting. Three anticoagulants commonly used in the hematology laboratory are heparin, sodium citrate, and ethylenediaminetetraacetic acid (EDTA).

Heparin: A substance produced naturally by basophils and mast cells. Heparin acts in the body as an antithrombin factor to prevent intravascular clotting. As an additive in blood collection, heparin is used in electrolyte studies and tests for arterial blood gases. Heparin also is used as an anticoagulant in the prevention and treatment of thrombosis and embolism.

Sodium citrate: A white granular powder, used as an anticoagulant in transfusions and coagulation studies.

EDTA: Used as an anticoagulant additive in hematology studies. It also is used to treat exposure to toxic chemicals; it chemically "grasps" toxic substances, thereby making them nonactive. Excessive EDTA produces a shrinkage of the erythrocytes.

Antiseptic: A cleaning product used on human tissue that inhibits the growth and reproduction of microorganisms. Some examples of antiseptics are 70% isopropyl alcohol, povidone-iodine (Betadine®), and benzalkonium chloride (Zephiran®).

NOTE: Red-stoppered tubes do not contain an anticoagulant, and should not be mixed after collection.

Betadine®: An antiseptic recommended for use in arterial blood gas studies and blood culture draws.

Zephiran®: A trade name for benzalkonium chloride, used in blood collection to detect alcohol levels.

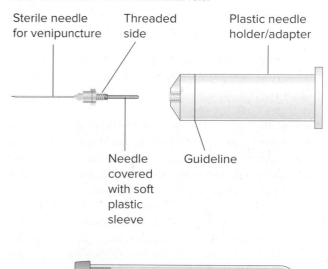

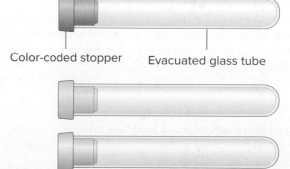

Figure 25-4 *The Vacutainer® system uses interchangeable collection tubes that allow you to draw several blood specimens from the same venipuncture site.*

Color	Additive	Test Types
Yellow	Sodium polyanetholesulfonate	Plasma cultures
Light blue	Sodium citrate (anticoagulant)	Coagulation studies
Red	None	Blood chemistries, AIDS, antibody tests, viral studies, serological tests, blood grouping and typing
Red/black (tiger stripes or marbled)	Silicone serum separator	Tests requiring blood serum
Green	Sodium heparin (anticoagulant)	Electrolyte studies, arterial blood gas tests
Lavender	EDTA (anticoagulant)	Hematology studies, such as complete blood count, WBC differential, and platelet count
Gray	Potassium oxalate or sodium fluoride (anticoagulant)	Blood glucose tests

Table 25-2

Labeling containers: After blood is drawn, all tubes, slides, and other containers should be labeled with the patient's name, the date and time of collection, the initials of the person who collected the specimen, and any other required information, such as the patient's identification code.

Tube size: Tubes range in size from 15 mL down. Most tubes used for adults range three–10 mL, and those for children range two–four mL. Microcapillary collection tubes hold less than one mL.

Order of draw tubes: The National Committee for Clinical Laboratory Standards publishes the recommended order of draw as follows: yellow, light blue, red, red/black (tiger stripes), green, lavender, and gray.

Tourniquet: A device used to control hemorrhage or to distend veins for the withdrawal of blood. It should not remain on the patient's arm longer than one minute. It is placed on the upper arm of the patient, three–four inches above the elbow. Latex-free tourniquets are the most commonly used.

Gloves: Made from a variety of materials, such as vinyl, latex, and nitrile. Latex gloves were formerly the most commonly used, but no longer, since many individuals are highly allergic to latex. Nitrile gloves are more tear-resistant and feel more comfortable on the hand.

Needle disposal: Needles must be properly disposed of in appropriate sharps containers. They should not be laid down or placed on any surface and should not be recapped except when absolutely necessary.

Procedures

Assembling equipment and supplies: After reviewing the test order, make sure that you have the appropriate equipment to collect the required samples.

Preparing patients: After greeting the patient, ask for the patient's full name to verify that the patient is the one listed on the order. Confirm that the patient has followed any pretest restrictions, such as fasting before the appointment.

Universal precautions: It is important to follow universal precautions during all phlebotomy procedures. Before collecting blood, make sure to wash your hands and put on examination gloves. When you have finished drawing blood, properly dispose of used supplies and disposable instruments, disinfect the area, remove the gloves, and wash your hands.

Steps in venipuncture or phlebotomy: The following steps describe how to perform venipuncture using the evacuation method.

1. Prepare the needle holder/adapter assembly, and push the collection tube into the open end of the needle holder/adapter. Do not puncture the stopper yet. You usually use a 19–23 gauge needle for venipuncture.

2. Ask the patient which arm he or she prefers you to use, and make sure that the arm is positioned slightly downward.

3. Apply tourniquet to the patient's upper arm.

4. Palpate the site, using your index finger to locate the vein.

5. Clean area with antiseptic or an antiseptic wipe. Use a circular motion to clean the area, starting at the center and working outward. Let the site dry.

6. Remove cap from outer point of the needle.

7. Ask the patient to make a fist.

8. Hold the patient's skin taut above and below the insertion site. Holding the needle at approximately a 15-degree angle, use a steady and quick motion to insert the needle into the vein to a depth of one inch.

9. Seat the collection tube firmly into place over the needle, puncturing the stopper.

10. Once blood is flowing steadily, ask the patient to release the fist, and untie the tourniquet. Switch tubes as needed, using a smooth and steady motion. Fill each tube until the blood stops running. An evacuation tube containing an additive must be filled completely. The last tube must be removed before removing the needle, or bruising will occur.

11. As you withdraw the needle in a smooth and steady motion, immediately activate the safety mechanism, then place a sterile gauze square over the insertion site. Have the patient hold the gauze in place and keep the arm straight and slightly elevated.

12. If the collection tubes contain additives, invert them slowly several times to mix the chemical with the blood.

13. Check the patient's condition and the puncture site for bleeding, and replace the gauze square with a sterile adhesive bandage.

Steps in capillary puncture: The following steps are taken in capillary puncture using the finger stick method.

1. Examine the patient's hand to determine which finger to use for the procedure. If necessary, warm the hands to improve circulation. Keep the hand below heart level.

2. Prepare the finger by gently rubbing it, and clean the area with a cotton ball and antiseptic or an antiseptic wipe.

3. Hold the patient's finger between the thumb and forefinger of one hand.

4. Hold the lancet at a right angle to the lateral aspect of the pad of the patient's finger (near the part that leaves a fingerprint).

5. Puncture the skin with a quick, sharp motion.

6. Allow a drop of blood to form. If it is slow in forming, apply steady pressure, but do not milk the finger.

7. Wipe away the first droplet of blood.

8. Fill the collection devices.

9. When the samples have been collected, wipe the patient's finger with a sterile gauze square.

10. Check the site for bleeding. If necessary, apply a sterile adhesive bandage.

Chain of custody: A means of ensuring that a specimen obtained from a patient is correctly identified, is under the uninterrupted control of authorized personnel, and has not been altered or replaced. It is established for blood samples drawn for drug and alcohol analysis as well as for specimens taken in cases of medico-legal importance such as rape. Because donating a specimen for drug and alcohol testing is potentially self-incriminating, the patient must sign a consent form for the testing.

Handling an exposure incident: Following universal precautions should reduce your risk of exposure, but accidents sometimes still happen. If you suffer a needlestick or other injury that results in exposure to blood or blood products from another person, report the incident to the appropriate staff members immediately. Wash the injured area carefully, and apply a sterile bandage. Record the time, date, and nature of the incident and the names of the people involved. Hepatitis B virus is the main blood-borne hazard for health-care workers.

Complications of Blood Collection

Syncope: Fainting, usually caused by pain, fright, and the sight of blood. Syncope lasts only one–two minutes. If fainting occurs, the procedure must be terminated immediately. The patient should be placed lying down, with legs elevated. The event should be completely documented on the laboratory log. Assistance should be called for, and the patient should never be left alone.

Failure to obtain blood: There are several factors that may make blood collection impossible. It is important to remain calm and to determine the cause of the problem. If you cannot collect a good sample on the second try, do not make a third attempt. Ask for assistance.

Scarred and sclerosed veins: Do not draw blood from injured or diseased areas.

Hematoma: A pooling of blood just under the skin. It is caused by blood leaking into the tissues (infiltration). When it happens, pressure should be applied to the area for three minutes, and then ice should be applied.

Hemorrhage: Excessive bleeding.

Petechiae: Tiny red spots appearing on the skin as a result of small hemorrhages within the dermal layer. They may be a complication of keeping a tourniquet in place for longer than two minutes, which can also cause hemolysis.

Testing Blood
Hematology

Hematological tests: May be performed on venous or capillary whole blood specimens. These tests include blood cell count, morphological studies, coagulation tests, and the erythrocyte sedimentation rate test. See Table 25-3 for normal ranges of selected blood tests.

Erythrocyte sedimentation rate (ESR, or sed rate) test: Measures the rate at which RBCs settle out in a tube of unclotted blood, expressed in millimeters per hour. The test determines the degree of inflammation in the body. For the ESR using the modified Westergen method, the test pipette must stand for 60 minutes.

Bleeding time test: Gives information about the integrity of the patient's platelet function. A prolonged bleeding time indicates such conditions as low platelet count and dysfunction of the platelets. Aspirin impairs the platelets' ability to form aggregates. Antihistamines also interfere with bleeding time.

Blood smears: Used to obtain a differential cell count and to reveal abnormal RBC morphology for anemia. To prepare a blood smear slide, apply a drop of blood to the slide, one inch from the frosted end, and use a spreader slide at a 30- to 35-degree angle to spread the blood droplet. See Figures 25-5, 25-6, and 25-7.

Test	Blood Component	Normal Range
Red blood cells	Whole blood	Men: 4.3–5.7×10^6 cells/μL
		Women: 3.8–5.1×10^6 cells/μL
White blood cells	Whole blood	4.5–11.0×10^3 cells/μL
Platelets	Whole blood	150–400×10^3 cells/μL
Hematocrit (Hct)	Whole blood	Men: 39–49% Women: 35–45%
Hemoglobin (Hb, Hgb)	Whole blood	Men: 13.2–17.3g/dL Women: 11.7–16.0 g/dL
Bleeding time	Whole blood	2–7 minutes
Cholesterol, total	Serum, plasma	Men: 158–277 mg/dL Women: 162–285 mg/dL
Glucose (fasting blood sugar [FBS])	Serum	74–120 mg/dL
Insulin	Serum	<17 μU/mL
Iron, total	Serum	Men: 65–175 μg/dL Women: 50–170 μg/dL
Uric acid	Serum	Men: 4.4–7.6 mg/dL Women: 2.3–6.6 mg/dL

Table 25-3

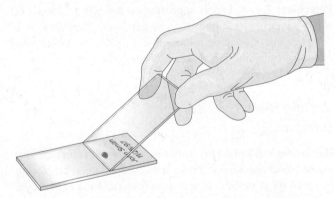

Figure 25-5 *Hold the spreader slide at a 30- to 35-degree angle. Pull the spreader slide toward the frosted end until it touches the drop of blood.*

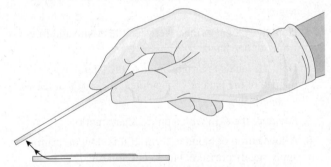

Figure 25-7 *Lift the spreader slide away from the smear slide, maintaining a 30- to 35-degree angle. The smear should be thicker on the frosted end of the slide.*

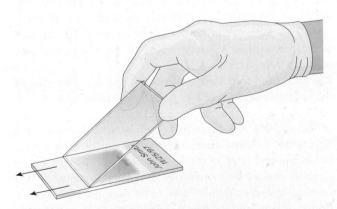

Figure 25-6 *When the drop covers most of the spreader slide edge, push the spreader slide back toward the unfrosted end of the smear slide.*

Prothrombin time (PT): A prolonged PT indicates deficiency in one of the clotting factors, as in liver disease, vitamin K deficiency, or anticoagulation therapy with the drug *warfarin sodium*.

Partial thromboplastin time (PTT): A test for detecting coagulation defects. It is one of the basic tests used to measure specific factor activity, and to detect hemophilias. It can be used to monitor the activity of the anticoagulant *heparin*.

Clotting time: The time required for blood to form a clot. Its chief application is in monitoring anticoagulant therapy. It is rarely used in clinical practice.

Stains: Used to selectively color microscopic objects and tissues for study. Common stains are termed *polychromatic* because they contain dyes that stain various cell components different colors. They usually contain *methylene blue* and *eosin* (a red-orange stain), each of which is attracted to different cell parts, helping them to be visualized more easily. The most common differential blood stain is *Wright's stain,* which usually contains mixtures of methylene blue, eosin Y, azure A, and thionin. Some common stains are listed in Table 25-4.

Morphological studies: Used in the examination of a blood smear for the purpose of recording the appearance and shape of cells, with special note made of abnormal cell size, shape, or content and abnormal organization of cells.

Coagulation tests: Used to identify bleeding problems, generally scheduled before surgery or to monitor therapeutic drug levels.

Hemoglobin (Hgb or Hb) tests: Used to measure the concentration of hemoglobin in the blood. Hb testing can be performed on either venous or capillary whole blood specimens. Among the types of hemoglobin are hemoglobin A, hemoglobin F, and hemoglobin S. Hemoglobin level is high at birth but declines during childhood. It then increases at different ages.

Hemoglobin A: Normal adult hemoglobin.

Hemoglobin F (HbF): Fetal hemoglobin, the normal hemoglobin of the fetus and the predominant hemoglobin variety in the fetus and neonate. Most HbF is replaced by hemoglobin A in the first days after birth.

Hemoglobin S: Sickle-shaped hemoglobin, found in sickle cell anemia and also in sickle cell trait. It is found primarily in persons of African descent. About 8% of African Americans in the United States are affected, and Hispanics of Caribbean ancestry are also commonly affected.

Blood count: The complete blood count (CBC) is the most common laboratory procedure ordered on blood. It includes the red blood count (RBC), white blood count (WBC), differential WBC, and platelet count, as well as a hematocrit determination and a hemoglobin determination.

Hematocrit (Hct): The relative volume of RBCs in a blood sample after the sample has been spun in a centrifuge (packed cell volume), expressed as a percentage. The erythrocytes collect at the bottom of the tube. Above the packed erythrocytes is a layer of leukocytes and thrombocytes. This layer is called the buffy coat. Above the buffy coat is the plasma, which is free of cell elements. The packed cell volume is reported as the *microhematocrit,* in percentage.

Serology

Serological tests: Used to detect the presence of specific substances in blood serum (e.g., disease antibodies, drugs, hormones, and vitamins) and to determine blood types. See Table 25-5.

Amylase test: Amylase is an enzyme of the exocrine pancreas. Its function is to break down starches into dextrin and maltose during the digestive processes. Blood serum is tested for increased amylase levels, which may occur in patients with a perforated ulcer, salivary gland disease, obstruction of the pancreas duct, or cancer of the pancreas. Decreased amylase levels are seen in patients with extensive destruction of the pancreas and hepatic insufficiency.

Western blot: Confirms the presence of HIV.

Radioimmunoassay (RIA): Uses radioisotopes to "tag" antibodies.

Enzyme-linked immunosorbent assay (ELISA): Used to diagnose HIV infection. Enzyme-labeled antigens and substances able to absorb antigens generate reactions to certain antibodies.

Immunofluorescent antibody (IFA) test: Dye that is visible when a sample is examined under a fluorescent microscope is used to color certain antibodies.

Rapid screening tests: Used for quick processing, include the following:

- Home early pregnancy tests
- HIV: Clearview HIV Stat-Pak® (Chembio Diagnostic Systems, Inc.); Uni-gold Recombigen HIV Test® (Trinity Biotech plc)
- *Helicobacter pylori:* Beckman Coulter ICON HP Test® (Princeton Biomed-tech Corp.); Rapid Response *H. pylori* Rapid Test Device® (Acon Laboratories, Inc.)
- Infectious mononucleosis: BioStar Acceava Mono II® (Acon Laboratories, Inc.); LifeSign Status Mono® (Princeton Biomed-tech Corp.)

AT A GLANCE Common Stains

Stain	Use
Acidic	To stain basic elements of cells
Basic	To stain the nucleic or acidic elements of cells
Contrast	To color one part of a tissue or cell
Differential (e.g., Gram's stain)	To differentiate among various types of bacteria
Giemsa's	To stain tissues that include blood cells, Negri bodies, and chromosomes
Silver	To stain cells in the diagnosis of *Legionella, Pseudomonas, Leptospira, H. pylori,* and fungi such as *Pneumocystis* and *Candida*.
Wright's	To stain blood smears

Table 25-4

Substance Identified or Quantified	Blood Component Tested	Indication, Disease, or Disorder
ABO antigens and Rh factor (indicated by clumping reactions that occur when the blood specimen is mixed with serum containing different antibodies)	Whole blood	Possible transfusion or transplant reaction; hemolytic disease of the newborn
Acetone	Serum, plasma	Diabetic conditions or fasting metabolic ketoacidosis
Antistreptolysin O (ASO) antibodies	Serum	Streptococcal infection (which may indicate rheumatic fever, glomerulonephritis, bacterial endocarditis, or scarlet fever)
Bilirubin	Serum	Liver disease, fructose intolerance, or hypothyroidism
Blood urea nitrogen (BUN)	Serum, plasma	Indicates kidney disorders
Cancer antigens and tumor-associated glycoprotein	Serum	Cancer of a specific type depending on the antigen found
Cholesterol	Serum, plasma	Hyperlipoproteinemia, coronary artery disease, or atherosclerosis
Creatine kinase	Serum	Muscular dystrophies, Reye's syndrome, heart disease (particularly myocardial infarction), shock, or some neoplasms
Epstein-Barr virus	Serum	Infectious mononucleosis
Erythrocyte (RBC) count	Whole blood	Anemia
Erythrocyte sedimentation rate (ESR)	Whole blood	Infectious diseases, malignant neoplasms, or sickle cell anemia
Leukocyte (WBC) count	Whole blood	Leukemia, infection, or leukocytosis
Phenylalanine	Plasma	Hyperphenylalaninemia, obesity, or phenylketonuria
Potassium and sodium	Serum	Fluid-electrolyte balance
Prostatic acid phosphatase (PAP)	Serum	Prostate cancer
Rheumatoid factor (RF)	Serum	Rheumatoid arthritis
Treponema pallidum antibodies	Plasma, serum, spinal fluid	Syphilis The most common tests are the VDRL (Venereal Disease Research Laboratories) test and the rapid plasma reagin (RPR) test.

Table 25-5

Blood Bank Tests (Immunohematology)

ABO blood group test: Determines blood groups and type. For a summary of the ABO system and Rh groups, see Table 25-6.

Rh blood groups: Blood that has the Rh (or D) antigen on the surface of its RBCs is Rh positive (Rh+), and blood that does not have the antigen is Rh negative (Rh−). If an individual with Rh− blood receives a transfusion of Rh+ blood, anti-Rh agglutinin forms, and subsequent transfusions may result in serious reactions.

Crossmatching: A test to establish blood compatibility before transfusion that simulates the transfusion in a test tube by mixing donor cells with recipient serum or plasma. A compatible crossmatch is one in which no reaction occurs between cells and serum at room and body temperature.

Type	Antigen on Erythrocytes	Serum Antibodies
A	A	Anti-B
B	B	Anti-A
AB	Both antigen A and antigen B	None
O	None	Both anti-A and anti-B
Rh+	D	No anti-D
Rh−	No D	Anti-D

Table 25-6

Universal donor blood: Uncrossmatched blood, which may be requested from a blood bank by a physician in emergency situations. This uncrossmatched blood is usually group O, Rh− with packed RBCs.

Clinical Chemistry

Clinical chemistry: The use of computerized instruments to perform one or more tests on a single blood sample. Tests are conducted for such substances as alcohol, potassium, sodium, cholesterol, lead, phenobarbital, and cocaine.

Glucose testing: Can be performed on whole blood, plasma, or serum, but plasma and serum free of hemolysis are preferred. Glucose concentration is stable for up to eight hours at room temperature and up to 72 hours under refrigeration. Blood should be centrifuged and separated from the clot and cells as soon as possible or within 30 minutes, unless a specific additive (such as fluoride) is used. If the blood must be stored for several hours, fluoride-oxalate is the anticoagulant mixture of choice.

Home testing: Glucose testing kits, which can be used at home by diabetic patients, are classified as *waived tests* since they are simple to use and have a relatively low risk of inaccurate results.

Glucose tolerance test: Performed by giving a certain amount of glucose to a patient, then drawing blood samples at specified intervals and measuring the blood glucose level in each sample. Patients with diabetes may have normal fasting blood glucose levels, but they may be unable to produce a sufficient amount of insulin when needed to metabolize normal loads of carbohydrates. In these cases, blood glucose levels rise to abnormally high levels and remain high for a long period of time. The patient should be instructed to eat a high-carbohydrate diet for three days before the test, and to fast for eight–12 hours before the appointment.

Hemoglobin A1c (HgBA1c): The HgBA1c test is a useful tool for monitoring the overall stability of the patient's blood glucose. When blood glucose levels are elevated, the glucose molecules bind with hemoglobin to form HgBA1c. Once HgBA1c is formed, it remains for the life of the RBC (90–120 days). The test may be sent to an outside reference laboratory, and some physicians' offices have the equipment necessary to perform this test in the office laboratory. Several FDA-approved home tests have recently become available. Testing of HgBA1c should always be done in conjunction with routine blood glucose monitoring.

Arterial blood gas: Oxygen and carbon dioxide in arterial blood are measured by various methods to assess the adequacy of ventilation and oxygenation and the acid-base balance. Oxygen saturation of hemoglobin is normally 95% or higher.

Arterial pH: The hydrogen ion concentration of arterial blood. The normal range is 7.35–7.45.

Neonatal blood collection: Neonatal screening tests are commonly conducted to detect increased bilirubin, phenylketonuria (PKU), and hypothyroidism. PKU and thyroid tests are required by law in the United States. The common site for collection of blood is the infant's foot. Care must be taken not to damage the heel bone, which could cause osteomyelitis in the newborn.

PKU screening: Tests the infant's ability to metabolize phenylalanine. Increased phenylalanine in the blood can result in brain damage and mental retardation.

Cholesterol tests: Routine metabolic chemistry tests that may use automated devices, and be performed in a medical facility or at home. They test for many blood chemicals, including total cholesterol, HDL cholesterol, glucose, and triglycerides, using a small sample of blood, which may be obtained via capillary puncture. FDA-approved tests include:

- CardioChek Analyzer® (Polymer Technology Systems, Inc.)
- Piccolo Lipid Panel Plus Reagent Disc® (Abaxis, Inc.)
- SpotChem HDL, Total Cholesterol, and Triglyceride® (Arkray, Inc.)

Blood-Testing Equipment

Microscope: The instrument most often used in the physician's office laboratory (POL). Microscopes are used to examine blood smears, perform blood-cell counts, and identify body-fluid samples. See Figure 25-8. In using a microscope, follow these steps:

1. Clean the lenses and oculars with lens paper.
2. Place the specimen slide on the stage, sliding the edges under the slide clips.

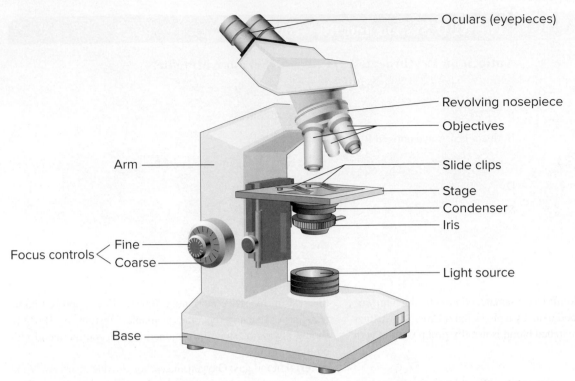

Figure 25-8 *The microscope is the most heavily used piece of equipment in the physician's office laboratory.*

3. Adjust the distance between the oculars so that you see a merged field.

4. Adjust the objectives so that the low-power objective points directly at the specimen slide.

5. Turn on the light, and adjust the amount of light illuminating the specimen.

6. Lower the body tube to move the objective closer to the specimen slide.

7. Use the coarse focus control to slowly adjust the image.

8. Use the fine focus control to adjust the image.

9. Switch to the high-power objective.

10. Apply immersion oil to the specimen slide.

11. Switch to the oil-immersion objective, and examine the specimen. Figure 25-9 shows the pattern to follow for counting leukocytes under the oil-immersion objective.

Objectives: The objectives of a microscope contain magnifying lenses that increase the magnification of the oculars by various amounts. A *scanning objective lens* has the lowest power, and usually adds magnification of 4 ×. A *small objective lens* usually adds magnification of 10 ×. The most powerful lens is referred to as a *large objective lens,* which adds magnification of 10 × to 40 ×. This lens may or may not be an *oil-immersion objective.*

Oil-immersion objective: This large objective lens is designed to be lowered into a drop of immersion oil placed directly over the prepared specimen under examination. This design eliminates the air space between the microscope slide and the objective, thereby reducing the loss of light and creating images that are sharper and brighter.

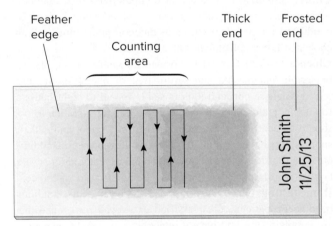

Figure 25-9 *Follow this pattern when counting leukocytes visible in the field under the oil-immersion objective of the microscope.*

Centrifuge: A laboratory machine used to separate particles of different densities within a liquid by spinning them at very high speeds.

Hemocytometer: A special microscope slide used primarily for counting blood cells that can also be used for counting platelets, sperm, and other cells. The most commonly used hemocytometer is the Neubauer type.

Blood chemistry analyzer: Uses a reflectance photometer to measure chemical substances, or *analytes,* in the blood. The photometer measures light intensity to determine exact amounts of analytes.

Incubator: Used to control and maintain temperature and condition of blood samples.

Conditions Identified by Blood Testing

Hyperglycemia: A higher-than-normal blood glucose level. The most common cause of hyperglycemia is diabetes mellitus. Other conditions that can cause hyperglycemia are hyperthyroidism, Cushing's syndrome, acromegaly, obesity, severe liver or kidney damage, alcoholism, and elevated levels of the hormones estrogen, epinephrine, or norepinephrine.

Hypoglycemia: Abnormally low levels of glucose in the blood, below 50 mg/dL. The most common cause of hypoglycemia is insulin overdose in patients with unstable insulin-dependent diabetes mellitus. The cause of a diabetic emergency may be unknown. The patient should be given sugar via fruit juices or candy.

Hemophilia: A hereditary disorder of clotting factors, in which blood fails to coagulate at a wound site.

Hyperlipidemia: A higher-than-normal level of lipids, especially cholesterol, in the blood.

Visual indications: Hyperlipidemia gives plasma or serum a milky, or turbid, appearance. Sometimes the plasma or serum will have a pale, watery appearance as a result of protein disorders or kidney disease. In certain types of cancers, the color of the serum may be green, attributable to heme (part of hemoglobin).

Extramedullary hematopoiesis: In abnormal circumstances, the spleen, liver, and lymph nodes revert back to producing immature blood cells. This reversion can be the result of aplastic anemia, infiltration by malignant cells, leukemia, or hemolytic anemias.

Anemia: A reduction in the number of circulating RBCs per cubic millimeter. Hemoglobin content is less than that required to provide the oxygen needed by the body.

Abnormal erythrocytes: Vary from the norm in terms of size, shape, and color. Normal mature erythrocytes are biconcave and disc shaped, and lack a nucleus.

Anisocytosis: An abnormal condition characterized by excessive inequality in the size of erythrocytes.

Macrocyte: An abnormally large erythrocyte.

Megalocyte: An erythrocyte that is larger than average.

Microcyte: An abnormally small erythrocyte.

Poikilocytosis: Variation in the shapes of erythrocytes.

Schistocyte or schizocyte: An erythrocyte that has been fragmented during circulation.

Ovalocyte: An erythrocyte that is oval in shape. It is also called an elliptocyte.

Spherocyte: An erythrocyte that is spheroid in shape, having a decreased ratio of surface area to volume.

Target cell: An abnormally thin RBC with a dark center and a surrounding ring of hemoglobin. Also called leptocytes, target cells occur in anemia and jaundice.

Sickle cell: An erythrocyte that is sickle or crescent shaped. Such cells are produced by the polymerization of hemoglobin and occur in hereditary anemias.

Hypochromia: A condition in which cells have decreased hemoglobin.

Polycythemia: An above-normal concentration of erythrocytes in the circulating blood. It is also called erythrocytosis.

Polycythemia vera: A blood dyscrasia (disease) characterized by abnormally increased levels of erythrocytes, leukocytes, and thrombocytes. It is also called erythremia.

Neutropenia: A severe decrease in the number of neutrophilic granulocytes in the peripheral blood.

Neutrophilia: A significant increase in the number of neutrophilic granulocytes in the peripheral blood.

Leukocytosis: An increase in the number of leukocytes in the blood, generally caused by infection and usually transient.

Leukemia: A neoplastic, proliferative disease characterized by an overproduction of immature or mature cells of various leukocyte types in the bone marrow or peripheral blood.

Lymphoma: A solid, malignant tumor of the lymph nodes and associated tissue or bone marrow.

Infectious mononucleosis (IM): An acute, infectious disease, commonly called mono or the kissing disease, in which there is an abnormally high number of mononuclear leukocytes in the blood. Most cases are caused by the Epstein-Barr virus. The most common serological test is the rapid slide test.

Hemolytic disease of the newborn: A neonatal disease generally caused by Rh incompatibility between mother and child, occurring when an Rh– woman carries an Rh+ fetus. Symptoms are anemia, jaundice, liver and spleen enlargement, and generalized edema. It can be controlled during pregnancy but may require intrauterine transfusion or early induced labor.

Bloodletting: The therapeutic opening of an artery or vein to withdraw blood from a particular area. Also called therapeutic phlebotomy, it is sometimes performed to treat polycythemia or congestive heart failure. One pint is collected and discarded.

Blood lavage: The removal of toxic elements from the blood by the injection of serum into the veins.

Alanine aminotransferase (ALT): An enzyme normally present in the serum and tissues of the body, especially the tissue of the liver. It is released into the serum as a result of tissue injury and increases in patients with acute liver damage.

Acid phosphatase (AP): An enzyme found in the kidneys, serum, semen, and prostate gland. It is elevated in the serum because of prostate cancer or trauma.

25.2 Collecting and Testing Urine

Role of the medical assistant: To help collect, process, and test urine specimens. These activities involve dealing with potentially infectious body waste, so following universal precautions is generally required.

Physical and Chemical Composition and Function

Urinary system or tract: Consists of two kidneys, two ureters, a bladder, and a urethra. The kidneys remove excess water from the body and waste products from the blood in the form of urine, which then drains through the ureters into the urinary bladder. The bladder stores urine until it leaves the body through the urethra.

Nephron: The basic unit of the kidney. See Figure 25-10. Each kidney contains approximately one million nephrons. Nephrons filter blood to produce urine. One of the main functions of the nephron is to remove waste material from the body.

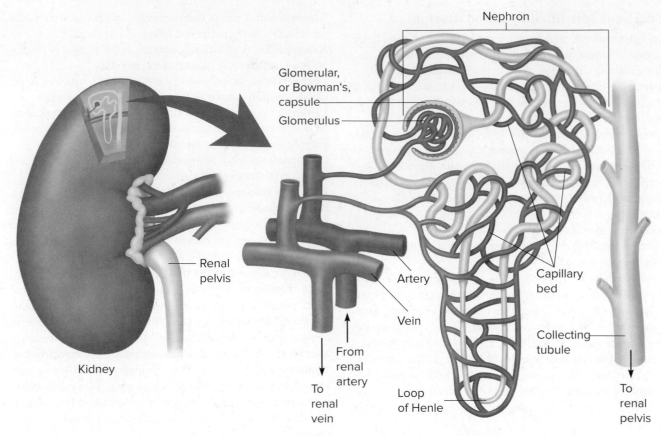

Figure 25-10 *Urine is formed in the nephron, a long tubular structure, during a complex filtering process.*

It also allows reabsorption of water and some electrolytes back into the blood.

Urinary meatus: The external opening of the urethra.

Chemical composition of urine: Approximately 95% water and 5% waste materials and other components, which include urea, ammonia, uric acid, creatinine, urobilinogen, and a few WBCs and RBCs. The presence of a few sperm cells in the urine of males is normal.

Urea: The end product of protein metabolism after ammonia is broken down by the liver.

Urochrome: The yellow pigment that gives urine its color. It is produced by the breakdown of hemoglobin.

Urination: The act of passing urine. It is also called micturition.

Urgency: An immediate need to urinate.

Urinary retention: The inability to empty the bladder.

Urinary frequency: Increased frequency can often be a symptom of a urinary tract infection, but there also may be other causes.

Incontinence: The inability to prevent release of urine. Some causes include an overfilling of the bladder and stress caused by laughing, sneezing, coughing, or lifting.

Enuresis: The involuntary discharge of urine after the age at which bladder control is normally established.

Nocturnal enuresis: Urinary incontinence during the night, also called bedwetting, which can be a symptom of a neurological disorder.

Dysuria: Painful or difficult urination, symptomatic of cystitis, infection, and many other conditions.

Polyuria: Increased output of urine.

Uropathy: Any disease or abnormal condition of any structure of the urinary tract.

Obtaining Specimens

Urine collection: Urine tests require 30–50 mL of the specimen. When it is collected, it must be properly labeled with the patient's name, the date, and the time. Urine tests for females should be avoided during menstruation. Any medication taken by the patient must be recorded on the laboratory requisition and the patient's chart. If urinalysis cannot be performed within 30 minutes after collection, the urine specimen must be stored in a refrigerator.

Home collection: Instruct patients on how to obtain the specimen. Tell them to urinate into an appropriate container, one that has a wide opening, and not to add anything else to the container. However, if you provide a container that contains preservative, caution them not to throw out the preservative. Instruct them to refrigerate the container and to keep the lid on it.

Random specimen: A single urine specimen taken at any time. A random specimen is the most common type of sample. If collection is done in a doctor's office, provide a urine specimen container, show the patient to the restroom, and ask the patient to void a few ounces of urine into the specimen container and

ADH	antidiuretic hormone		RBCs	red blood cells
BIL; bili; BR	bilirubin		SPG; sp gr; sp.gr.	specific gravity
BJP	Bence Jones proteins		U/A	urinalysis
Ca	calcium		UBG	urobilinogen
CC	clean catch (urine)		U/C	urine culture
CCMS	clean catch, midstream (urine)		UC	urinary catheter
CL VOID	clean voided specimen (urine)		UC&S	urine culture and sensitivity
CrCl	creatinine clearance		UcaV	urinary calcium volume
CSU	catheter specimen (urine)		UCRE	urine creatinine
Cys	cysteine		UFC	urinary free cortisol
CYS	cystoscopy		UK	urine potassium
EMU	early morning urine(s)		Una	urinary sodium
HCG; hcg; hCG	human chorionic gonadotropin		Uosm	urine osmolarity
IVP	intravenous pyelogram		UTI	urinary tract infection
K	potassium		UUN	urinary urea nitrogen
pH	hydrogen ion concentration		UV	urinary volume
PKD	polycystic kidney disease		Vol	volume
PKU	phenylketonuria		WBCs	white blood cells

Table 25-7

leave it on the sink. Transport the specimen to the laboratory immediately, or refrigerate the specimen.

Clean-catch midstream specimen: A method of urine collection that may be ordered to diagnose urinary tract infections or to evaluate the effectiveness of drug therapy. The purpose of this type of collection is to obtain a urine specimen that is free from contamination. Patients completing this procedure independently need written instructions on how to make sure that the container and the urine specimen remain uncontaminated.

Timed specimen: Collected over a predetermined time period to obtain more specific information. Such specimens are sometimes collected two hours after a meal to test for diabetes. The patient should discard the first specimen and then collect all urine for the specified time, making sure that the urine does not mix with stool or toilet paper. The sample should be kept refrigerated until it is brought to the doctor's office or laboratory.

24-hour specimen: Collected to measure the amount of urine output in a 24-hour period. The urine will be tested for substances that are released sporadically into the urine. It is extremely important to avoid using a bedpan, urinal, or toilet tissue, which could retain the substances for which the test is being done. The first specimen should be discarded. Over the next 24 hours, the patient should urinate directly into the small collection container and then pour the urine into the large container. Between two collections, the small container must be sanitized with soap and warm water. This type of collection is helpful in diagnosing renal disease, dehydration, urinary tract obstructions, and pheochromocytoma.

First-voided morning specimen: Collected after a night's sleep. It contains greater concentrations of substances that collect over time than do specimens taken during the day. A urine specimen container or clean, dry jar is used. It is best for pregnancy testing, microscopic examination, and culturing.

Catheterization: Insertion of a sterile plastic tube into the bladder to withdraw urine. It is used to obtain a sterile urine specimen from a patient, to obtain a specimen from a patient who cannot void naturally, or to measure the amount of residual urine in the bladder after normal voiding, among other reasons. Catheterization may cause infection.

Drainage catheter: Used to withdraw fluids.

Splinting catheter: Used after plastic repair of a ureter.

Urinalysis

Urinalysis: The examination of urine to obtain information about body health and disease, done as part of a general physical examination or for a specific reason. The testing may be physical, chemical, or microscopic. Table 25-7 lists abbreviations common to urine analysis and testing, and Table 25-8 lists normal values for tests done on urine.

Test	Value
Acetone	None
Albumin, qualitative	Negative
Albumin, quantitative	10–140 mg/L (24 hours)
Bacteria (culture)	< 10,000 colonies/mL
Blood, occult	Negative
Calcium, quantitative	100–300 mg/24 hours
Color	Pale yellow to dark amber
Creatine, nonpregnant women or in men	< 6% of creatinine
Creatine, pregnant women	≤ 12% of creatinine
Creatinine, men	1.0–1.9 g/24 hours
Creatinine, women	0.8–1.7 g/24 hours
Crystals	Negative
Ketones	Negative
Lead	0.021–0.038 mg/L
Odor	Distinctly aromatic
pH	4.5–8.0
Phenylpyruvic acid	Negative
Protein	Negative
Specific gravity, single specimen	1.005–1.030
Specific gravity, 24-hour specimen	1.015–1.025
Turbidity	Clear
Volume, adult females	600–1600 mL/24 hours
Volume, adult males	800–1800 mL/24 hours
White blood cells	0–8/high-power field

Table 25-8

Physical testing of urine: Provides information about color, volume, odor, and specific gravity.

Color: Normal urine ranges from pale yellow to dark amber, depending on food and fluid intake, medications and vitamin supplements, and waste products present in the urine.

Volume: With a timed specimen, urine volume is measured by pouring the entire collection into a large, graduated cylinder. It is usually not accurate enough to use the markings on the side of the collection container. After measuring and recording the volume, a portion of the well-mixed specimen *(aliquot)* is removed for testing.

Clarity: Urine can be clear, or it can range from slightly cloudy to very cloudy. Cloudiness is also known as turbidity and sometimes indicates an abnormal condition. Causes of urine color and cloudiness are listed in Table 25-9.

Urine volume: Normal adult urine output is 600–1800 mL per 24-hour period, with an average of 1250 mL per 24 hours.

Oliguria: Decreased output of urine, often resulting from dehydration, decreased fluid intake, shock, or renal disease.

Anuria: The complete suppression of urine formation by the kidney. It may be a result of renal or urethral obstruction or renal failure.

Urine odor: Can provide clues about the body's condition. Diseases, the presence of bacteria, and certain foods can change the odor.

Urine specific gravity: A measure of the amount or concentration of a substance dissolved in urine. It is calculated by

Color and Turbidity	Pathological Causes	Other Causes
Colorless or pale straw color (dilute)	Diabetes, anxiety, chronic renal disease	Diuretic therapy, excessive fluid intake (water, beer, coffee)
Cloudy	Infection, inflammation, glomerular nephritis	Vegetarian diet
Milky white	Fats, pus	Amorphous phosphates, spermatozoa
Dark yellow, dark amber (concentrated)	Acute febrile disease, vomiting or diarrhea (fluid loss or dehydration)	Low fluid intake, excessive sweating
Orange-yellow, orange-red, orange-brown	Excessive RBC destruction, bile duct obstruction, diminished liver-cell function, bilirubin	Drugs (such as pyridium and rifampin), dyes

Table 25-9

dividing the weight of the sample by the weight of an equal amount of distilled water. The specific gravity of normal urine ranges from 1.005 to 1.030. The specific gravity of urine is lower in cases of chronic kidney disease, diabetes insipidus, overhydration, and systemic lupus.

Measuring specific gravity: Three methods are used to measure specific gravity: urinometer, refractometer, and reagent strip (dipstick).

Urinometer: A sealed glass float with a calibrated scale on the stem that measures specific gravity. At least 15 mL of urine is required. See Figure 25-11.

Refractometer: An optical device that measures the refraction of light as it passes through a liquid. The degree of refraction is proportional to the amount of dissolved material in the liquid. It is faster and easier to use than the urinometer and requires only a drop of urine. It must be calibrated daily. See Figure 25-12.

Reagent strips, or dipsticks: Plastic strips to which one or more pads containing chemicals are attached. The pads react to substances in the urine and change color; a chart enables you to interpret the color changes. They are available for many tests: specific gravity, pH, protein, glucose, ketones, leukocytes, erythrocytes,

nitrite, bilirubin, urobilinogen, and phenylketones. Quality control of urine dipsticks should be performed.

Chemical testing of urine specimens: Usually performed with reagent strips. These tests can measure liver or kidney function, metabolism of carbohydrates, acid-base balance, and urinary pH. They also show the presence of drugs or infections, ketone bodies, blood, hemoglobin, myoglobin, bilirubin, urobilinogen, glucose, protein, nitrite, phenylketones, and leukocytes.

Using reagent strips: It is important to follow the directions of the manufacturer. Keep strips in tightly closed containers in a cool, dry area, and do not remove them until immediately before testing. Never use expired strips. A dipstick may be used only once.

Figure 25-11 *Read the value on the scale where the bottom of the meniscus touches the stem.*

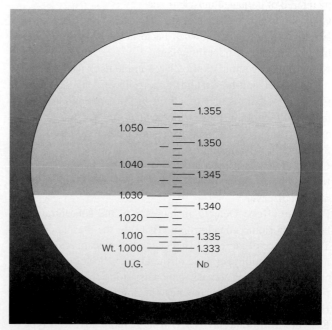

Figure 25-12 *A refractometer uses light refraction to measure specific gravity.*

Urinary pH: A measure of the acidity or alkalinity (hydrogen ion concentration) of urine. The normal pH of urine is 4.5–8.0.

Proteinuria: The presence of protein, such as albumin, in the urine. Protein is not normally found in the urine. Its presence may signal renal disease, heart failure, hypertension, or fever, or it may be the result of heavy exercise.

Uremia: A high level of urea in the blood. Excessive amounts of urea and other nitrogenous waste products in the blood are seen in renal failure.

Uremic: Pertaining to a toxic level of urea in the blood.

Uric acid: The end product of the metabolism of purine, an important constituent of nucleic acids. A high level of uric acid in the urine may be associated with urinary calculi or gout.

Urobilinogen: A colorless compound formed in the intestines after the breakdown of bilirubin by bacteria. Some of this substance is excreted in feces, and some is reabsorbed and excreted again in bile or urine.

Urobilin: A brown pigment formed by the oxidation of urobilinogen. It is normally found in feces and in small amounts in urine.

Bilirubin: An orange-colored pigment in bile. Jaundice is a result of the accumulation in tissues of excess bilirubin in the blood.

Pyuria: The presence of pus in the urine, which may be evidence of renal disease.

Hematuria: The presence of blood in the urine, which may be a result of menstruation, urinary tract infection, or trauma or bleeding in the kidneys.

Hemoglobinuria: The presence of free hemoglobin in the urine, caused by a transfusion or drug reaction, malaria, snakebite, or severe burn.

Leukocyte esterase test: A method of screening for a substance that suggests the presence of white blood cells in the urine; this may mean there is a urinary tract infection.

Myoglobinuria: The presence of myoglobin in the urine, caused by injured or damaged muscle tissue.

Glycosuria: The presence of sugar (glucose) in the urine.

Nitrite: Occurs in urine when bacteria break down nitrate. It indicates a urinary tract infection.

Ketosis: An accumulation of large amounts of ketone bodies in the tissues and body fluids as a result of dehydration, starvation, hyperemesis, dry mouth, dry skin, uncontrolled diabetes, or taking too much aspirin. Ketones are sometimes present after general anesthesia has been administered. Ketones are the by-products of fat metabolism.

Creatinine: A waste product of the metabolism of creatine. Increased quantities are found in the urine in advanced stages of renal disease.

Pregnancy test: Detects an increase in the concentration of human chorionic gonadotropin (HCG) in the plasma or urine. The presence of increased HCG can also indicate ectopic pregnancy; a hydatidiform mole of the uterus; choriocarcinoma; or cancer of the lung, breast, pancreas, stomach, or colon. The first-voided morning urine has the highest concentration of HCG.

Enzyme immunoassay (EIA) test: A more advanced type of pregnancy testing that uses either urine or serum. In this test, a sample is added through a chamber window where it migrates through the membrane and reacts with the reagents to produce a reaction. The test is easy to set up and interpret, and is designed with a control feature incorporated into the reagent pack for quality assurance of the test results.

STD testing: In response to increasing numbers of sexually transmitted diseases, the CDC recommends that all sexually active females between the ages of 15 and 25 be screened annually for chlamydia. To accomplish this, several tests called Nucleic Acid Amplification Tests (NAATs) have recently been developed. These tests use urine samples to detect the presence of chlamydia or gonorrhea. By amplifying nucleic acids specific to these organisms, the test can detect the presence of very small numbers of bacteria.

Microscopic examination of urine: May show formed elements and also can determine the presence of cells, casts, crystals, bacteria, and other microorganisms. The first step is to use a centrifuge to obtain sediment for analysis. See Figures 25-13 and 25-14.

Crystals: Commonly found in urine specimens. They usually do not indicate a significant disorder. They are found in large numbers in patients with renal stones.

Urinary casts: Cylinder-shaped elements that form when protein accumulates in the kidney tubules and is washed down into the urine.

Mucous threads: Found in normal urine. Increased amounts usually indicate urinary tract inflammation. They are examined under low-power magnification.

Erythrocytes: Though found in normal urine in small amounts, increased erythrocytes may be caused by inflammation, injury, or disease. They are examined under high-power magnification, counted, and reported as *range/high-power field (hpf)*.

Leukocytes: If found in higher than normal amounts in urine sediment, this usually indicates a urinary infection or

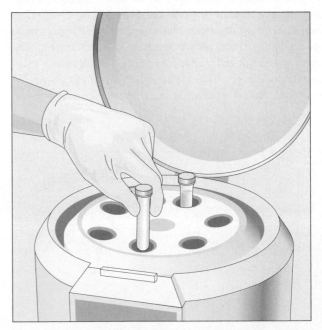

Figure 25-13 *The centrifuge must be balanced by placing test tubes on opposite sides.*

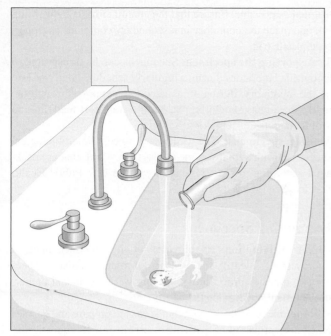

Figure 25-14 *Make sure that you do not lose any sediment when you pour off the urine.*

inflammation. They are counted and reported the same way as erythrocytes.

Epithelial cells: While most epithelial cells in urine are the result of normal sloughing of epithelial tissue, if these cells are present in large numbers, they may indicate nephrotic syndrome or a urinary tract infection. The type of epithelial cells present help to identify the level and extent of infection.

Special Considerations

Pregnant patients: Pregnancy normally increases urinary frequency. Pregnant women are also prone to urinary tract infections. At each prenatal visit, they must have their urine checked for abnormal levels of glucose (indicative of diabetes) and abnormal levels of protein (preeclampsia or renal problems).

Elderly patients: Bladder muscles weaken with age, often leading to incomplete bladder emptying and chronic urine retention, which can cause urinary tract infections, nocturia, and incontinence.

Pediatric patients: Ask whether there are any problems with diaper rash (indicative of renal dysfunction), excessive thirst (possible diabetes), crying during urination (urinary tract infection), or bedwetting or enuresis (stress or urinary tract infections).

25.3 Medical Microbiology

Diagnosing infections: There are six steps in diagnosing infections: examining the patient, obtaining one or more specimens, examining the specimen, culturing the specimen, determining the culture's antibiotic sensitivity, and treating the patient.

Aerobic cultures: Bacterial cultures performed to identify bacteria that grow only in the presence of oxygen.

Anaerobic cultures: Bacterial cultures performed to identify bacteria that grow only in the absence of oxygen.

Collecting Specimens

Guidelines for collecting specimens: Following these guidelines will make it possible to collect specimens properly.

- Try to avoid causing the patient harm, discomfort, or undue embarrassment.
- If the patient is to collect the specimen, provide clear, detailed instructions and the proper container.
- Collect the material from a site where the organism is most likely to be found and where contamination is least likely to occur.
- Obtain the specimen at a time that allows optimal chance of recovery of the microorganism.
- Use appropriate collection devices, specimen containers, transport systems, and culture media. Follow aseptic techniques.
- Obtain a sufficient quantity of the specimen.
- Obtain the specimen before antimicrobial therapy begins.
- Label the container, and include the proper requisition form.

Throat culture: A frequently performed microbiological procedure that is often performed when the patient shows signs or symptoms of an upper respiratory, throat, or sinus infection. In most cases, a throat culture is obtained to determine whether the patient has strep throat. Left untreated, strep throat can lead to rheumatic fever. To obtain sterile specimens, such as those used for throat cultures, a sterile swab is used. When collecting a specimen for throat culture, the pharynx should be swabbed. See Figure 25-15.

Sputum specimen: The patient should cough deeply and expectorate mucus from the lungs into a sterile container. The patient should be instructed to avoid contaminating the specimen with saliva. Follow universal precautions when handling sputum specimens, and wear a face shield or mask and goggles.

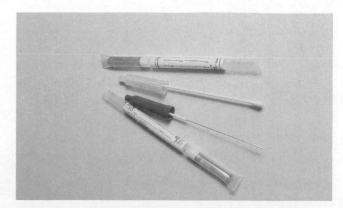

Figure 25-15 *Sterile swabs vary in size and in material.*
© Image Source/Jupiter Images RF

Spinal fluid specimens: Via lumbar puncture, under sterile conditions, spinal fluid is obtained. A needle is inserted into the subarachnoid space, usually between the third and fourth lumbar vertebrae. When normal, *cerebrospinal fluid* is clear and colorless.

Wound specimens: The procedure for obtaining specimens from infected wounds is similar to that for a throat culture. Obtain representative material from a deep area and a surface area without contaminating the swab by touching areas outside the site.

Stool culture: Ordered if the physician suspects that the patient has certain diseases such as cancer or colitis or bacterial, protozoal, or parasitic infections. Patients can collect stool specimens on a clean paper plate, in a clean waxed-paper carton, or in a collection container or collection tissue. Collection containers for stool cultures do not have to be sterile. The container must be clean, and the stool should not be contaminated with urine.

Fecal occult blood specimens: Tested as part of early screening for colon cancer. The presence of blood in the stool may indicate colorectal cancer, hemorrhoids, or gastric ulcers. Based on the *guaiac reagent,* which turns blue when oxidized in the presence of blood, tests of fecal occult blood are referred to as *guaiac tests.* Prior to stool collection, red meat should be avoided in the diet, because it can cause false-positive results.

Melena: Abnormal black tarry stools containing digested blood.

O and P specimen: A type of stool sample examined for the presence of parasites and their ova (eggs). Both a fresh and a preserved specimen are required.

Preparing specimens for an outside laboratory: If testing is to be done by an outside laboratory, be sure to follow the collection procedures and use the collection device required by the laboratory. Maintain the samples in a state as close to their original as possible. Ensure that the container has a tight-fitting lid, and place the container in a secondary container or zipper-type plastic bag.

Transporting the specimen: Specimens can be transported to an outside laboratory during a regularly scheduled daily pickup by the laboratory, during an as-needed pickup, or through the mail. Specimens should be placed in a transport medium and sent to an outside laboratory.

Mailing specimens: The USPS will accept microbiological specimens with a total volume of less than 50 mL that are packaged according to strict regulations of the U.S. Public Health Service. See Figure 25-16.

Examining Specimens

Direct examination: Examination of the specimen under a microscope to identify the presence of microorganisms. There are two types of procedure: preparing wet mounts and preparing potassium hydroxide (KOH) mounts.

Wet mount: A type of mount that is easy to prepare and enables quick determination of many microorganisms. It requires mixing a small amount of the specimen with a drop of normal saline (0.9% sodium chloride) on a glass slide. Then a coverslip is placed over the mixture. The physician can examine the slide directly under the microscope.

Potassium hydroxide (KOH) mount: A type of mount used for identification of a fungal infection of the skin, nails, or hair. The procedure involves the following steps:

1. Suspend the specimen in a drop of 10% KOH on a glass slide.
2. Apply a coverslip.
3. Let the specimen sit for 30 minutes at room temperature.
4. Examine the slide under the microscope.

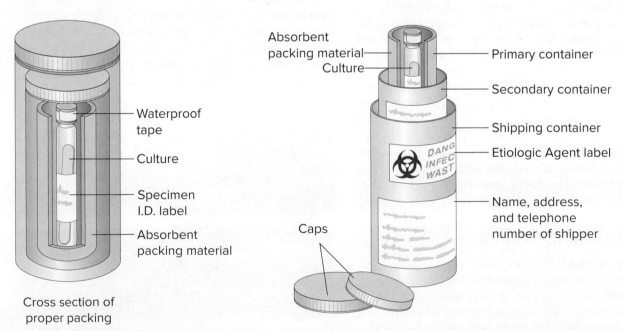

Cross section of proper packing

Figure 25-16 *When packaging and labeling a specimen for mail delivery, you must follow the procedures set by the CDC, based on U.S. Public Health Service regulations.*

Stained specimens: Microorganisms can be seen more clearly when stained with a dye or group of dyes.

Smear: The first step in preparing a stained specimen is to prepare a smear. Apply a small amount of the specimen to a glass slide. Allow the sample to dry, then briefly heat the slide to fix the sample to the slide. Stain the smear. Heating is the most effective method of affixing a bacterial smear.

Gram's stain: The stain most commonly used in examining bacteriological specimens. It involves a simple procedure, shown in Figure 25-17. If the bacteria have a deep purple color, they are gram positive. If the bacteria exhibit a pink or red color, they are gram negative. Gram-stained specimens are first examined using the low-power 10x objective, followed by higher powered objectives if necessary.

Acid-fast: Not readily susceptible to decolorization by acids during the staining procedure. The acid-fast nature of certain microorganisms, such as those of the genus *Mycobacterium*, allows microscopic examination and differentiation.

Culture Media

Culture media: Liquid, semisolid, and solid substances used to foster the growth of bacteria. Semisolid media are most commonly used in medical offices.

Agar: A gelatin-like substance extracted from algae that gives a semisolid culture medium its consistency.

Petri dish or plate: A covered glass or plastic dish that holds the culture medium. Handle Petri dishes only on the outside, so as to avoid contaminating them. Store them with the bottom (agar side) up.

Culturette®Collection and Transport System: A sterile, self-contained unit that holds a polyester swab and a small, thin-walled glass vial of transport medium in a plastic sleeve. It is used for obtaining and transporting specimens. (It is manufactured by Becton Dickinson Microbiology Systems.)

Selective culture media: Culture media that allow the growth of only certain kinds of bacteria. They are commonly used for

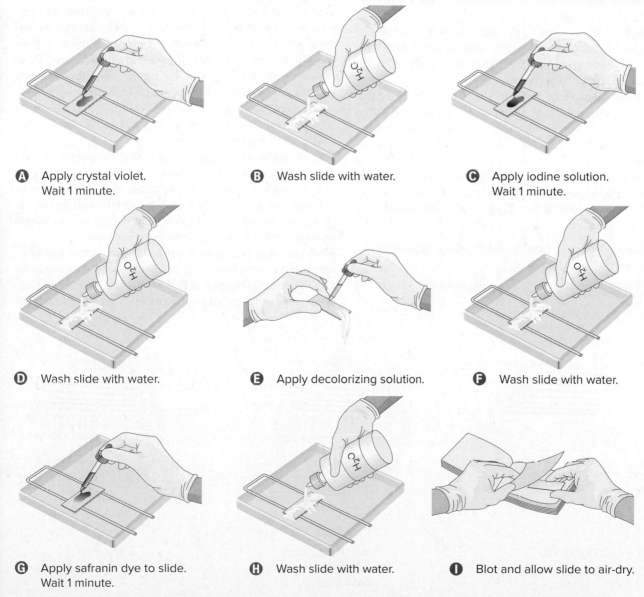

A Apply crystal violet. Wait 1 minute.

B Wash slide with water.

C Apply iodine solution. Wait 1 minute.

D Wash slide with water.

E Apply decolorizing solution.

F Wash slide with water.

G Apply safranin dye to slide. Wait 1 minute.

H Wash slide with water.

I Blot and allow slide to air-dry.

Figure 25-17 *The procedure for performing a Gram's stain on a microbiologic specimen involves applying a series of stains, water washes, and alcohol in a specific order, for precise periods of time.*

specimens that normally contain bacteria, such as stools or vaginal samples.

Nonselective culture media: Media that support the growth of most organisms. For example, blood agar is a nonselective culture medium used to culture a throat swab specimen, such as for *Streptococcus pyogenes,* which causes "strep throat."

Special culture units: Commercially prepared units with specific purposes, such as performing rapid urine cultures or culturing vaginal specimens.

Preparing the plate: Before inoculating a culture plate, label it on the bottom (agar side) with the patient's name, doctor's name, source of the sample, date and time of inoculation, and your initials.

Bacitracin: An antibiotic used in cultures to give an early indication of the presence of group A streptococci.

Qualitative analysis: The determination of the type of pathogen by its appearance. Inoculate the plate as shown in Figure 25-18.

Quantitative analysis: The determination of the number of bacteria present in a sample.

Incubation: After inoculating the plate, put it in an incubator set at 35°–37°C, with the bottom (agar side) up, for 24–48 hours.

Colony: A visible growth on a culture plate, usually resulting from a single type of bacteria.

Culture isolation: Once isolated, the pathogenic-appearing colony is transferred from the primary culture plate. The secondary culture plate is incubated at 37°C to allow a pure culture to grow. A pure culture contains only a single type of organism.

Sensitivity testing: Determines an organism's susceptibility to specific antibiotics in order to enable the doctor to decide which one to use to treat the infection. The test involves the following steps:

1. Suspend a sample of the isolated pathogen in a small amount of liquid medium.

2. Streak the pathogen evenly on the surface of a culture plate.

3. Place small disks of filter paper containing various antimicrobial agents on top of the plate, using sterile forceps or a special dispenser.

4. Incubate the plate at 37°C for one day.

A clear zone around a disk indicates an effective antimicrobial agent, whereas growth next to a disk indicates an ineffective agent.

Quality control: All staining reagents should be checked frequently for effectiveness. All slides must be checked. All devices with temperature controls should be checked every day. All reagents and media must be used before the expiration date and evaluated for sterility. Equipment such as refrigerators, freezers, and incubators should be properly monitored and maintained.

Clinical Laboratory Improvement Amendments of 1988 (CLIA '88): A law enacted by Congress placing all laboratory facilities involved with human health and disease under federal regulations administered by the Health Care Financing Administration (HCFA) and the CDC. As a result, laboratories must meet complex standards, and medical assistants may perform only certain types of tests. The amendments classify and regulate laboratories based on the complexity of the procedures being performed, and establish personnel qualifications. These rules apply to all testing sites, but several procedures and tests have waivers from these regulations. CLIA came about because congressional investigation of *physician office laboratories (POLs)* found some POLs to be deficient in the services and results that they provided.

Waived tests: FDA-approved laboratory examinations and procedures that may be performed at home, or that have an insignificant risk of an erroneous result. This may be because of simple, accurate methodologies that significantly reduce the chance of user error, or because even if they are performed incorrectly, they pose no real risk of patient harm.

Moderate- and high-complexity tests: Three out of four laboratory tests are categorized by the FDA as *moderate-complexity tests.* Some are performed in POLs, and include Gram staining, hematology and chemistry testing using an automated analyzer,

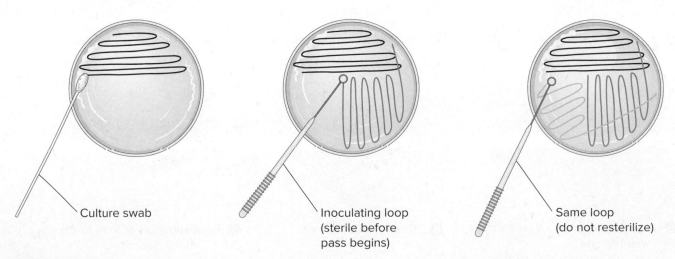

Culture swab

Inoculating loop (sterile before pass begins)

Same loop (do not resterilize)

Figure 25-18 *When inoculating a plate for qualitative analysis, roll and streak the culture swab or inoculating loop of specimen material across one-third of the surface of the culture plate. Begin the next pass with a sterile loop.*

and microscopic urine sediment analyses. *High-complexity tests* are usually not performed in a POL, and include blood typing and cross-matching, cytologic testing, and the Papanicolaou (Pap) smear. Any lab performing moderate- or high-complexity testing must meet CLIA regulations and can be inspected every two years. These labs must follow strict written quality control and quality assurance procedures and maintain high proficiency levels.

STRATEGIES FOR SUCCESS

▶ *Test-Taking Skills*

Use your anxiety, or overcome it!
Some anxiety is to be expected in any test-taking situation, and often the rush of adrenaline can help keep you energized and focused. However, if you feel that your anxiety is getting in the way of your doing well, learn to control it. Take deep breaths and think positively. Budget your time, but do not let excessive worry over the time limit interfere with your performance. You have studied, and you know your material; now all you need to do is to recall it. You may miss some questions, and some questions may be difficult, but if you keep focused, you can pass the certification test.

Instructions:

Answer the following questions.

1. Which cells play a vital role in internal respiration?

   A. bone marrow cells
   B. erythrocytes
   C. leukocytes
   D. mast cells
   E. basophils

2. What is the longest time a tourniquet should remain on a patient's arm?

   A. one minute
   B. two minutes
   C. three minutes
   D. four minutes
   E. five minutes

3. Which of the following devices might be used to collect blood from fragile veins?

   A. a finger stick lancet
   B. a Vacutainer® system
   C. a butterfly needle
   D. an automatic puncturing device
   E. none of these

4. To test for substances that are sporadically released into urine, a physician might order which type of urine specimen?

   A. 24-hour
   B. clean catch
   C. random
   D. first voided
   E. timed

5. If a urinalysis cannot be performed within 30 minutes after collection, the urine specimen must be stored

   A. in an incubator.
   B. in a freezer.
   C. at room temperature.
   D. in a refrigerator.

6. The quality control log

   A. lists specimens sent to another laboratory for testing.
   B. shows when the testing equipment was last calibrated.
   C. shows all the procedures completed during the workday.
   D. shows the quality testing performed on every batch of reagent product.
   E. documents maintenance done on laboratory equipment.

7. The color code for an evacuation tube that does *not* contain an additive is

   A. red.
   B. lavender.
   C. gray.
   D. red and black.
   E. yellow.

8. Which of the following describes a centrifuge?

   A. machine used to count blood cells
   B. machine used to separate particles
   C. machine used to heat cultures
   D. machine used to analyze specimens
   E. machine used to clean laboratory equipment

9. A home diabetes test is an example of

   A. a POL.
   B. a red blood cell index.
   C. Wright's stain.
   D. a waived test.
   E. an aliquot.

10. Albumin found in urine might indicate

   A. renal disease.
   B. heart failure.
   C. hypertension.
   D. fever.
   E. all of these

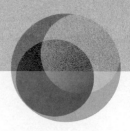

CMA Questions for the end of Section 3 (Chapters 16–25, mixed).

1. How long is the hepatitis B virus capable of surviving in a dried state on environmental surfaces?

    A. one day
    B. one week
    C. two days
    D. two weeks
    E. one month

2. Which of the following is a definite means of transmission of HIV?

    A. saliva
    B. tears
    C. intact skin
    D. blood
    E. hair

3. Medical asepsis is defined as which of the following?

    A. growth of organisms after they leave the body
    B. growth of organisms before they enter the body
    C. destruction of organisms after they leave the body
    D. destruction of organisms before they enter the body
    E. growth of organisms on medical equipment

4. Which of the following is one of the six Cs of charting?

    A. clerical
    B. clients words
    C. consult
    D. counsel
    E. court

5. Minor cauterization procedures are performed in the medical office by all of the following means *except*

    A. lasers.
    B. hemostats.
    C. hot instruments.
    D. electric currents.
    E. caustic agents.

6. Which of the following instruments is used to drain an abscess?

    A. tissue forceps
    B. tenaculum
    C. curette
    D. needle holder
    E. scalpel

7. Which of the following is not considered a vital sign?

    A. blood pressure
    B. pulse rate
    C. body temperature
    D. respiration
    E. weight

8. Which of the following areas of the body is the site at which the popliteal pulse is detected?

    A. knee
    B. ankle
    C. forearm
    D. foot
    E. brachial artery

9. The difference between the apical pulse rate and the radial pulse rate is called

    A. pulse deficit.
    B. apical pulse.
    C. radial pulse.
    D. femoral pulse.
    E. pulse pressure.

10. The formula that explains the composition of the drug is known as its

    A. generic name.
    B. chemical name.
    C. trade name.
    D. brand name.
    E. biological name.

11. A chemical substance that interferes with the development of bacterial organisms is

    A. anti-inflammatory.
    B. antiviral.
    C. antisecretory.
    D. antiepileptic.
    E. antibiotic.

12. What drug is prescribed for the treatment of manic episodes?

    A. idoxuridine
    B. lithium
    C. baclofen
    D. zolpidem
    E. ampicillin

13. Which of the following is a common route for the administration of parenteral medications?

    A. topical
    B. transdermal
    C. injection
    D. rectal
    E. oral

14. The doctor has ordered 120 mg of a drug that comes only
in 30-mg tablets. How many tablets constitute a dose?

    A. 3
    B. 4
    C. 6
    D. 12
    E. 15

15. A suppository must be inserted

    A. 0.5 inch above the internal anal sphincter.
    B. one inch above the external anal sphincter.
    C. two inches above the external anal sphincter.
    D. one–two inches above the internal anal sphincter.
    E. four–five inches above the internal anal sphincter.

16. Which of the following is not necessary in administering
an ECG?

    A. sterilizing the leads
    B. activating the standardization control
    C. cleaning the patient's skin
    D. selecting the speed
    E. activating the standardization control *and* selecting
       the speed

17. The QRS complex represents

    A. contraction of the atria.
    B. recovery of the atria.
    C. contraction of the heart.
    D. recovery of the ventricles.
    E. contraction of the ventricles.

18. When ventricular rhythm is extremely slow and irregular,
and it becomes slower to the point of asystole, it is called

    A. bigeminy.
    B. sinus rhythm.
    C. agonal rhythm.
    D. heart rhythm.
    E. acardiac rhythm.

19. A measurement of the actual absorbed dose of radiation is
called

    A. rem.
    B. rad.
    C. roentgen.
    D. contrast media.
    E. ray.

20. Before a mammogram, the patient should

    A. drink coffee.
    B. use body lotion.
    C. avoid wearing deodorant.
    D. fast after midnight.
    E. avoid exercise.

21. A radiological study of the spinal cord is called a

    A. mammography.
    B. myelography.
    C. thermography.
    D. cholangiography.
    E. arthrography.

22. How long does diathermy usually last?

    A. 5–10 minutes
    B. 10–15 minutes
    C. 15–30 minutes
    D. 60–90 minutes
    E. two–three hours

23. Electromyography is the process of electrically recording
muscle

    A. contraction.
    B. relaxation.
    C. action potentials.
    D. energy production.
    E. flexion.

24. A slow gait used by persons who can bear weight on both
legs is referred to as a

    A. crutch gait.
    B. two-point gait.
    C. three-point gait.
    D. four-point gait.
    E. five-point gait.

25. In emergency childbirth, at what point should the umbilical cord be tied and cut?

   A. when the infant is fully out of the birth canal
   B. within 10 minutes of birth
   C. when the infant starts breathing
   D. when the mother and baby get to the hospital
   E. when the baby is ready to nurse

26. Which of the following is a correct way to treat a snakebite?

   A. administer activated charcoal
   B. walk the patient to a hospital
   C. suction the wound and apply ice
   D. immobilize the bitten area and wash it with soap and water
   E. cut out the affected area

27. Chest pain might indicate

   A. cocaine use.
   B. myocardial infarction.
   C. epistaxis.
   D. myocardial infarction *and* epistaxis.
   E. cocaine use *and* myocardial infarction.

28. Dysuria is

   A. inability to retain urine.
   B. painful or difficult urination.
   C. increased output of urine.
   D. decreased output of urine.
   E. micturition.

29. Which of the following stains is specific to blood?

   A. contrast
   B. grams
   C. Wright's
   D. basic
   E. agar

30. Urine that is too acidic could indicate

   A. urinary tract infection.
   B. renal failure.
   C. diabetes.
   D. gout.
   E. incontinence.

SECTION 3 RMA REVIEW

RMA Questions for the end of Section 3 (Chapters 16–25, mixed).

1. The nicotine patch, which is indicated to aid in smoking cessation, is an example of which of the following routes of administration?
   A. subcutaneous
   B. intramuscular
   C. transdermal
   D. intravenous

2. Postprandial serum glucose levels are measured after
   A. eating.
   B. fasting.
   C. drinking.
   D. exercising.

3. Surgical asepsis is most appropriate during which of the following procedures?
   A. pulmonary function test
   B. stool guaiac test
   C. pap smear
   D. endometrial biopsy

4. The hepatitis B vaccine is administered in a series of how many injections?
   A. two
   B. three
   C. four
   D. five

5. Which of the following tubes is required when drawing blood to measure prothrombin time?
   A. sodium citrate (light blue)
   B. sodium heparin (green)
   C. potassium oxalate (gray)
   D. EDTA (lavender)

6. Tapping with the fingers, particularly in the abdomen, back, and chest is called
   A. inspection.
   B. palpation.
   C. percussion.
   D. auscultation.

7. The knee-chest position is used for examination of the
   A. rectal and vaginal area.
   B. lower back.
   C. abdomen.
   D. head and neck.

8. Which of the following types of drugs is used to prevent disease?
   A. therapeutic
   B. prophylactic
   C. diagnostic
   D. prognostic

9. Which of the following is the most common initial site for venipuncture?
   A. back of the hand
   B. wrist
   C. ankle
   D. forearm

10. Which of the following parts of a compound microscope contains the light source?
    A. base
    B. stage
    C. turret
    D. ocular

11. How many feet from the Snellen eye chart should a patient be placed for a distance visual acuity test?
    A. 10
    B. 15
    C. 20
    D. 30

12. Which of the following arteries is used to obtain a pulse from the antecubital space?
    A. popliteal
    B. carotid
    C. temporal
    D. brachial

13. Drugs classified as which of the following have no prescriptive use?
    A. Schedule I
    B. Schedule II
    C. Schedule III
    D. Schedule IV

14. During urinalysis, which of the following can be measured with a urinometer, a refractometer, or a reagent strip?
    A. protein
    B. ketones
    C. glucose
    D. specific gravity

15. The P wave on an electrocardiogram represents which of the following?

    A. ventricular depolarization
    B. atrial depolarization
    C. atrial repolarization
    D. ventricular repolarization

16 Which of the following is the most common type of hearing loss in adults?

    A. low frequency
    B. mid frequency
    C. high frequency
    D. multitonal

17 Which of the following diagnostic studies uses high-frequency sound waves to produce an image of a patient's internal organs?

    A. magnetic resonance imaging (MRI)
    B. ultrasonography
    C. fluoroscopy
    D. computer tomography (CT)

18. Which of the following drugs is prescribed for a patient who has pain after a surgical procedure?

    A. prednisone (Deltasone®)
    B. hydrocodone with APAP (Vicodin®)
    C. albuterol (Proventil®)
    D. furosemide (Lasix®)

19. Which of the following terms refers to the amount of gas left in the lungs after a person exhales as much as possible?

    A. residual volume
    B. tidal volume
    C. forced expiratory volume
    D. expiratory reserve volume

20. When performing electrocardiography, which of the following chest leads should be placed on the fourth intercostal space, right sternal border?

    A. V_1
    B. V_2
    C. V_3
    D. V_4

21. When collecting a specimen for throat culture, a medical assistant should swab which of the following structures?

    A. tongue
    B. hard palate
    C. buccal mucosa
    D. pharynx

22. Which of the following drugs is used to prevent or relieve nausea and vomiting?

    A. antipyretic
    B. antiemetic
    C. antianemic
    D. antifungal

23. To determine the erythrocyte sedimentation rate using the modified Westergren method, the test pipette must stand for how many minutes?

    A. 15
    B. 30
    C. 45
    D. 60

24. A sweet and fruity odor in the urine may indicate the presence of

    A. ketones.
    B. protein.
    C. nitrites.
    D. bilirubin.

25. When observing a patient's gait, which of the following should be noted?

    A. weight
    B. skin color
    C. style of walking
    D. mental orientation

26. Which of the following is the most effective method of affixing a bacterial smear to a slide?

    A. drying
    B. heating
    C. staining
    D. placing under a light

27. In a patient with impaired platelet function, the result of which of the following tests is most likely to be increased?

    A. bleeding time
    B. prothrombin
    C. partial thromboplastin time
    D. clot lysis time

28. Which of the following is used to determine the total number of white blood cells in the urine?

    A. urinometer
    B. chemical strip
    C. refractometer
    D. microscope

29. Which of the following drugs is used to treat osteoporosis?

    A. Zoloft® (sertraline)
    B. Fosamax® (alendronate)
    C. Synthroid® (levothyroxine)
    D. Saphris® (asenapine)

30. A myelogram is an X-ray of which of the following?

    A. gallbladder
    B. kidneys
    C. spinal canal
    D. fallopian tubes

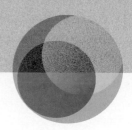

CCMA Questions for the end of Section 3 (Chapters 16–25, mixed).

1. Which of the following is the most appropriate site for intramuscular injections in infants?

    A. gluteus maximus
    B. dorsogluteal
    C. deltoid
    D. vastus lateralis

2. Which of the following actions is the universal sign for choking?

    A. Run to the nearest exit.
    B. Place hands over the neck.
    C. Get into the hands-and-knees position.
    D. Call for help.

3. Which of the following is the normal range for rates of respiration per minute in healthy adults?

    A. 8–12
    B. 12–15
    C. 12–20
    D. 20–40

4. Which of the following types of forceps is used to clamp blood vessels?

    A. tissue
    B. hemostat
    C. dressing
    D. sponge

5. How often must the medical assistant calibrate the spirometer?

    A. daily
    B. weekly
    C. biweekly
    D. monthly

6. A three-hour glucose tolerance test should be performed after a patient has fasted for how many hours?

    A. 4
    B. 6
    C. 12
    D. 16

7. Which of the following angles of insertion is correct when administering a Mantoux test?

    A. 10 degrees
    B. 25 degrees
    C. 45 degrees
    D. 90 degrees

8. Which of the following muscles is most appropriate for the administration of a two-mL intramuscular injection in an adult?

    A. rectus abdominis
    B. vastus lateralis
    C. deltoid
    D. latissimus dorsi

9. Which of the following is the most common type of urine specimen collected in the medical office?

    A. random
    B. postprandial
    C. timed
    D. first morning

10. On an electrocardiogram, repolarization of the ventricle and ventricular recovery is represented by which of the following waves?

    A. P
    B. Q
    C. R
    D. T

11. Which of the following is the process of listening for sounds within the body?

    A. inspection
    B. auscultation
    C. percussion
    D. mensuration

12. Which of the following instruments is used during auditory testing?

    A. reflex hammer
    B. tongue blade
    C. tuning fork
    D. tape measure

13. Which of the following is an instrument used to explore wounds?

    A. probe
    B. speculum
    C. retractor
    D. curette

14. Which of the following is an instrument that measures oxygen concentration in arterial blood?

    A. spirometer
    B. oximeter
    C. nebulizer
    D. nasal cannula

15. Which of the following positions is most appropriate for a patient who is undergoing a rectal examination?

    A. Sims'
    B. lithotomy
    C. prone
    D. Fowler's

16. Which of the following X-ray studies is performed after a contrast medium is injected into a patient's bile ducts?

    A. pyelography
    B. myelography
    C. arthrography
    D. cholangiography

17. For sterile packs, which of the following is the maximum shelf life from the date of sterilization?

    A. 10 days
    B. 15 days
    C. 25 days
    D. 30 days

18. Which of the following radiologic procedures is contraindicated in a man with a cardiac pacemaker?

    A. nuclear scan
    B. magnetic resonance imaging (MRI)
    C. fluoroscopy
    D. computed tomography (CT) scan

19. Which of the following instruments is most appropriate for draining a paronychia?

    A. scalpel
    B. tenaculum
    C. speculum
    D. biopsy forceps

20. A 56-year-old woman has acute pain in the lower back. Which of the following positions is most appropriate for examination of this patient?

    A. lithotomy
    B. prone
    C. Fowler's
    D. sitting

21. Which of the following needle gauges is most commonly used with an evacuated system?

    A. 18
    B. 21
    C. 23
    D. 25

22. A second-degree burn extends to which of the following levels of tissue?

    A. dermis
    B. epidermis
    C. subcutaneous tissue
    D. muscle

23. A newborn's pulse is most accurately measured at which of the following sites?

    A. side of the neck
    B. side of the wrist
    C. over the apex of the heart
    D. inside of the forearm

24. Which of the following is a physical therapy modality that uses acoustic vibrations to stimulate tissue?

    A. ultrasound
    B. ultraviolet light
    C. electric stimulation
    D. traction

25. Which of the following equipment is used during a neurologic examination?

    A. stethoscope
    B. tonometer
    C. tenaculum
    D. percussion hammer

26. A patient with which of the following conditions is in most urgent need of treatment?

    A. vertigo
    B. abdominal cramps
    C. profuse bleeding
    D. swollen legs

27. The hemoglobin level multiplied by three is approximately equal to the

    A. platelet count.
    B. hematocrit.
    C. red blood cell count.
    D. mean corpuscular volume.

28. Which of the following types of fractures is characterized by fragments of bone protruding through the skin?

    A. impacted
    B. greenstick
    C. comminuted
    D. compound

29. The most appropriate site for capillary puncture in adults is the

    A. tip of the middle finger.
    B. side of the heel pad.
    C. great toe.
    D. earlobe.

30. Which of the following classes of drugs causes relaxation of the blood vessels?

    A. hemostatic
    B. vasopressor
    C. vasodilator
    D. anticoagulant

NCMA Questions for the end of Section 3 (Chapters 16–25, mixed).

1. An established patient with diabetes mellitus collapses in the medical office. After determining that the patient is unconscious, the medical assistant should immediately administer

   A. insulin, subcutaneously.
   B. oxygen by inhalation.
   C. glucose, sublingually.
   D. epinephrine, intramuscularly.

2. Measurement of which of the following is the most effective method to monitor a patient who takes warfarin (Coumadin®)?

   A. clotting time
   B. prothrombin time (PT)
   C. partial thromboplastin time (PTT)
   D. bleeding time

3. Health-care workers who perform X-ray studies must wear which of the following to detect and record the amount of exposure to radiation?

   A. photometer
   B. densitometer
   C. dosimeter
   D. sensitometer

4. Which of the following thermometers can be used with uncooperative patients of any age?

   A. oral electronic
   B. rectal electronic
   C. disposable oral chemical
   D. tympanic membrane electronic

5. Which of the following are denoted by the graduations on an insulin syringe?

   A. minims
   B. cubic centimeters
   C. milliliters
   D. units

6. While performing electrocardiography, the medical assistant notes that the line on the paper is too dark. Which of the following should be adjusted?

   A. marker
   B. paper speed
   C. stylus heat
   D. electrode placement

7. Which of the following parts of a prescription include the name and quantity of the medication prescribed?

   A. signature
   B. subscription
   C. inscription
   D. superscription

8. A pregnant woman has had hyperemesis for the past 48 hours. She says her mouth is dry, and on examination, her skin is dry and pale. Which of the following is the most likely abnormal finding on urine dipstick testing?

   A. ketones
   B. nitrites
   C. bilirubin
   D. blood

9. Which of the following medications is most appropriate for a seven-year-old child during an acute attack of asthma?

   A. prednisone, sublingually
   B. albuterol (Ventolin®) by nebulizer
   C. ampicillin, intravenously
   D. aminophylline, by rectal suppository

10. To prevent a false-positive result when testing for occult blood in the stool, patients should be instructed to omit which of the following from their diet for three days before stool collection?

    A. whole milk
    B. green vegetables
    C. red meat
    D. coffee

11. Which of the following types of urine collection is most appropriate for pregnancy testing?

    A. first-voided morning specimen
    B. 24-hour specimen
    C. random specimen
    D. timed specimen

12. Which of the following classes of controlled substances is dispensed by written prescription only?

    A. Schedule I
    B. Schedule II
    C. Schedule III
    D. Schedule IV

13. Before administration of penicillin, which of the following is the most important aspect of a patient's medical history?

    A. history of present illness
    B. current medications
    C. social history
    D. allergies

14. On urinalysis, a positive result of a leukocyte esterase test is most indicative of which of the following?

    A. hemolytic reaction
    B. urinary tract infection
    C. dehydration
    D. muscle injury

15. While having blood drawn, a patient says he "feels faint." Which of the following adverse reactions is most likely to occur in this patient?

    A. myocardial infarction
    B. seizure
    C. syncope
    D. anaphylaxis

16. Which of the following medications is most appropriate for a patient with depression?

    A. simvastatin (Zocor®)
    B. sertraline (Zoloft®)
    C. rifampin (Rifadin®)
    D. zolpidem (Ambien®)

17. A healthy patient has a random serum glucose level of 153 mg/dL on finger stick. What is the first question the medical assistant should ask the patient?

    A. "How often do you exercise?"
    B. "When did you last eat or drink?"
    C. "Are you taking antibiotics?"
    D. "Do you have a family history of diabetes?"

18. To perform irrigation of the ear in an adult patient, the ear canal should be straightened by gently pulling the earlobe in which of the following directions?

    A. up and out
    B. up and back
    C. down and back
    D. down and out

19. Which of the following is the most appropriate first step in management after a patient faints?

    A. Perform cardiopulmonary resuscitation (CPR).
    B. Lay the patient flat, with the legs elevated.
    C. Transport the patient to the nearest emergency department.
    D. Call an ambulance.

20. For subcutaneous injection of medication in an infant, which of the following is the maximum amount that should be administered?

    A. 0.5 mL
    B. 1 mL
    C. 1.5 mL
    D. 2 mL

21. When sending a specimen for throat culture to an outside laboratory, which of the following should be used?

    A. fixative solution
    B. saline solution
    C. transport medium
    D. agar medium

22. Which of the following types of drugs is used to reduce body temperature in a patient with fever?

    A. antitussive
    B. antipyretic
    C. antiemetic
    D. antibiotic

23. The anticoagulant EDTA is most appropriate for a blood specimen that has been collected for

    A. a complete blood count (CBC).
    B. coagulation studies.
    C. plasma toxicology.
    D. blood culture.

24. Which of the following is the most appropriate distance visual acuity chart for an adult patient who does not speak English?

    A. Snellen E chart
    B. Snellen chart
    C. Snellen object chart
    D. Rosenbaum chart

25. Which of the following substances is considered a Schedule II drug?

    A. tramadol (Ultram®)
    B. diazepam (Valium®)
    C. hydrocodone with APAP (Vicodin®)
    D. celecoxib (Celebrex®)

26. An infant, at birth, can safely receive which of the following immunizations?

    A. varicella-zoster virus vaccine
    B. measles, mumps, and rubella vaccine
    C. poliovirus vaccine
    D. hepatitis B vaccine

27. Which of the following types of injections requires a 23-gauge needle that is one inch in length, and a syringe calibrated for three mL?

    A. intravenous
    B. intramuscular
    C. intradermal
    D. intrathecal

28. Which of the following is both an analgesic and an anti-inflammatory drug?

    A. morphine
    B. amoxicillin
    C. acetaminophen with codeine
    D. ibuprofen

29. Which of the following describes the difference between systolic and diastolic blood pressure?

    A. pulse pressure
    B. pulse deficit
    C. elastic pulse
    D. bounding pulse

30. Red, dry skin, a weak pulse, and dyspnea are most characteristic of which of the following conditions?

    A. shock
    B. heat exhaustion
    C. heat stroke
    D. hypothermia

PRACTICE EXAMS

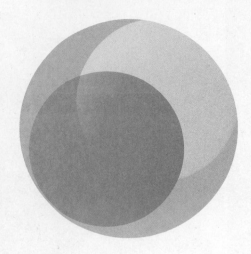

PRACTICE EXAM 1 - CMA

1. Which of the following is the primary benefit of numeric filing?

   A. Patient confidentiality is preserved.
   B. Only the patients' names must be shown on the labels of the files.
   C. Files may be stored either vertically or horizontally.
   D. Color coding is not necessary.
   E. Less storage space is required.

2. If a patient is unresponsive, which of the following should be assessed first?

   A. blood pressure   D. muscle tone
   B. pulse   E. respiration
   C. pupils

3. The receptionist who is responsible for opening the medical office must arrive how long before office hours begin?

   A. 45–60 minutes   D. 5–10 minutes
   B. 30–45 minutes   E. more than 60 minutes
   C. 15–20 minutes

4. Which of the following information is obtained from a completed daysheet?

   A. credit bureau accounts
   B. annual gross income of a medical practice
   C. amount in a petty cash fund
   D. accounts receivable data
   E. withheld payroll taxes

5. Which of the following organisms commonly causes toxic shock syndrome?

   A. *Mycobacterium leprae*
   B. *Staphylococcus aureus*
   C. *Haemophilus ducreyi*
   D. *Neisseria meningitides*
   E. *Neisseria gonorrhoeae*

6. Which of the following white blood cells is the smallest in size?

   A. eosinophils   D. neutrophils
   B. monocytes   E. lymphocytes
   C. basophils

7. A patient must pay $400 per year for medical expenses before the insurance company will begin to cover any expenses. Which of the following terms describes this payment?

   A. premium   D. coinsurance
   B. fee for service   E. deductible
   C. copayment

8. Pulmonary arteries

   A. send blood toward the heart.
   B. transfer oxygenated blood away from the heart.
   C. transfer low-oxygen blood to the lungs.
   D. are very small vessels that connect with veins.
   E. transfer blood to the brain.

9. Which of the following is the most effective way to educate new patients about office policies?

   A. Distribute patient information packets.
   B. Distribute office procedure manuals.
   C. Distribute videotapes.
   D. Distribute newsletters.
   E. Make appointments for formal patient orientation sessions.

10. The term *cryptorchidism* means

    A. inflammation of the penis.
    B. undescended testicle.
    C. ligation of the vas deferens.
    D. herniation of the scrotum.
    E. decreased sperm count.

11. When collecting a specimen for throat culture, a medical assistant should swab which of the following structures?

    A. gums   D. buccal mucosa
    B. pharynx   E. hard palate
    C. tongue

12. Which of the following is the most appropriate study to detect breast abscesses?

    A. stereoscopy   D. MUGA scan
    B. thermography   E. MRI
    C. myelography

13. A disadvantage of single-entry bookkeeping is that it

    A. is the most expensive system to set up.
    B. is hard to learn.
    C. makes errors hard to spot.
    D. is time consuming.
    E. is rare in medical practices.

14. A scheduling method in which patients sign in and are seen on a first-come, first-served basis is known as which of the following?

    A. double booking
    B. open hours
    C. stream
    D. wave
    E. clustering

15. Which of the following causes would give plasma or serum a milky appearance?

    A. hyperlipidemia
    B. kidney disease
    C. cancer
    D. protein disorder
    E. vegetarian diet

16. Which of the following is a type of mail service that guarantees delivery by 3:00 p.m. the following day?

    A. Certified
    B. Priority
    C. Express
    D. Registered
    E. Special Delivery

17. Which of the following words is misspelled?

    A. nueron
    B. malaise
    C. humerus
    D. desiccation
    E. glaucoma

18. The underlined portion of the word hypolipemia represents which of the following word parts?

    A. prefix
    B. root
    C. suffix
    D. combining form
    E. none of these

19. *Legionella pneumophila* is a bacterium that is primarily intracellular and is detected by which of the following?

    A. gram stain
    B. iodine
    C. silver stain
    D. crystal violet
    E. dark-field microscopy

20. Which of the following converts printed matter into a form that can be read by a computer?

    A. scanner
    B. keyboard
    C. monitor
    D. printer
    E. mouse

21. The main body part involved in the metabolism of drugs is the

    A. stomach.
    B. kidneys.
    C. small intestine.
    D. large intestine.
    E. liver.

22. Which of the following refers to the process of determining the circumference of an infant's head?

    A. mensuration
    B. manipulation
    C. palpation
    D. auscultation
    E. inspection

23. Depakene® is a type of

    A. antipsychotic.
    B. antidepressant.
    C. antiepileptic.
    D. antibiotic.
    E. antivenereal.

24. Which of the following parts of a prescription provides directions to the pharmacist?

    A. inscription
    B. subscription
    C. signature
    D. superscription
    E. repetatur

25. An eye examination using a Snellen eye chart tests for which of the following?

    A. peripheral vision
    B. intraocular pressure
    C. extraocular muscle movement
    D. color perception
    E. distance visual acuity

26. The first cervical vertebra is the

    A. sternum.
    B. axis.
    C. scapula.
    D. atlas.
    E. clavicle.

27. You are alone, providing CPR for a very small three-year-old child. Which of the following describes the correct technique to follow in performing chest compressions on this child?

    A. Use both hands, one on top of the other.
    B. Use the heel of one hand.
    C. Use the tips of two fingers.
    D. Use the palm and fingers of one hand.
    E. Use the tips of three fingers.

28. A record must be maintained for all drugs dispensed in the medical office that are classified in which of the following schedules?

    A. II
    B. III
    C. IV
    D. all of these

29. Who should correct an error in a patient's chart?

    A. the medical office manager
    B. the person who originally charted the entry
    C. the medical records manager
    D. the patient's attending physician
    E. the attorney for the practice

30. Which of the following types of mail provides proof that a letter has been received?

    A. First class
    B. Certified
    C. Priority
    D. Bulk

31. According to the American Association of Medical Assistants (AAMA), how often is recertification of the medical assistant (CMA) credential required?

    A. every two years
    B. every three years
    C. every five years
    E. every seven years
    D. every six years

32. The combined contraceptive pill contains

    A. estrogen only.
    B. progesterone only.
    C. both estrogen and progesterone.
    D. progesterone and testosterone.
    E. none of these.

33. An amount that constitutes an addition to revenue is called

    A. debit.   D. equity.
    B. credit.   E. charge.
    C. payables.

34. The type of listening that occurs when the medical assistant does not offer advice or give assistance is

    A. social.   D. critical.
    B. active.   E. passive.
    C. emotional.

35. Which of the following is a type of memory used in computers?

    A. CPU   D. VDT
    B. DOS   E. RAM
    C. DPI

36. During a surgical procedure, tissue is cauterized to accomplish which of the following?

    A. removal of contaminated tissue
    B. burning or cutting of tissues
    C. preparation of a specimen
    D. inspection of the wound for necrosis
    E. prevention of the patient syncope

37. Which of the following parts of a prescription indicates the number of tablets to be dispensed?

    A. subscription   D. inscription
    B. superscription E. none of these
    C. signature

38. An ICD-10-CM code may contain up to how many digits?

    A. two   D. seven
    B. three   E. nine
    C. four

39. The sudden onset of a disease marked by intensity is described as

    A. critical.   D. morbid.
    B. aplastic.   E. acute.
    C. chronic.

40. The amylase test is used for disorders related to the

    A. heart.
    B. brain.
    C. pancreas.
    D. lymphatic system.
    E. endocrine system.

41. A substance that is released from an injured cell is called a(n)

    A. antihistamine.   D. anticoagulant.
    B. histamine.   E. ampule.
    C. antibiotic.

42. To comply with Medicare guidelines, the physician must write off which of the following charges?

    A. prevailing charges
    B. limiting charges
    C. disallowed charges
    D. coinsurance
    E. deductible

43. Which of the following is the recommended screening test for tuberculosis?

    A. patch   D. hemoccult
    B. Schiller's   E. radioallergosorbent test
    C. Mantoux

44. Distention of the pelvis and calyces of the kidney by urine is referred to as

    A. nephrotic syndrome.
    B. pyelonephrosis.
    C. hydronephrosis.
    D. polycystic renal disease.
    E. chronic glomerulonephritis.

45. Which of the following types of medications may need to be refrigerated when stored?

    A. nasal sprays
    B. antihistamine tablets
    C. normal saline
    D. antibiotics

46. A disbursement journal is a summary of

    A. all daily transactions.
    B. accounts paid out.
    C. patient receipts.
    D. refunds.

47. The physician has just arrived and several patients are waiting to be seen. Which of the following patients should the physician see first?

    A. a patient scheduled for evaluation of burning when urinating
    B. a patient scheduled for rechecking of blood pressure
    C. a patient scheduled for cryosurgery
    D. a walk-in patient with a swollen ankle
    E. a walk-in patient complaining of pain radiating to the left arm

48. For a multipage letter, the medical assistant should use

   A. three-inch margins.
   B. letterhead for the first page and blank paper for all other pages.
   C. letterhead for all pages, always.
   D. double or triple spacing throughout.
   E. blank paper for all pages.

49. Which of the following medications is used to treat patients with hypertension?

   A. paroxetine (Paxil®)
   B. lansoprazole (Prevacid®)
   C. alendronate (Fosamax®)
   D. hydralazine (Apresoline®)
   E. atorvastatin (Lipitor®)

50. Which of the following pieces of incoming mail should be delivered directly to the physician?

   A. an office supply catalog
   B. a magazine for the office waiting room
   C. a letter marked "confidential"
   D. an insurance form to be completed
   E. a check from a patient

51. In an emergency situation, patients with which of the following conditions should be treated first?

   A. multiple fractures
   B. severe sprain
   C. eye injury
   D. shock
   E. first-degree burns

52. The white and outermost layer of the eye is called the

   A. retina.   D. vitreous humor.
   B. iris.   E. sclera.
   C. ciliary body.

53. If a drop of blood does not form after capillary puncture, which of the following should be done?

   A. Puncture the skin again.
   B. Push repeatedly on the finger as if milking it.
   C. Apply a tourniquet.
   D. Apply steady pressure.
   E. Wait until a drop forms.

54. Which of the following is an appropriate collection technique?

   A. calling patients at work to remind them of their financial obligation and to offer to work with them to help pay their debt
   B. threatening legal action, even though your office rarely undertakes legal action to collect, because the threat makes patients more likely to pay quickly
   C. calling patients at home after 10 p.m
   D. sending a payment reminder in the form of a statement or letter when the account is 30 days past due
   E. None of these is an appropriate collection technique.

55. The outermost layer of the cell is known as

   A. ectoplasm.   C. endoplasm.
   B. protoplasm.   D. envelope.

56. A patient has a sudden decrease in blood pressure after an acute hemorrhage. The primary cause is a decrease in which of the following?

   A. blood vessel elasticity   D. peripheral resistance
   B. blood volume   E. heart rate
   C. blood viscosity

57. The sympathetic action of the pupil of the eye is

   A. constriction.
   B. dilation.
   C. stimulation.
   D. maintaining a constant size.
   E. none of these.

58. The prefix *milli-* means

   A. one-thousandth.
   B. many.
   C. one.
   D. one hundredth.
   E. one-tenth.

59. Which of the following tests may indicate a kidney disorder?

   A. measurement of T3 and T4
   B. blood urea nitrogen
   C. antinuclear antibody
   D. luteinizing hormone
   E. guaiac test

60. Furosemide is prescribed for

   A. congestive heart failure (CHF).
   B. nephrotic syndrome.
   C. hypercalcemia.
   D. none of these.
   E. all of these

61. Which of the following is performed to detect the presence of human chorionic gonadotropin?

   A. urine pregnancy test
   B. complete blood cell count
   C. measurement of blood urea nitrogen level
   D. measurement of fasting serum glucose level
   E. measurement of Rh factor and ABO

62. Deficiency of which of the following may cause rickets?

   A. potassium   D. iron
   B. protein   E. calcium
   C. folic acid

63. Which of the following computer menu selections changes the typeface in a document?

   A. graphics   D. edit
   B. tools   E. font
   C. view

64. When dealing with a seriously ill patient, you should

    A. trivialize the patient's feelings.
    B. judge the patient's statements.
    C. avoid empty promises.
    D. abandon the patient.
    E. isolate the patient.

65. Which of the following instruments is used to expand and separate the walls of a cavity to make examination possible?

    A. sound
    B. hemostat
    C. tenaculum
    D. tonometer
    E. speculum

66. The most common type of anemia is

    A. sickle cell.
    B. pernicious.
    C. folic acid deficiency.
    D. iron deficiency.
    E. none of these.

67. The subject line of a letter appears

    A. two lines below the last line of the body.
    B. two lines below the salutation.
    C. one line above the outside address.
    D. one line above the inside address.
    E. one line below the date.

68. A medical assistant should do all of the following when answering the telephone *except*

    A. give the caller the medical assistant's name first and then the name of the office.
    B. identify the caller.
    C. ask, "How may I help you?".
    D. hold the phone's mouthpiece an inch away from the mouth.
    E. use words appropriate to the situation, but avoid using technical terms.

69. The thalamus

    A. controls body temperature.
    B. acts as a relay station for sensory impulses.
    C. is the center of the brain for memory and visual recognition.
    D. connects the two hemispheres of the brain.
    E. has no brain function.

70. Standard letterhead is

    A. used in general business correspondence.
    B. 5.5 × 8.5 inches in size.
    C. used for social correspondence.
    D. not used in the medical office.
    E. none of these

71. Which of the following prefixes means "bad, difficult, painful"?

    A. ex-
    B. dis-
    C. dys-
    D. dia-
    E. meta-

72. Which of the following bookkeeping terms refers to charges on the patient's account?

    A. credits
    B. equities
    C. debits
    D. assets
    E. liabilities

73. Which of the following diagnostic studies uses high-frequency sound waves to produce an image of a patient's internal organs?

    A. positron emission tomography (PET) scan
    B. magnetic resonance imaging (MRI)
    C. computed tomography (CT)
    D. ultrasonography
    E. fluoroscopy

74. Which of the following medications is most appropriate for a patient with depression?

    A. Cardura
    B. Fuzeon
    C. Zocor
    D. Zoloft
    E. Bactroban

75. Which of the following terms refers to the balance due to a creditor on a current account?

    A. collection ratio
    B. aging analysis
    C. accounts payable
    D. income statement
    E. balance sheet

76. Which of the following items is a capital purchase for the medical office?

    A. gowns
    B. cleaning supplies
    C. surgical scissors
    D. autoclave
    E. bandages

77. Which of the following classes of drugs is most appropriate for a patient with a persistent cough?

    A. antidotes
    B. antivirals
    C. antitussives
    D. antibiotics
    E. antidepressants

78. A patient should be advised to bring an insurance card to each appointment for which of the following reasons?

    A. to identify changes in the patient's current insurance coverage
    B. to confirm the patient's employment
    C. to verify the correct spelling of the patient's name
    D. to streamline the processing of insurance claims

79. Which of the following types of tinea is known as "jock itch"?

    A. tinea capitis
    B. tinea corporis
    C. tinea inguinal
    D. tinea cruris
    E. tinea pedis

80. Which of the following suffixes means "beginning, origin, production"?

    A. -iasis
    B. -genic
    C. -genetic
    D. both -genic and -genetic
    E. none of these

81. A 26-year-old woman has swallowed an overdose of pre-scribed sleeping pills. She is now unresponsive. When you open her airway, you find that she is gasping for breath and is not breathing normally at all. Using a pocket mask, you provide two rescue breaths and check for signs of circulation, including her pulse, which is rapid but weak. What should you do next?

A. Provide rescue breathing at a rate of one breath every five seconds.
B. Begin chest compressions because her pulse is weak.
C. Place the victim in the recovery position.
D. Perform CPR for one minute with chest compressions only.
E. Give two more rescue breaths, place the victim in the recovery position, and then perform CPR for two minutes.

82. Which of the following is used in preparing a blood smear slide?

A. hemoclip
B. microhematocrit tube
C. lens paper
D. automatic puncturing device
E. spreader slide

83. A physician may order a stool culture if he or she suspects

A. cancer.
B. protozoal infection.
C. bacterial infection.
D. colitis.
E. any of these.

84. Which of the following can increase blood pressure?

A. fear of medical personnel
B. age younger than 20 years
C. use of calcium channel blockers
D. height greater than six feet
E. dehydration

85. Which of the following cells can release histamine and heparin?

A. lymphocytes
B. Kupffer cells
C. erythrocytes
D. neurons
E. mast cells

86. The suffix -kinesia means

A. mind.
B. muscle.
C. pain.
D. touch.
E. movement.

87. Which of the following terms describes the technique used when the medical assistant repeats this back to the patient: "So you have a lot of difficulty sleeping because of your pain?"

A. paraphrasing
B. compensation
C. displacement
D. rationalization
E. projection

88. The most common causative organism of meningitis in adults is

A. *Herpes zoster.*
B. *Streptococcus pneumoniae.*
C. *Poliovirus.*
D. *Neisseria meningitides.*
E. *Escherichia coli.*

89. Lidocaine is a type of

A. antibiotic.
B. antiarrhythmic.
C. diuretic.
D. general anesthetic.
E. antihypnotic.

90. In sickle cell anemia, what component is abnormal that causes the erythrocytes to change shape?

A. hemoglobin
B. hematocrit
C. lymphocytes
D. intrinsic factor
E. erythropoietin

91. Operative Procedure: Left thyroid lobectomy with removal of the isthmus. A medical assistant preparing an insurance claim for this operative procedure should select coding for which of the following body systems?

A. respiratory
B. endocrine
C. reproductive
D. integumentary
E. digestive

92. The medical assistant calls the endocrinologist to sched-ule an appointment for a patient who has type 1 diabetes mellitus. To avoid hypoglycemia in the patient, which of the following appointment times should the medical assistant request?

A. first appointment in the morning
B. last appointment before lunch
C. a midafternoon appointment
D. last appointment of the day

93. Which of the following is the recommended age to admin-ister the first *Haemophilus influenzae* type B immuniza-tion to a child?

A. 2 months
B. 6 months
C. 12 months
D. 15 months

94. The combining form *xer/o* refers to something

A. dry.
B. yellow.
C. multiple.
D. pertaining to hair.
E. pertaining to X-rays.

95. Which of the following is the route of administration for parenteral medications?

A. oral
B. instillation
C. injection
D. inhalation
E. transdermal

96. Which of the following positions is most commonly used for pelvic examination?

    A. lithotomy
    B. Trendelenburg's
    C. jackknife
    D. Fowler's
    E. Sims'

97. According to the Patient's Bill of Rights, which of the following is a patient right?

    A. to waive payment if treatment is unsatisfactory
    B. to expect continuity of care
    C. to participate in research without informed consent
    D. to obtain information about family members' health care
    E. to be provided with sample medications

98. Which of the following branches off the trachea and passes into the lungs?

    A. bronchus
    B. hypothalamus
    C. epiglottis
    D. pancreas
    E. spleen

99. Which of the following checks is drawn by the bank and made payable out of the bank's account?

    A. limited
    B. certified
    C. voucher
    D. counter
    E. cashier's

100. Which of the following is the most appropriate response by a medical assistant who answers a prank telephone call?

    A. Place the caller on hold.
    B. Keep the caller on the telephone and trace the call.
    C. Tell the caller that the police will be called.
    D. Blow a whistle into the mouthpiece.
    E. Hang up the telephone.

101. An area of dead cells due to a lack of oxygen is called

    A. ischemia.
    B. infarction.
    C. atresia.
    D. gangrene.
    E. placenta previa.

102. In the matrix scheduling system, medical assistants should block off

    A. physicians' lunch hours.
    B. visits with drug company representatives.
    C. time for performing hospital rounds.
    D. none of these
    E. all of these

103. Medical assistants should take all of the following actions when opening mail *except*

    A. annotate mail with comments in the margin.
    B. open the physician's personal mail.
    C. date all opened mail.
    D. transmit letters to the physician with the most important ones on the top.
    E. check for enclosures.

104. Which of the following words is misspelled?

    A. vacsine
    B. sphincter
    C. parietal
    D. osseous
    E. asthma

105. Which of the following drug types is used to reduce cholesterol?

    A. hypolipidemic
    B. anticoagulant
    C. antiarrhythmic
    D. cholinergic
    E. antisecretory

106. The combining form *ot/o* means

    A. hearing.
    B. seeing.
    C. light.
    D. eye.
    E. ear.

107. Which of the following *International Classifications of Diseases, Clinical Modification (ICD-CM)* code ranges should be used to indicate the cause of injury, such as a fall?

    A. F01–F99
    B. C00–D49
    C. D50–D89
    D. P00–P96
    E. S00–T88

108. Which of the following medical records should be filed first in a terminal-digit numeric series?

    A. 12-34-52
    B. 14-52-46
    C. 24-61-35
    D. 65-43-21
    E. 24-53-16

109. Which of the following is a type of tickler file?

    A. numerical
    B. subject
    C. alphabetical
    D. geographical
    E. chronological

110. According to U.S. Postal Service guidelines, which of the following is the correct state abbreviation for an envelope addressed to Boston?

    A. MA
    B. MT
    C. MS
    D. ME
    E. MD

111. The proofreader's mark that resembles an equal sign means which of the following?

    A. delete
    B. insert hyphen
    C. insert space
    D. close up space
    E. center

112. Which of the following is the correct spelling for the term describing absence or abnormal cessation of menses?

    A. ammenorrhea
    B. amennorrhea
    C. ammennorhea
    D. amenorrhea
    E. amenorhea

113. Which of the following medical terms is commonly known as "crossed eyes"?

    A. nystagmus
    B. strabismus
    C. myopia
    D. presbyopia
    E. astigmatism

114. Which of the following basic computer software operations obtains a saved file?

  A. retrieving file
  B. merging file
  C. editing
  D. formatting file
  E. creating file

115. Cromolyn is used to treat

  A. asthma.
  B. allergies.
  C. viral infections.
  D. tuberculosis.
  E. pneumonia.

116. You are providing rescue breathing to an unresponsive, nonbreathing child who shows signs of circulation. How often should you provide rescue breaths for this child?

  A. once every six–eight seconds (eight–ten breaths per minute)
  B. once every four seconds (15 breaths per minute)
  C. once every five seconds (12 breaths per minute)
  D. once every 10 seconds (six breaths per minute)
  E. once every 12 seconds (five breaths per minute)

117. Butenafine is prescribed to treat

  A. depression.
  B. constipation.
  C. osteoporosis.
  D. athlete's foot.
  E. obesity.

118. Which of the following steps must be taken to recall a mailed letter?

  A. Contact the postmaster general.
  B. Call the post office.
  C. Ask the mail carrier to return the letter.
  D. E-mail the application to the postmaster.

119. If a patient weighs 165 pounds, how much does he or she weigh in kilograms?

  A. 35 kg
  B. 54 kg
  C. 62 kg
  D. 75 kg
  E. 86 kg

120. Which of the following actions is most appropriate to ensure the security of electronic medical records?

  A. changing users' login codes and passwords annually
  B. restricting access to information based on each user's job function
  C. storing backup disks in the safety of the medical office
  D. creating users' passwords with letters for encryption
  E. locating computer terminals centrally within the medical office

121. The production of heat needed to use food is called

  A. catabolism.
  B. thermogenesis.
  C. anabolism.
  D. metabolism.
  E. none of these

122. Scheduling two or more patients in the same slot is known as

  A. wave scheduling.
  B. open hours.
  C. modified wave scheduling.
  D. double booking.
  E. none of these.

123. Serum sickness is what type of sensitivity?

  A. I
  B. II
  C. III
  D. IV
  E. V

124. The combining form *cheillo* means

  A. cheek.
  B. lip.
  C. gum.
  D. tongue.
  E. mouth.

125. Which of the following devices is used to keep irregular flows of alternating current electricity from damaging computer components?

  A. spark arrester
  B. surge protector
  C. battery backup
  D. grounding floor mat

126. Which of the following is the body's initial response to any injury?

  A. sneezing
  B. fever
  C. inflammation
  D. bleeding
  E. burning

127. Which of the following is collected for a leukocyte count?

  A. plasma
  B. clotted blood
  C. whole blood
  D. serum
  E. buffy coat

128. When practicing sterile technique, the medical assistant should use which of the following instruments to set up a sterile field?

  A. towel clamp
  B. thumb forceps
  C. retractor
  D. needle holder
  E. transfer forceps

129. Standard precautions require that examination rooms, equipment, blood spills, and other potentially infectious materials be cleaned with which of the following?

  A. soap and water
  B. povidone-iodine
  C. bleach
  D. hydrogen peroxide
  E. isopropyl alcohol

130. Which of the following is a general term for measuring weight and height?

  A. auscultation
  B. palpation
  C. manipulation
  D. inspection
  E. mensuration

131. Which of the following is the portion of a centrifuged urine sample used for microscopic examination?

  A. sediment
  B. supernatant
  C. artifacts
  D. casts
  E. crystals

132. A daysheet provides complete and up-to-date information about

    A. income taxes.
    B. accounts receivable.
    C. accounts payable.
    D. accounts forwarded to a collection agency.

133. Which of the following is the most important consideration when scheduling patient appointments?

    A. scheduling preferences of the physician
    B. availability of the medical equipment
    C. urgency of patient need
    D. convenience of the patient

134. What action should a medical assistant take if a caller wants to talk to a physician but refuses to identify him- or herself?

    A. Hang up.
    B. Transfer the call to the physician anyway.
    C. Advise the person that the physician is not in the office and to call back later.
    D. Ask the person to write a letter to the physician and mark it "personal.".
    E. Transfer the call to another medical assistant.

135. Which of the following procedures requires that surgical asepsis be maintained?

    A. using a spirometer
    B. cleaning a colonoscope
    C. performing a dipstick urinalysis
    D. applying casting materials to a patient with a closed fracture
    E. aspiration of fluid from a cyst in the breast

136. Which of the following muscles is located in the torso?

    A. masseter   D. gastrocnemius
    B. triceps   E. soleus
    C. external oblique

137. Which of the following thermometers can be used to obtain the fastest accurate reading?

    A. rectal electronic
    B. oral electronic
    C. disposable oral chemical
    D. tympanic membrane electronic
    E. none of these

138. When performing electrocardiography, which of the following chest leads should be placed at the fifth intercostal space at the junction of the left midclavicular line?

    A. V_1 D. V_4
    B. V_2 E. V_5
    C. V_3

139. Biohazardous waste must be collected in impermeable polyethylene bags that are which of the following colors?

    A. yellow   D. blue
    B. red   E. green
    C. black

140. A synapse is

    A. the junction between two neurons.
    B. the junction between two bones.
    C. the main part of the neuron.
    D. a type of nerve cell that supports, protects, and nourishes the neuron.
    E. a type of bone cell that supports, protects, and nourishes the bone.

141. Which of the following is the *best* use of computers in the medical office?

    A. to set up networks
    B. accessing patient records
    C. to avoid repetitive strain injuries
    D. to avoid eye strain
    E. to order supplies

142. Sensitivity testing is used to determine

    A. a pathogen's susceptibility to antibiotics.
    B. a patient's susceptibility to antibiotics.
    C. a patient's susceptibility to a pathogen.
    D. a pathogen's susceptibility to antiseptic agents.
    E. none of these

143. Drugs that increase urine secretion are

    A. laxatives.   D. cromolyns.
    B. diuretics.   E. uremics.
    C. hypolipidemics.

144. The condition in which one of the sex chromosomes is missing is called

    A. Klinefelter's syndrome. D. tetralogy of fallot.
    B. Turner's syndrome.   E. Peyronie's disease.
    C. Down syndrome.

145. Which of the following terms refers to an advance directive made by an individual that specifies his or her end-of-life wishes?

    A. hospice   C. living will
    B. implied contract D. euthanasia

146. When a urine culture is being performed, the urine should be incubated on the culture dishes for how many hours?

    A. 6   C. 18
    B. 12   D. 24

147. The physician prescribes Prozac 60 mg per day for 30 days. Prozac is available in 20-mg tablets. Which of the following is the correct number to be dispensed?

    A. 30   D. 120
    B. 60   E. 180
    C. 90

148. The proofreaders' mark "#" represents which of the following?

    A. delete   D. add a space
    B. spell out   E. align this line
    C. transpose

149. The anticoagulant EDTA is most appropriate for a blood specimen that has been collected for

    A. glucose-tolerance tests.
    B. complete blood cell counts.
    C. blood cultures.
    D. plasma toxicology.
    E. coagulation studies.

150. Which of the following terms means "fainting"?

    A. volvulus
    B. fibrillation
    C. epistaxis
    D. syncope
    E. cachexia

151. Which of the following injections is administered under the skin and into the fat layer?

    A. intramuscular
    B. subcutaneous
    C. intravenous
    D. intradermal
    E. intracavity

152. A telephone feature that answers calls and has a recording that identifies services available by pressing a specific number is known as which of the following?

    A. voice mail
    B. answering service
    C. automated routing unit
    D. fax transmission
    E. all of these

153. An 18-month-old girl was taken to her pediatrician for a vaccine. Which of the following terms most likely relates to her reaction to the nurse with the needle?

    A. acceptance
    B. anxiety
    C. aggression
    D. anger
    E. alertness

154. Which of the following words is misspelled?

    A. peritoneum
    B. dissect
    C. homerous
    D. mctastasis
    E. none of these

155. All but which of the following are characteristics of the endocrine system?

    A. It is responsible for many conscious and unconscious activities.
    B. Its response is slow and prolonged when compared with that of the nervous system.
    C. Endocrine glands are ductless and release hormones into the bloodstream.
    D. It controls many body functions, such as blood pressure, heart rate, and sexual characteristics.
    E. The endocrine system produces hormones that affect activities such as growth, metabolism, and reproduction.

156. Which of the following is the most likely adverse effect in a patient who takes a beta-adrenergic blocking agent?

    A. polyuria
    B. photosensitivity
    C. bradycardia
    D. agitation
    E. anorexia

157. Through the U.S. Postal Service, a package of books that weighs 90 pounds

    A. can be sent Standard Mail (B).
    B. can be sent Priority Mail.
    C. cannot be sent because it exceeds weight limits.
    D. can be sent Express Mail.
    E. can be sent Standard Mail (A).

158. Which of the following types of insurance covers medical expenses for patients who are injured "in their home"?

    A. special risk
    B. workers' compensation
    C. disability protection
    D. overhead
    E. liability

159. Which of the following is a mechanism involved in healing ulcers?

    A. reduction of gastric acidity
    B. enhancement of mucosal defenses
    C. increase of gastric acidity
    D. reduction of gastric acidity *and* enhancement of mucosal defenses
    E. none of these

160. Fluoxetine is a type of

    A. antipsychotic.
    B. antihypertensive.
    C. analgesic.
    D. antidepressant.
    E. hypolipidemic.

161. The abbreviation NP stands for

    A. neurological performance.
    B. no-show patient.
    C. new practice.
    D. new physical.
    E. new patient.

162. Which of the following statements is true about a typical purchasing procedure in a medical office?

    A. An authorized person should be in charge of purchasing.
    B. Receipts of goods should be recorded.
    C. High-quality goods should be ordered at the lowest price.
    D. Shipments should be checked against packing slips.
    E. all of these

163. Thrombophlebitis occurs most commonly in the

    A. lower legs.
    B. lower arms.
    C. lower abdomen.
    D. neck.
    E. lungs.

164. The part of the brain responsible for visual recognition is the

    A. occipital lobe.
    B. temporal lobe.
    C. parietal lobe.
    D. Broca's area.
    E. pons.

165. Which of the following is a horizontal plane that divides the body into upper and lower portions?

    A. sagittal
    B. midsagittal
    C. transverse
    D. frontal
    E. coronal

166. Which of the following provides detailed information about the potential hazards of chemicals used in the physician's office?

    A. *Physicians' Desk Reference*
    B. Safety Data Sheets
    C. office policy manual
    D. controlled substances log
    E. incident report

167. Epinephrine is a(n)

    A. adrenergic.
    B. adrenergic blocker.
    C. cholinergic.
    D. cholinergic blocker.

168. Which of the following body systems contains the cervix and fallopian tubes?

    A. urinary
    B. integumentary
    C. reproductive
    D. cardiovascular
    E. endocrine

169. Which of the following is a type of hormone?

    A. chyme
    B. globulin
    C. bile
    D. secretin
    E. agglutinin

170. In a medical record, dyspepsia should be recorded under which of the following body systems?

    A. digestive
    B. urinary
    C. respiratory
    D. circulatory
    E. lymphatic

171. Which of the following is the study of death and dying?

    A. euthanasia
    B. serology
    C. oncology
    D. thanatology
    E. scientology

172. A medical assistant is paid biweekly and earns a regular rate of $10.50/hour. Her employer pays 1.5 times the regular rate for any hours exceeding 80 within a two-week time period. During the past two weeks, she worked 82 hours. Which of the following represents her gross earnings for this biweekly time period?

    A. $840.00
    B. $861.00
    C. $871.50
    D. $880.00
    E. $884.50

173. Which of the following terms is spelled correctly?

    A. lythiasis
    B. litthiasis
    C. lithiasis
    D. lithisis
    E. lithiosis

174. Certified mail is used to send

    A. all office mailings.
    B. hazardous materials.
    C. documents, contracts, and bankbooks.
    D. appointment reminders.
    E. results of medical tests.

175. Type A blood has

    A. A antigen on the red blood cells and A antibodies in plasma.
    B. B antigen on the red blood cells and A antibodies in plasma.
    C. A antigen on the red blood cells and anti-B antibodies in plasma.
    D. both A and B antigens on red blood cells and no antibodies in plasma.
    E. no antigens on red blood cells and both A and B antibodies in plasma.

176. The three bones in the middle ear that amplify vibration are called

    A. auditory ossicles.
    B. cochlea.
    C. organs of Corti.
    D. vestibule.
    E. malleus.

177. You are babysitting your infant nephew. You are alone and find the infant unresponsive. Which of the following is the best action?

    A. Check for signs of circulation and, if there are none, call 9-1-1.
    B. Call 9-1-1 immediately to ensure that advanced life support is on the way, and then return to the infant to begin the ABCs of CPR.
    C. Give two rescue breaths; if there is no response to the rescue breaths, call 9-1-1.
    D. Begin the ABCs of CPR and then call 9-1-1 after one minute of rescue support.
    E. Check for signs of circulation, give two rescue breaths, and then call 9-1-1.

178. Which of the following should be placed on top of a stack of incoming mail for the physician's attention?

    A. medical journal
    B. patient payment
    C. seminar brochure
    D. contribution request
    E. consultant's report

179. What is the function of the hormone calcitonin, which is released from the thyroid gland?

    A. It increases sodium and potassium in the blood.
    B. It increases reabsorption of water in kidney tubules.
    C. It increases plasma calcium concentrations.
    D. It decreases secretion of milk in nursing mothers.
    E. It decreases plasma calcium concentrations.

180. A patient with Addison's disease should be examined by which of the following types of specialists?

    A. neurologist
    B. radiologist
    C. nephrologist
    D. endocrinologist
    E. immunologist

PRACTICE EXAM 2 - RMA

1. Which of the following must be on file in a medical office that uses hazardous materials?

   A. proof of medical waste disposal
   B. material safety data sheets
   C. blood-borne pathogens standard
   D. chemical hygiene plan

2. The patient's first impression of the medical office is most often determined by the

   A. physician.   C. phlebotomist.
   B. office manager.   D. receptionist, on the phone.

3. A colposcopy is an examination that is performed to visualize tissue in which of the following body systems?

   A. reproductive   C. digestive
   B. urinary   D. endocrine

4. Which of the following suffixes means "digestion"?

   A. -chezia   C. -pepsia
   B. -phagia   D. -phasia

5. Which of the following is the symbol for potassium?

   A. Hg   C. Na
   B. K   D. Si

6. A symbol on the computer monitor that shows the location where the next character will appear when typed or inserted is called the

   A. router.   C. browser.
   B. cursor.   D. motherboard.

7. Which of the following filing systems is most appropriate for a practice with more than 15,000 active patient records?

   A. subject   C. alphabetic
   B. geographic   D. numeric

8. Which is the easiest filing system for locating a misfiled record?

   A. color coding   C. subject filing
   B. chronological filing D. alphanumeric filing

9. Which of the following pieces of incoming mail should be delivered directly to the physician?

   A. an office supply catalog
   B. a meeting notice from a medical society
   C. an insurance form to be completed
   D. a check from a patient

10. Hematemesis should be recorded under which of the following body systems?

    A. respiratory   C. gastrointestinal
    B. integumentary   D. urinary

11. Which of the following infectious microorganisms can be seen only with an electron microscope?

    A. protozoa   C. fungi
    B. viruses   D. bacteria

12. Which of the following classes of drugs may be used to treat vomiting?

    A. hemostatic   C. vasodilator
    B. anticoagulant   D. antiemetic

13. Which of the following terms describes the process that reduces the number of microorganisms to a safe level?

    A. sterilization   C. disinfection
    B. sanitization   D. asepsis

14. Which of the following terms describes a diagnosis based on a comparison of signs and symptoms of similar disease?

    A. differential   C. tentative
    B. preoperative   D. admitting

15. How often should the medical assistant inventory the supplies that are stored in examination rooms?

    A. once a day
    B. once a week
    C. once a month
    D. twice a month

16. When direct pressure does not effectively control bleeding from a wrist wound, pressure should be applied at which of the following arteries?

    A. brachial
    B. radial
    C. femoral
    D. carotid

17. Allergen extracts are administered by which of the following routes?

    A. oral
    B. subcutaneous
    C. intramuscular
    D. intradermal

18. When processing a specimen for detection of *Streptococcus*, which of the following culture mediums should be used?

    A. MacConkey
    B. mannitol salt
    C. blood agar
    D. Thayer-Martin

19. The MRI report states, "The patient has a tear of the medial meniscus." The patient has a tear of the

    A. lining of the uterus.
    B. fibrocartilage of the knee.
    C. membrane of the spinal cord.
    D. cortex of the brain.

20. Which of the following word-processing functions is used to align the right margin of a document?

    A. justification
    B. indentation
    C. tabulation
    D. hyphenation

21. Which of the following postal services provides insurance coverage for valuable items?

    A. Restricted Delivery
    B. Certified Mail
    C. Return Receipt
    D. Registered Mail

22. When coding an insurance claim for a thoracentesis, according to *Current Procedural Terminology* (CPT), the code should be listed under which of the following body systems?

    A. integumentary
    B. respiratory
    C. musculoskeletal
    D. cardiovascular

23. Which of the following is the most common mode of transmission of *Chlamydia trachomatis*?

    A. ingestion
    B. airborne
    C. direct contact
    D. blood-borne

24. Which of the following equipment is used to stop the heart from quivering by delivering an electric shock?

    A. ultrasonograph
    B. electrocardiograph
    C. echocardiograph
    D. defibrillator

25. Which of the following used items is classified as contaminated waste?

    A. elastic bandage used to wrap a wrist
    B. disposable suture removal kit
    C. otoscope speculum
    D. goggles

26. Cystoscopy is used to examine which of the following body structures?

    A. bladder
    B. rectum
    C. knee joint
    D. nasal cavity

27. Which of the following medications is most appropriate for patients who have osteoarthritis?

    A. cephalexin (Biocef®)
    B. cefprozil (Cefzil®)
    C. cefuroxime (Ceftin®)
    D. celecoxib (Celebrex®)

28. Which of the following is used to screen for occult blood in the stool?

    A. prothrombin time
    B. hematocrit determination
    C. guaiac test
    D. blood smear

29. In which of the following situations should surgical asepsis be used?

    A. performing a physical examination
    B. inserting a urinary catheter
    C. applying a dermal patch
    D. measuring blood pressure

30. Which of the following requires the patient's written consent before reporting to proper authorities?

    A. stillbirth
    B. substance abuse
    C. gunshot wound
    D. rape

31. Gustatory sensors detect which of the following senses?

    A. taste
    B. hunger
    C. smell
    D. pain

32. Inflammation of the joints between the vertebrae in the spine is known as

    A. tendinitis.
    B. myositis.
    C. spondylitis.
    D. hidradenitis.

33. An aggressive person who becomes a boxer is utilizing the Freudian defense mechanism known as

    A. sublimation.
    B. regression.
    C. rationalization.
    D. projection.

34. Which of the following suffixes means "drooping, prolapse, falling"?

    A. -philia
    B. -phobia
    C. -plasty
    D. -ptosis

35. Which of the following terms refers to an order to appear in court with a patient's medical records?

    A. subpoena duces tecum   C. res ipsa loquitur

    B. respondeat superior   D. res judicata

36. Which of the following types of information is most likely to be dictated in an ambulatory care facility?

    A. pathology report   C. autopsy report

    B. operative report   D. progress note

37. To comply with Medicare guidelines, the physician must write off which of the following?

    A. prevailing charge   C. deductible

    B. disallowed charges   D. limiting charge

38. Which of the following items is part of a single-entry bookkeeping system?

    A. pegboard   C. ledger

    B. receipt   D. computer software

39. Which of the following products is used to absorb poison after vomiting has stopped?

    A. sorbitol   C. ipecac

    B. ibuprofen   D. activated charcoal

40. The chain of infection starts at which of the following levels?

    A. transmission   C. susceptible host

    B. reservoir host   D. means of entry

41. According to standard precautions, medical assistants should first wash which of the following after handling body fluids?

    A. mask   C. face

    B. gloves   D. hands

42. Which of the following legal documents applies to anatomical gifts?

    A. living will   C. uniform donor card

    B. power of attorney   D. advance directive

43. A medical assistant who releases a patient's medical record without authorization from the patient can be charged with which of the following?

    A. defamation of character   C. negligence

    B. invasion of privacy   D. assault

44. Which of the following checks is drawn by the bank, payable from the bank's account, and signed by an authorized bank official?

    A. cashier's   C. voucher

    B. certified   D. limited

45. Which of the following should be inventoried as capital equipment?

    A. wall clock   C. garbage can

    B. coffee maker   D. photocopier

46. Which of the following is used for inpatient hospital care?

    A. Uniform Ambulatory Care Data Set

    B. Uniform Hospital Discharge Data Set

    C. Minimum Data Set for Long-Term Care

    D. Essential Medical Data Set

47. Which of the following elements in urine sediments are counted and reported as range/hpf?

    A. erythrocytes   C. bacteria

    B. mucus   D. crystals

48. Biohazardous materials must be disposed of in containers labeled with a symbol of which color?

    A. yellow-gray   C. black-white

    B. orange-red   D. blue-green

49. Chemical substances that are broken down by fatty acids in the liver are called

    A. triglyceride.   C. ketosis.

    B. cholesterol.   D. urea.

50. An immature erythrocyte is known as

    A. a reticulocyte.   C. anisocytosis.

    B. poikilocytosis.   D. pinocytosis.

51. Listening to sounds with a stethoscope is referred to as

    A. percussion.   C. palpation.

    B. inspection.   D. auscultation.

52. Which of the following microorganisms appear as grapelike clusters when stained and viewed through a microscope?

    A. vibrio   C. staphylococci

    B. streptococci   D. bacilli

53. Before reading the prescription to the patient, the medical assistant should ask the physician to do which of the following?

    A. verify the number of refills

    B. verify the number of tablets to be dispensed

    C. replace the trade name with the generic name

    D. clarify the route of administration

54. The Occupational Safety and Health Act is primarily designed to protect which of the following individuals who enters the medical office?

    A. patient   C. employer

    B. vendor   D. employee

55. Artificial surfactants are administered to premature infants to help prevent their lungs from

    A. infection.   C. dropping.

    B. collapsing.   D. inspiration.

56. When a medication irritates subcutaneous tissue, which of the following types of injections should be administered?

    A. subcutaneous   C. intravenous
    B. Z-track   D. intradermal

57. Which of the following types of membranes lines the joints?

    A. mucous   C. synovial
    B. fibrous   D. arachnoid

58. Which of the following documents is most appropriate for verifying a supply order when supplies are received?

    A. packing slip   C. billing invoice
    B. purchase order   D. inventory record

59. Which of the following bones is most likely to be fractured in a patient who sustained a wrist injury?

    A. tibia   C. olecranon
    B. humerus   D. radius

60. Which of the following is classified as the universal donor blood type?

    A. A negative   C. O negative
    B. AB negative   D. B negative

61. Which of the following is the functional unit of the kidney that forms urine by the process of filtration, reabsorption, and secretion?

    A. renal pelvis   C. medulla
    B. cortex   D. nephron

62. Which of the following diagnostic procedures is used to visually examine the stomach?

    A. gastroscopy   C. choledochoscopy
    B. cystoscopy   D. colonoscopy

63. The chemical known as deoxyribonucleic acid (DNA) is stored in which of the following parts of a cell?

    A. ribosomes   C. mitochondria
    B. nucleus   D. cytoplasm

64. Which of the following is a fungal infection of the skin?

    A. urticaria   C. ringworm
    B. impetigo   D. psoriasis

65. Which of the following terms is the plural of lumen?

    A. luminous   C. luminance
    B. luminal   D. lumina

66. Which of the following terms means "surgical removal of an ovary"?

    A. oophorrhaphy   C. oophoropexy
    B. oophorotomy   D. oophorectomy

67. Which of the following endocrine glands secretes glucagon?

    A. parathyroid   C. pituitary
    B. pancreas   D. adrenal

68. Which of the following is an appropriate step before applying sterile surgical gloves?

    A. removing jewelry from hands and wrists
    B. rinsing hands with warm water
    C. putting on a laboratory coat
    D. applying moisturizing lotion

69. A standard tab key on a computer will move the cursor how many spaces?

    A. one   C. five
    B. three   D. seven

70. Which of the following bookkeeping terms refers to a chronologic history of the financial transactions of a patient's account?

    A. ledger   C. balance sheet
    B. daysheet   D. charge slip

71. Which of the following describes the conscious awareness of one's own feelings and the feelings of others?

    A. sublimation   C. perception
    B. regression   D. projection

72. Which of the following is a computer output device?

    A. mouse   C. printer
    B. hard drive   D. CD-ROM

73. Which of the following is the primary organ responsible for absorption of nutrients?

    A. stomach   C. esophagus
    B. small intestine   D. large intestine

74. Which of the following computer terms describes a collection of related files that serves as a foundation for retrieval?

    A. network   C. database
    B. software   D. batch

75. Low power, high power, and oil immersion describe which of the following parts of a compound microscope?

    A. monocular lens   C. binocular lenses
    B. objective lenses   D. condenser

76. Which of the following is the most common cause of burning during urination in men?

    A. pyelonephritis   C. enuresis
    B. epididymitis   D. urethritis

77. Which of the following terms describes a forward curvature of the lumbar spine (swayback)?

    A. lordosis   C. spina bifida
    B. scoliosis   D. kyphosis

78. When a patient is deceased, which of the following is the most appropriate medical record classification?

    A. released   C. inactive
    B. active   D. closed

79. A patient who has been advised to maintain a 1000-calorie diet on a long-term basis should eliminate which of the following foods?

A. kale
B. whole milk
C. apples
D. sweet potatoes

80. Which of the following terms describes erythrocytes that have decreased hemoglobin?

A. hypochromic
B. normochromic
C. anisochromic
D. microcytic

81. The basic building blocks of the body are

A. organs.
B. muscles.
C. tissues.
D. cells.

82. Which of the following is used to send and receive messages through a computer network?

A. scanner
B. e-mail
C. dialogue box
D. toolbar

83. Which of the following types of epithelial cells forms a protective cover on the skin?

A. cuboidal
B. columnar
C. squamous
D. transitional

84. A urine sample that cannot be processed immediately should be placed in which of the following?

A. incubator
B. freezer
C. refrigerator
D. centrifuge

85. Which of the following schedules of controlled substances is considered to have a moderate potential for abuse?

A. I
B. II
C. III
D. IV

86. Which of the following microscopic objectives should be used first to examine a Gram-stained specimen?

A. 10×
B. 20×
C. 40×
D. 100×

87. Which of the following conditions is caused by the lack of melanin pigment in the skin, hair, and eyes?

A. keratosis
B. leukoplakia
C. albinism
D. hyperkinesia

88. Which of the following is the hardest substance in the body, covering the crowns of the teeth?

A. dentin
B. enamel
C. periodontal ligament
D. cement

89. Which of the following basic food groups contains the greatest amount of ascorbic acid?

A. meat and poultry
B. milk and cheese
C. breads
D. fruits

90. Which of the following methods of examination is used to assess organ location and size?

A. mensuration
B. percussion
C. palpation
D. auscultation

91. In patients with liver disease, which of the following serum levels is most likely to be increased?

A. hemoglobin
B. alanine aminotransferase (ALT)
C. albumin
D. acid phosphatase

92. Which of the following vitamins aids in blood clotting?

A. C
B. K
C. E
D. B_{12}

93. Which of the following best describes respirations that are increased in rate and depth?

A. hyperpnea
B. hypervolemia
C. hypercapnia
D. hyperpyrexia

94. Which of the following is the definition of the term "encephalitis"?

A. swelling of the spinal cord
B. swelling of the brain
C. inflammation of the spinal cord
D. inflammation of the brain

95. The left common carotid artery is a branch of which area of the aorta?

A. descending
B. arch
C. ascending
D. thoracic

96. Which of the following leads of the electrocardiograph is bipolar?

A. standard
B. augmented
C. precordial
D. intra-atrial

97. Which of the following cranial nerves is called "abducens"?

A. II
B. IV
C. VI
D. VIII

98. Which of the following is a hereditary disease that causes copper accumulation in the brain?

A. Tay-Sachs disease
B. Wilson's disease
C. Hirschsprung's disease
D. Paget's disease

99. Toxic shock syndrome is an acute infection commonly caused by which of the following bacteria?

A. *Klebsiella pneumonia*
B. *Neisseria gonorrhoeae*
C. *Staphylococcus aureus*
D. *Chlamydia trachomatis*

100. Which of the following abbreviations means "after meals"?

    A. hs
    B. ac
    C. qd
    D. pc

101. The thoracic cavity is separated from the abdominopelvic cavity by the

    A. mediastinum.
    B. stomach.
    C. diaphragm.
    D. liver.

102. Which of the following reagents should be used to prepare a blood smear for identification of white blood cells?

    A. crystal violet
    B. Wright's
    C. methylene blue
    D. acid-fast

103. According to the National Fire Protection Association, which of the following colored labels indicates "unstable, may react if mixed with water"?

    A. red
    B. white
    C. yellow
    D. blue

104. Which of the following is the most appropriate position for examination of a patient with dyspnea?

    A. supine
    B. Sims'
    C. knee-chest
    D. Fowler's

105. Which of the following terms means "take-home pay"?

    A. income tax
    B. net income
    C. income statement
    D. gross income

106. The scheduling process of screening and treating patients with the most serious problems first is known as which of the following?

    A. cluster
    B. open book
    C. triage
    D. categorization

107. Which of the following letter formats is the most common type used in medical practices?

    A. full block
    B. simplified
    C. modified block
    D. indented

108. Which of the following hereditary diseases or conditions may result in brain damage?

    A. color blindness
    B. phenylketonuria
    C. albinism
    D. classic hemophilia

109. Which of the following vitamin deficiencies may cause rickets?

    A. B_6
    B. K
    C. D
    D. B_1

110. Which of the following terms means a legal proceeding by which a case is transferred from a lower to a higher court for rehearing?

    A. subpoena
    B. appeal
    C. summons
    D. testimony

111. Which of the following best describes "liabilities" in the double-entry accounting system?

    A. services provided to patients
    B. assets that have a dollar value
    C. amounts owed by the medical practice to creditors
    D. amounts owed to the medical practice by patients

112. Which of the following proofreaders' marks means "insert a space"?

    A. #
    B.]
    C. Sp
    D. fl

113. Volume 2 of the ICD-CM coding system contains which of the following?

    A. tabular index to diseases
    B. list of modifiers to specify coding
    C. alphabetic index to diseases
    D. list of procedures and treatments

114. A patient who has a legal will dies. Which of the following persons may authorize release of medical records?

    A. the patient's next of kin
    B. the patient's attorney
    C. the hospital chief of staff
    D. the insurance carrier

115. Which of the following drugs is an example of diuretics?

    A. meperidine (Demerol®)
    B. haloperidol (Haldol®)
    C. furosemide (Lasix®)
    D. clozapine (Clozaril®)

116. Which of the following waves on the electrocardiograph represents the recovery of the ventricles?

    A. P
    B. QRS
    C. R
    D. T

117. The American Cancer Society recommends annual mammograms for women at low risk after what age?

    A. 30 years
    B. 35 years
    C. 40 years
    D. 45 years

118. Which of the following types of incoming mail requires immediate attention?

    A. payments from patients
    B. physician's personal letters
    C. utility bills
    D. certified letters

119. Which of the following terms describes an agent that inhibits or prevents perspiration?

    A. anicteric
    B. androgenic
    C. anhidrotic
    D. amitosis

120. The violation of narcotics laws by a health-care provider is classified as which of the following?

    A. felony
    B. defamation of character
    C. misdemeanor
    D. breach of contract

121. Which of the following terms means "surgical removal of the colon"?

    A. colotomy   C. colectomy

    B. colostomy   D. cholecystectomy

122. Which of the following laboratory studies is specifically ordered to diagnose a condition associated with the male reproductive system?

    A. CBC   C. CEA

    B. HIV   D. PSA

123. Which of the following is a flat, bladelzike bone that forms the midanterior portion of the upper trunk?

    A. sternum   C. scapula

    B. clavicle   D. xiphoid process

124. Which of the following terms describes a record of all outstanding accounts and the amounts that are due?

    A. daysheet   C. adjustment

    B. credit balance   D. accounts receivable

125. After the death of a patient, the patient's medical record legally belongs to which of the following entities?

    A. patient's family   C. patient's attorney

    B. patient's physician D. medical examiner

126. Which of the following microorganisms may cause syphilis?

    A. *Chlamydia trachomatis* bacterium

    B. *Treponema pallidum*

    C. human papillomavirus

    D. herpes simplex virus

127. Which of the following is caused by a deficiency of vitamin C?

    A. pernicious anemia   C. scurvy

    B. osteomalacia   D. spina bifida in a fetus

128. Accounts of patients who are poor, uninsured, or underinsured are called

    A. hardship cases.   C. delinquent.

    B. single entry.   D. open book.

129. Which of the following drugs may cause birth defects?

    A. placebos   C. diuretics

    B. teratogens   D. levothyroxine

130. Which of the following terms means "preparing items for filing by removing loose pieces of tape or paper clips"?

    A. indexing   C. annotating

    B. coding   D. sorting

131. Drugs classified in which of the following schedules under the Controlled Substances Act have the LEAST potential for abuse?

    A. II   C. IV

    B. III   D. V

132. Which of the following is the most important aspect of infection control procedures?

    A. hand washing   C. disinfection

    B. decontamination D. sterilization

133. Which of the following abbreviations is written in the appointment book to indicate that a patient did not show up?

    A. FU   C. NP

    B. CX   D. NS

134. Which of the following is caused by an excess of growth hormone in an adult?

    A. gigantism   C. acromegaly

    B. dwarfism   D. myxedema

135. In capillary puncture, which of the following blood values is higher?

    A. calcium   C. potassium

    B. glucose   D. total protein

136. Which of the following sterilization methods is most effective for surgical instruments?

    A. chemical   C. steam

    B. radiation   D. gas

137. According to tort law, the performance of an act that is wholly wrongful and unlawful is classified as which of the following?

    A. malfeasance   C. misdemeanor

    B. misfeasance   D. nonfeasance

138. Which of the following refers to a combination of activities designed to ensure reliable and valid test results?

    A. sensitivity training C. safety education

    B. standard precautions D. quality control

139. Which of the following types of medications are most likely to be stored on a crash cart?

    A. vasodilators   C. antibiotics

    B. narcotics   D. antipyretics

140. Which of the following terms describes the organs and tissues separating the lungs?

    A. myocardium   C. mediastinum

    B. diaphragm   D. endocardium

141. Which of the following information included in a patient's medical record is subjective information?

    A. patient's family history C. treatments prescribed

    B. radiology reports   D. laboratory results

142. Which of the following abbreviations means "instructions to the patient"?

    A. Rx   C. stat

    B. X   D. sig:

143. How long are employee health records required to be kept?

    A. six months
    B. one year
    C. three years
    D. five years

144. Which of the following abbreviations means "before meals"?

    A. pc
    B. ac
    C. hs
    D. qh

145. Which of the following is a salicylate?

    A. Motrin®
    B. Nuprin®
    C. Anacin®
    D. Advil®

146. Round bacteria that grow in chains are called

    A. streptococci.
    B. staphylococci.
    C. diplococci.
    D. bacilli.

147. Which of the following instruments is used to perform the Weber test for hearing assessment?

    A. tympanometer
    B. audiometer
    C. otoscope
    D. tuning fork

148. Which of the following chambers of the heart is the largest and most powerful?

    A. left ventricle
    B. left atrium
    C. right ventricle
    D. right atrium

149. Which of the following combining forms refers to a portion of the elbow?

    A. femor/o
    B. calcane/o
    C. olecran/o
    D. ibi/o

150. Which of the following is also called "tic douloureux"?

    A. Bell's palsy
    B. trigeminal neuralgia
    C. quadriplegia
    D. amyotrophic lateral sclerosis

151. Which of the following types of viral hepatitis is transmitted via the fecal-oral route?

    A. hepatitis B
    B. hepatitis C
    C. hepatitis D
    D. hepatitis A

152. Which of the following diseases or conditions is transmitted by eating raw or undercooked pork from infected pigs?

    A. trichinosis
    B. siderosis
    C. botulism
    D. hypersomnia

153. Which of the following is the act of releasing or transferring information so that the information is outside the party that holds it?

    A. fraud
    B. abuse
    C. disclosure
    D. ownership

154. Rapport involves

    A. silence.
    B. repeating.
    C. a direct, confrontational relationship.
    D. a positive and harmonious relationship.

155. Which of the following positions is used for treatment of patients who are in shock?

    A. lithotomy
    B. Trendelenburg's
    C. dorsal recumbent
    D. sitting

156. Which of the following is also called shingles?

    A. herpes simplex type I
    B. herpes simplex type II
    C. herpes zoster
    D. rubeola

157. The number of organisms required to cause a disease in a susceptible host is known as

    A. an infective dose.
    B. a pathogen.
    C. virulence.
    D. parasitism.

158. Which of the following ICD-9-CM codes indicates the cause of an accident?

    A. P00-P96
    B. 140-239
    C. 800-999
    D. 290-319

159. The notation "WL:CM" appears at the bottom of a letter written to a patient. The initials "CM" represent which of the following individuals?

    A. the patient
    B. the typist
    C. the physician
    D. the consultant

160. Which of the following methods of measuring a patient's body temperature is the most accurate?

    A. oral
    B. axillary
    C. tympanic
    D. rectal

161. Which of the following organisms is a type of protozoan?

    A. *Trichomonas vaginalis*
    B. *Neisseria gonorrhoeae*
    C. *Gardnerella vaginalis*
    D. *Candida albicans*

162. Which of the following is the correct route of administration for measles, mumps, and rubella (MMR)?

    A. intravenous
    B. intradermal
    C. subcutaneous
    D. intramuscular

163. Which of the following routes of administration allows a drug to enter the bloodstream immediately?

    A. subcutaneous
    B. sublingual
    C. transdermal
    D. oral

164. Which of the following agencies regulates the disposal of infectious waste outside the workplace?

    A.   Occupational Safety and Health Administration (OSHA)
    B.   Centers for Disease Control and Prevention (CDC)
    C.   Association for Professionals in Infection Control (APIC)
    D.   Environmental Protection Agency (EPA)

165. Which of the following abbreviations is used for diagnosis of a disease?

    A.   Dx   C.   Tx
    B.   Hx   D.   Rx

166. Which of the following is used for measuring tension or pressure of the intraocular region?

    A.   Snellen chart   C.   tonometer
    B.   Wood's light   D.   ophthalmoscope

167. Which of the following examinations is used for the lower rectum and anal canal?

    A.   colonoscopy   C.   sigmoidoscopy
    B.   proctoscopy   D.   colposcopy

168. Which of the following suffixes means "attraction"?

    A.   -plasia   C.   -phobia
    B.   -ptosis   D.   -philia

169. When using a terminal digit filing system, which of the following records should be filed first?

    A.   022232   C.   091433
    B.   042555   D.   110562

170. Which of the following is a *unicellular* exocrine gland?

    A.   fat cell   C.   goblet cell
    B.   neuron   D.   phagocyte

171. Which of the following antibiotics are bactericidal?

    A.   penicillins   C.   tetracyclines
    B.   sulfonamides   D.   clindamycin and spectinomycin

172. Which of the following waves represents the slow recovery of Purkinje fibers?

    A.   T wave   C.   U wave
    B.   P wave   D.   R wave

173. A medical record is most defensible in a court of law if it includes which of the following?

    A.   complete laboratory results
    B.   names of consulting physicians
    C.   signature of the primary care physician
    D.   accurate documentation of care

174. Which of the following drugs may cause the urine to become orange-red in color?

    A.   rifampin   C.   lithium
    B.   penicillin   D.   levodopa

175. Consent is unnecessary

    A.   if the situation involves a minor in a foster home.
    B.   if the patient is mentally incompetent.
    C.   if the patient is an emancipated minor.
    D.   in an emergency situation.

176. Which of the following is also called "grinder's disease"?

    A.   histoplasmosis   C.   asbestosis
    B.   silicosis   D.   anthrocosis

177. Atomic weight is determined by the number of

    A.   protons and electrons.   C.   electrons and neutrons.
    B.   protons and neutrons.   D.   protons only.

178. Which of the following medical terms is misspelled?

    A.   embarrass   C.   exhileration
    B.   entrepreneur   D.   emphasis

179. Which of the following are the most commonly used suture sizes?

    A.   2-0 through 3-0   C.   2-0 through 6-0
    B.   2-0 through 4-0   D.   2-0 through 11-0

180. Which of the following fractures most commonly occur in children?

    A.   comminuted   C.   spiral
    B.   greenstick   D.   impacted

181. Which of the following hormones increases blood glucose?

    A.   insulin   C.   growth hormone
    B.   thymosin   D.   glucagon

182. Which of the following terms describes hearing loss because of the aging process?

    A.   presbycusis   C.   otitis media
    B.   otosclerosis   D.   cerumen impaction

183. The patient lies on the left side with the left leg slightly bent, and the left arm placed behind the back so that the patient's weight is resting primarily on the chest. This is an example of which of the following positions?

    A.   Fowler's   C.   Sims'
    B.   lithotomy   D.   prone

184. Surgical hand washing is performed

    A.   for 10 minutes with a clean hand brush.
    B.   for 10 minutes with a sterile hand brush.
    C.   with a nail brush and germicidal soap.
    D.   by scrubbing for two minutes.

185. Which of the following parts of a business letter is keyed on the second line below the salutation?

    A.   subject line   C.   enclosure notation
    B.   reference initials   D.   complimentary close

186. Two patients are scheduled for an appointment at the same time on the same day. This is an example of which of the following scheduling systems?

    A. categorization   C. double booking
    B. modified wave   D. stream

187. The coronal plane is also called the

    A. frontal plane.   C. transverse plane.
    B. sagittal plane.   D. midsagittal plane.

188. Which of the following is an example of sublimation?

    A. A rape victim cannot recall the crime.
    B. An athlete who did not win the game says, "It makes you a better player to lose."
    C. An aggressive person becomes a boxer.
    D. A compulsive gambler refuses to believe his behavior is hurting anyone.

189. Which of the following infestations is transmitted by eating raw or undercooked pork from infected pigs?

    A. trichinosis   C. encephalitis
    B. Paget's disease   D. botulism

190. Which of the following arteries is most commonly used to monitor lower limb circulation?

    A. common iliac   C. femoral
    B. dorsalis pedis   D. popliteal

191. The doctor has ordered 120 mg of a drug that comes only in 30-mg tablets. How many tablets constitute a dose?

    A. 3   C. 6
    B. 4   D. 15

192. Which of the following vaccines can be given at birth?

    A. mumps   C. varicella
    B. tetanus   D. hepatitis B

193. Which of the following suffixes means "abnormal fear"?

    A. -philia   C. -plasia
    B. -phobia   D. -pathy

194. A drug combined with an oil base, resulting in a semi-solid preparation is a(n)

    A. suppository.   C. ointment.
    B. liniment.   D. cream.

195. Which of the following types of urine specimen collection contains greater concentrations of substances?

    A. first-voided morning C. timed
    B. 24-hour   D. random

196. Which of the following is the most secure service offered by the U.S. Postal Service?

    A. Mail Tracing   C. First-Class Mail
    B. Priority Mail   D. Registered Mail

197. With an angry patient, you should always

    A. stay very close to the patient while talking.
    B. learn how to cause anger.
    C. remain calm.
    D. defend yourself.

198. A participating provider in a managed health-care program must write off

    A. disallowed charges.   C. deductibles.
    B. copayments.   D. coinsurance.

199. Amantadine is classified as an

    A. anti-inflammatory.   C. antifungal.
    B. antiepileptic.   D. antiviral.

200. OSHA standards require which of the following?

    A. cleaning only after procedures
    B. cleaning only when needed
    C. a written schedule for cleaning
    D. hourly cleaning

201. The prefix *epi-* means

    A. upon.   C. good.
    B. within.   D. off.

202. The living together of two microorganisms of different species is called

    A. mutualism.   C. parasitism.
    B. symbiosis.   D. commensalism.

203. Weight gain during pregnancy

    A. should both be avoided and treated with a low-fat diet.
    B. should be avoided.
    C. is recommended to be anywhere 24–35 pounds.
    D. is treated with a low-fat diet.

204. Scheduling patients so that two come in at the beginning of each hour, and the others are scheduled every 10–20 minutes is called

    A. modified wave scheduling.
    B. advance scheduling.
    C. appointment time pattern.
    D. wave scheduling.

205. Heparin is produced naturally in the blood circulation by which of the following cells?

    A. basophils   C. mast cells
    B. eosinophils   D. monocytes

206. The positive electrodes of an ECG lead are called

    A. baselines.   C. intra-atrial leads.
    B. anodes.   D. cations.

207. Which of the following medical record filing systems best provides confidentiality of patient information?

A. tickler
B. numeric
C. alphabetic
D. geographic

208. The goal of a medical assistant to treat patients so that they become comfortable and at ease is achieved by

A. good attitude.
B. patient confidentiality.
C. therapeutic communication.
D. good appointment scheduling.

209. Which of the following abbreviations is used for treatment of a disease?

A. Rx
B. Tx
C. Dx
D. Hx

210. The gastrocnemius muscle is located in which of the following parts of the body?

A. neck
B. chest
C. abdomen
D. lower leg

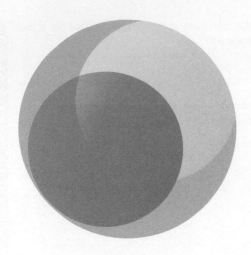

PRACTICE EXAM 3 - CCMA

1. Voucher checks are commonly used for
   A. payroll.
   B. payment collection.
   C. internal billing.
   D. cycle billing.

2. From which of the following is agar extracted?
   A. algae
   B. bacteria
   C. fungi
   D. protozoa

3. When addressing an envelope, the word "confidential" should be placed
   A. two lines below the address.
   B. two lines below the return address.
   C. one line below the address.
   D. one line above the city and state.

4. The ledger provides up-to-date financial information pertaining to which of the following?
   A. pharmaceutical representatives
   B. insurance companies
   C. physicians
   D. patients

5. Which of the following abbreviations is used in a prescription to indicate that a medication should be taken orally before meals?
   A. PO ac
   B. PO hs
   C. PO qd
   D. PO pc

6. Which of the following is caused by accumulation of uric acid in the blood?
   A. gout
   B. Lyme disease
   C. Wilson's disease
   D. Crohn's disease

7. Which of the following is the most appropriate medical record classification for a deceased patient?
   A. inactive
   B. closed
   C. active
   D. transferred

8. A microbe that lives only in the absence of oxygen is called a(n)
   A. cilia.
   B. flagella.
   C. virus.
   D. obligate anaerobe.

9. Medicare Part C involves which of the following?
   A. prescription drugs
   B. private health plans
   C. hospitalization
   D. indigent people

10. Which of the following is the most appropriate initial action for the medical assistant when a patient is referred to the medical office?
    A. Schedule an appointment for the patient in one week.
    B. Determine the urgency of the patient's appointment.
    C. Discuss the case with the referring physician.
    D. Ask the patient for more information about his or her insurance coverage.

11. Which of the following is a safety hazard in a medical office?
    A. dosimeter
    B. lead apron
    C. aneroid sphygmomanometer
    D. mercury thermometer

12. Antiemetics are indicated for which of the following conditions?
    A. diarrhea
    B. seizures
    C. vomiting
    D. congestion

13. The placement of the subject line in a letter should be in the
    A. special notations.
    B. closing.
    C. heading.
    D. opening.

14. Which of the following is used to indicate that a patient's medical record is stored in two locations?
    A. cross-reference guide
    B. color coding
    C. tickler file
    D. outguide

15. Which of the following is the most appropriate method to remove sterile forceps from a sterile package?

    A. by the tip, handles up
    B. by the hinged joint
    C. by the handles, tip up
    D. by the tip, handles down

16. The process in which molecules, ions, or particles move from an area of higher concentration to an area of lower concentration is known as

    A. diffusion.
    B. filtration.
    C. osmosis.
    D. pinocytosis.

17. Which of the following is the correct spelling for the term that means "characterized by an exaggerated reaction to an antigen or toxin"?

    A. anafilactic
    B. anaphilactic
    C. annaphylactic
    D. anaphylactic

18. The Occupational and Safety Administration (OSHA) requires that health-care workers be tested annually for which of the following communicable diseases?

    A. epidemic parotitis
    B. hepatitis B
    C. tuberculosis
    D. rubeola

19. Which of the following is an instrument that measures and records the volume of air that moves in and out of the lungs?

    A. spirometer
    B. electrocardiogram
    C. tonometer
    D. spirogram

20. Which of the following actions by the medical assistant is most likely to protect the physician if a caller to the office were to take legal action?

    A. answering all calls promptly
    B. using technical terms on the phone
    C. avoiding lengthy phone conversations
    D. proper documentation of calls

21. Which of the following is a hereditary disorder of clotting factors?

    A. poikilocytosis
    B. pernicious anemia
    C. polycythemia
    D. hemophilia

22. In an electrocardiogram, what does the QRS complex represent?

    A. depolarization of the atria
    B. repolarization of the atria
    C. repolarization of the ventricles
    D. depolarization of the ventricles

23. The gallbladder is normally located in which of the following abdominal quadrants?

    A. left lower
    B. right lower
    C. right upper
    D. left upper

24. Nonabsorbable suture material is used for which of the following types of tissue?

    A. nerve
    B. muscle
    C. fascia
    D. skin

25. Which psychologist believed that as people age, they also go through psychosocial changes?

    A. Kübler-Ross
    B. Maslow
    C. Erickson
    D. Jung

26. Which of the following types of filing systems requires a cross-reference file?

    A. geographic
    B. alphabetic
    C. subject
    D. numeric

27. The plan that covers spouses of veterans with permanent disabilities is called

    A. TRICARE.
    B. CHAMPUS.
    C. Blue Cross and Blue Shield.
    D. CHAMPVA.

28. The central processing unit (CPU) is a type of

    A. motherboard.
    B. microprocessor.
    C. RAM.
    D. ROM.

29. Which of the following is an example of a medical aseptic technique?

    A. use of a disinfectant
    B. surgical scrubbing
    C. autoclaving with steam
    D. gas sterilization

30. A patient scheduled for which of the following services is most likely to need the longest appointment time?

    A. postoperative visit
    B. complete physical examination
    C. prenatal checkup
    D. annual pelvic examination

31. Which of the following information provided on a patient registration form is demographic information?

    A. name and address of referring physician
    B. effective date of insurance policy
    C. postsurgical history
    D. patient's place of employment

32. Disorders that involve an apparent, abrupt, and repeated shifting from one "personality" to another are referred to as

    A. obsessive-compulsive.
    B. dissociative.
    C. panic anxiety.
    D. personality.

33. The physician uses six packs of 5-0 sutures daily during a five-day workweek. One box of sutures contains 32 packs. How many boxes of sutures are ordered each month?

    A. two
    B. three
    C. four
    D. five

34. If a fracture is at the distal end of the tibia and fibula, it is called a

    A. Wilson's fracture.
    B. greenstick fracture.
    C. Pott's fracture.
    D. comminuted fracture.

35. Which of the following combining forms is matched correctly with its meaning?

    A. hypo- / above
    B. latero- / below
    C. antero- / back
    D. peri- / around

36. On a urinalysis reagent strip, infection is indicated by the presence of which of the following?

  A. urobilinogen C. bilirubin
  B. leukocytes D. ketones

37. Dry scaling and fissuring of the lips is called

  A. xerosis. C. keratosis.
  B. xanthoma. D. cheilosis.

38. Which of the following is a bactericidal antibiotic?

  A. cephalosporin C. tetracycline
  B. aminoglycoside D. vancomycin

39. The artificial breaking of adhesions of an ankylosed joint is known as

  A. arthroclasia. C. rachischisis.
  B. arthrodesis. D. spondylitis.

40. Which of the following may result from sunburn over time?

  A. sebaceous nevus C. Kaposi's sarcoma
  B. epidermal nevus D. malignant melanoma

41. Which of the following should replace a patient's medical record when the record is removed from the filing system?

  A. Post-it note C. outguide
  B. index card D. cross-reference card

42. Which of the following is *not* a computer input device?

  A. trackball C. mouse
  B. printer D. keyboard

43. Which of the following is an advantage of metered mail?

  A. traceable C. faster processing
  B. insured D. less expensive

44. Which of the following is a chest pain symptom that results from a temporary loss of oxygen to the heart muscle?

  A. intermittent claudication
  B. angina pectoris
  C. atrial fibrillation
  D. carotid artery bruit

45. What is the term for a court order that requires a witness to appear in court with a patient's medical record?

  A. *Qui facit per alium* C. *Res ipsa loquitur*
  B. *Subpoena duces tecum* D. *Respondeat superior*

46. When scheduling an appointment, which of the following should be considered?

  A. demographics C. analyzing patient flow
  B. cancellations D. inactive files

47. Which of the following terms best describes the awareness and insight one person has for another's feelings and emotions?

  A. sympathy C. apathy
  B. sensitivity D. empathy

48. When a false statement is made under oath, it is referred to legally as

  A. a verdict. C. libel.
  B. perjury. D. slander.

49. Which of the following medical terms is spelled correctly?

  A. ostoarthritis C. mylogram
  B. proteinuria D. cholocystitis

50. Retinol and carotene are referred to as which of the following vitamins?

  A. vitamin K C. vitamin A
  B. vitamin D D. vitamin E

51. Which of the following types of casts are most commonly seen during microscopic examinations of urine?

  A. waxy C. hyaline
  B. granular D. cellular

52. Drugs classified as which of the following have no prescriptive use?

  A. Schedule I C. Schedule III
  B. Schedule II D. Schedule IV

53. Which of the following terms describes the strength of a drug required to produce the desired effect?

  A. tolerance C. additive action
  B. cumulation D. potency

54. "Have you had this problem before?" is an example of which of the following types of questions?

  A. closed ended C. hypothetical
  B. leading D. exploratory

55. A deceitful practice undertaken to induce someone to part with something of value is known as

  A. invasion of privacy. C. fraud.
  B. libel. D. defamation.

56. Office policy regarding the length of time for retaining patient files should be based on the

  A. statute of limitations.
  B. number of inactive files.
  C. number of active files.
  D. availability of storage space.

57. Which of the following positions is most appropriate for a patient with hypotension?

  A. Trendelenburg's C. Fowler's
  B. dorsal recumbent D. supine

58. Amounts of salary held out of payroll checks for the purpose of paying government taxes for employees refers to

  A. withholding. C. employee earnings.
  B. net earnings. D. payroll.

59. Which of the following is a "write it once" bookkeeping system?

  A. double entry C. pegboard
  B. single entry D. journal

60. The abbreviation that means "left eye" is

    A. OP.   C. OU.
    B. OC.   D. OS.

61. Cyanocobalamin is another name for which of the following vitamins?

    A. vitamin B_1 C. vitamin B_9
    B. vitamin B_2 D. vitamin B_{12}

62. Retinol (vitamin A) deficiency can cause all of the following, except

    A. amenorrhea.   C. night blindness.
    B. infection.   D. xerophthalmia.

63. Encouraging patients to think through and answer their own questions and concerns is a technique called

    A. restating.   C. reflecting.
    B. reassuring.   D. rapport.

64. The best description of the term "erythropoietin" is

    A. a hormone that stimulates red blood cell formation.
    B. a disorder that causes an abnormal decrease of red blood cells.
    C. a disorder that causes redness of the skin.
    D. abnormal shape of red blood cells.

65. Which of the following is a licensed ambulatory health-care worker?

    A. phlebotomist   C. medical assistant
    B. nurse practitioner D. cytotechnologist

66. Which of the following terms means "administering medication via a route other than the alimentary canal"?

    A. pectoral   C. paramesial
    B. popliteal   D. parenteral

67. A group of bacteria considered to be the smallest free-living organisms is known as

    A. rickettsia.   C. cycobacteria.
    B. chlamydia.   D. mycoplasma.

68. Which of the following instruments is used to examine a patient's blood pressure?

    A. spirometer   C. ophthalmoscope
    B. sphygmomanometer   D. otoscope

69. In the chain of infection, a person with a compromised immune system would be which of the following links?

    A. portal of entry   C. infectious agent
    B. means of transmission D. susceptible host

70. The patient history and physical report begins with which of the following types of information?

    A. review of systems C. allergies
    B. present illness   D. chief complaint

71. "The matter speaks for itself" is communicated as

    A. *res ipsa loquitur.*   C. *res judicata.*
    B. *quid pro quo.*   D. *respondeat superior.*

72. Which of the following information should be excluded from a résumé?

    A. names of references
    B. professional licenses or certification
    C. extracurricular activities
    D. foreign language abilities

73. Which of the following is governed by the Uniform Anatomical Gift Act?

    A. blood transfusions
    B. medical experimentation
    C. organ donations
    D. death certificates

74. The physician has agreed to accept a new patient. A contract will exist when the patient

    A. calls for information about the practice.
    B. provides medical records from the previous physician.
    C. is examined by the physician.
    D. arrives at the office.

75. Which of the following types of medical insurance is an example of "fee for service"?

    A. Medicare Part D   C. Medicaid
    B. Medicare Part A   D. Blue Cross Blue Shield

76. Which of the following radiographic records is obtained after a contrast medium is injected into a patient's joint?

    A. myelogram   C. hysterogram
    B. cytogram   D. arthrogram

77. In the modified-block style of letter writing, all lines begin where (with the exception of the date line, complimentary closing, and keyed signature)?

    A. in the center   C. at the right margin
    B. at the left margin D. at a justified position

78. Which of the following is the primary purpose of a computer password?

    A. to store information
    B. to start and shut down the computer
    C. to prevent unauthorized access to data
    D. to back up computer files

79. Which of the following types of drugs is used as an anticoagulant?

    A. xylocaine   C. zocor
    B. dilantin   D. coumadin

80. The suffix -*rrhexis* means

    A. repair.   C. stasis.
    B. rupture.   D. nose.

81. A vacutainer tube with which of the following colored stoppers contains no additives?

    A. green   C. yellow
    B. red   D. blue

82. The difference between systolic and diastolic pressure is referred to as

    A. pulse pressure.   C. bounding pulse.
    B. pulse deficit.   D. unequal pressure.

83. In the term *urethrostenosis*, the suffix *-stenosis* means

    A. softening.   C. resembling.
    B. narrowing.   D. enlarging.

84. Which of the following terms refers to the rule and principles of conduct that are required of citizens by legislative enactments?

    A. philosophy   C. ethics
    B. morals   D. laws

85. Which of the following is included in a memorandum?

    A. signature   C. subject line
    B. salutation   D. inside address

86. Who believed that the basic needs of humans must be met before upper-level functioning can occur?

    A. Maslow   C. Piaget
    B. Kübler-Ross   D. Salk

87. Which of the following medical terms describes the surgical formation of a temporary opening in a joint for drainage purposes?

    A. arthrotomy   C. arthrostomy
    B. arthroscopy   D. arthrectomy

88. Which of the following topics is included in an office procedures manual?

    A. paid holiday and vacation time
    B. documentation requirements for patient care
    C. annual employment evaluations
    D. performance expectations based on job description

89. Which of the following is the most appropriate turn-around time for payment of an account?

    A. 7 days   C. 30 days
    B. 15 days   D. 60 days

90. Which of the following foods is chemically broken down by saliva?

    A. nucleic acids   C. carbohydrates
    B. proteins   D. lipids

91. Which of the following is the causative agent of candidiasis?

    A. virus   C. yeast
    B. protozoa   D. bacteria

92. Which of the following suffixes means "to crush"?

    A. -tripsy   C. -tresia
    B. -tropic   D. -tomy

93. The *Current Procedural Terminology* (CPT) coding system is based on a main number with how many digits?

    A. three   C. five
    B. four   D. six

94. Which of the following shows the state of finances of a business?

    A. balance sheet   C. daysheet
    B. trial balance   D. patient ledger

95. Which of the following computer terms is defined as "an accumulation of data to be processed"?

    A. interface   C. memory
    B. menu   D. batch

96. The most widely used filing system for medical practices is called

    A. chronological filing.
    B. alphanumerical filing.
    C. subject filing.
    D. color-coded filing.

97. Stretching of the stomach is called

    A. gastritis.   C. splenomegaly.
    B. stomatitis.   D. gastrectasia.

98. When performing a hemoccult test, which color is a positive indicator of blood?

    A. green   C. orange
    B. yellow   D. blue

99. Which of the following terms means "preparing items for filing by removing loose pieces of tape or paper clips"?

    A. indexing   C. sorting
    B. annotating   D. coding

100. The need for increasing doses of medication to maintain the desired therapeutic effect is a result of

    A. synergism.   C. tolerance.
    B. cumulative action.   D. trigger action.

101. How often must employers file Federal Tax Form 941?

    A. every two weeks   C. every four months
    B. every three months   D. every six months

102. Which type of endorsement should be used on a check that is being mailed to the bank for deposit?

    A. conditional   C. blank
    B. qualified   D. restrictive

103. The root word *enter* refers to the

    A. stomach.   C. intestines.
    B. spleen.   D. liver.

104. Which of the following computer pointing devices is the most commonly used?

    A. touch pad   C. modem
    B. trackball   D. mouse

105. The obturator foramen is located in which of the following bones?

    A. hipbone   C. knee
    B. skull   D. face

106. The pectoralis major muscle is in which part of the body?

    A. chest   C. thigh
    B. abdomen   D. skull

107. Which of the following medical terms is spelled correctly?

    A. percardiectomy   C. thromboctomy
    B. phlebitis   D. venipuncture

108. Repair of a rupture in the liver is referred to as

    A. hepatorrhaphy.   C. hepatorrhexis.
    B. cystorrhaphy.   D. hepatomegaly.

109. Which of the following vitamins is necessary for hemoglobin synthesis?

    A. vitamin B$_{12}$ C. vitamin D
    B. vitamin C   D. vitamin E

110. In an adult patient, which of the following arteries is used to obtain a blood pressure reading?

    A. carotid   C. brachial
    B. subclavian   D. ulna

111. Restriction of sodium in the diet is very common for patients with all of the disorders or conditions *except*

    A. hypertension.
    B. renal disease with edema.
    C. congestive heart failure.
    D. cirrhosis.

112. Which type of gastric cells secrete pepsinogen?

    A. goblet cells   C. chief cells
    B. parietal cells   D. intrinsic cells

113. Which of the following instruments is most appropriate for retinal testing?

    A. tonometer   C. gonioscope
    B. pen light   D. ophthalmoscope

114. The degree of pathogenicity or relative power of an organism to produce a disease is called

    A. contagion.   C. pathogenesis.
    B. purulence.   D. virulence.

115. The deltoid muscle is commonly used for injection of all of the following *except*

    A. tetanus boosters in adults.
    B. rabies vaccines after exposure.
    C. penicillin.
    D. vitamin B$_{12.}$

116. Which of the following specialists is most likely to interpret the results of magnetic resonance imaging (MRI)?

    A. gynecologist   C. hematologist
    B. radiologist   D. oncologist

117. Which of the following is included in a patient's vital signs?

    A. visual acuity   C. respiration rate
    B. reflexes   D. chest circumference

118. Which of the following terms is used to describe a software application that allows users to locate and display websites?

    A. flash   C. browser
    B. banner   D. cookie

119. Which of the following terms describes the process of linking two or more computers?

    A. compressing   C. networking
    B. configuring   D. encrypting

120. *Choroid* refers to the anatomy of the

    A. ear   C. brain.
    B. eye.   D. liver.

121. Safety regulations require a medical assistant to wear a dosimeter when using which of the following pieces of equipment?

    A. spirometer   C. electromyography
    B. ultrasound   D. radiograph

122. The presence of which of the following substances in urine most likely indicates increased metabolism of fat?

    A. ketones   C. hemoglobin
    B. glucose   D. bilirubin

123. Which of the following portions of the brain controls memory, judgment, and emotion?

    A. medulla oblongata   C. cerebellum
    B. thalamus   D. cerebrum

124. Which of the following is an abnormality of the digestive system?

    A. blepharoptosis   C. diaphoresis
    B. cholelithiasis   D. atelectasis

125. The physician prescribes 0.7 gram of aspirin for a patient. Aspirin is available in 350-mg tablets. How many tablets should the patient receive?

    A. 0.5   C. 1.5
    B. 1   D. 2

126. Which of the following is the most appropriate initial step before applying sterile surgical gloves?

    A. removing jewelry from hands and wrists
    B. rinsing hands with warm water
    C. applying hand moisturizer
    D. putting on a laboratory coat

127. The primary purpose of cardiopulmonary resuscitation (CPR) is to

    A. supply oxygen to vital tissue.
    B. restore the normal acid-base balance.
    C. restore palpable peripheral pulse.
    D. increase the blood pressure.

128. The suffix *-phasia* means

    A. swallowing.   C. phasing.
    B. breathing.   D. speech.

129. What defense mechanism involves a self-justifying explanation that is substituted for an unacceptable one?
    A. rationalization   C. sublimation
    B. projection   D. repression

130. An official paper ordering a person to appear in court under penalty for failure to do so is called a
    A. felony.   C. plaintiff.
    B. subpoena.   D. slander.

131. Which of the following is a form used to identify the number of withholding allowances chosen by an employee?
    A. I-9   C. W-2
    B. 1099   D. W-4

132. When are business accounts considered to be "in balance"?
    A. when there are more payables than assets
    B. when total ending balances of patient ledgers equal the total accounts receivable
    C. when there are more assets than payables
    D. when computer posting has occurred

133. Which of the following morphologic structures is characteristic of bacilli?
    A. rod   C. sphere
    B. ova   D. cluster

134. Which of the following is the insurance program that provides for the medically indigent?
    A. CHAMPUS/TRICARE   C. Medicaid
    B. CHAMPVA   D. Medicare

135. Which of the following is a document that shows how the amount of the benefit was determined?
    A. Medicare audit form
    B. explanation of benefits form
    C. patient encounter form
    D. coordination of benefits

136. Which of the following procedures is performed to view a cross section of an organ?
    A. pyelography   C. hysterography
    B. ultrasonography   D. tomography

137. Which of the following in the urine indicates a urinary tract infection?
    A. ketones   C. urobilin
    B. nitrite   D. bilirubin

138. Wilms' tumor is seen in children younger than five years of age in which of the following organs?
    A. lungs   C. liver
    B. brain   D. kidneys

139. Which of the following terms best describes signs and symptoms that come and go?
    A. latent   C. acute
    B. intermittent   D. cardinal

140. Which of the following procedures is performed by an orthopedist?
    A. bronchoscopy   C. arthroscopy
    B. laparoscopy   D. colonoscopy

141. Which of the following is an abbreviation representing a prescription written for a patient?
    A. Rx   C. Px
    B. Tx   D. Hx

142. Which of the following classes of mail should be used to send an item that has significant monetary value?
    A. Priority   C. First Class
    B. Express   D. Registered

143. The corpus luteum secretes which of the following hormones?
    A. prolactin   C. estrogen
    B. testosterone   D. progesterone

144. Teaching patients how to perform a procedure is best accomplished by which of the following?
    A. lecture   C. brochure
    B. video   D. demonstration

145. An organism that contains a membrane-bound nucleus with chromosomes is called a
    A. eukaryote.   C. virus.
    B. prokaryote.   D. mold.

146. Which of the following bones is located in the foot?
    A. tibia   C. metacarpal
    B. mandible   D. metatarsal

147. Malabsorption of vitamin B_{12} results in
    A. goiter.   C. rickets.
    B. scurvy.   D. pernicious anemia.

148. If the average adult's respirations are 12–20 per minute, and the average pulse rate is 60–100 per minute, which of the following is the closest ratio of respiration to pulse?
    A. 1 : 3   C. 1 : 8
    B. 1 : 5   D. 1 : 10

149. Which of the following word-processing functions is most appropriate for the medical assistant to use when verifying the accuracy of words in a business letter?
    A. find and replace   C. spell check
    B. autocorrect   D. word count

150. If Medicare sends a check for payment to the medical office, the physician is considered which one of the following parties?
    A. registered   C. accepting
    B. sponsoring   D. participating

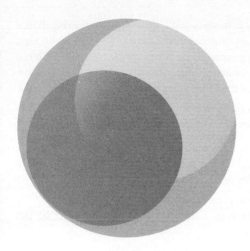

PRACTICE EXAM 4 - NCMA

1. Which of the following is caused by an enzyme deficiency, causes abnormal lipid metabolism in the brain, and affects people of the Ashkenazi Jewish population?

   A. Tay-Sachs disease
   B. Turner's syndrome
   C. Klinefelter's syndrome
   D. myelomeningocele

2. Which of the following is a doctrine that holds physician employers responsible for the actions of their employees?

   A. *res ipsa loquitur*
   B. *respondeat superior*
   C. manifestation of assent
   D. *locum tenens*

3. Practice expenses for the month of June are $8,500. Revenue for the same month is $16,180. The practice has total assets of $283,000 and liabilities of $55,000. What is the net income for the practice for the month of June?

   A. $7,680
   B. $24,680
   C. $38,000
   D. $228,000

4. The code for intravenous administration of chemotherapy is found in which of the following sections of the *Current Procedural Terminology* (CPT) manual?

   A. surgery
   B. medicine
   C. pathology and laboratory
   D. evaluation and management

5. Which of the following is a breathing pattern marked by a period of apnea lasting 10–60 seconds, followed by gradually increasing depth and frequency of respiration?

   A. eupnea
   B. dyspnea
   C. hypoxia
   D. Cheyne-Stokes

6. When injecting a medication, which of the following parts of the needle allows the medication to flow from the syringe to the needle?

   A. shaft
   B. lumen
   C. bevel
   D. hilt

7. A pediatrician is unexpectedly delayed, and there are patients in the waiting room. Which of the following is the most appropriate action for the medical assistant to take?

   A. Tell the patients to leave and come back when the physician is available.
   B. Ignore the delay and explain it to individual patients if they ask.
   C. Explain the delay to the patients and estimate how long the physician will be unavailable.
   D. Ask the patients to wait until the physician is available to avoid rescheduling their appointments.

8. The physician orders promethazine (Phenergan) 25 mg intramuscularly for a patient with nausea. The bottle of promethazine is labeled "50 mg per ml." How much of the drug should be administered to the patient?

   A. 0.5 mL
   B. 1 mL
   C. 1.5 mL
   D. 2 mL

9. What should you offer to do immediately after a patient calls to cancel an appointment?

   A. Notify the patient that next time there will be a penalty for rescheduling.
   B. Refer the patient to another physician.
   C. Offer to reschedule the appointment.
   D. Create a new matrix.

10. When using standard-sized letterhead to prepare a full-page business letter, the left and right margins should each be how many inches wide?

    A. 0.5
    B. 1
    C. 1.5
    D. 2

11. Which of the following is a type of reimbursement by a health maintenance organization (HMO) to a group of physicians on a per-person-per-month contract?

    A. managed care
    B. fee-for-service
    C. capitation
    D. copayment

12. The medical assistant is giving instructions to a patient. Which of the following types of body language on the part of the patient most effectively communicates understanding of the instructions?

    A. touch
    B. facial expression
    C. eye contact
    D. personal space

13. A 67-year-old deaf woman is scheduled for an appointment and is sitting in the waiting room. When the medical assistant is ready to escort the patient to an examination room, which of the following is the most appropriate method of getting her attention?

    A. calling her name loudly from the doorway
    B. gently touching her shoulder
    C. asking the interpreter to go find her
    D. asking the other patients in the waiting room if they know who she is

14. Which of the following portions of a blood smear should be used to perform the differential blood cell count?

    A. feathered edges of the smear
    B. thickest area of the smear
    C. middle area of the smear
    D. complete smear

15. When a physician offers open office hours, which of the following best describes when patients are seen by the physician?

    A. in 15-minute intervals
    B. at the time of their appointment
    C. at the physician's discretion
    D. in the order of their arrival

16. A 53-year-old woman comes to the medical clinic because she has a headache. Her blood pressure is 120/75 mm Hg, her pulse is 130 bpm, her temperature is 37.3°C (99.2°F), and her respirations are 18/min. Which of the following terms would most likely be documented in the patient's chart?

    A. hypertension
    B. hypotension
    C. bradypnea
    D. tachycardia

17. Quality-control tests are performed daily in laboratories for which of the following reasons?

    A. to pass inspection by the Occupational Safety and Health Administration (OSHA)
    B. to determine whether test results are accurate
    C. to comply with local health department regulations
    D. to comply with state regulations

18. Which of the following additives is used as an anticoagulant in a blood specimen collected to determine a complete blood cell count?

    A. thrombin
    B. EDTA
    C. sodium heparin
    D. sodium citrate

19. Which of the following protects a computer monitor's screen from "burning in" by changing the display at short intervals?

    A. password
    B. screen saver
    C. terminal
    D. surge protector

20. A 71-year-old woman with weak leg muscles is advised to use axillary crutches. She can bear weight on both legs, but she has poor balance. When instructing her in the use of axillary crutches, the medical assistant should show her which of the following crutch-gait patterns?

    A. two-point
    B. three-point
    C. four-point alternating
    D. five-point

21. A 13-year-old boy with type 1 diabetes mellitus needs to modify his lifestyle. Which of the following is the most effective way for the medical assistant to educate him?

    A. Tell him to call the office if he has questions.
    B. Explain type 1 diabetes mellitus on a level he can understand.
    C. Refer him to a registered dietitian.
    D. Give him a brochure on type 1 diabetes mellitus.

22. When a child is covered by separate insurance policies through each parent, the policy of which parent is considered primary?

    A. either parent
    B. the father
    C. the mother
    D. the parent whose birthday falls first

23. If a patient is chronically late and requires more of the physician's time than most patients, when should this patient's appointment be scheduled?

    A. first appointment of the day
    B. last appointment of the day
    C. last appointment before lunch
    D. first appointment after lunch

24. A physician advises a 28-year-old patient to increase his daily intake of complex carbohydrates. To do this, it is most appropriate to increase intake of which of the following foods?

    A. fruits
    B. fish
    C. peas
    D. breads

25. A 14-year-old boy has an obvious bone deformity of the thigh. An X-ray study of which of the following bones should be ordered?

    A. fibula
    B. femur
    C. tibia
    D. humerus

26. A blood sample is collected from a patient, and the plasma is pink to red in color. Which of the following is the most likely cause?

    A. polycythemia
    B. agglutination
    C. hemolysis
    D. lipema

27. How should a medical assistant conduct a patient interview when the patient is an eight-year-old boy who has severe bruises on the right leg?

    A. Finish the child's sentences.
    B. Ask leading questions.
    C. Ask closed-ended questions.
    D. Allow the child to answer each question in his own words.

28. Which of the following has jurisdiction over the manufacture and distribution of controlled substances in the United States?

    A. Drug Enforcement Administration (DEA)
    B. American Medical Association (AMA)
    C. Federal Trade Commission (FTC)
    D. Food and Drug Administration (FDA)

29. Which of the following is the most appropriate reference for a medical assistant to identify the action of a particular medication?

    A. *The American Hospital Formulary*
    B. *United States Pharmacopeia*
    C. *The Physicians' Desk Reference* (PDR)
    D. *Family Physician's Compendium of Drug Therapy*

30. A medical assistant earns $15.00 per hour and works 40 hours during a one-week pay period. Federal taxes for the Federal Insurance Contributions Act (FICA) are withheld at 7.65%. How much money will be withheld from her gross earnings for a one-week pay period?

    A. $22.65   C. $45.90
    B. $34.60   D. $57.30

31. When submitting an insurance claim, which of the following International Classification of Diseases, Clinical Modification (ICD-CM) codes should be placed on the form first?

    A. principal diagnosis
    B. ruled-out conditions
    C. conditions previously treated
    D. conditions that coexist at the time of the visit

32. Physicians who administer controlled substances are required to register with which of the following organizations?

    A. Federal Trade Commission (FTC)
    B. Drug Enforcement Administration (DEA)
    C. Food and Drug Administration (FDA)
    D. U.S. Public Health Service (PHS)

33. A patient calls the office and angrily states that he is dissatisfied with his medical care. Which of the following is the most appropriate initial response?

    A. Suggest that he calm down and call back later.
    B. Tell him the physician will return his call.
    C. Ask him to describe the problem.
    D. Apologize and suggest that he change physicians.

34. A patient known to have terminal cancer arrives at the office. He is depressed and annoyed at having to wait to see the physician. Which of the following is the most appropriate approach to this patient?

    A. Listen to him and be sensitive to whether he indicates a need to talk.
    B. Put your arm around him and indicate to him that you know how he must feel.
    C. Leave him alone until it is time for him to see the physician.
    D. Offer him a beverage and a nonmedical magazine while he waits.

35. Which of the following activities related to scheduling surgical procedures is most likely to be the medical assistant's responsibility?

    A. determining what preoperative laboratory tests should be ordered
    B. obtaining the patient's consent for surgery
    C. ordering postoperative care for the patient
    D. ensuring that the arrangements concerning surgery are confirmed with the patient

36. Private medical records for an individual patient should be kept separate from the individual's

    A. CHAMPUS records.
    B. Medicare records.
    C. Medicaid records.
    D. workers' compensation records.

37. When screening telephone calls, which of the following patients should be referred to an emergency department?

    A. a 37-year-old woman with intermittent nosebleeds
    B. a 12-year-old girl who has leg pain after falling while playing football
    C. a 14-year-old boy with asthma who has mild difficulty breathing
    D. a woman at 27 weeks' gestation with moderate vaginal bleeding

38. The combining form *enter/o* refers to the

    A. spleen.   C. gallbladder.
    B. intestines.   D. kidneys.

39. A patient who only speaks Japanese is scheduled for a routine annual examination in 10 days. Her 12-year-old daughter will accompany her to the office. Who is the most appropriate individual to facilitate communication between this patient and the physician?

    A. the receptionist, who speaks some Japanese
    B. a Japanese teacher from a local high school
    C. the patient's 12-year-old daughter, who speaks both Japanese and English
    D. a professional interpreter

40. The physician orders 75 mg of medication to be given intramuscularly. The medication is available in 50-mg/mL vials. The medical assistant should administer

    A. 0.50 mL.   C. 1.0 mL.
    B. 0.75 mL.   D. 1.5 mL.

41. Which of the following body systems in the *Current Procedural Terminology* (CPT) includes the code for a mastectomy?

    A. integumentary   C. endocrine
    B. female reproductive D. musculoskeletal

42. A patient is most likely to experience dyspepsia in which of the following anatomic regions?

    A. epigastric   C. umbilical
    B. inguinal   D. hypochondriac

43. Which of the following conditions is characterized by opacity of the lens of the eye?

    A. nystagmus   C. glaucoma
    B. myopia   D. cataract

44. Which of the following expenses is most likely to be paid with petty cash?

    A. postage due   C. laboratory supplies
    B. repair of a photocopier D. employee holiday party

45. Which of the following terms means "deciding where to file a letter or paper"?

    A. indexing   C. sorting
    B. storing   D. conditioning

46. A telephone feature that answers calls and has a recording that identifies services available by pressing a specific number is known as which of the following?

    A. voice mail   C. answering service
    B. automated routing unit D. fax transmission

47. When an intradermal injection is correctly administered, which of the following should appear?

    A. small papule   C. small pustule
    B. small wheal   D. large bulla

48. Which of the following scalpel blade numbers is often used in performing minor surgeries?

    A. 5   C. 15
    B. 10   D. 20

49. Which of the following cells in the digestive system secretes intrinsic factor?

    A. parietal   C. mucous
    B. chief   D. goblet

50. If a flat line on an ECG tracing occurs on more than one lead, which of the following may have occurred?

    A. The patient is in cardiac arrest.
    B. The wires may have been switched.
    C. The electrocardiograph unit is faulty.
    D. The electrocardiograph connections are faulty.

51. Which of the following requires physicians' offices that perform nonwaived tests to participate in a recognized proficiency testing program?

    A. Occupational Safety and Health Act (OSHA)
    B. Health Care Quality Improvement Act (HCQIA)
    C. Food and Drug Act (FDA)
    D. Clinical Laboratory Improvement Amendments of 1988 (CLIA '88)

52. Which of the following is the most confidential method to notify a patient about an upcoming appointment?

    A. Use an appointment reminder service.
    B. Leave a message on the patient's answering machine.
    C. Send an e-mail message.
    D. Mail a postcard.

53. In the medical office, the statute of limitations for a patient's medical records applies to which of the following?

    A. length of time for retention
    B. standard of care
    C. termination of services
    D. charge for care

54. Which of the following instruments is used to visualize the lower digestive tract?

    A. otoscope   C. sigmoidoscope
    B. cystoscope   D. ophthalmoscope

55. The prefix *peri-* means

    A. before.   C. near.
    B. around.   D. large.

56. In a medical malpractice suit, which of the following terms represents the legal defense that "unreasonable patient behavior helped cause the injury"?

    A. statute of limitations C. assumption of risk
    B. informed consent   D. contributory negligence

57. According to U.S. Postal Service guidelines, which of the following is the correct state abbreviation for an envelope addressed to Boston?

    A. Mass   C. MT
    B. MA   D. MS

58. Which of the following serum levels is included in a lipid profile?

    A. potassium   C. sodium
    B. albumin   D. cholesterol

59. Hemolysis is most likely to be caused when performing venipuncture with a needle of which of the following gauges?

    A. 18   C. 23
    B. 21   D. 25

60. When using an autoclave for sterilization of instruments that have been sanitized and wrapped, which of the following is the required exposure time?

    A. 10 minutes   C. 25 minutes
    B. 15 minutes   D. 30 minutes

61. Measurement of which of the following laboratory values is most appropriate to assess renal function?

    A. creatinine   C. ketones
    B. uric acid   D. glucose

62. A patient has had pain in the quadriceps since she started an exercise program two days ago. Which of the following is the most likely result of applying heat to the affected areas?

    A. prevention of swelling C. decreased inflammation
    B. decreased blood flow   D. relaxation of muscles

63. Which of the following words means "mental deterioration due to organic brain disease"?

    A. dysphoria   C. depression
    B. dementia   D. hypomania

64. A patient has been instructed to exercise his arm for five minutes several times a day. He tells the medical assistant he could not do the exercises since his last appointment because he had to go to work. Which of the following defense mechanisms is he using?

A. displacement
B. regression
C. projection
D. repression

65. Which of the following involves the scheduling of appointments for a certain amount of time, based on patient need?

A. double booking
B. cluster
C. advance
D. streaming

66. Which of the following is the most common cancer in males between the ages of 20 and 35?

A. thyroid
B. testicular
C. pancreatic
D. prostate

67. Which of the following identifies the subjects to be covered during a meeting?

A. portfolio
B. minutes
C. agenda
D. abstract

68. Which of the following is the minimum amount of time that must elapse after a patient has eaten before spirometry can be performed?

A. 15 minutes
B. 30 minutes
C. 45 minutes
D. 60 minutes

69. Which of the following postal services provides insurance coverage for valuable items?

A. Certified Mail
B. Registered Mail
C. Restricted Delivery
D. Return Receipt Requested

70. The Occupational Safety and Health Administration (OSHA) mandates the use of which of the following protective equipment by health-care professionals whose work exposes them to patients with tuberculosis?

A. filter mask
B. goggles and head cover
C. gloves and gown
D. head and face mask

71. During which step of filing should medical assistants prepare a fax for inclusion in a patient's medical record?

A. conditioning
B. sorting
C. releasing
D. inspecting

72. Which of the following cytoplasmic organelles digests material that comes into the cell?

A. mitochondrion
B. lysosome
C. ribosome
D. centriole

73. Amino acids are the primary building blocks of which of the following nutrients?

A. vitamins
B. carbohydrates
C. proteins
D. lipids

74. The metabolism of most drugs is a function of which of the following organs?

A. kidneys
B. liver
C. lungs
D. brain

75. Which of the following is the most effective method to educate a patient about sexually transmitted infections?

A. Give the patient a video to view.
B. Give the patient a brochure to read.
C. Refer the patient to the Department of Health.
D. Conduct a face-to-face discussion with the patient.

76. A patient with severe depression states that he does not want to see a psychiatrist because his insurance will not cover mental health. This patient should be referred to which of the following?

A. sheriff's department
B. local department of social services
C. his insurance provider
D. The American Red Cross

77. Which of the following terms best describes the method used in surgery to prevent contamination of a wound and operative site?

A. disinfection
B. sanitization
C. aseptic technique
D. decontamination

78. Which of the following used items is classified as contaminated waste?

A. disposable suture removal kit
B. elastic bandage that was used for an ankle sprain
C. gown
D. goggles

79. Which of the following parts of a business letter is keyed on the second line below the salutation?

A. enclosure notation
B. complimentary close
C. subject line
D. reference initials

80. The physician orders phenytoin (Dilantin) for a child who weighs 18 kg. If the recommended dosage is five mg/kg per day in three equal doses, how much of the drug should be administered to the child in each dose?

A. 15 mg
B. 27 mg
C. 30 mg
D. 90 mg

81. Diabetes mellitus is a disorder that originates in which of the following organ systems?

A. reproductive
B. endocrine
C. integumentary
D. urinary

82. Which of the following components of an insurance policy specifies the maximum amount that can be reimbursed for the performance of a specific procedure?

A. fee-for-service reimbursement
B. reasonable fee
C. fee schedule
D. allowable charge

83. Which of the following is the most important consideration in maintaining examination rooms?

    A. physician's preference
    B. patient flow management
    C. patient comfort and safety
    D. convenience for the medical assistant

84. Which of the following is the route of administration of a drug that is placed between the gums and the cheek?

    A. buccal   C. sublingual
    B. topical   D. transdermal

85. A patient who comes into the office is angry and distraught. Which of the following is the most appropriate first step when interacting with this patient?

    A. Tell the patient that the physician will be with him shortly.
    B. Escort the patient to a private area.
    C. Ask the patient to calm down.
    D. Ask the patient to have a seat and wait for the physician.

86. How many digits are contained in an International Classification of Diseases, Clinical Modification (ICD-CM) code that is listed at the highest level of specificity?

    A. three   C. five
    B. four   D. six

87. Which of the following is a useful telephone technique for collecting payments?

    A. Review the value of the medical treatment received.
    B. Suggest alternative payment methods.
    C. Describe the financial status of the medical practice.
    D. Allow the patient time to offer explanations.

88. A woman at 36 weeks' gestation has abdominal pain, uterine tenderness, and tetanic uterine contraction. The patient complains of a sudden massive hemorrhage. These findings are most consistent with which of the following conditions?

    A. preeclampsia   C. ectopic pregnancy
    B. placenta previa   D. abruptio placentae

89. What is the purpose of a living will?

    A. to establish a durable power of attorney
    B. to allow a family member to act as a health-care surrogate or proxy
    C. to protect the attending physician from liability
    D. to enable a patient to refuse life support

90. Which of the following diseases is caused by a bacterium?

    A. rabies   C. diphtheria
    B. chickenpox   D. hepatitis B

91. Which of the following situations causes incomplete sterilization in an autoclave?

    A. keeping the temperature too high
    B. allowing air to enter the chamber
    C. venting after the pressure is equalized
    D. using distilled water in the reservoir

92. Which of the following is involved with the breathing maneuver used in which a patient is instructed to take a deep breath until the lungs are filled with air, and then to blow all the air out of the lungs until no more can be expelled?

    A. forced vital capacity
    B. functional residual volume
    C. expiratory reserve volume
    D. inspiration capacity

93. Which of the following muscles is located in the torso?

    A. soleus   C. external oblique
    B. gastrocnemius   D. masseter

94. Which of the following is *not* an element of the "six rights" of proper drug administration?

    A. route   C. time
    B. room   D. patient

95. In infants, which of the following is the most appropriate site to perform a puncture to obtain a capillary blood specimen?

    A. middle finger   C. thumb
    B. earlobe   D. heel

96. Which of the following procedures is performed to view a cross section of an organ?

    A. ultrasonography   C. hysterography
    B. tomography   D. pyelography

97. Which of the following is a parasitic infection associated with AIDS?

    A. Epstein-Barr virus   C. cytomegalovirus
    B. cryptococcosis   D. toxoplasmosis

98. A medical office schedules two patients at the beginning of each hour, followed by single appointments every 20 minutes during the rest of the hour. This is an example of which of the following types of appointment scheduling?

    A. modified wave   C. stream
    B. clustering   D. open hours

99. Which of the following is a microprocessor?

    A. monitor   C. hard drive
    B. keyboard   D. central processing unit

100. Which of the following laboratory tests is most appropriate to detect tuberculosis?

    A. modified Allen   C. D-dimer
    B. Mantoux   D. Dick

101. Office policy manuals contain which of the following types of information?

    A. names and positions of each employee
    B. employee health records
    C. employer insurance contributions
    D. employee salaries

102. The medical assistant demonstrates the proper procedure for administering an insulin injection, and then asks the patient to perform the procedure. This represents which of the following educational processes?

    A. planning
    B. implementation
    C. documentation
    D. assessment

103. Which of the following terms describes the dose required to sustain a level of narcotics in a patient's blood to control pain caused by cancer?

    A. maintenance
    B. maximum
    C. therapeutic
    D. loading

104. Which of the following is the most appropriate method of maintaining an airway in an unconscious adult who does not have a neck or spinal injury?

    A. jaw-thrust maneuver
    B. turning the patient on his or her side
    C. head-tilt, chin-lift maneuver
    D. placing your thumb in the patient's mouth and lifting the lower jaw

105. Which of the following is the purpose of the film badge worn by a health-care provider when performing an X-ray study?

    A. estimation of the number of X-ray studies performed monthly
    B. detection and recording of the amount of exposure to radiation
    C. protection from exposure to radiation
    D. personal identification

106. It is important to leave time to complete forms for patients who are

    A. minors.
    B. rich.
    C. new.
    D. poor.

107. Which one of these is a correct complimentary closing?

    A. Very best
    B. Thanks
    C. Always
    D. Best regards

108. How long is the hepatitis B virus capable of surviving in a dried state on environmental surfaces?

    A. one week
    B. two weeks
    C. three weeks
    D. one month

109. Kaposi's sarcoma is a malignancy of which of the following organs?

    A. skin and lungs
    B. skin and kidneys
    C. skin and lymph nodes
    D. skin and bones

110. Which of the following instructions is most appropriate for a patient who has just had an arm cast applied?

    A. Sprinkle powder in the cast if itching is present.
    B. Observe the fingers for changes in temperature.
    C. Rest the arm at waist level.
    D. Clean the cast by washing it gently with soap and water.

111. Which of the following terms best describes the flattened, funnel-shaped expansion end of the proximal ureter?

    A. nephron
    B. cortex
    C. medulla
    D. renal pelvis

112. Which of the following can convert nonelectronic graphics and text into a computerized format?

    A. scanner
    B. modem
    C. printer
    D. fax machine

113. The physician will be away from the medical office for one week. A substitute physician will be working in his place. Which of the following terms is used to describe the substitute physician?

    A. *res ipsa loquitur*
    B. *qui facit per alium facit per se*
    C. *locum tenens*
    D. *respondeat superior*

114. To avoid purchasing unnecessary medical office supplies, which of the following is the most appropriate action by the medical assistant?

    A. Take inventory of supplies frequently.
    B. Get permission from the physician.
    C. Examine previous purchase orders before ordering supplies.
    D. Balance the bank statement before ordering supplies.

115. Good interpersonal skills include

    A. selective hearing.
    B. getting very close to the patient.
    C. demonstrating respect.
    D. having only the physician talk to the patient.

116. A prefilled syringe is also known as a

    A. hypodermic syringe.
    B. cartridge.
    C. tuberculin syringe.
    D. flange.

117. Minor cauterization procedures are performed in the medical office by all of the following means *except*

    A. electric currents.
    B. caustic agents.
    C. hemostats.
    D. lasers.

118. Blood pressure readings should routinely be started at the age of

    A. 5 years.
    B. 10 years.
    C. 15 years.
    D. 20 years.

119. Which of the following terms means a tightness and narrowing of the prepuce on the penis that prevents the retraction of the foreskin over the glans penis, which may obstruct urine flow?

    A. emission
    B. acrosome
    C. tunica albuginea
    D. phimosis

120. Codeine is an example of what kind of drug?

    A. sedative
    B. antiepileptic drug
    C. narcotic analgesic
    D. antidepressant

121. When a venipuncture is performed in the antecubital space for intravenous therapy, the angle of the needle in relationship to the arm should be at which of the following degrees?

    A. 15
    B. 25
    C. 45
    D. 90

122. According to the National Childhood Vaccine Injury Act, which of the following must be documented in a child's permanent medical record?

    A. manufacturer and lot number of the vaccine
    B. receipt of informed consent
    C. vaccine information sheets
    D. patient's signature

123. Amoxicillin (Amoxil) is prescribed for a patient, and the dose is 250 mg qid by mouth. The medication is available as 500 mg per 10 mL, oral suspension. What is the correct daily dose?

    A. 10 mL
    B. 15 mL
    C. 20 mL
    D. 25 mL

124. Which of the following psychological theories was developed by Abraham Maslow?

    A. hierarchy of needs
    B. stages of grief
    C. negative reinforcement
    D. conditional response

125. The process of food digestion begins in which of the following parts of the digestive system?

    A. stomach
    B. mouth
    C. duodenum
    D. ileum

126. Which of the following terms describes "difficulty in seeing objects that are near"?

    A. strabismus
    B. hyperopia
    C. astigmatism
    D. myopia

127. Patient consent is required to release which of the following information from a medical record?

    A. history of drug or alcohol abuse
    B. history of communicable disease
    C. history of committing child abuse
    D. history of being stabbed

128. Which of the following endocrine glands is considered to be the master gland of the body?

    A. thymus
    B. adrenal
    C. mammary
    D. pituitary

129. Which of the following is included in the "S" portion of a SOAP chart note?

    A. temperature of 39.4°C (103.0°F)
    B. cardiac arrhythmia
    C. headache of four days' duration
    D. edema of the feet

130. Which of the following is a contaminant that is commonly found in midstream clean-catch urine specimens collected by young women who are menstruating?

    A. blood cells
    B. mucous cells
    C. epithelial cells
    D. fecal material

131. The medical assistant enters the examination room and finds the patient lying on the floor and unresponsive. After initiating the emergency response protocol, which of the following should the medical assistant do next?

    A. start chest compressions
    B. check the patient's pulse
    C. assess the patient for bleeding
    D. check the patient's airway

132. Which of the following is most likely to reduce bruising after venipuncture?

    A. placing a bandage over the puncture site
    B. applying pressure to the puncture site
    C. applying ice to the puncture site
    D. wiping the puncture site with alcohol

133. Which of the following terms refers to a constant involuntary movement of one or both eyes?

    A. strabismus
    B. amblyopia
    C. nystagmus
    D. hyperopia

134. Exchange transfusions are often performed on newborns with hemolytic disease and high serum levels of which of the following substances?

    A. creatinine
    B. glucose
    C. albumin
    D. bilirubin

135. Swelling and pain around the site of intravenous insertion is a sign of which of the following?

    A. infiltration
    B. erythema
    C. nerve damage
    D. sepsis

136. Which of the following is known as a statement of financial condition?

    A. daysheet
    B. patient ledger
    C. balance sheet
    D. trial balance

137. According to standard precautions, surfaces contaminated with blood or body fluid should be cleaned with which of the following agents?

    A. peroxide
    B. alcohol
    C. soap
    D. bleach

138. Which of the following skin tumors is often caused by overexposure to sunlight?

    A. Kaposi's sarcoma
    B. malignant melanoma
    C. sebaceous nevus
    D. epidermal nevus

139. Which of the following glands is located in the chest?

    A. pituitary
    B. thyroid
    C. thymus
    D. adrenal

140. Which of the following radiologic procedures is most appropriate for studying esophageal function?

    A. fluoroscopy
    B. xeroradiography
    C. magnetic resonance imaging (MRI)
    D. computed tomography (CT) scan

141. The medical assistant writes a business letter and revises it for accuracy, logical flow, conciseness, clarity, and tone. Which of the following best describes this process?

A. proofreading   C. editing
B. word processing   D. formatting

142. Which of the following is a federal health insurance plan?

A. indemnity
B. Medicare
C. Health maintenance organization (HMO)
D. Preferred provider organization (PPO)

143. Which of the following terms describes the sac in which the heart is enclosed?

A. myocardium   C. pericardium
B. endocardium   D. epithelium

144. For a patient who is covered by Medicare only, and has paid the annual deductible, which of the following is the maximum percentage of allowable charges he is required to pay to a physician who participates in Medicare Part B?

A. 10%   C. 30%
B. 20%   D. 50%

145. In a medical office, computer spreadsheet programs are most often used for which of the following tasks?

A. tracking accounts payable
B. scheduling appointments
C. maintaining medical records
D. composing letters

146. Which of the following is the most important guideline to follow when performing routine urinalysis?

A. Centrifuge the specimen before chemical testing.
B. Use the same pipette for each specimen.
C. Handle the specimen as if it were infectious.
D. Allow the specimen to sit at room temperature.

147. Which of the following parts of the brain controls emotions?

A. cerebrellum   C. pons
B. hypothalamus   D. medulla oblongata

148. A medical assistant who works for a dermatologist orders patch test kits that are available in quantities of five kits per box. The physician currently uses two kits per week. How many boxes should be ordered for an eight-week supply?

A. four   C. eight
B. six   D. ten

149. Which of the following is used to document a patient's illness on an insurance claim form?

A. Resource-based relative value scale (RBRVS)
B. Current Procedural Terminology (CPT)
C. International Classification of Diseases, Clinical Modification (ICD-CM)
D. Diagnosis-related groups (DRGs)

150. Which of the following types of medical supplies has the shortest shelf life?

A. tongue blades   C. alcohol pads
B. hydrogen peroxide   D. biohazard bags

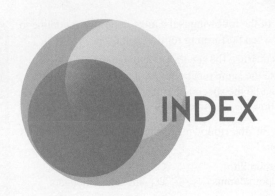

INDEX

4 Ds of negligence, 115
5 Cs of communication, 165
6 Cs of charting, 159, 252
7 rights of drug administration, 306
9s, rule of, in burns, 348f
940 federal employer's tax return
form, 197f

A

Abbreviations
appointments, 157t
blood testing, 363t–364t
cardiovascular system, 24t–25t
common, 16t–17t
digestive system, 27t
ear, 31t
endocrine system, 29t
eye, 30t–31t
household measurement system,
304t
integumentary system, 19t
metric system, 304t
musculoskeletal system, 21t
nervous system, 23t
pharmaceutical, 16
reproductive system, 34t–35t
respiratory system, 26t
urinary system, 32t–33t
urine analysis and testing, 377t
ABCs (airway, breathing, circulation),
emergency assessment, 345t.
See also C-A-B
Abortion, 123
Accessibility, 253
Accounting
balances, 188–189
bookkeeping systems, 185–186
definition, 185
posting to records, 186–188
Accounts payable, 194
payroll, 194–195, 195f
tax, 195–199
Accounts receivable, age-analysis, 193f

Adaptation, 98
Addiction, 101
Administrative supplies, 183, 184t
Adrenal glands, 61f
Advance directives, 124
AIDS (acquired immunodeficiency
syndrome), 242
opportunistic infections, 243
stages, 243
AIDS-related complex (ARC), 243
Alcoholic solutions, 284
Alphabetical filing system, 160
ALS (amyotrophic lateral sclerosis,
Lou Gehrig's disease), 75
Alveoli, 59f
American Association of Medical
Assistants (AAMA), 4–5
American Registry of Medical
Assistants (ARMA), 5
Amino acids, 105, 105t
Analgesics, 292
Anaphylactic shock, 352
Anatomy, definition, 39
Anemia, 375
Anesthetics, 292
Aneurysm, 77
Angiography, 323, 328t, 329
Angry patients, communication with,
169
Anorexia nervosa, 111
Antiallergic drugs, 297
Antianginal drugs (vasodilators), 294,
295t
Antiarrhythmic drugs, 296, 296t
Antibiotics, 287–289
Anticoagulant drugs, 296–297
Antidepressant drugs, 291
Antiepileptic drugs, 292, 292t
Antifungal drugs, 289, 289t
Antihistamines, 297
Antihypertensive drugs, 294, 295t
Antiparkinsonian drugs, 292
Antipsychotic drugs, 291, 291t

Antitubercular agents, 288–289
Antiviral agents, 289
Apothecaries' system, 16, 304
metric conversion, 305t
Appointment book, 155, 156f
Appointment card, 157
Appointments
abbreviations, 157t
scheduling, 157–158, 178
types, 155, 157
Arteriosclerosis, 76
Arthrography, 328t, 329
Arthroplasty, 74
Artificial insemination, 123
ARU (automated response unit)
telephone systems, 150
Asepsis
medical, 243
surgical, 243, 262
Aseptic hand-washing, 244, 244t
Aseptic precautions, 244
Assertiveness skills, 168
Asthma
drugs, 297
emergencies, 356
medications, 297, 297t
Atrophy, definition, 74
Attention deficit/hyperactivity
disorder (ADHD), 99
Auditing, definition, 185
Authorizing processing rules,
referrals, 208
Autism, 99
Autoclave, 245, 262
Automatic external defibrillator
(AED), 353–354
Autonomic nervous system, 52
medications, 294, 294t

B

Bacteria, 85
shapes and arrangements, 86f
Bactericidal antibiotics, 287–288, 287t

central, 50–51
cranial nerves, 50, 51t
diseases and disorders, 74–76
head injuries, 351
medications, 290–294, 290t–294t
peripheral, 50
somatic, 50
spinal cord, 50
spinal nerves, 52
Neurology tests, 261
Neuron, 48
Neurotransmitters, 49
Niacin (vitamin B₃), 106, 106t
Non-participating (nonPAR) provider, 203
Medicare payments to, 211t
Nonopioid analgesics, 293t
Nonspecific defense mechanism, 69–70
Nonsteroidal anti-inflammatory drugs (NSAIDs), 293t
Nonverbal clues, 252
Nonverbal communication, 166
Normal flora, 92
Normal ranges
blood pressure, 272t
selected blood tests, 370t
standard urine values, 378t
vital signs, 268t
Nosocomial, definition, 69
NPP (notice of privacy practices), HIPAA, 122
Nuclear medicine (radionuclide imaging), 329, 329t
Numerical filing system, 160
Nutrition, 104
breastfeeding, 109
carbohydrates, 104
diet needs and guidelines, 108–111, 108f
food-related diseases, 111
lipids, 104–105
normal-range blood tests, 105t
during pregnancy, 109
protein, 105
serving sizes, 109t
vitamins, 106–107, 107t
water, 104

O

Obesity, 104
Obsessive-compulsive disorders, 99
Occult blood specimen, 382
Occult blood tests, 260
Olfaction, 52
Open hours, 158
Ophthalmoscope, 254f

Opioid analgesics, 293t
Opportunistic infections, 243
Organelles, 41
Orthopedic injuries, 351
Orthostatic hypotension, 272
OSHA (Occupational Safety and Health Administration), 245
Blood-Borne Pathogens Standard (1991), 245
infectious waste disposal penalties, 246t
requirements, 245–247
Osteoporosis, 335
Output devices, 176
Ovaries, 63b, 65

P

P-R interval, ECG tracing, 321f, 322
P wave, ECG tracing, 321, 321f
Pacemaker, 318, 323
Palliative care, 124
Pantothenic acid (vitamin B complex), 106, 106t
Pap (Papanicolau) test/smear, 261
Paraplegia, 336
Parasympathetic nervous system medications, 294
Parenteral drug administration, 307
Parkinson's disease, 75
Participating (PAR) provider, 203
Medicare payments to, 211t
Patch test, 260
Pathology, definition, 69
Patient education, 152
cane use, 339, 340t
crutches use, 339
walker use, 340, 340t
wheelchair use, 340
Patient interview, 251
Patient ledger card, 186, 187f
Patient registration form, 158
Patient Self-Determination Act, 124
Patient's Bill of Rights, 118, 118t
Patient's Bill of Rights, 118, 118t, 251
PDA (personal digital assistant), 174
Pediatric drug dose calculation, 306
Pegboard bookkeeping system, 186
Penicillins, 287, 287t
Peripheral nervous system, 50, 52
Personal protective equipment (PPE), 345
Personal space, and communication, 169
PET (positron emission tomography) scan, 329, 329t
Petri dish, 383
Pharmacology

abbreviations, 16
terms, 277, 280
Pharynx, 59f
Phenobarbital, 292t
Phenylketonuria (PKU), definition, 70
PHI (protected health information), HIPAA, 121, 179
Phlebotomy, 365
Phosphorus (P), 107
Physical examination, 252–253
cardiovascular system, 257
ear, 257, 258f
equipment, 253–255, 254f
eye, 255–257, 257f
gastrointestinal system, 259–260, 259f
gynecology and obstetrics, 260
infants and children, 261
neurology tests, 261
positioning and draping, 255, 256f
respiratory system, 258–259
urinary system, 260
Physical therapy
mobility-assisting devices, 339–340
patient assessment, 336
terminology, 335–336
treatment, 336–339
Physician-assisted suicide, 124
Physiology, definition, 39
PKU (phenylketonuria) screening, 373
Platelets (thrombocytes), 361f, 362
Plural forms, 14
Pneumococcal conjugate (PCV13), vaccine, 312
Pneumococcal polysaccharide (PPSV23) vaccine, 312–313
Pneumocystis carinii pneumonia, 243
Pneumothorax, definition, 78
Poisoning emergencies, 357
Poisons and antidotes, 286, 286t
Policies and procedures, 162
POMR documentation system, 120, 159
Positioning
and draping, 255, 256f
for radiography, 330, 331f
Positive communication, 166
Post-traumatic stress disorder (PTSD), 101
Potassium (K), 108
PPO (preferred provider organization), 207
Prefixes
endocrine system, 28t
metric system, 304t
nervous system, 22t